MICHIGAN MANUAL OF PLASTIC SURGERY

Third Edition

Editors

David L. Brown, MD, FACS
William C. Grabb Professor
Section of Plastic Surgery
Department of Surgery
University of Michigan Medical School
Ann Arbor, Michigan

Widya Adidharma, MD
Resident
Section of Plastic Surgery
Department of Surgery
University of Michigan Medical School
Ann Arbor, Michigan

Geoffrey E. Hespe, MD
Resident
Section of Plastic Surgery
Department of Surgery
University of Michigan Medical School
Ann Arbor, Michigan

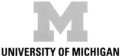

**UNIVERSITY OF MICHIGAN
MEDICAL SCHOOL**
MICHIGAN MEDICINE

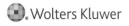

Philadelphia • Baltimore • New York • London
Buenos Aires • Hong Kong • Sydney • Tokyo

**Written by Residents and Faculty
from Michigan Medicine**

Acquisitions Editor: Tulie McKay
Senior Development Editor: Ashley Fischer
Editorial Coordinator: Priyanka Alagar
Marketing Manager: Kirstin Watrud
Production Project Manager: Nancy Devaux
Senior Production Project Manager: Catherine Ott
Manager, Graphic Arts & Design: Stephen Druding
Manufacturing Coordinator: Lisa Bowling
Prepress Vendor: Straive

Third Edition

9 8 7 6 5 4 3 2 1

Printed in Singapore

Cataloging-in-Publication Data available on request from the Publisher

ISBN-13: 978-1-9751-9739-1

shop.lww.com

MK0823

I would like to dedicate this third edition to the incredible residents and students who I am privileged to work with on a daily basis. They keep me on my toes and stimulate all of us to ask more questions about the world around us. The work on this manuscript would not have been possible without my family—their love and support are the most important things in my life.
–D.L.B.

I would like to dedicate this textbook to my mentors, whom inspire my passion for plastic surgery and have helped shape my academic journey. I also thank my parents, Hertanto and Mari, whose unwavering encouragement has been invaluable throughout my life. To my mentees, thank you for inspiring me with your enthusiasm and curiosity. And most importantly, to my husband, Kyle, who has been my number one supporter and constant source of love and motivation.
–W.A.

To every future student, resident, and APP who will use this book to provide excellent care to their patients: this edition is dedicated to you. To my mentors, thank you for your constant support and guidance. I am forever grateful for your wisdom, encouragement, and belief in me. But above all, I owe everything to my family. Mom and dad, your love and support have been the foundation of my success. And to my wife Anasta, your unwavering love and encouragement has made everything possible. You inspire me daily with your strength and kindness. I am so lucky to have you in my life and would not be where I am today without you.
–G.E.H.

About the Editors

David L. Brown is the William C. Grabb Professor of Plastic Surgery in the Section of Plastic Surgery at the University of Michigan. He received his BA at Wittenberg University in Springfield, Ohio; his MD at Vanderbilt University in Nashville, Tennessee; General Surgery training at the University of Cincinnati; Plastic Surgery Fellowship at the University of Michigan in Ann Arbor; and Microvascular Reconstruction Fellowship at St. Vincent's Hospital and the University of Melbourne, Australia. He passionately believes that education and training of the next generation of physicians is our greatest gift to the specialty.

Widya Adidharma is a plastic surgery resident at the University of Michigan in the Section of Plastic Surgery. She received her BS at Michigan State University and MD at the University of Washington School of Medicine. She is passionate about advancing the field of plastic surgery through her involvement in research and education. During her residency, she is completing a 2-year postdoctoral research fellowship with the University of Michigan Neuromuscular Lab developing innovative surgical interventions for the restoration of sensory feedback and bidirectional sensorimotor signaling after amputation injury. She is planning on pursuing a career as a surgeon-scientist with a focus on translational research and peripheral nerve and hand surgery.

Geoffrey E. Hespe is a chief integrated plastic surgery resident at the University of Michigan. He received his BS with honors from the University of Richmond, followed by his MD with distinction in research from Rutgers-Robert Wood Johnson Medical School. During medical school, he completed a 2-year research fellowship at Memorial Sloan Kettering Cancer Center investigating lymphedema and the effects of obesity on the lymphatic system. He is planning on returning to Memorial Sloan Kettering Cancer Center to complete a microsurgery fellowship following graduation, with a future career as a surgeon-scientist focusing on complex reconstructive surgery and basic science research.

Section Editors

Megan Lane, MD
Resident
Section of Plastic Surgery
Department of Surgery
University of Michigan Medical School
Ann Arbor, Michigan

Rami D. Sherif, MD
Resident
Section of Plastic Surgery
Department of Surgery
University of Michigan Medical School
Ann Arbor, Michigan

Sherry Tang, MD
Resident
Section of Plastic Surgery
Department of Surgery
University of Michigan Medical School
Ann Arbor, Michigan

Chien-Wei Wang, MD
Resident
Section of Plastic Surgery
Department of Surgery
University of Michigan Medical School
Ann Arbor, Michigan

Christine S. Wang, MD
Resident
Section of Plastic Surgery
Department of Surgery
University of Michigan Medical School
Ann Arbor, Michigan

Contributors

Widya Adidharma, MD
Resident
Section of Plastic Surgery
Department of Surgery
University of Michigan Medical School
Ann Arbor, Michigan

Brigit Baglien, MD
Resident
Section of Plastic Surgery
Department of Surgery
University of Michigan Medical School
Ann Arbor, Michigan

Emily Barrett, MD
Resident
Department of Surgery
University of Michigan Medical School
Ann Arbor, Michigan

Christopher J. Breuler, MD
Resident
Section of Plastic Surgery
Department of Surgery
University of Michigan Medical School
Ann Arbor, Michigan

Naomi Briones, MD, MAT
Resident
Department of Dermatology
University of Michigan Medical School
Ann Arbor, Michigan

Lauren Bruce, BA
Medical Student
University of Michigan Medical School
Ann Arbor, Michigan

Katherine L. Burke, MD
Postdoctoral Research Fellow
Section of Plastic Surgery
Department of Surgery
University of Michigan Medical School
Ann Arbor, Michigan

Ayana K. Cole-Price, MD, MSc
Resident
Section of Plastic Surgery
Department of Surgery
University of Michigan Medical School
Ann Arbor, Michigan

Atticus Coscia, MD
Resident
Department of Orthopaedic Surgery
University of Michigan Medical School
Ann Arbor, Michigan

Ryan O. Davenport, MD
Resident
Department of Orthopaedic Surgery
University of Michigan Medical School
Ann Arbor, Michigan

Paul Gagnet, MD
Resident
Department of Orthopaedic Surgery
University of Michigan Medical School
Ann Arbor, Michigan

Rebecca W. Gao, MD, MS
Resident
Department of Otolaryngology–Head
and Neck Surgery
University of Michigan Medical School
Ann Arbor, Michigan

Davin C. Gong, MD
Resident
Department of Orthopaedic Surgery
University of Michigan Medical School
Ann Arbor, Michigan

Caleb Haley, MD
Resident
Section of Plastic Surgery
Department of Surgery
University of Michigan Medical School
Ann Arbor, Michigan

Geoffrey E. Hespe, MD
Resident
Section of Plastic Surgery
Department of Surgery
University of Michigan Medical School
Ann Arbor, Michigan

Hossein E. Jazayeri, DMD
Resident
Department of Oral and Maxillofacial
    Surgery
University of Michigan Medical School
Ann Arbor, Michigan

Peter M. Kally, MD
Oculoplastic Surgery Fellow
Consultants in Ophthalmic and Facial
    Plastic Surgery, PC
Southfield, Michigan

Meera Kattapuram, BA
Medical Student
University of Michigan Medical School
Ann Arbor, Michigan

Sarah Hart Kennedy, MD
Resident
Section of Plastic Surgery
Department of Surgery
University of Michigan Medical School
Ann Arbor, Michigan

Alexander N. Khouri, MD
Resident
Section of Plastic Surgery
Department of Surgery
University of Michigan Medical School
Ann Arbor, Michigan

Jane S. Kim, MD
Clinical Lecturer, Ophthalmology
Fellow, Oculofacial and Orbital Surgery
    (ASOPRS)
University of Michigan Medical Center/
    Kellogg Eye Center
Ann Arbor, Michigan

Evangeline F. Kobayashi, MD
Resident
Department of Orthopaedic Surgery
University of Michigan Medical School
Ann Arbor, Michigan

Megan Lane, MD
Resident
Section of Plastic Surgery
Department of Surgery
University of Michigan Medical School
Ann Arbor, Michigan

Kory LaPree, DO
Resident
Department of Anesthesiology
University of Michigan Medical School
Ann Arbor, Michigan

Kyle R. Latack, MD
Resident
Department of Obstetrics and Gynecol-
    ogy
University of Michigan Medical School
Ann Arbor, Michigan

Jennifer C. Lee, MSE
Medical Student
University of Michigan Medical School
Ann Arbor, Michigan

Alexandra O. Luby, MD, MS
Resident
Section of Plastic Surgery
Department of Surgery
University of Michigan Medical School
Ann Arbor, Michigan

Katelyn G. Makar, MD, MS
Assistant Professor
Department of Plastic Surgery
Indiana University School of Medicine
Indianapolis, Indiana

Jaclyn T. Mauch, MD, MBE
Resident
Section of Plastic Surgery
Department of Surgery
University of Michigan Medical School
Ann Arbor, Michigan

Humza N. Mirza, MS
Medical Student
University of Michigan Medical School
Ann Arbor, Michigan

Connor Mullen, MD
Resident
Section of Plastic Surgery
Department of Surgery
University of Michigan Medical School
Ann Arbor, Michigan

Stefano Muscatelli, MD
Resident
Department Orthopaedic Surgery
University of Michigan Medical School
Ann Arbor, Michigan

Paige L. Myers, MD
Clinical Assistant Professor
Section of Plastic Surgery
Department of Surgery
University of Michigan Medical School
Ann Arbor, Michigan

Shay Nguyen, BS
Medical Student
University of Michigan Medical School
Ann Arbor, Michigan

Cecilia M. Pesavento, BS, MBA
Medical Student
University of Michigan Medical School
Ann Arbor, Michigan

Galina G. Primeau, MD
Resident
Section of Plastic Surgery
Department of Surgery
University of Michigan Medical School
Ann Arbor, Michigan

Matthew T. Rasmussen, MD
Resident
Department of Orthopaedic Surgery
University of Michigan Medical School
Ann Arbor, Michigan

Stacia M. Ruse, MD
Resident
Department of Orthopaedic surgery
University of Michigan Medical School
Ann Arbor, Michigan

Gina N. Sacks, MD
Resident
Section of Plastic Surgery
Department of Surgery
University of Michigan Medical School
Ann Arbor, Michigan

Shahan Saleem, MBBS, FCPS
Consultant Plastic Surgeon
Department of Plastic Surgery
Jinnah Burn and Reconstructive Surgery
   Center
Jinnah Hospital
Lahore, Pakistan

Rami D. Sherif, MD
Resident
Section of Plastic Surgery
Department of Surgery
University of Michigan Medical School
Ann Arbor, Michigan

Alexandria Sherwood, MD
Resident
Department of Orthopaedic Surgery
University of Michigan Medical School
Ann Arbor, Michigan

Amy L. Strong, MD, PhD, MPH
Resident
Section of Plastic Surgery
Department of Surgery
University of Michigan Medical School
Ann Arbor, Michigan

Shelby Svientek, MD
Resident
Section of Plastic Surgery
Department of Surgery
University of Michigan Medical School
Ann Arbor, Michigan

Sherry Tang, MD
Resident
Section of Plastic Surgery
Department of Surgery
University of Michigan Medical School
Ann Arbor, Michigan

Jennifer Waljee, MD, MPH, MSc
Associate Professor of Surgery
Section of Plastic Surgery
Department of Surgery
University of Michigan Medical School
Ann Arbor, Michigan

Chien-Wei Wang, MD
Resident
Section of Plastic Surgery
Department of Surgery
University of Michigan Medical School
Ann Arbor, Michigan

Christine S. Wang, MD
Resident
Section of Plastic Surgery
Department of Surgery
University of Michigan Medical School
Ann Arbor, Michigan

Ayobami L. Ward, MD
Resident
Department of Neurosurgery
University of Michigan Medical School
Ann Arbor, Michigan

Johnny Yanjun Xie, MD
Resident
Department of Otolaryngology–Head
 and Neck Surgery
University of Michigan Medical School
Ann Arbor, Michigan

Alisa Yamasaki, MD
Clinical Instructor
Division of Facial Plastic and Reconstruc-
 tive Surgery
Department of Otolaryngology–Head
 and Neck Surgery
University of Michigan Medical School
Ann Arbor, Michigan

Alfred P. Yoon, MD
Resident
Section of Plastic Surgery
Department of Surgery
University of Michigan Medical School
Ann Arbor, Michigan

Foreword

It is with great pleasure that I write the Foreword for the third edition of the *Michigan Manual of Plastic Surgery*. The *Michigan Manual of Plastic Surgery* has become the go-to reference guide for medical students, physician assistants, nurses, residents, and medical practitioners from around the world, as they provide care for their patients. It highlights all of the critical aspects of plastic surgery in a compact, information rich, visually pleasing, and yet surprisingly comprehensive book. It provides each physician and surgeon exactly what they need to know in sufficient depth and breadth to be highly valuable throughout the entire duration of a patient's care from their initial outpatient evaluation through the successful completion of their care. In addition, the *Michigan Manual of Plastic Surgery* has been written entirely by residents and fellows in plastic surgery and related specialties. As such, the *Michigan Manual of Plastic Surgery* has a focus, structure, and approach, which is perfectly suited to the people who need to access this information the most. It doesn't require reading exhaustively detailed chapters to glean the critical information they need on each topic. Instead, the nicely crafted *Michigan Manual of Plastic Surgery* has a visually pleasing presentation style with readily accessible information, which is designed to provide "on-time" learning, whether it is the night before an operation, during an outpatient clinic visit, on the hospital wards, or between cases in the operating room. The first two editions of the *Michigan Manual of Plastic Surgery* have been highly successful and have helped countless health care providers and learners. I am very excited about the enhancements and additions made by Drs. David Brown, Widya Adidharma, and Geoffrey Hespe to make the third edition even more valuable. The editors have significantly improved and updated the content of the book, revamped the layout to enhance readability, created new chapters on hot topics in plastic surgery (ie, lymphedema surgery, gender affirmation surgery, and neuroma surgery), and added beautiful illustrations and figures to enhance the visual learning experience. The third edition will also be available electronically for ease of accessibility to the content of the book. If you prefer a copy of the book in your hands, the third edition of the *Michigan Manual of Plastic Surgery* will still fit in your white coat so the information is no further than a pocket away. I am excited about the release of the third edition of the *Michigan Manual of Plastic Surgery*, the most comprehensive, portable plastic surgery textbook available. I am sure you will find it an incredibly valuable resource to provide "just-in-time" information as you care for your patients.

Paul S. Cederna, MD, FACS
Chief, Section of Plastic Surgery
Robert Oneal Collegiate Professor of Plastic Surgery
Professor, Department of Biomedical Engineering
University of Michigan Medical School
Ann Arbor, Michigan

Preface

We are excited to present the third edition of the *Michigan Manual of Plastic Surgery*, the world's only pocket-sized, yet comprehensive treatise on this vast subject.

As in the first edition, we sought to present the entire scope of contemporary plastic surgery in an easily accessible format. We have produced this handbook primarily for medical students and surgical residents to facilitate clinical consultations and pre-, intra-, and postoperative care. The content and format are also an excellent reference for practitioners in the multitude of other fields with which plastic surgery interacts, who need ready access to basic, practical information. Additionally, we trust that the *Michigan Manual* will provide a succinct review for the in-service and written board examinations. To aid in review for such examinations, we have placed an * in front of material that is commonly tested. Additionally, we have included questions that are commonly asked in the operating room at the end of each chapter to prepare for each case. We have also included key references for additional reading on each topic.

This book was written and edited by residents at the University of Michigan. We wish to thank our section editors, Megan Lane, Rami D. Sherif, Sherry Tang, Christine S. Wang, and Chien-Wei Wang, for their contributions.

We hope that you find this handbook helpful in your quest for improving your knowledge base of plastic surgery. We are delighted to contribute to the education of those dedicated to caring for plastic surgery patients. Never stop learning!

David L. Brown, MD, FACS
Widya Adidharma, MD
Geoffrey E. Hespe, MD

Contents

SECTION I: GENERAL
Section Editor: Christine S. Wang

SECTION II: CRANIOFACIAL
Section Editor: Chien-Wei Wang

SECTION III: UPPER EXTREMITY
Section Editor: Megan Lane

SECTION IV: BREAST AND BODY RECONSTRUCTION
Section Editor: Sherry Tang

SECTION V: AESTHETICS
Section Editor: Rami D. Sherif

SECTION VI: OTHER

1 Complex Wound Care

Brigit Baglien

ANATOMY

- **Collagen:** most abundant connective tissue protein in mammals
  - Twenty types of collagen; most abundant types are as follows
    - *Type I: skin, tendon, bone, and mature scar; have a 4:1 ratio of type I:III
    - Type II: cartilage and cornea
    - Type III: blood vessels and immature scar
    - Type IV: basement membrane
  - Composed of high concentration of hydroxyproline and hydroxylysine amino acids.
- **Skin Layers and Structures (Fig. 1-1A and B):** ordered from superficial to deep layers
  - **Epidermis:** derived from ectoderm—stratified, keratinized, and avascular layer
    - Stratum corneum: acellular layer of keratin.
    - Stratum lucidum: dead cells without nuclei.
    - Stratum granulosum: cytoplasmic granules contribute to keratin formation.
    - Stratum spinosum: desmosomes connect cells and create a shiny appearance.
    - Stratum basale (aka germinativum): melanocytes produce melanin, which is taken up by the predominant keratinocytes.
  - **Dermis:** derived from mesoderm
    - **Papillary:** loose vascular tissue
    - **Reticular:** dense, more vascular layer
    - Contains fibroblasts, adipocytes, macrophages, collagen, and ground substance
  - **Adnexa:** sources of reepithelialization in partial-thickness wounds
    - **Hair follicles** (ectodermal origin)
      - Ingrowth of epidermis into dermis and subcutaneous tissue
      - Associated sebaceous glands secrete into the hair follicle
      - Remains intact when harvesting split-thickness skin grafts
    - **Eccrine sweat glands** (ectodermal origin)
      - Coiled structures located throughout the body with high concentrations in the palms and soles that secrete primarily water and salt via a single duct into the epidermis
      - Not present in split-thickness skin grafts
    - **Apocrine sweat glands** (ectodermal origin)
      - Located in axillary, inguinal, and areolar regions, secrete watery fluid higher in protein into hair follicles. Associated with malodorous sweating
- **Muscle:** derived from paraxial mesoderm; classified as smooth, skeletal, and cardiac muscles
  - Microscopic: sarcomere unit—bundles of myofibers (composed of actin and myosin filaments) form muscle fibers.
  - Macroscopic: organized groups of muscle fibers form fascicles; bundles of fascicles form muscles.
  - Neuromuscular junction: "motor endplate" consists of sarcolemmal folds within which acetylcholine receptors reside.

---

*Denotes common in-service examination topics.

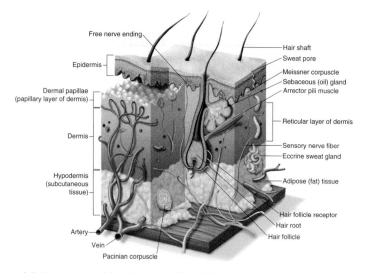

Figure 1-1 Cross section of the skin. (From Chung KC, ed. *Grabb and Smith's Plastic Surgery.* 8th ed. Wolters Kluwer; 2020. Figure 45.1)

- **Bone:** derived from lateral plate mesoderm (except for skull bones derived from neural crest)
  - ○ **Cross-sectional anatomy**
    - ▪ Outer layer: fibrous periosteum and osteogenic periosteum
    - ▪ Mature compact (cortical) bone: 80% of total bone mass; lamellar structure that is permeated by elaborate interconnecting vascular canals (haversian canals)
    - ▪ Immature compact (cortical) bone: woven structure of collagen fibrils that is replaced by mature bone through remodeling
    - ▪ Trabecular (cancellous) bone: 20% of total bone mass, but much greater surface area due to lower density; bony matrix organized into a matrix (trabeculae) along lines of stress. Develops into compact bone via osteoblasts along the trabeculae
- **Tendon:** derived from lateral plate mesoderm
  - ○ **Organizational anatomy**
    - ▪ Collagen is arranged longitudinally into fibrils.
    - ▪ Fibrils and fibroblasts are organized into fascicles, which are grouped into tendons.
- **Cartilage:** derived from lateral plate mesoderm, the cartilage consists of extracellular matrix (ECM) composed of collagen fibers, ground substance, and elastin, and is classified into elastic cartilage, hyaline cartilage, and fibrocartilage, depending on the proportion of each component.
- **Nerve:** peripheral nerves have neural crest origin.
  - ○ **Organizational anatomy**
    - ▪ A nerve describes a bundle of axons traveling together peripherally.
    - ▪ The nerve is covered by the *epineurium.*
    - ▪ Bundles of axons are called fascicles and are wrapped in the *perineurium.*
    - ▪ The majority of axons are myelinated, and individual axons are enveloped in the *endoneurium.*

WOUND HEALING

NORMAL WOUND HEALING

- **Skin and Subcutaneous Tissue**
  - ○ **Wound healing categories**
    - ▪ **Primary intention**
      - □ *Immediate primary closure of a surgical incision (epithelialization occurs in ~24 hours).
      - □ Delayed closure of a surgical incision (usually to either allow clearance of infection or resolution of edema) is known as "delayed primary closure."
    - ▪ **Secondary intention**
      - □ Full-thickness wound healing by a combination of migration of fibroblasts and keratinocytes from the wound periphery leading to wound contraction
  - ○ **Phases of wound healing**
    - ▪ **Inflammatory phase** (first minutes to first week)
      - □ **Vasoconstriction of vessels:** occurs for first 10 minutes following injury.
      - □ *Coagulation: Platelets arrive and degranulate, releasing thromboxane A2 that causes transient vasoconstriction to facilitate hemostasis with thrombus formation. Platelet-derived growth factor (PDGF) is released, acting as a potent chemotaxin and mitogen for fibroblasts and macrophages.
      - □ **Vasodilation and increased permeability:** small vessels dilate in response to prostaglandins to allow white blood cells (WBCs) (neutrophils, plasma cells, and monocytes) attracted by the leukotrienes, complement, and cytokines (interleukin-1 [IL-1], tumor necrosis factor-α [TNF-α], TGF-β, epidermal growth factor (EGF), and platelet factor 4 [PF4]) to enter.
      - □ **Cellular response.**
        - ▪ **Neutrophils**
          - • *Dominant cell type at 24 hours, first to respond
          - • Approach injury site by chemoattractants via circulatory system
          - • Undergo margination and diapedesis
          - • Migrate through interstitium by chemotaxis to injury site
        - ▪ *Macrophages (transformed monocytes) are the dominant cell type at 2-3 days, most important for releasing cytokines to attract fibroblasts and releasing growth factors (PDGF and TGF-β1).
    - ▪ **Proliferative phase** (aka "fibroblastic phase," approximately days 3-21)
      - □ *Fibroblasts are the predominant cell population at 3-5 days and transform into myofibroblasts to promote wound contraction.
      - □ High rate of collagen type III and I synthesis from days 5 to 21.
      - □ Tensile strength begins at days 4-5.
      - □ Fibroblasts form ECM by synthesizing proteoglycan and fibronectin.
      - □ *Keratinocytes migrate into the wound due to loss of contact inhibition secondary to wound.
      - □ *Neovascularization occurs under the influence of vascular endothelial growth factor (VEGF) expression.
    - ▪ **Remodeling (maturation) phase** (approximately week 3 to 1 year)
      - □ Collagen replaces proteoglycan/fibronectin and reorganizes creating stronger cross-links.
      - □ *Equilibrium between collagen breakdown and synthesis by weeks 3-5.
      - □ Matrix metalloproteinases (MMPs) and tissue inhibitors of metalloproteinases (TIMPs) remodel the collagen matrix.
      - □ The wound achieves 5% of its tensile strength at 1 week, 20% at 3 weeks, 50% at 4 weeks, and 80% after 6 weeks to a year after repair. Maximum tensile strength of a wound reaches only approximately 80% of noninjured skin.
      - □ *Final ratio of type I:type III collagen is 4:1.

- **Epithelialization**
  - Mobilization: due to loss of contact inhibition in keratinocytes.
  - Migration: cells migrate across the wound until contact inhibition is reestablished when touch cells of opposite wound edge.
  - Mitosis: cells further back from wound edge proliferate to bridge wound.
  - Differentiation: after migration ceases, epithelial layers are reestablished from basal layer to stratum corneum.
- **Contraction** (occurs with full-thickness injury *through dermis*)
  - Fibroblasts differentiate into myofibroblasts and are present throughout granulating wound.
  - Myofibroblasts appear at day 3 and reach the maximum level at days 10-21.
  - Amount of secondary contraction is dependent upon the amount of dermis within the wound; more dermis equals less secondary contraction.
- **Muscle Healing**
  - **Phases of muscle healing** (phases overlap with each other)
    - **Destructive phase** (days 0-7 following injury)
      - Myoblasts join with each other to form myotubes, which then fuse to form new myofibers.
      - Analogous to inflammatory phase of skin healing with cytokine release and initial response with neutrophils followed by macrophages.
    - **Repair phase** (starting at day 3 and lasting up to several weeks)
      - Regeneration of disrupted myofibers
      - Production of connective tissue scar
    - **Remodeling phase** (occurs concomitantly with repair phase)
      - Vascular ingrowth (to feed the upregulated metabolism of regeneration).
      - Regeneration of intramuscular nerves is necessary for functional regeneration.
      - Adhesion of myofibers to ECM.
- **Bone Healing**
  - **Bone healing categories**
    - **Primary** (direct) bone healing in the setting of absolute stability created by rigid surgical fixation
      - Minimal callus formation (bypasses the stage of woven bone formation)
      - Lamellar bone formation parallel to the long axis of the bone
    - **Secondary** (indirect) bone healing by external splint/cast fixation (nonrigid fixation)
      - Healing with callus formation; amount of callus correlates with the amount of instability encountered during healing.
      - Immobilization is important to allow for healing.
  - **Phases of bone healing**
    - **Inflammatory phase** (from time of fracture to start of bone formation at 7-10 days)
      - Initial platelet degranulation and contained hematoma aids in healing.
      - Inflammatory response as detailed in previous section; osteoclasts break down necrotic bone edges, releasing osteogenic cytokines.
    - **Reparative phase** (starting during the first week and lasting up to several months)
      - Inflammatory debris is cleared by macrophages.
      - Acid tide—acidic local environment stimulates osteoclasts.
      - Vascular ingrowth from periosteum and endosteum.
      - pH rises at approximately day 10 with the presence of increased alkaline phosphatase, leading to the formation of newly woven bone at the edges.
      - At approximately 3 weeks, callus fills in between the edges (starts as soft callus populated by chondrocytes, which gradually calcifies into

hard callus by endochondral ossification); continued bone formation by osteoblasts leads to bony edge unification.
- **Remodeling phase** (starting at 2-3 months and continuing for years)
  - Woven bone is slowly replaced by the lamellar bone according to the Wolff law; medullary canal is restored.
  - "Clinical healing" (defined as the state of adequate stability and resolution of pain to allow protected motion) occurs in most bones by 4-6 weeks. Radiographic healing may lag by 6 months.

- **Tendon Healing**
  - **Mechanisms of tendon healing**
    - **Intrinsic healing**
      - Tendon's innate capacity to heal (operative repair aims to maximize this type of healing)
      - Mediated by tenocytes/fibroblasts that arise from the tendon and epitenon
      - Relies on synovial diffusion for nutrition
      - Enhanced by mobilization
    - **Extrinsic healing**
      - Surrounding soft tissue's tendency to repair damaged tendon.
      - Infiltration of inflammatory cells and fibroblasts overlying the sheath.
      - Immobilization leads to the formation of adhesions, limiting range of motion (early mobilization minimizes adhesions caused by extrinsic healing).
  - **Phases of healing**
    - **Inflammatory phase** (within first few days, peaking at 3 days)
      - Tendon defect fills with hematoma, tissue debris, and fluid.
      - Increased phagocytic activity clears necrotic debris.
    - **Proliferative phase** (starting at approximately day 5 and lasting up to several weeks)
      - Fibroblasts are the predominant cell type, proliferating from epitenon and endotenon.
      - Collagen deposited, vascular ingrowth occurs.
      - Strength of repair begins and increases at ~2-3 weeks; synovial sheath is reconstituted at 3 weeks.
    - **Remodeling phase** (starting at several weeks after injury and lasting up to 1 year after)
      - Collagen fibers initially deposited perpendicular to tendon axis realign to the long axis of the tendon by 8 weeks.

- **Cartilage Healing**
  - Avascular tissue without intrinsic healing potential
  - Healing initiated by damage to the surrounding tissue (eg, perichondrium and subchondral bone)
  - **Extra-articular cartilage vs intra-articular cartilage healing**
    - **Extra-articular cartilage** (eg, auricular and nasal) injury
      - Tissue injury response generated by perichondrium with fibroblast influx and scar formation (but not true regeneration of cartilage)
    - **Intra-articular cartilage injury**
      - Superficial (without violation of subchondral bone)—no blood-carrying progenitor cells are released, thus no repair occurs.
      - Full-thickness (through cartilage and into subchondral bone)—allows influx of progenitor cells and formation of fibrocartilage. Fibrocartilage is less organized, more vascular, less tolerant of mechanical force, and more susceptible to degradation compared with normal cartilage. Fibrocartilage eventually breaks down, resulting in an arthritic joint.

- **Nerve Healing**
  - Response to injury **see Chapter 45: Nerve Injuries, Neuromas, and Compression Syndromes** for classifications of nerve injuries.

- Trauma to vasa nervorum and surrounding tissue leads to inflammatory response.
- If the injury is close to the neuron cell body, the entire neuron may die (eg, brachial plexus avulsion injuries).
- Typical injuries to *nerves* in peripheral locations (eg, complex forearm laceration) will affect connective tissues (Schwann cells) and the axon but not the actual neuronal cell body.
- *Wallerian degeneration: Schwann cells will die, and the distal axon degrades. This can extend up to 2 cm proximal to the injury site.
- Axon degradation and clearing of debris takes 15-30 days and precedes nerve regeneration.
- **Axonal regrowth** occurs in response to neurotrophins (eg, brain-derived neurotrophic factors, ciliary neurotrophic factor, and nerve growth factor) secreted by target cells (postsynaptic neurons or muscle cells) and by Schwann cells.
- Macrophages secrete interleukins that induce Schwann cell proliferation.
- Schwann cells along the distal axonal tract express laminins and adhesion molecules, which help guide the regenerating axon.
- Axonal sprouts from the proximal cut end must enter the distal tract to regrow. If budding axons cannot cross the gap, regeneration does not occur.
- Muscles innervated by the injured nerve will atrophy (70% loss at 2 months). Some muscle fibers die at 6-12 months if there is no regeneration of nerve. Motor endplates remain open for approximately 1 year (variable) before fibrosis develops, and reinnervation is then unlikely.
- *Once growth is initiated, axons extend by ~1 mm a day.

PATHOLOGIC WOUND HEALING

- **Wound Failure (Skin, Subcutaneous Tissue, Fascia, Muscle)**
  - **Acute wound failure (dehiscence):** postoperative separation of the surgical incision
    - Occurs when the load applied to the wound exceeds the strength of the suture line and provisional matrix
    - Most commonly happens at 7-10 days postoperatively, can happen any time from day 1 to more than 20 days after surgery
  - **Chronic wound failure** (nonhealing wounds)
    - Failure to achieve anatomic/functional integrity over 3 months.
    - Chronic wounds can development into squamous cell carcinoma (aka Marjolin ulcer).
    - Associated physiologic derangements.
      - *Abnormal ECM dynamics: increased MMPs, decreased TIMPs
  - **Associated factors for acute and chronic wound failure (see Table 1-1)**
    - *Radiation therapy leads to vascular fibrosis (relative ischemia) and decreases mitotic potential of fibroblasts (also consider possibility of osteoradionecrosis of the bone).
    - Diabetes (microvascular and macrovascular diseases leading to local ischemia; glycosylation of hemoglobin impairs oxygen delivery; impaired neutrophil function; peripheral neuropathy).
    - Advanced age (shortened inflammatory phase causing decreased strength of healing).
    - Malnutrition.
      - **Vitamin C**
        - *Role in collagen cross-linking by hydroxylation of proline and lysine.
        - *Lack of vitamin C leads to "scurvy": low collagen tensile strength manifests in collagen-containing tissues (skin, dentition, bone, and blood vessels) as hemorrhage (petechiae and swollen gums), loss of dentition, and impaired bone healing.

TABLE 1-1 Factors Affecting Acute and Chronic Wound Healing

Factors affecting wound dehiscence			Factors affecting bone malunion or nonunion		
Surgeon	Systemic	Local	Surgeon	Systemic	Local
Technical error	Advanced age	Hematoma	Technical error	Anemia	Soft tissue crush
Emergency surgery	Chronic steroids	Seroma	Emergency surgery	Malnutrition	Tissue interposition into fracture
	Malnutrition	Infection		Vitamin D deficiency	Inadequate reduction
	Radiation therapy	Edema		Growth hormone deficiency	Inadequate immobilization
	Chemotherapy	Excessive tension		NSAIDs	Rigid fixation with gap
	Systemic disease (hereditary healing disorders, renal failure, diabetes)	Previous wound dehiscence		Systemic disease (hereditary healing disorders, renal failure, diabetes)	Open, segmental, or articular fractures
		Venous insufficiency		Smoking	Pathologic fractures
	Smoking	Infected foreign body		Steroids	Infection

◻ Folate and vitamin B$_6$ (pyridoxine): DNA synthesis and cellular proliferation
◻ Vitamin E: strong antioxidant and immune modulator
◻ Zinc: cofactor for numerous metalloenzymes and proteins; necessary for protein and nucleic acid synthesis
◻ Nutrition historically assessed in the acute phase with prealbumin level (normal >17 g/dL, 3-day half-life) and in the chronic phase with albumin level (normal >3.5 g/dL, 20-day half-life)
  ▪ More recent literature suggests that these are more representative of inflammation than nutrition.
▪ Chemotherapy: Most detrimental agents are doxorubicin, cyclophosphamide, methotrexate, bis-chloroethylnitrosourea (BCNU), and nitrogen mustard.
▪ Glucocorticoids.
  ◻ Inhibit the inflammatory phase and collagen synthesis of fibroblasts, leading to decreased wound strength
  ◻ *Can reverse effect with oral vitamin A to augment epithelialization and fibroblast proliferation
▪ Anemia by itself does not impair wound healing.
• Bone
  ○ Types of bone healing pathology
    ▪ **Delayed union:** When clinical healing is delayed beyond the usual expected time with radiographic evidence of inadequate osteocyte activity and deficient callus formation.
    ▪ **Nonunion:** When there is no evidence of clinical or radiographic healing beyond the usual healing time, often with a mobile area fibrous scar and interposed tissue in the gap (pseudoarthrosis).
  ○ Factors detrimental to bone healing (see Table 1-1)
• Tendon
  ○ **Immobilization after primary tendon repair**
    ▪ Extrinsic healing predominates with tendon sheath adhesion formation.
    ▪ Disorganized collagen fibrils and decreased strength of repair.
    ▪ Poor tendon healing can be attributable to gapping from poor surgical technique.
  ○ **Overuse tendinosis:** painful condition beginning with repetitive microtrauma to tendon without allowing appropriate time to heal; characterized by degenerative changes in tendon
• Nerve
  ○ **Neuroma**—painful regrowth of nerve in a scarred area of previous injury
  ○ **Failure of axonal regeneration** (regeneration decreases with age)
    ▪ Degeneration of sensory receptors (for sensory nerves)
    ▪ Fibrosis of motor endplates (for motor nerves)
  ○ **Cross-innervation** (eg, facial synkinesis, gustatory sweating [Frey syndrome])

SCARRING

NORMAL SCARRING

• Visible scar is the normal end point for all full-thickness skin injuries. No such thing as scarless surgery.
• Factors That Lead to Less Conspicuous Scars
  ○ Older age
  ○ Lighter colored skin
  ○ Surgical incision as opposed to traumatic laceration
  ○ Placement of incision or laceration within (parallel to) relaxed skin tension line
  ○ Minimal tension following closure (eg, eyelids)
  ○ Optimal surgical technique (eg, atraumatic manipulation, skin edge eversion, and removal of suture in 5-7 days on face)

PATHOLOGIC SCARRING

- **Hypertrophic Scar**
  - ○ **Definition:** an abnormal wound healing end point in response to trauma, inflammation, burn, or surgery
    - Raised, erythematous, and often pruritic.
    - *Remains within the boundaries of original wound.
    - Upregulated fibrogenic cytokines (TGF-β isoforms, PDGF, and insulinlike growth factor 1 [IGF-1]) lead to higher levels of collagen synthesis.
  - ○ **Etiology**
    - Major factors
      - □ Extent/depth of trauma (most commonly with burns)
      - □ Inflammation, infection
      - □ Prolonged open wound (>21 days, most commonly with burns)
    - Contributing factors
      - □ Tension on wound
      - □ Darker skin tone
  - ○ **Natural history**
    - Becomes apparent at ~6-8 weeks after injury
    - Worsens over 6 months
    - May cause contractures at joints
    - May take 1-2 years to mature (scar typically will become less red, less tender, and less pruritic)
  - ○ **Histologic characteristics** (under standard light microscopy, hypertrophic scar and keloid are indistinguishable)
    - Cigar-shaped nodules of blood vessels, fibroblasts, and collagen fibers that are arranged parallel to epidermis and oriented along tension lines vs normal skin, which has the basketlike woven pattern of collagen fibers
    - *Presence of α-smooth muscle actin producing myofibroblasts (not present in keloids)
    - Primarily composed of well-organized type III collagen
  - ○ **Treatment approach**
    - Nonoperative
      - □ **Pressure garments**
        - Commonly used for hypertrophic burn scars
        - Induces local tissue hypoxia, reduces fibroblast proliferation and collagen synthesis
        - Compression of 24-30 mm Hg to be effective
      - □ **Silicone sheeting and topical silicone gel**
        - Unclear mechanism of action—thought to increase hydration of remodeling scar
        - Require application at least 12 hours per day for at least 3 months to be effective
      - □ **Corticosteroid injection**
    - Surgical excision
      - □ Attention to atraumatic technique, excision of inflamed tissue, avoidance of nidus for inflammation (eg, trapped hair or unnecessary deep resorbable suture), and tension-free closure.
      - □ Z-plasty tissue rearrangements to release contractures.
      - □ May require graft or flap reconstruction for coverage.
      - □ Fractional ablative CO_2 laser can be helpful adjunct as well as pulse dye lasers to remove the redness of scars.
- **Keloids**
  - ○ **Definition:** an abnormal wound healing end point in response to trauma, inflammation, burns, or surgery

- May start as a raised, erythematous, and pruritic lesion
- *Evolves into an enlarging mass that extends beyond the original boundaries of the wound
- Higher level of collagen synthesis compared with hypertrophic scars due to upregulated fibrogenic cytokines (TGF-β isoforms, PDGF, and IGF-1) and increased number of receptors for these cytokines within keloidal fibroblasts
- *Increased fibroblast proliferation
- *Absence of myofibroblasts and decreased density of blood vessels in comparison to hypertrophic scars
- Decreased expression of MMPs (that degrade ECM), increased ATP
  - **Etiology**
    - Major factors
      - Darker skin tone
      - Genetic predisposition
    - Contributing factors
      - Age (peak just after puberty)
      - Hormones (keloids worsen during puberty and pregnancy; postmenopausal women experience softening and flattening of keloids)
  - **Natural history:** evolves over time without a significant regression or quiescent phase
  - **Histologic characteristics** (under light microscopy, hypertrophic scar and keloid are indistinguishable)
    - *Thick and large collagen fibers haphazardly packed closely together comprised of both type I and type III collagen
  - **Treatment approach:** Nonoperative and operative interventions are required, and an extremely high rate of recurrence persists (50%-80%).
    - **Nonoperative**
      - Pressure devices (eg, pressure clip for earlobe) (preventative measure)
      - Silicone sheeting and topical silicone gel (preventative measure)
      - Corticosteroid injection (recurrence 15.4%)
      - 5-fluorouracil (5-FU) injection (chemotherapeutic drug) (recurrence rate 19%)
    - **Surgical**
      - Attention to atraumatic technique, excision of inflamed tissue, avoidance of nidus for inflammation (eg, trapped hair or unnecessary deep resorbable suture), and tension-free closure
      - Excision ± skin graft depending on the size of the lesion
      - Radiation therapy performed within 1-3 days after excision, ideally within 24 hours (recurrence rate 14%)

MANAGEMENT OF WOUNDS

INITIAL WOUND ASSESSMENT

- **Acute vs chronic (see Fig. 1-2)**
  - Origin and duration of wound
    - Traumatic vs atraumatic
      - Zone of injury is larger in high- vs low-impact traumas
      - Assessment for other associated injuries
  - Extent of contamination
    - Antibiotics are not needed for most wounds unless they demonstrate signs of active infection (eg, cellulitis in chronic venous stasis ulcers).
    - Bite wounds are always contaminated and have a high likelihood of infection.
      - Assume that the contamination is polymicrobial, and always treat with antibiotics that cover Gram-positive and anaerobic organisms (eg, ampicillin/sulbactam or amoxicillin/clavulanate, ciprofloxacin + clindamycin if allergic to penicillin)

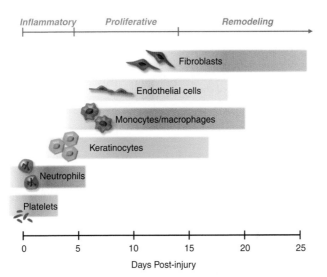

Figure 1-2 The phases of wound healing. (From Thorne CH, Gurtner GC, Kevin Chung KC, et al., eds. *Grabb and Smith's Plastic Surgery*. 7th ed. Wolters Kluwer; 2014. Figure 2.2.)

- □ Consider bacteria specific to type of bite:
  - Human bites: *Eikenella corrodens*
  - Cat bites: *Pasteurella multocida*
- □ Tetanus prophylaxis (**Table 1-2**)
- ○ Size of wound
- ○ Extent of exposed tissue: dermis, subcutaneous tissue, fascia, muscle, bone
  - >85% chance of osteomyelitis in wounds with exposed bone
- **Assessment of patient-specific local and systemic factors**
  - ○ Presence of ischemia-reperfusion injury
  - ○ Hypoxia of the wound bed
  - ○ Bacterial load of the wound
    - Contaminated: Bacteria present without proliferation.
    - Colonized: Bacteria present and proliferating but without causing host response.
    - Critically colonized: Bacteria present, proliferating, and causing host response but not enough to overcome host's resistance.
    - Infected: Expanding bacterial counts that have overcome the host's ability to respond.

TABLE 1-2 Tetanus Prophylaxis Guidelines

Tetanus toxoid history	Clean, minor wounds	Contaminated or major wounds
<3 doses or unknown	Tetanus toxoid	Tetanus toxoid Tetanus immunoglobulin
≥3 doses	Nothing (except tetanus toxoid if >10 y since last booster)	Nothing (except tetanus toxoid if >10 y since last booster; consider immunoglobulin if toxoid is not administered)

From CDC Guidelines, 1998.

PHYSICAL EXAMINATION

- **General Assessment**
  - ○ Overall health of the patient
  - ○ Quality of tissue surrounding the wound
    - ▪ Presence/absence of
      - □ Radiation-induced chronic skin changes
      - □ Edema
      - □ Color: dependent rubor vs erythema
      - □ Induration/focal fluid collections
      - □ Hemorrhage
      - □ Foreign bodies
      - □ Other wounds in the area
  - ○ **Condition of wound bed**
    - ▪ Location: Evaluate the area for excess pressure or dependent positioning.
    - ▪ Depth: Evaluate for damage to surrounding structures, including blood vessels, nerves, bone, muscle, and subcutaneous tissues.
    - ▪ Characteristics of wound bed
      - □ Amount of granulation tissue vs fibrinous exudate
      - □ Odor
      - □ Exposed structures
      - □ Foreign bodies
      - □ Sinus tract/tunnel formation
      - □ Drainage
  - ○ **Neurosensory examination**
    - ▪ Gross sensation based on dermatomes involved
    - ▪ Two-point discrimination: normal two point <5 mm
    - ▪ Vibration sensation
  - ○ **Vascular examination**
    - ▪ The presence of both palpable peripheral pulses and Doppler signals in vascular territories adjacent to the wound
    - ▪ Temperature of extremity or digit
    - ▪ Skin changes consistent with venous stasis, peripheral arterial disease, and/or lymphedema
- **Laboratory/Radiographic Testing**
  - ○ **Complete blood count (CBC):** evaluate for elevated WBC count and anemia.
  - ○ **Albumin: evaluate for malnutrition if <3.5 g/dL.**
  - ○ **Erythrocyte sedimentation rate and C-reactive protein:** may signal the presence or recurrence of osteomyelitis but are nonspecific inflammatory markers that may be elevated in any proinflammatory state, so should be interpreted in the context of the entire clinical picture.
  - ○ **Hemoglobin A1C.**
  - ○ **Creatinine**
    - ▪ Renal failure may predispose patients to chronic wounds and poor wound healing.
    - ▪ Calciphylaxis is an important underlying cause of chronic wounds in patients with end-stage renal disease.
  - ○ **Plain films:** Assess for fractures, orthopedic plates/screws, foreign bodies, and osteomyelitis.
  - ○ **Computed tomography (CT):** Assess for abscesses, chronic sinuses, extent of wound, and involved structures
  - ○ **Magnetic resonance imaging (MRI):** To evaluate the extent of osteomyelitis, especially if spine is involved.
  - ○ **Ankle-brachial indices**
    - ▪ >1.2: calcified vessels (eg, diabetes)
    - ▪ 0.9-1.2: normal
    - ▪ 0.5-0.9: mixed arterial/venous disease

- <0.5: critical stenosis, symptomatic claudication
- <0.2: ischemia and gangrene
  - **Angiography:** to evaluate the extent of vascular disease or vascular injury
    - If there is evidence of significant peripheral vascular disease, wounds should not be débrided until revascularization procedures are complete to optimize wound healing.
    - Exception: Wounds must be débrided regardless of vascular status if there are signs of overt infection (eg, "wet" suppurative gangrene).
  - **Biopsy/cultures**
    - Help target antibiotic regimens and durations; should only be taken after appropriate débridement.
    - Evaluate for malignancy for atypical or chronic nonhealing wounds.
    - Quantification of bacterial colonies helps in diagnosis and in following progression of treatment.

DÉBRIDEMENT

- **Surgical, Enzymatic (Collagenase), Mechanical (Versajet, Waterpik), and Autolytic**
  - **Reduces bioburden** by removing inflammatory component of wound, biofilms, fibrinous tissue, which contains cytotoxic mediators that inhibit wound healing.
  - Promotes wound healing by converting a chronic wound into an acute wound to promote keratinocyte migration.
  - **Vital structures** (eg, nerve, tendon, bone, and vessels) should not be débrided whenever possible unless gross infection or ischemia is present.

DRESSINGS

- **Goals**
  - Protect the wound from the external environment and mechanical forces.
  - Absorb secretions/maintain a clean environment.
  - **Promote granulation** tissue formation and reepithelialization: Moist environment leads to increased granulation tissue formation and tissue reepithelialization as compared with dry environment and can promote débridement during dressing changes.
  - Optimize patient comfort.
- **Type of Dressings**
  - **Nonocclusive dressings** (eg, Gauze)
    - Permeable to both gas particles and fluids
    - **Typically utilized for "wet to dry" dressing**
      - Allowing the gauze to dry prior to removal results in mechanical débridement of the wound during each dressing change.
      - Removal of the dry gauze also creates a mild proinflammatory state, which can help with wound healing.
      - Coarse gauze provides greater débridement compared with fine gauze.
    - **"Wet to wet" dressing:** Used over exposed tendon, bone, and neurovascular structures to minimize desiccation.
  - **Semiocclusive dressings** (eg, Tegaderm)
    - Sheet dressings that are impermeable to fluids but allow passage of gas molecules.
    - Typically used to cover skin graft donor sites and for fingertip amputations to keep area moist and promote healing.
    - Must be cautious in using on areas of thin/fragile skin.
    - Should not be used in contaminated wounds.
  - **Occlusive dressings**
    - **Hydrogel** (eg, AquaSorb and Hydrosorb).
    - Composed of complex polysaccharides, nonadhesive.
    - Use in wounds with mild, superficially exudative regions and in painful wounds.

- Rehydrate wounds and maintain moisture independent from the moisture that is inherently present in the wound.
- Can be used in infected wound beds.
  ○ **Hydrocolloids** (eg, Duoderm)
  - Comes in paste, powder, and sheet forms.
  - Fully adhesive, minimally absorptive.
  - Cannot use in infected wounds.
  - Induces autolytic débridement within wound.
  - Use in mild, superficially exudative wounds.
  ○ **Foam** (eg, Mepilex)
  - Usually composed of nonadhering polyurethane.
  - Highly absorptive, but nonhydrating.
  - Use in moderately to heavily exudative wounds.
  ○ **Alginates** (eg, Algiderm, Aquacel)
  - Derived from seaweed.
  - Comes in ribbon/rope forms.
  - Can absorb 20× the dry weight of the dressing.
  - Use in highly exudative wounds.
  ○ **Antimicrobial dressings**
  - Silver-coated or -impregnated dressings (eg, Silverlon)
  - Xeroform: 3% bismuth tribromophenate-impregnated gauze
  ○ **Negative pressure wound therapy**
  - Consists of using a sponge, occlusive dressing, and vacuum
    □ Reduces edema
    □ Removes excess interstitial fluid from the wound bed, decreasing interstitial pressure and promoting improved blood flow from wound bed capillaries
    □ Vacuum imparts strain on cells within wound, activating molecular changes including upregulation of the VEGF pathway and angiogenesis
    □ Does not auto-débride wounds but induces tissue deformation
  - *Must not use over
    □ Normal skin
    □ Infected tissues
    □ Tissues harboring malignant cells
    □ Inadequately débrided wounds
    □ Neurovascular structures

SURGICAL WOUNDS

- **Classification of Surgical Wounds**
  ○ **Clean (class I):** nontraumatic; no entry into respiratory, gastrointestinal (GI), genitourinary (GU) systems prior to incision; no break in sterile technique (<2% risk of infection)
  ○ **Clean-contaminated (class II):** nontraumatic; minor breaks in sterile technique; entry into GU, GI, and/or respiratory tracts, but without significant spillage (<10% risk of infection)
  ○ **Contaminated (class III):** traumatic, may include gross entry and spillage from GI or GU systems, involves grossly infected tissues/fluid (~20% risk of infection)
  ○ **Dirty (class IV):** traumatic, dirty wound, significant devitalized tissue, fecal matter, foreign bodies, evidence of perforated viscus, and inflammation (40% risk of infection)
- **General Considerations When Creating Incisions and for Wound Closure**
  ○ **Type of skin and location on the body**
  - Specific areas are prone to scar widening and hypertrophy (eg, shoulder/ sternal areas, high-tension, lots of motion), whereas others tend to heal more favorably (eg, eyelid and dorsum of the hand).

- Hair-bearing skin: Scalp incisions are typically beveled to allow for hair growth after incision has healed by avoiding disruption of the hair follicles.
- Extremity
  - Longitudinal incisions are preferred to avoid crossing joint surfaces to minimize tension and lessen the chance of mobility-limiting scar contracture.
  - Excisional and incisional biopsies should always be oriented longitudinally in order to prevent later morbidity and complexity if additional resection and reconstruction is required (eg, sarcoma).
- Hand incisions
  - Midaxial or volar zigzag (Bruner) incisions are preferred to approach the digit volarly.
  - S-shaped, C-shaped, or curvilinear incisions are preferred to approach the digit dorsally.
- Direction and length of the incision
  - **Langer lines of tension (relaxed skin tension lines):** Incisions that are able to be planned should be made parallel to the relaxed skin tension lines.
- Surgical technique
  - Minimize damage to skin edges with atraumatic technique
  - Débridement of necrotic or foreign material
  - Tension-free closure
  - Wound edge eversion
  - Placement of suture that should not leave permanent suture marks
  - Prompt removal of sutures
    - Face: 5-7 days
    - Hand/foot: 10-14 days
    - Trunk/breast: 7-10 days
- **Types of Closure**
  - **Primary closure:** Tissues are reapproximated (using sutures, staples, etc.) on initial presentation.
    - Edges must be under minimal tension.
    - Wound cannot be infected.
  - **Secondary intention closure:** Wound heals with time through accumulation of granulation tissue, usually with frequent dressing changes.
  - **Delayed primary closure:** Wound initially heals through secondary intention. Once wound bed is clean and under minimal tension, wound edges can be reapproximated using primary closure techniques.
- **Closure Materials (See Table 1-3)**
  - Suture
    - Classified as absorbable vs nonabsorbable; monofilament vs braided; synthetic vs natural
      - **Absorbable**
        - Lose at least 50% of strength in 4 weeks
        - Often used in children/unreliable patients to avoid suture removal
      - **Nonabsorbable:** Permanent, body induces a cell-mediated reaction around the suture, which eventually encapsulates the suture.
      - **Monofilament vs braided:** Braided sutures have greater knot security and flexibility but has slightly increased risk of infection and greater friction through tissue.
      - **Synthetic vs natural:** Silk and gut are the only natural sutures available; the rest are synthetic.
  - Staples
    - Quick closure
    - Good for hair-bearing regions
    - Use forceps to initiate wound eversion and staple in place
  - Surgical adhesives

TABLE 1-3 Commonly Used Suture Materials

	Suture types	Configuration	Time to 50% original strength	Unique features and typical uses
Absorbable	Plain gut: enzyme-mediated hydrolysis in 60 d	Monofilament (natural)	5–7 d	Composed of bovine intestinal submucosa/serosa. Can be used as a skin closure suture as it dissolves rapidly with minimal scarring
	Chromic gut	Monofilament (natural)	14 d	Often used for oral and nasal mucosa, palmar hand incisions
	Polyglycolic acid (Vicryl): absorbed within 90 d	Braided (synthetic)	2–3 wk	Often used for dermal apposition
	Polydioxanone (PDS): completely absorbed in 6 mo	Monofilament (synthetic)	4 wk	Can be used for dermal apposition or for subcuticular closure
	Poliglecaprone 25 (Monocryl): completely absorbed in 3 mo	Monofilament (synthetic)	3 wk	Can be used for dermal apposition or for subcuticular closure
	Polyglyconate (Maxon)	Braided (synthetic)	4 wk	
Nonabsorbable	Nylon	Monofilament (synthetic)		Has a low coefficient of friction, minimally reactive, maintains tensile strength >2 y. Most commonly used externally for skin closure but can also be used internally (eg, rhinoplasty and otoplasty)
	Polypropylene (Prolene)	Monofilament (synthetic)		Used for suturing vascular anastomoses, dermal closures of the face
	Silk	Braided (natural)	Starts losing strength in 2 y	Commonly used for vascular ligation but can be a nidus for infection
	Braided polyester (Ethibond)	Braided (synthetic)		Minimal breakdown in strength, even after 2 y. Commonly used for tendon repairs

- Cyanoacrylate (Dermabond)
  - Used in conjunction with a proper closure initiated by suture material, which is under minimal tension
  - Pros: decreased time for closure, improved cosmetic outcome, possible decreased risk of infection due to decrease in suture use
  - Cons: must have a tension-free closure, must not be used on mucosal surfaces. Increased risk of wound dehiscence
- **Surgical tapes** (eg, Steri-Strips): can be used in conjunction with sutures or alone if the closure is completely tension free
- **Methods of Wound Closure (See Fig. 1-3)**
  - **Simple interrupted:** Needle is placed perpendicular to the skin and drawn into the targeted layers of tissue on one side, then out through the same layers/levels of tissue on the opposite side, then tied in place.

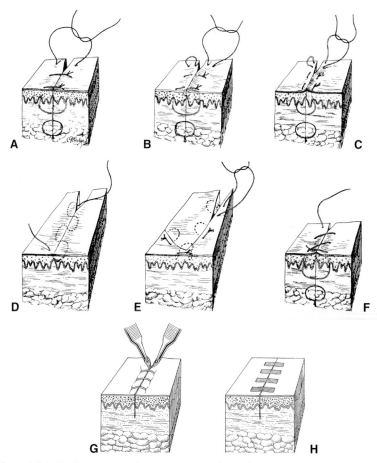

Figure 1-3 A. Simple interrupted closure. **B.** Interrupted vertical mattress pattern. **C.** Interrupted horizontal mattress pattern. **D.** Running subcuticular (intracuticular) sutures. **E.** Half-buried horizontal mattress (applicable in corners). **F.** Simple running ("over-and-over") suture. **G.** Stapled closure. **H.** Steri-Strips (adhesive tape).

- The needle pathway allows the width of the suture at the base to be wider than at the epidermal entrance to allow eversion of the skin edges.
- Place sutures 5-7 mm apart and 1-2 mm from the skin edges to allow for appropriate wound closure.

o **Vertical/horizontal mattress suture**
- Good for glabrous skin and wounds under tension.
- Horizontal mattress causes more hypoxia to tissues than vertical mattress.

o **Subcuticular:** avoids marks on the external surface of the incision to result in a more favorable scar; allows for reapproximation of the epidermis.

o **Running suture:** best used when wound edges are already somewhat approximated, faster closure. Use locking running stitch if hemostasis is needed.

PEARLS

1. Scars typically widen over time. Some areas, such as the back or the legs, where the tension is higher, are especially prone to scar widening.
2. Nicotine in any form (smoking, patches, and gum) impairs wound healing significantly due to vasoconstrictive effects.
3. Macrophages are critical cells in wound healing and initiate the growth factor cascade, fibroblast proliferation, and collagen formation.
4. Prior to considering scar revision, at least 1 year should pass to allow for complete scar remodeling.
5. Antibiotic ointments (eg, Bacitracin) should only be used for 2-3 days as patients can develop hypersensitivity and rash that may be mistaken for cellulitis/infection.
6. Absorbable suture should be used in children whenever possible or when suture removal is anticipated to be difficult or may disrupt closure.
7. Topical skin adhesives can be used in conjunction with sutures that have achieved epithelial continuity.

QUESTIONS YOU WILL BE ASKED

1. What is the difference between wound contraction and wound contracture?
   Wound contraction is a part of secondary healing beginning a few days after injury as myofibroblasts contract and reduce the size of the wound to be epithelialized. Wound contractures occur when bands of collagen are deposited at the site of hypertrophic scar formation; these are termed "contractures" when they impair functionality (eg, hands) or range of motion (eg, axillae and neck).
2. What is the difference between hypertrophic scar and keloid?
   Hypertrophic scar does not extend beyond the borders of the original wound, whereas keloids grow well beyond these borders; histologically, these two fibroproliferative disorders are different, but they are indistinguishable under standard H&E preparation on light microscopy. They have different type I:type III collagen ratios. Hypertrophic scars produce smooth muscle actin by myofibroblasts, whereas keloids do not.
3. What are the factors that impair wound healing?
   Systemic conditions (eg, diabetes, autoimmune conditions, and medications), ischemia, pressure injury, infection, malignancy, foreign body, venous insufficiency, irradiation, hypoxia, smoking, advanced age, and malnutrition.
4. What is the timing of wound healing and what is the final tensile strength a wound achieves?
   The wound achieves 5% of its tensile strength at 1 week, 20% at 3 weeks, and 80% after 6 weeks. Maximum tensile strength of a wound reaches only ~80% of noninjured skin.

5. Describe the classification of sutures and what factors of a wound/incision affect the choice of suture.

   Sutures are classified as absorbable vs nonabsorbable, natural vs synthetic, and braided vs monofilament. The suture chosen should effectively minimize tension on the closure, promote eversion of the skin edges, and remain in place for the optimal length of time necessary to maintain a strong and durable closure while minimizing the body's inflammatory response to the suture itself to optimize the appearance of the scar.

6. Describe the timing of suture removal for the extremities, face, and trunk.

   Extremities: 10-14 days; face: 5-7 days; trunk/breast: 7-10 days.

7. What are the contraindications to wound VAC therapy?

   Do not use a wound VAC over normal skin, infected tissues, tissues harboring malignant cells, inadequately débrided wounds, or directly on top of neurovascular structures.

8. What dressings are good for highly exudative wounds?

   Alginates and foam (eg, Mepilex) are good for highly exudative wounds and can decrease dressing change frequency.

9. Describe the treatment of animal/human bite wounds.

   Bite wounds should be washed out aggressively and thoroughly on presentation given the predisposition of such wounds for infection. If closure is needed, tissues should be loosely approximated to allow for egress of débris and infected fluid. Antibiotics that provide coverage against anaerobic and Gram-positive organisms, namely *Eikenella corrodens* and group A *Streptococcus*, should be prescribed. Amoxicillin-clavulanate has good activity against common oral pathogens. Patients should be followed closely to monitor for signs of infection.

Recommended Readings
1. Broughton G, Janis JE, Attinger CE. The basic science of wound healing. *Plast Reconstr Surg.* 2006;117(7 Suppl):12S-34S.
2. Garner WL, Rahban SR. Fibroproliferative scars. *Clin Plast Surg.* 2003;30(1):77-89.
3. Janis J, Harrison B. Wound Healing: Part II. Clinical Applications. *Plast Reconstr Surg.* 2014;133(3):383e-392e.
4. Janis J, Harrison B. Wound Healing: Part I. Basic Science. *Plast Reconstr Surg.* 2016;138(3S):9S-17S.
5. Leach J. Proper handling of soft tissue in the acute phase. *Facial Plast Surg.* 2001;17(4):227-238.
6. Maggi SP, Lowe JB III, Mackinnon SE. Pathophysiology of nerve injury. *Clin Plast Surg.* 2003;30(2):109-126.
7. Ueno C, Hunt TK, Hopf HW. Using physiology to improve surgical wound outcomes. *Plast Reconstr Surg.* 2006;117(7 Suppl):59S-71S.

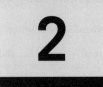

2 Grafts

Jennifer C. Lee and Widya Adidharma

BASIS OF RECONSTRUCTION

- **Reconstructive Goals**
  - Restore form and function to the defect.
  - Minimize donor site morbidity.
- **Reconstructive Ladder (Fig. 2-1)**
  - Systematic approach to facilitate decision-making for reconstruction of defects.
  - Least complicated technique is generally chosen to address the reconstructive goals.
- **Reconstructive Elevator**
  - Sometimes, the best solution is not the simplest.
  - Option is chosen that will give patient best aesthetic and functional result, often requiring a "jump" in the ladder (eg, free flap may be the best first choice if superior result is unmatched by other options, even if simpler option can also be used).
  - In reality, this is the method in which flap selection is typically done.

OVERVIEW

- Unlike flaps (**Chapter 3: Flaps**), grafts do not bring independent blood supply to a recipient bed.
  - *Autograft: from same individual
  - *Allograft: from another individual of same species (ie, homograft/cadaver graft)
  - *Xenograft: from another species (ie, heterograft)
- Skin, dermis, fat, bone, tendon, cartilage, nerve, fascia, or combinations of tissues can be transferred as grafts.

EVALUATION

- **History**
  - **Assess for factors that impact graft survival (anything that would influence new vascular growth into the graft):** systemic diseases/conditions (nutritional status, diabetes, anticoagulants, immunosuppression, and nicotine), local conditions (prior radiation and venous/arterial insufficiency), and anticipated compliance
- **Physical Exam**
  - **Recipient site considerations**
    - Wound site preparation removes devitalized tissue and contamination, which is critical to success of graft.
      - □ Viability: adequate blood supply, no devitalized tissue.
      - □ Hemostasis: hematoma is a major cause of graft failure.
      - □ Bacterial load: contamination prevents graft survival.
    - *Perform recipient site tissue culture if history or concern for infection (counts $<10^5$ CFU/g tissue for most pathogens required before grafting).

---

*Denotes common in-service examination topics.

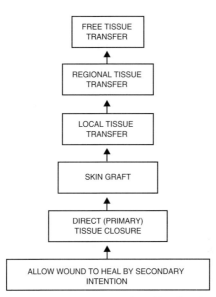

Figure 2-1 Reconstructive ladder. (From Thorne CH, ed. *Grabb and Smith's Plastic Surgery*. 7th ed. Wolters Kluwer; 2014. **Figure 1.21.**)

- o **Donor site considerations:** defect is best replaced with like tissue. For example, an eyelid skin defect requires a thin skin graft best harvested from "like" tissue, such as preauricular or cervical thin skin, rather than thicker skin of inguinal region.
  - ■ Also consider donor site availability
  - ■ Location based on patient preference for location of scar, ease of donor site care, anticipated match of donor skin to recipient site, availability of sufficient quantity of tissue, decreased donor site morbidity

TYPES OF GRAFTS

SKIN GRAFTS
- **General Indications**
  - o Primary closure not feasible
  - o Lack of adjacent tissue for coverage (poor quality, insufficient quantity, and inferior aesthetic appearance)
  - o Uncertain tumor clearance
  - o Patients with significant comorbid conditions who may not tolerate the potential risks or complications of more complex reconstructive options
  - o Benefits compared to healing by secondary intention: quicker healing, decreased scar contraction, improved aesthetic appearance, and less fluid loss
- **General Contraindications**
  - o Infected recipient bed.
  - o Unreliable vascularization from recipient bed (eg, history of radiation).
  - o Repeated motion or trauma to recipient bed.
  - o Exposed white/avascular structures (tendon, nerve, bone, and cartilage) in recipient bed; grafts can technically be placed on paratenon, periosteum, and perichondrium but typically do not provide durable coverage.

- Anticipated staged reconstruction beneath recipient bed (nerve, tendon reconstruction).
- **Classification.** Full-thickness (FTSG) vs split-thickness skin graft (STSG) (**Table 2-1**)
- **Application Principles**
  - **Harvest graft based on the size of defect**
    - Harvesting STSG: think about harvest technique, thickness, and mesh vs not mesh
      - Harvest techniques: free hand knife, drum dermatome, air- or electricity-driven dermatome (most common method). Can use mineral oil to facilitate smooth harvest.
        - Can use tumescence to flatten out area of harvest as well as to decrease blood loss from donor site.
      - Most grafts are 12/1000-18/1000 inches thick (infants, elderly, and immunocompromised patients may have thin skin, thus should consider patient and recipient site needs when choosing thickness).
      - Meshed vs sheet grafts.

TABLE 2-1 Comparison Between Split-Thickness and Full-Thickness Skin Grafts

	Split-thickness grafts	Full-thickness grafts
Components	Include epidermis and part of dermis; thicker grafts contain more donor characteristics	Include epidermis and entire dermis
Harvest sites	Anterolateral thigh, back, abdomen, upper inner arm, and scalp	Preauricular and supraclavicular for head and neck recipient sites; groin, lower abdomen, and medial forearm for hand recipient sites (choose based on texture, thickness, pigmentation, and presence/absence of hair)
Indications	Resurface large wounds, cavities, mucosal defects, muscle flap coverage, flap donor site closure, and temporary closure of wounds after tumor extirpation pending margin clearance with less donor site morbidity compared with other reconstructive options	Limited to small, uncontaminated and well-vascularized wounds, generally preferred in cosmetic or functionally sensitive sites (eg, joints, hands, and face); preferable when color match, thickness, and resistance to contraction are important qualities
Contraction	Greater secondary contraction/less primary	Greater primary contraction/less secondary
Donor site	Donor site heals by reepithelialization, reharvesting after healing possible (back = best site for reharvesting)	Donor site typically closed primarily
Availability	Greater quantity available, thus used to resurface larger wounds	Less quantity available, thus use is limited to smaller, cosmetic/functionally sensitive wounds
Hair	Hair growth through graft not possible	Hair growth through graft possible (growth assumes characteristics of donor site)
Growth potential	Limited ability to grow in pediatric patients	Retain ability to grow in pediatric patients
Pigmentation	Less predictable pigmentations	More predictable pigmentation

- Meshed grafts
  - □ Increase surface area of graft while decreasing harvest area.
  - □ Improve contour of grafts over irregular surfaces.
  - □ Allow for drainage of exudate and blood.
  - □ Increased secondary contraction (may be desired in some locations but should be avoided over joints and face).
  - □ The larger the meshing, the worse the aesthetic outcome, though interstices will fill in over time.
- Sheet (unmeshed) grafts
  - □ Provide superior aesthetic benefit
  - □ Used in face and hands
  - □ May need pie crusting (small holes) depending on graft size to allow egress of fluid or blood
  - □ Harvesting FTSG
- Harvest of FTSGs usually done in ellipse shape to facilitate primary closure of donor site.
- Aggressive defatting of donor skin critical to improve initial survival.
- Tissue expansion of lower abdomen or groin prior to FTSGs can be used to allow for primary closure of larger graft harvest.
  - ○ Graft is secured to skin edges and base of recipient bed with staples, suture (usually chromic or absorbable monofilament), or fibrin glue.
  - ○ Excess harvested skin may be stored on donor site or at 4 °C for several weeks (viability of graft decreases with time) to use for delayed application.
- **Graft Survival and Healing**
  - ○ *Imbibition (first 24-48 hours): plasma imbibition (diffusion) responsible for skin graft survival until angiogenesis occurs → thinner grafts more likely to survive
  - ○ *Inosculation (48-72 hours): process of capillaries joining between skin graft and recipient bed
  - ○ **Revascularization (4-7 days):** ingrowth of capillaries into graft
  - ○ **Primary contraction**
    - Occurs at the time of graft harvest/application
    - Due to elastin fibers in dermis
    - Greater in FTSGs (>40%) compared with STSGs (<20%); depends on the amount of dermis in the graft
  - ○ **Secondary contraction**
    - Occurs after graft take during healing phase of graft over 6-18 months.
    - Greater in STSGs. Dermal components of FTSGs suppress myofibroblast activities responsible for secondary contraction.
  - ○ **Regeneration of dermal appendages**
    - More likely to regenerate in thicker grafts.
    - Sweating assumes characteristics of recipient site when glands are reinnervated.
    - Sebaceous glands retain characteristics of donor site.
  - ○ **Reinnervation**
    - Begins 2-4 weeks after grafting. Process takes several months to years.
    - Assumes characteristics of recipient site.
    - Reinnervation incomplete and some degree of decreased sensation will persist.
    - STSGs regain sensation quicker, but FTSGs regain more complete innervation.
    - Pain returns first, then touch, and then temperature.
- **Complications**
  - ○ Graft failure
    - Poor recipient bed vascularization due to smoking, radiation, and other clinical factors
    - Inadequate revascularization of skin graft due to hematoma, seroma, or poor graft fixation
    - Skin graft infection

- ○ Pigment changes (donor and recipient sites); permanent hyperpigmentation may result from early sun exposure before full maturation.
- ○ Scar contraction, hypertrophic scarring, and graft instability.
- **Postoperative Considerations**
  - ○ **Graft donor site care**
    - Options: occlusive dressings (eg, Duoderm), semi-occlusive dressings (eg, Tegaderm), and semi-open dressings (eg, Xeroform and Mepilex).
    - **Semi-occlusive dressings encourage faster reepithelialization, least painful, nearly maintenance free, and keep wound moist.**
    - Semi-open dressings reliable but require daily drying (except for Mepilex).
    - Watch for infection that can convert a donor site wound from partial- to full-thickness injury.
  - ○ **Graft dressing and bolster**
    - Key to bolster is ability to keep the graft in contact with the donor site (tie over or staple into place). Should provide uniform pressure to prevent seroma, hematoma, and shear.
    - Many bolster/dressing options: nonadherent contact layer (Xeroform). This is followed by Reston dressing, cotton balls wrapped in xeroform, Una boot wrap for extremities, or a negative pressure wound therapy device.
    - Bolster not used when graft placed over a transferred muscle flap (eg, soleus flap for lower extremity defect) due to undesired compression and need to check flap viability.
    - Elevate and immobilize recipient site if possible.
    - Dressing left undisturbed for 4-5 days unless it shows signs of infection to allow for graft to take.
    - After bolster removal, bid to qd Xeroform dressing changes ± antibiotic ointment until healing is complete (~2-3 weeks) to prevent desiccation.
    - Graft is fragile for several weeks and should be protected from shear forces and edema even after initial bolster is removed.

BONE GRAFTS

- **Indications**
  - ○ Promote and enhance bone healing: delayed union, nonunion, osteotomies, or other sites of poor healing potential
  - ○ Bridge bony defects: fill cortical defects (comminuted fractures and tumor excision), provide continuity
  - ○ Arthrodesis: replacement of native joint with bone graft
    - Provide structural support to implanted devices
- **Classifications (See Table 2-2)**
- **Donor Sites:** selection depends on quantity, type, vascularity of bone desired, donor site morbidity, and patient characteristics
  - ○ **Ilium:** large quantity cancellous and corticocancellous bone; inner or both tables of iliac crest available for harvest with additional cancellous bone available by curettage; vascularized graft based on deep circumflex iliac artery can be used
    - Advantages: little aesthetic deficit, limited use of cortical bone in patients <10 years old due to incomplete ossification
    - Disadvantage: donor site pain
  - ○ **Cranium** (along the origin of temporalis muscle if possible where calvarium thickest): large quantity of cortical bone (outer table used in adults; both inner and outer tables used in children due to osteogenic potential of dura)
    - Advantages: low graft resorption, low donor morbidity, and good aesthetic result
    - Disadvantages: brittleness, larger bone grafts require formal craniotomy
  - ○ **Ribs (11th and 12th):** cortical bone that is more porous and malleable than graft from other sources
    - Advantages: malleable, can split in half
    - Disadvantages: difficult fixation due to porosity

TABLE 2-2 Classification of Bone Grafts

	By composition		
	Cortical	**Cancellous**	**Corticocancellous**
Composition	Nonporous, lamellar bone	Porous, trabecular bone	Theoretically provides benefits of both
Considerations	Support of major bony defects, more osteogenesis, more structural support, less easily remodeled	Stimulate healing or bony ingrowth, more osteoinductive and osteoconductive, quicker revascularization	

	By vascular supply		
	Nonvascularized	**Pedicle vascularized**	**Free vascularized**
Composition	Transfer without vascular pedicle	Transfer with vascular pedicle	Transfer of large segment of bone
Considerations	Scaffolding for vascular and cellular ingrowth; ingrowth eventually resorbs and replaces graft (creeping substitution or osteoconduction)		Promotes healing at recipient site; retains epiphyseal growth

	By origin		
	Autograft	**Allograft**	**Other bone graft substitutes**
Composition	Self-tissue sources	Cadaver tissue sources	Examples include bone morphogenic protein (BMP), ceramics, and mineral composites
Consideration	Maximal healing potential, increased surgical time, no risk of viral transmission	Readily available, avoids donor site morbidity, increased time for incorporation due to immunogenicity	Minimal structural integrity

- o **Fibula:** pedicled or free graft based on peroneal artery and venae comitantes; bridges defects in long bones. Important to leave cuff of fibula proximal proximally and distally (~6 cm) to allow for joint stability.
  - ▪ Advantages: good graft length, long pedicle, and little functional deficit
  - ▪ Disadvantages: limited size
- o **Other sites:** distal radius, proximal ulna for cortical and cancellous bone
- **Harvesting and Recipient Site Preparation Tips**
  - o Minimize time between harvest and placement.
  - o Graft should be kept wrapped in blood-soaked sponges.
  - o Use copious irrigation during sawing and drilling to reduce mechanical and thermal damage to bone.
  - o Bone edges at recipient site should be freshened to bleeding edges to ensure potential for revascularization of graft.

- **Graft Survival and Healing**
  - *Osteoconduction: scaffold or template function that graft provides to allow ingrowth of capillaries, osteoprogenitor cells, and matrix components from host tissue (eg, nonvascularized bone graft).
  - *Osteoinduction: growth factors (BMPs) present within graft recruit host stem cells to form bone-producing cells (osteoblasts) (eg, cancellous bone).
  - *Osteogenesis: production of new bone by cells in graft that survive transplantation (eg, vascularized bone graft).
- **Complications**
  - Harvest site: infection, fracture, pain, wound dehiscence, damage to local structures
  - Grafted site: infection, damage to local structures, partial or total loss of graft due to resorption
  - Costochondral bone grafts retain ability to grow and may grow excessively

CARTILAGE GRAFTS

- **Indications**
  - Structural support and augmentation: ear reconstruction, eyelid and tracheal support
  - Contour deformity: correction of nasal deformity (eg, saddle nose) and inverted nipples, alternative to bone graft in facial contour deformities
  - Joint repair and resurfacing: spacer in temporomandibular joint (TMJ) repair, fill defects in articular cartilage
- **Classifications (see Table 2-3)**
- **Donor Sites**
  - Ear (concha): elastic cartilage source, possesses natural curvature, used for eyelid support and nipple reconstruction, TMJ, and orbital floor repair
    - Advantages: easily accessible, abundant
    - Disadvantages: curvature not always desirable

TABLE 2-3 Classification of Cartilage Graft

	By matrix characteristics		
	Hyaline	Elastic	Fibrocartilage
Sources	Trachea, larynx, nasal septum, nasal ala, and ribs	External ear, external auditory meatus, eustachian tube, and epiglottis	Pubic symphysis, intervertebral disks, ligamentous, and tendinous insertions
Considerations	Offers support through rigidity	More malleable, elastic, more resistant to repeated bending than hyaline cartilage	Resists tensile and compressive forces, lacks flexibility
	By source		
	Autogenous	Homologous (cadaveric)	
Considerations	Primary and preferred source	Produces relatively small immune response (chondrocytes surrounded by nonreactive extracellular matrix); freeze-dried/preserved cartilage reduces further inflammation/disease transfer; more absorption compared with autogenous cartilage	

- ○ **Nasal septum:** straight, rigid, hyaline cartilage source, used for nasal or lower eyelid reconstruction
    - ▪ Advantages: easily accessible
    - ▪ Disadvantages: limited availability, overresection results in saddle-nose deformity
- ○ **Costal cartilage:** abundant source of hyaline cartilage, used for reconstructions requiring large amount of cartilage (total auricular reconstruction, tracheal reconstruction)
    - ▪ Advantages: large quantity graft material, reliable, and distant recipient site allows two-team harvest approach
    - ▪ Disadvantages: tend to warp with time, donor site morbidity (pneumothorax and pain)
- **Graft Survival and Healing**
    - ○ Chondrocytes and extracellular matrix survive and maintain cartilage characteristics
    - ○ Survives by osmosis from well-vascularized recipient site (avascular)
    - ○ Limited inflammatory reaction with little graft resorption (<20% in autografts)
    - ○ Requires coverage to prevent desiccation and infection
    - ○ Scoring allows graft to be shaped (bending away from scored side)
    - ○ Symmetric carving, K-wire stabilization, harvest without perichondrium, making central rather than peripheral cuts, and waiting at least 30 minutes after carving before placement at recipient site can be employed to decrease warping

FAT GRAFTING

(See Chapter 6: Fat Grafting.)

COMPOSITE GRAFTS

- **Composed of two or more tissue components** (eg, skin or mucosa with cartilage, skin with fat, and full-thickness eyelid)
- **Indications**
    - ○ Nasal ala: prevent alar collapse
    - ○ Nasal sidewall: prevent nasal valve obstruction
    - ○ Nasal tip: provide structural integrity
    - ○ Ear (anterior helical root): repair substantial auricular defects, restoration of ear structure for glasses or hearing aid placement
    - ○ Eyelid: prevent ectropion and lid contraction from loss of tarsal plate
- **Donor Sites:** septal cartilage, auricular cartilage, and costal cartilage
- **Graft Survival and Healing**
    - ○ Survival occurs via imbibition, inosculation, and then revascularization.
    - ○ Initial survival dependent on revascularization solely from wound edges; thus, no portion of the graft should be >1 cm from wound edges.
    - ○ Metabolic demand of graft limits size that will survive to 1.0-1.5 cm width.
    - ○ More prone to graft loss than other graft types.

PEARLS

1. The dermal side of skin graft can be distinguished from epidermal surface by its shiny appearance (graft placed shiny side [dermis] down).
2. Donor scars for harvesting of FTSGs should be oriented parallel to relaxed skin tension lines.
3. Harvest of FTSGs from the volar wrist should never be performed due to social stigma of wrist scar.
4. Patients should be warned that composite grafts often initially appear cyanotic.

QUESTIONS YOU WILL BE ASKED

1. Name the stages and timing of skin graft healing?

   Imbibition (24-48 hours), inosculation (48-72 hours), and revascularization (4-7 days).

2. After skin grafting, does the donor or recipient site determine characteristics of hair growth, sweating, and sensibility?

   Hair growth assumes characteristics of the donor site, but only has potential to return after FTSG, sweating assumes characteristics of recipient site when glands are reinnervated, and sensibility is incomplete and assumes characteristics of recipient site.

3. What is the difference between primary and secondary contraction and which type of skin graft is primarily affected by each?

   Primary contraction occurs immediately at the time of graft harvest/application due to elastin fibers in dermis, greater in FTSGs; secondary contraction occurs during the healing phase of graft over 6-18 months, greater in STSGs.

4. Draw the layers of skin from epidermis to subcutaneous fat.

   See Figure 1-1.

Recommended Readings

1. Azoury SC, Shakir S, Bucky LP, Percec I. Modern fat grafting techniques to the face and neck. *Plast Reconstr Surg.* 2021;148(4):620e-633e.
2. Coleman SR. Facial augmentation with structural fat grafting. *Clin Plast Surg.* 2006;33(4):567-577.
3. Hallock GG, Morris SF. Skin grafts and local flaps. *Plast Reconstr Surg.* 2011;127(1):5e-22e.

3 Flaps

Jennifer C. Lee and Widya Adidharma

OVERVIEW

- **Definitions**
  - **Angiosome:** unit of skin and deeper structures supplied by a source vessel; makes up the entire surface area of the body
  - **Perforator:** a blood vessel that branches off a major named vessel (or source vessel), supplying a particular tissue territory, or angiosome
  - **Flap:** a volume of tissue that is transferred with its own blood supply (in contrast to graft, which is revascularized from recipient bed)
  - **Pedicle:** blood supply to a flap or segment of tissue
  - **Pedicled flap:** a flap that remains attached to its native vascular supply when transferred
  - **Free flap:** a flap that is fully detached from its vascular supply and reconnected to recipient vessels using microvascular techniques
- **Flap Selection Considerations**
  - Patient factors: goals of intervention, expectations, donor site morbidity, comorbidities, history of radiation, cost of care
  - Surgical considerations: defect location and size, missing and exposed structures, viability of surrounding tissue (eg, previous radiation, vascular disease, tissue necrosis), available donor sites, donor site morbidity, pedicle length and caliber, technical demand, availability of microsurgery equipment and team

FLAP CLASSIFICATION

Flaps can be classified by blood supply, method of transfer, and tissue composition

BLOOD SUPPLY

- **Random pattern flap:** raised without regard to any named blood supply, relying on blood flow through subdermal plexus (eg, bilobed flap)
- **Axial flaps:** raised on dominant (named) arterial supply (eg, radial artery flap)
- **Reverse flow flaps:** dominant supply is divided, flap left to survive on intact distally based vessels that form connections to another blood supply system (eg, reverse sural)
- **Perforator flap:** blood supply is a perforator from a dominant feeding vessel
  - "Direct" vs "indirect" perforators (**Fig. 3-1**)
    - Direct perforators course from the source vessel to the skin without first supplying any other deep structure. Examples: an axial vessel, a direct cutaneous vessel (Mathes and Nahai Type A), or a septocutaneous vessel (Mathes and Nahai Type B).
    - Indirect perforators first pass through an intermediary structure before ultimately reaching the subdermal plexus. Example: a muscle or musculocutaneous perforator (Mathes and Nahai Type C), in which the source vessel to the skin passes through and arises from the underlying muscle.
  - **Branching patterns** of musculocutaneous perforators

---

*Denotes common in-service examination topics.

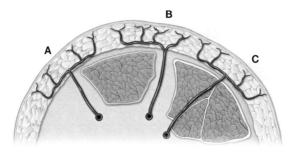

Figure 3-1 Mathes and Nahai classification of fasciocutaneous flaps. Type A: direct cutaneous perforator; type B: septocutaneous perforator; type C: musculocutaneous perforator.

- **Type 1 perforators** pass almost directly from deep fascia to subdermal plexus without branching.
- **Type 2 perforators** branch in the adipose tissue just before reaching the subdermal plexus, with branches then running parallel to the flap surface.
- **Type 3 perforators** follow deep fascia for an indeterminate distance before eventually proceeding into subcutaneous tissues.
  - ○ Advantages of perforator flaps
    - Reduced donor site morbidity
    - Reduced postoperative pain
    - Faster recovery, shorter hospital stay
    - Less difficult to tailor or thin the flap for covering or filling defects
    - Longer pedicle than with the parent musculocutaneous flap

METHOD OF TRANSFER

- **Local flap:** shares side with the defect
  - ○ Common types of local flaps (**Table 3-1**).
  - ○ *Z-plasty: increasing angle of limbs increases percent gain in length along the central limb (Table 3-2).
    - Multiple Z-plasties can be designed in series (**Fig. 3-2**).
- **Regional flaps:** in same region of the body as the defect, but does not share defect margin
  - ○ **Interpolated pedicle:** two-stage technique where a pedicle is kept intact initially between the flap and defect in the first stage before being removed in the second stage
  - ○ **Island pedicle:** all borders incised with no attachments to the donor site while maintaining original blood supply
- **Distal flap (free flap):** not in the region of the defect; detached from original blood supply at donor site and reattached to blood vessels in defect site

TISSUE COMPOSITION (TABLE 3-3)

- **Cutaneous flap**
  - ○ Blood supply: dependent on blood supply from fasciocutaneous plexus
  - ○ Flap design
    - Method of transfer: advancement, pivotal, or hinge
    - Random pattern flaps
      - □ *Size limited to length to width ratio ~2:1 in lower extremity and up to 4:1 in head and neck.
      - □ Ischemia can be expected when the recommended length to width ratio dimensions are exceeded without performing a flap delay.
- **Fascial and fasciocutaneous flap**
  - ○ Blood supply: Mathes and Nahai classification (see Fig. 3-1)
  - ○ Flap design
    - Includes deep fascia, incorporating rich vascular fascial plexus that reach the skin via direct or indirect perforators.

TABLE 3-1 Common Local Flap Methods of Transfer

	Technique	Considerations	Figure
Advancement: moved by sliding or stretching flap toward the defect; requires skin laxity			
Single/ bipedicle flap	Raised as square or rectangle → undermined and advanced	Bürow triangles made at base to facilitate advancement	Fig. A
V-Y	Raised in V shape → advanced to fill defect → closed in Y shape	The triangle of skin should have length 2-3× the diameter of the defect and width equal to the defect's greatest width	Fig. B
Rotation: moved in a curvilinear arc around a fixed point at base of pedicle			
Rotation flap	Raised in semicircle	Bürow triangle at defect margin may facilitate closure	Fig. C

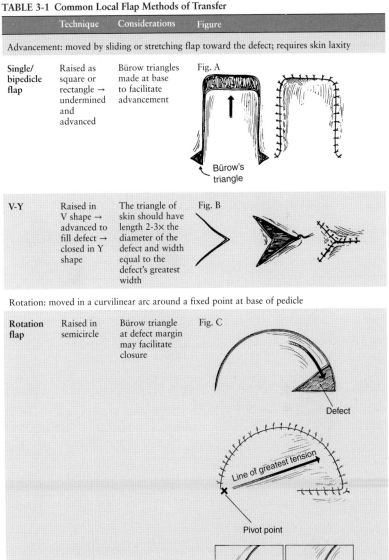

Bürow's triangle

Defect

Line of greatest tension

Pivot point

Backcut   Bürow triangle

(continued)

TABLE 3-1 Common Local Flap Methods of Transfer (*Continued*)

	Technique	Considerations	Figure
Transposition flap: moved in a linear fashion around a fixed point at base of pedicle			
Rhomboid (Limberg) flap	Defect made into rhombic shape; 60° and 120° angles	Four flaps can be designed around every defect	Fig. D
Bilobed flap	Two flaps raised 45°- 50° apart next to defect	Useful for nasal tip and ala	Fig. E
Z-plasty	Central limb oriented along direction of desired lengthening	Lengthens scar contractures, changes scar direction, etc.	Fig. F

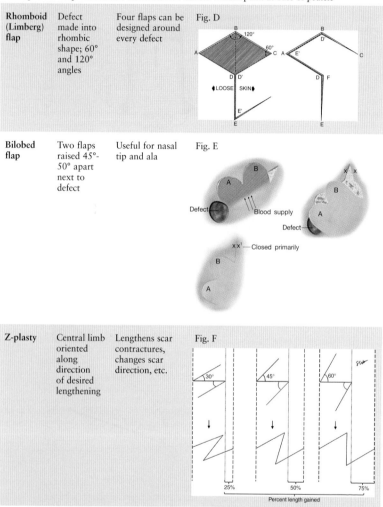

A. Single pedicled advancement flap with Bürow triangles. (Modified from Thorne CH, Gurtner GC, Chung KC, Gosain A, Mehrara B,Rubin P, Spear SL, eds. *Grabb and Smith's Plastic Surgery*. 7th ed. Wolters Kluwer; 2014. Figure 1.10.) B. V–Y advancement flap. C. Rotation advancement flap. D. Rhomboid flap. E. Bilobed flap. (From Hawn MT, ed. *Operative Techniques in Surgery*. 2nd ed. Wolters Kluwer; 2023. Figure 5.29.8.). F. Z-plasty.

- Type A and B pedicles are relatively constant in location; type C pedicles have more variability in location.
- Fascia-only flaps advantageous because donor site can be closed primarily; fasciocutaneous flaps may or may not require skin graft to close donor site.
- Can be used as pedicled or free flaps.
  ○ **Workhorse fasciocutaneous flaps (Table 3-4)**

TABLE 3-2 Z-plasty Angles and Theoretical Gain in Length of Central Limb*

Angle of Z-plasty limbs (°)	Gain in length (%)
30	25
45	50
60	75
75	100
90	120

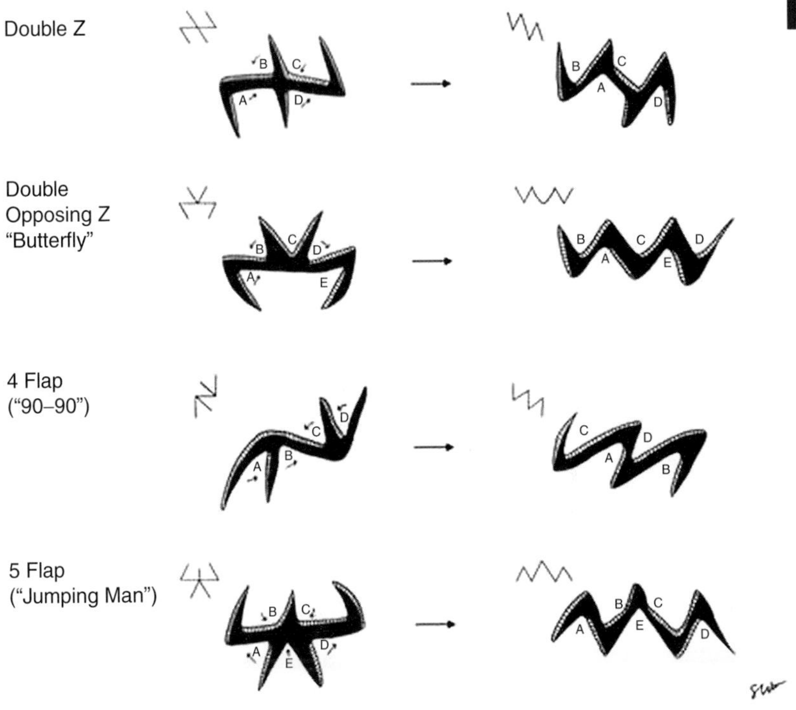
Double Z
B
C
A
D
B
C
A
D
Double
Opposing Z
"Butterfly"
B
C
D
A
E
B
C
D
A
E
4 Flap
("90–90")
D
C
A
B
C
D
A
B
5 Flap
("Jumping Man")
B
C
A
E
D
B
C
A
E
D

Figure 3-2 Multiple Z-plasties.

TABLE 3-3 Indications of Flaps of Different Tissue Composition*

	Indications
Cutaneous flaps (skin and sub-q)	• Similar, adjacent tissue • Coverage of bone, tendon
Fascial and fasciocutaneous flaps	• Thin, pliable coverage • Easier to elevate during reoperative procedures • Gliding surface for tendon coverage
Muscle and musculocutaneous flaps	• Eradication of dead space • Robust blood supply • Restoration of motor function (functional transfer)

TABLE 3-4 Workhorse Fasciocutaneous Flap*

Name	Class	Arc of rotation (pedicled)	Maximum size (cm)	Pedicle	Sensory nerve
Anterolateral thigh flap	Type C	Hip, thigh, groin, lower abdomen, perineum	18 × 25	Lateral circumflex femoral (descending branch)	Lateral femoral cutaneous
Groin flap	Type A	Abdominal wall, perineum, hand, forearm	25 × 10	Superficial circumflex iliac	Lateral cutaneous of T12
Lateral arm flap	Type B	Anterior, posterior shoulder	15 × 8	Posterior radial collateral	Posterior brachial cutaneous
Posterior interosseous flap	Type B	Elbow, antecubital fossa, proximal volar forearm	18 × 8	Posterior interosseous	Medial and dorsal antebrachial cutaneous
Radial forearm flap	Type B	Anterior, posterior forearm, elbow, upper arm	10 × 40	Radial	Medial and lateral antebrachial cutaneous
Reverse sural flap	Type A	Foot, heel, ankle, inferior one-third lower leg	8 × 12	Median superficial sural (via peroneal perforators)	Sural
Scapular/parascapular flap	Type B	Shoulder, axilla, thoracic wall	20 × 7	Circumflex scapular (transverse and descending branches, respectively)	Intercostals (3-5)
Temporoparietal fascia flap	Type A	Ear, ipsilateral face, floor of mouth	12 × 9	Superficial temporal	Auriculotemporal

- Muscle/musculocutaneous flap
  - Blood supply/Mathes and Nahai classification (Fig. 3-3)
    - *Type I*: single vascular pedicle (eg, gastrocnemius, tensor fascia lata)
    - *Type II*: single dominant pedicle and one or more minor pedicles; flap cannot survive on minor pedicles alone; most common type of muscle in body (eg, soleus, gracilis, rectus femoris, biceps femoris)
    - *Type III*: two dominant pedicles; flap can survive on either pedicle alone (eg, rectus abdominis, gluteus maximus)
    - *Type IV*: segmental pedicles; multiple pedicles enter along course of muscle, each supplies a portion of the flap; least reliable type (eg, sartorius, tibialis anterior)
    - *Type V*: one dominant pedicle and secondary segmental pedicles; flap can survive on segmental pedicles alone (eg, latissimus dorsi, pectoralis major)
  - Flap design
    - Skin island is designed to include skin perforators arising from the source artery.
    - Musculocutaneous perforators typically located near entry of dominant pedicle into hilum of the muscle.
    - All or part of muscle can be used as a flap.
    - May also include bone, motor nerve, or sensory nerve in transfer (depending on donor muscle).
    - Functional muscle is sacrificed, thus donor morbidity must be considered when selecting flap.
  - Workhorse musculocutaneous flaps (Table 3-5)

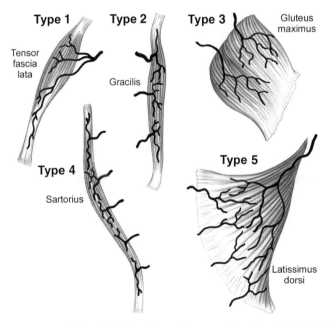

Figure 3-3 Mathes and Nahai classification of musculocutaneous flaps. (From Mathes SJ , Nahai F. Classification of the vascular anatomy of muscles: experimental and clinical correlation. *Plast Reconstr Surg*. 1981;67(2):177-187.)

TABLE 3-5 Workhorse Musculocutaneous Flaps

Name	Class	Arc of rotation (pedicled)	Maximum size (cm)	Dominant pedicle(s)	Regional artery	Minor pedicles	Sensory or motor nerves
Gastrocnemius (medial and lateral) flap	Type I	Suprapatellar, knee, upper one-third of tibia	20×8	Medial and lateral sural	Popliteal	None	S: saphenous, sural M: tibial
Gracilis flap	Type II	Groin, perineum, vagina, anus, ischium	6×24	Medial femoral circumflex (ascending branch)	Profunda femoris	Branches of superficial femoral	S: anterior femoral cutaneous, obturator M: obturator
Gluteus maximus flap	Type III	Sacrum, ischium	24×24	Superior and inferior gluteal	Internal iliac	None	S: L1-S3 M: inferior gluteal
Latissimus dorsi flap	Type V	Neck, occiput, parietal scalp, face, chest, abdomen, upper arm, elbow	25×35	Thoracodorsal	Subscapular	Perforators off of posterior intercostals or lumbar artery	S: intercostals M: thoracodorsal
Pectoralis major flap	Type V	Lower 1/2 face, neck, chest, neck, upper arm	15×23	Thoracoacromial	Subclavian	1. Pec branch of lateral thoracic 2. Internal mammary perforators	S: intercostals (2-7) M: medial and lateral pectoral
Rectus abdominis flap	Type III	Anterior thorax, inferior trunk, groin, perineum	25×6	Superior and inferior epigastric	Sup: internal mammary Inf: external iliac	None	S: intercostals (7-12) M: intercostals (7-12)
Soleus flap	Type II	Middle and lower 1/3 of leg	8×28	Proximal 2 branches of post-tibial and peroneal		Segmental branch off postibial	S: none M: posterior tibial, medial popliteal
Trapezius flap	Type II	Posterior skull, cervical and thoracic vertebra	20×8	Transverse cervical artery	Thyrocervical trunk (80%); subclavian (20%)	Dorsal scapular artery	S: #3,4 cervical nerves and branch of intercostal M: Spinal Accessory Nerve (CN XI)

- Other flap types include osseous/osteocutaneous/osteomusculocutaneous flap and omental flaps.
- Perforator considerations
  - Can identify perforators preoperatively by color duplex ultrasound, computerized tomography (CT) angiogram, or handheld audible Doppler
  - Can increase length of pedicle by dissecting perforator back to its origin

FLAP MODIFICATIONS

- **Flap Delay**
  - Staged technique to augment flap circulation and improve flap survival.
  - Flap is partially or entirely elevated, or selected pedicles are divided in one or more procedures; flap is brought back to in situ position in staged procedure before definitive flap elevation and transfer ~2 weeks after delay procedure.
  - Allows harvest of larger flap because areas farthest from blood supply (random-supply component) have improved perfusion following delay.
  - Physiology of improved perfusion with delay
    - Decrease in sympathetic tone from transection of sympathetic fibers.
    - *Dilation of previously closed choke vessels increases the area of tissue supplied by the dominant pedicle.
    - Relative tissue ischemia stimulates angiogenesis, increasing flap vascularity.
- **Crane Principle**
  - Pedicled flap used to lift, transport, and deposit subcutaneous tissue to recipient bed.
  - Flap is raised and transferred to recipient bed.
  - After 10-21 days, new blood vessels have grown in the recipient bed, which will support a skin graft. In the next stage, the top layer (superficial one-half to three-fourths) is raised and returned to original donor site.
  - Viable subcutaneous tissue is left behind and can be covered with skin graft.
  - Provides coverage to local or regional area without significant donor site morbidity.
- **Prelamination**
  - Introduction of additional tissue layers into flap prior to transfer to create multilayer composite flap; allows tissue to have time to mature before transfer
  - Indication: allows custom-made flaps for specialized areas of the body with 3D structure (eg, central face, penis)
  - Two-stage process
    - Stage 1: modify donor flap by introducing additional tissue layer into vascularized tissue before transfer to recipient site (eg, introduce cartilage and/or skin grafts to forehead flap before transfer to the defect).
    - Stage 2: raise flap en bloc as composite flap and transfer to recipient site after ~2-4 weeks (shorter maturation time than prefabrication because vascular supply is not altered).
- **Supercharging**
  - Enhances blood supply of a pedicled free flap by performing additional microvascular anastomosis to free flaps.
  - Example: transverse rectus abdominis musculocutaneous flap with classic superior epigastric artery pedicle that also has deep inferior epigastric artery anastomosed to vessels in the axilla, neck, or chest to enhance blood supply.
- **Composite Flaps**
  - **Angiosome principle** provides basis for transfer of composite flaps that contain combinations of multiple tissue types (eg, skin, muscle, bone, nerve, and/or tendon).
  - Tissues supplied by single source artery can be transferred together.
  - Useful when reconstruction of multiple tissue components is needed.

○ **Vascularized bone flaps**
  ▪ **Blood supply classification** (Serafin)
    □ Direct (endosteal) circulation
    □ Indirect (periosteal) circulation
  ▪ **Commonly transferred bones and their vascular pedicles**
    □ Radius: radial artery
    □ Fibula: peroneal artery
    □ Scapula: circumflex scapular or thoracodorsal artery
    □ Iliac crest: deep circumflex iliac artery
    □ Great toe/second toe transfer: first dorsal metatarsal artery
○ **Innervated flaps**
  ▪ Motor nerve and/or sensory nerves are preserved or coapted to appropriate nerve near the recipient site.
  ▪ Common functional muscle flap transfer and their motor nerve
    □ Gracilis with obturator nerve
    □ Latissimus with thoracodorsal nerve
    □ Pectoralis minor with medial and lateral pectoral nerve
  ▪ Common sensory flaps with their sensory nerves
    □ Lateral arm flap with posterior brachial cutaneous nerve
    □ Radial forearm flap with medial and/or lateral antebrachial cutaneous nerves
    □ Dorsalis pedis flap with deep peroneal nerve and/or superficial peroneal nerve
• **Chimeric vs Conjoined (Siamese) Flap**
  ○ **Chimeric flap:** has multiple territories, each with independent vascular supply (perforators or named branches), but territories are NOT connected except by connection to common source vessel.
  ○ **Conjoined flap:** has multiple territories, each with independent vascular supply, but territories remain connected.

POSTOPERATIVE MANAGEMENT

• **Flap Monitoring**
  ○ *Evidence of arterial or venous insufficiency in immediate post-op period requires immediate exploration (Table 3-6).
    ▪ If venous congested, unwrap, release sutures and consider leech therapy (patient must be on third-generation cephalosporin, quinolone or trimethoprim/sulfamethoxazole against *Aeromonas*)
  ○ *Clinical evaluation: gold standard method of flap assessment
    ▪ Temperature: should be body temperature
    ▪ Color: should be pink
    ▪ Capillary refill: should be ~2-3 seconds
    ▪ Bleeding: upon introduction of fine-gauge needle, bright-red bleeding should be present
    ▪ Firmness: should be soft, with some appreciable turgor

TABLE 3-6 Signs of Arterial and Venous Insufficiency

Signs of arterial insufficiency	Signs of venous insufficiency
Cool temperature	Increased temperature
White color	Blue to purple color
Slow capillary refill >2 s	Brisk capillary refill <2 s
Slow or absent pinpoint bleeding	Brisk pinpoint bleeding, dark in color
Low turgor	Increased turgor, tense, swollen

- Additional methods of flap monitoring
  - Doppler (implanted or external)
  - Near-infrared spectroscopy for tissue oxygen saturation (Vioptix)—measures tissue oxygen saturation (StO_2)
  - Fluorescein dye
  - pH or temperature sensors
- **Risk Factors for Flap Vascular Compromise**
  - Tight dressings and/or splints
  - Tight sutures
  - Patient position or motion that puts pressure on flap
  - Hematoma (increases tissue pressure and interferes with perfusion)
  - Kinking of flap, pedicle, or both (may be influenced by flap design, pedicle length, interpositional vein graft length)
  - Poor surgical technique
  - Systemic patient factors: use of vasoconstrictive pharmaceutical agents (vasopressors, nicotine, caffeine, etc.), hypovolemia, anemia, inadequate blood pressure

PEARLS

1. In most situations, follow the reconstructive ladder when deciding if a flap is needed for your reconstruction and what type of flap
2. Always consider both patient factors (I.e. patient comorbidities and goals) and surgical factors (I.e. defect characteristics and donor site considerations) when deciding the appropriate flap
3. Know how to evaluate a flap postoperatively and be able to detect flap compromise

QUESTIONS YOU WILL BE ASKED

1. What is the most common (Mathes and Nahai) type of muscle flap in the body?
   Type II (major and minor pedicle).
2. What is the physiology behind improved perfusion after flap delay?
   Flap perfusion is increased through (1) decrease in sympathetic tone from transection of sympathetic fibers; (2) dilation of previously closed choke vessels, which increases the area of tissue supplied by dominant pedicle; and (3) relative tissue ischemia stimulates angiogenesis, increasing flap vascularity before transfer.
3. What is the pedicle to the flap?
   Table 3-3.
4. What is difference between a type II and type V flap?
   Type II flap has secondary pedicle that cannot support the flap alone. Type V flap can be transferred on the secondary pedicles which are segmental.

Recommended Readings
1. Brown E, Suh HP, Han HH, Pak CJ, Hong JP. Best new flaps and tips for success in microsurgery. *Plast Reconstr Surg.* 2020;146(6):796e-807e.
2. Ghali S, Butler PE, Tepper OM, Gurtner GC. Vascular delay revisited. *Plast Reconstr Surg.* 2007;119(6):1735-1744.
3. Hallock GG, Morris SF. Skin grafts and local flaps. *Plast Reconstr Surg.* 2011;127(1):5e-22e.
4. Taylor GI. The angiosomes of the body and their supply to perforator flaps. *Clin Plast Surg.* 2003;30(3):331-342.
5. Wei F-C, Mardini S. *Flaps and Reconstructive Surgery.* Elsevier; 2017.

Vascularized Composite Allotransplantation

Sherry Tang

OVERVIEW

DEFINITIONS

- **Vascularized composite allografts (VCAs)** or **composite tissue allografts** are "composite" grafts made of multiple tissue types that are transplanted together as a single functional unit. This may consist of skin, bone, tendon, muscle, nerves, vessels, and fat.
- **Autotransplantation:** Tissues of an individual are moved to another location on the same individual.
- **Allotransplantation:** Tissues are transplanted from one individual to another individual of the same species.

TRANSPLANTATION IMMUNOLOGY

- Alloimmune Response
  - **Major histocompatibility complex (MHC)** and **human leukocyte antigens (HLAs)**
    - MHC complex is a cell surface glycoprotein that functions to distinguish between self- and non–self-antigens. It plays an important role in the alloimmune response and adaptive immunity.
    - Two classes: MHC class I and MHC class II.
      - MHC class I molecules are expressed on all nucleated cells.
        - HLA-A, HLA-B, HLA-C
      - MHC class II molecules are only expressed on antigen-presenting cells (APCs).
        - HLA-DP, HLA-DO, HLA-DR
    - Each MHC is associated with a group of HLA genes, which determine the compatibility of all organ and tissue transplants.
  - **Initiation of an alloimmune response**
    - Dendritic cells (DCs), which are APCs in the peripheral tissue, first acquire donor antigen in the peripheral tissues and express donor MHC alloantigen on their cell surface.
    - DCs then migrate to lymphoid tissue via lymphatics, where the donor MHC alloantigen that is on the surface of DCs interacts with T-cell receptors (TCRs) on the recipient naive T cell. In addition, a CD3 complex facilitates this interaction between DCs and T cells, forming signal 1.
    - APCs also provide costimulatory signals, referred to as signal 2, to fully activate T cells. The B7/CD28 and CD40/CD154 pathways are two costimulatory signal pathways in transplantation.
    - Once a naive T cell receives both signal 1 and signal 2, intracellular signal transduction pathways are activated, which leads to increased expression of cytokines that initiate T-cell proliferation and development of effector T cells. This is referred to as signal 3.
  - **T regulatory cells**
    - CD4+CD25+FoxP3+ cell population

---

*Denotes common in-service examination topics.

- May be induced or native (derived in thymus)
- Inhibit effector T cells, mitigating rejection or graft vs host disease
  □ Express cytotoxic lymphocyte antigen 4 (CTLA4).
  □ CTLA4 can bind to costimulatory molecules (CD80 and CD86) to activate indoleamine 2,3-dioxygenase (IDO) to deprive local environment of tryptophan and produce kynurenines, attenuating T-cell proliferation.
  □ Produces IL-10 (immunosuppressive cytokine), which inhibits APC activity and promotes T-cell conversion to T regulatory cells.
- Believed to exert their effects in the lymph node and allograft.
- *Types of Rejection
  ○ **Hyperacute rejection** occurs within minutes to hours after transplantation. It is mediated by preexisting antibodies to HLA or ABO antigens. Can lead to microthrombi, vascular occlusion, and necrosis of allograft.
  ○ **Acute rejection** occurs in days to weeks after transplantation. It is caused by HLA mismatch and mediated by effector T cells.
  ○ **Chronic rejection** occurs in months to years after transplantation and is the major cause of long-term graft loss. It is characterized by intimal proliferation of vessels, skin and muscular atrophy, and **fibrosis of deep tissues.**
- **Skin Immunogenicity in VCA**
  ○ Skin is a major component of most VCA grafts.
  ○ **Skin is the most immunogenic** of all types of a tissue due to a higher presence of effector T cells and the ability for endothelial cells to recruit immune cells and upregulate MHC class II molecule, inflammatory markers, costimulatory, and vasoactive molecules.
  ○ Approximately 80% of all face and upper extremity transplants have signs of acute rejection within 1 year, compared to 10% in kidney transplants.
  ○ **Acute rejection appears to affect the skin first.** It manifests as erythematous macules and diffuse redness. Histologic analysis shows lymphocytic infiltrate consisting of T cells. It is graded according to the Banff score (**Table 4-1**).
    ■ Treatment: Increase oral or IV steroids, polyclonal or monoclonal antibodies, and topical immunosuppressants.
  ○ **Split tolerance phenomenon** has been reported, in which there is rejection of the skin but no other types of tissue within the graft.
- **Immunosuppression**
  ○ **Immunosuppression medications** are required to prevent both acute and chronic rejection. The immunosuppressive protocols used for VCA are based on those used in solid organ transplantation.
  ○ **Two phases of immunosuppression**
    ■ Induction immunosuppression uses polyclonal antithymocyte antibody and basiliximab to deplete recipient T cells.

TABLE 4-1 Banff Score for Acute Rejection

Grade	Degree of rejection	Pathology findings
Grade 0	No rejection	None or rare inflammatory infiltrates
Grade 1	Mild rejection	Mild perivascular infiltration. No involvement of overlying epidermis
Grade 2	Moderate rejection	Moderate to severe perivascular inflammation with or without mild epidermal and adnexal involvement. No epidermal dyskeratosis or apoptosis
Grade 3	Severe rejection	Dense dermal inflammation associated with epidermal involvement (keratinocyte vacuolization, apoptosis, and necrosis)
Grade 4	Necrosis	Necrosis of epidermis or other skin structures

- Maintenance immunosuppression uses a triple therapy with tacrolimus, mycophenolate mofetil, and prednisone.
  - **Risks associated with immunosuppression**
    - Tacrolimus is associated with elevated serum creatinine levels.
    - Prednisone is associated with hypertension, diabetes, dyslipidemia, and risk of malignancy.
    - Opportunistic infection including CMV, EBC, HSV, *Pneumocystis jirovecii*, bacterial, and fungal infections.
  - Minimization protocols using tacrolimus and mycophenolate have been studied, but this is associated with increased acute rejection episodes.
  - **Topical tacrolimus and clobetasol** have been successful in treating lower-grade rejection (Banff grades 1-2). Some animal studies have demonstrated that topical immunosuppression can be superior to systemic immunosuppression in certain cases.
- **Tolerance induction** is an area of active research in preclinical models. It relies on achieving **mixed chimerism**, in which the immune cells of both recipient and donor can exist in the recipient without destructive immunologic responses.
  - Donor hematopoietic stem cells (HSCs) are isolated from the donor bone marrow.
  - The recipient is conditioned using whole-body irradiation, T-cell depletion, and costimulatory blockade.
  - Donor HSCs are injected into the recipient and migrate to the thymus, where both recipient and donor cells undergo clonal deletion to achieve central tolerance.
  - Stable engraftment of donor HSCs ensures mixed chimerism and allows tolerance of donor VCAs.
- **Graft vs Host Disease (GVHD)**
  - Multisystem complication associated with HSC transplantation and has been observed in VCA when combined with stem cell transplants in preclinical models.
  - Donor T cells attack the host.
  - Clinical findings
    - Acute GVHD: onset <100 days. Maculopapular rash, abdominal pain with diarrhea, elevated serum bilirubin.
    - Chronic GVHD: onset >100 days. May resemble autoimmune disorders. GI sclerosis, elevated bilirubin, skin manifestation such as cutaneous scleroderma, bronchiolitis obliterans.
- **Ischemia-Reperfusion Injury**
  - Maximum ischemic time has not been established for VCAs but prolonged ischemic time can negatively impact success.
  - Prolonged ischemia followed by reperfusion results in production of reactive oxygen species, which leads to oxidization of proteins and upregulation of heat shock proteins.
  - Heat shock proteins activate toll-like receptors and may mediate innate immune responses.

TYPES OF ALLOTRANSPLANTATION IN PLASTIC SURGERY

HAND AND UPPER EXTREMITY TRANSPLANTATION

- **Background**
  - The first hand transplantation was performed in Ecuador in 1964, ending in rejection 2 weeks postoperatively. Subsequent hand transplant in France in 1998 lost after 2.5 years due to medication noncompliance.
  - Over 150 upper limb transplants in 100 patients in 45 centers worldwide since 1998.

- **Indications and Patient Selection**
  - Unilateral or bilateral upper limb loss causing significant loss of quality of life.
  - Age over 18. Some centers may consider pediatric patients at a minimum of age 8 years with bilateral upper limb loss.
  - Trial of prostheses.
  - Lack of significant coexisting medical or psychosocial issues.
  - Patient must demonstrate compliance, motivation, and ability to successfully manage a VCA allograft.
  - ABO crossmatch is performed; however, most hand transplants to date have been performed despite HLA mismatch.
- **Surgical Procedure**
- **Surgical planning**
  - Requires a multidisciplinary team consisting of plastic, orthopedic and transplant surgery, transplantation medicine, anesthesiology, organ procurement organization, nursing, occupational and physical therapy, psychology, and social work.
  - Surgical rehearsals, check lists, and adjunctive planning tools such as CT virtual surgical planning and 3D printer models are useful.
  - **Donor procedure**
    - Donor limb evaluation: limb and bone size, skin color and tone, gender, absence of tattoos, limb quality (trauma, joint mobility, vessel patency, age).
    - Upper extremity procurement from deceased donor requires amputation of the allograft proximal to the level of the defect in the recipient.
    - The amputated allograft is flushed with cold preservation solution to avoid warm ischemia, wrapped in moist sterile gauze, placed in a sealed plastic bag, and transported on ice in a cooler.
    - A prosthesis is fitted to the deceased donor to avoid donor disfigurement after amputation of the allograft.
    - Deceased donor will also likely be donor for solid organs so careful coordination with solid organ transplant procurement team(s) is required.
    - Once back at the recipient operation room, all key structures are identified and tagged.
  - **Recipient procedure**
    - The recipient stump is dissected under tourniquet and the bony stump is prepared. All key structures are identified and tagged.
    - Transplantation then proceeds in the order of bony fixation, tendon/muscle repair, nerve repair, and vascular repair. Depending on the level of transplant and cold ischemia time, vascular repair can be performed earlier to avoid ischemia-reperfusion injury.
- **Rehabilitation**
  - Rehabilitation is similar to that after replantation. Generally, begin therapy within 2-3 days after surgery with passive motion and custom splint fitting. Active motion may be started within weeks after surgery. Therapy is intense during the first year and then gradually taper.
  - Steroid use as part of immunosuppression impedes healing and may place tendon repair at risk if active motion is started too early postoperatively.
- **Outcomes**
  - Patient survival rate for isolated unilateral or bilateral hand transplantations: 96.7% at 1, 5, and 10 years after transplantation
  - Graft survival rate: 90.4% at 1 year and 86.6% at 5 and 10 years
  - Functional outcome
    - Standardizing functional outcome measures is challenging due to nonuniversally agreed outcomes measures, the variability in levels of transplantation, and the long time required to reach maximal functional improvement.
    - Outcome measures include the Hand Transplant Scoring System, the Sollerman test, and the Disabilities of the Arm, Shoulder, and Hand test.

- In general, more distal transplants have the best absolute function with sensory and motor recovery.
- International Registry on Hand and Composite Tissue Transplantation report in 2010
  □ All patients developed protective sensation, 90% developed had protective sensibility, and 84% had discriminative sensibility.
  □ Majority developed intrinsic muscle reinnervation at 9-15 months postoperatively.
  □ Quality of life reported to be improved in 75% of patients.
- Hand and upper extremity transplantations are no longer considered "experimental." With the appropriate patient selection, this can be considered the most suitable treatment.

FACE TRANSPLANTATION

- **Background**
  - First face transplant in November 2005 in France.
  - More than 40 face transplantations documented worldwide since 2005.
- **Indications and Patient Selection**
  - No consensus on inclusion and exclusion criteria. Assessment tools such as the Cleveland Clinic FACES Score have been developed to identify ideal candidates.
  - Significant facial deformity after conventional autologous reconstruction has been tried with unsatisfactory results.
  - Facial deformity has been due to trauma (animal bites, gunshot wounds), congenital deformities, burns, and cancer defects. Gun shot and burn patients make up 2/3 of all face transplant recipients.
  - Consideration has been given to skin color and HLA matching.
- **Surgical Procedure**
  - **Surgical planning**
    - CT or MRI help determine amount of missing tissue.
    - Dental occlusion and orthognathic planning can help determine facial width and position.
  - **Donor procedure**
    - Surgical procedure is dependent on the structures required for transplantation.
      □ May include bone, muscle, nerve, mucosa, and skin.
      □ May include various aesthetic units, including nose, lips, and cheeks.
    - Facial artery or external carotid arteries are used as pedicles.
    - Facial nerve is transected at the level of the facial nerve trunk or more distally to perform neurorrhaphy with the recipient facial nerve.
    - Ischemia time ideally <4 hours, but no proven correlation between prolonged ischemia time and frequency of acute rejection episodes.
  - **Recipient procedure**
    - Recipient vessels and facial nerve trunks are identified.
    - Microvascular anastomosis performed between donor and recipient vessels.
    - Facial nerves are connected.
    - Sensory nerves (eg, trigeminal branches) are connected if available.
- **Rehabilitation**
  - Facial muscle reeducation, speech, and swallow therapy start immediately after surgery.
- **Outcomes**
  - Patient survival rate: 96.6% at 1 year and 96.2% at 5 years
    - Graft survival rate:
      □ 96.6% at 1 and 5 years
      □ 80% of patients have at least one episode of acute rejection within the first year with the majority of rejections episodes being steroid sensitive

- Functional outcome
  - No standard functional outcomes measure given variability in injuries and face transplant protocols. Functional success is determined by restoration of breathing, eating, tasting, smelling, talking, facial expressions, and sensation.
  - Motor recovery detectable 6-8 months after surgery.
  - Sensory recovery detectable as early as 3 months after surgery.
  - Improvement in quality of life is variable and is influenced by pretransplant mental disorder and risk factors.
  - Most patients are able to accept their new faces without issues relating to facial identity. However, lack of acceptance of the transplanted face increases risk of psychological problems, including suicide attempts.
  - Studies have demonstrated accelerated facial aging associated with reduction of bone and nonfat subcutaneous soft tissues.

ABDOMINAL WALL TRANSPLANTATION

- **Background**
  - Involves transplantation of the abdominal wall to close the abdomen.
  - All cases reported to date have been in conjunction with intestinal or multivisceral transplantation in both pediatric and adult patients.
- **Indications and Patient Selection**
  - Traditional methods of abdominal wall closure are not possible following intestinal or multivisceral transplantation.
  - Desire to avoid donor site morbidity associated with autologous free flap.
  - Need to avoid risk of infection with open abdomen or prosthetics.
  - Need to prevent abdominal compartment syndrome by achieving tension-free closure.
- **Surgical Procedure**
  - **Surgical planning**
    - Composite tissue allograft to assess abdominal wall vessels.
    - ABO matching is common. Some studies report that HLA matching may not be needed but sample sizes are small.
    - Donor abdominal wall is typically harvested from the same donor as the solid organ/intestinal grafts.
  - **Surgical technique**
    - Partial thickness grafts involve donor rectus fascia only.
      - Nonvascularized: rectus fascia incorporated as scar tissue overtime.
      - Vascularized: rectus fascia harvested en bloc with falciform ligament and liver grafts. Uses hepatic artery as blood supply.
    - Full thickness grafts may involve peritoneum, rectus muscle, oblique muscle, transversalis muscle, subcutaneous fat, and skin (vascularized myocutaneous abdominal wall flap).
      - Flap pedicle based off the deep inferior epigastric vessels, deep circumflex iliac vessels, internal mammary vessels, or various intra-abdominal vessels.
      - Direct orthotopic revascularization: anastomosis is done directly after completion of visceral transplantation.
      - Indirect orthotopic revascularization: used in cases of prolonged cold ischemia time over 5 hours. The abdominal wall graft is first revascularized to the recipient's forearm vessels. Then following completion of the visceral transplant, the graft is disconnected from the forearm and revascularized to the recipient abdominal vessels.
- **Outcomes**
  - An area of ongoing research.
  - Abdominal wall transplant skin is a good monitor for visceral graft rejection.
  - Skin changes occur prior to bowel or organ dysfunction so patients can be treated earlier.
  - Potentially higher rate of graft vs host disease.
  - Some studies suggest no increased risk of rejection when abdominal wall transplant is included with intestinal transplant.

○ Neurotization of abdominal wall grafts has not been performed but cadaveric study shows adequate length and caliber of thoracolumbar nerves to achieve tension-free coaptation.

GENITOURINARY TRANSPLANTATION

- **Background**
  - ○ Goal of penile transplantation is to restore urinary and sexual function.
  - ○ Five total penis/genitourinary transplants attempted worldwide since 2006. Two in the United States, two in South Africa, and one in China.
- **Indications and Patient Selection**
  - ○ Loss of phallus due to trauma, cancer, or infection.
  - ○ Lack of donor site for phalloplasty using autologous tissue such as the radial forearm free flap.
  - ○ Extensive perineal loss at the recipient site.
- **Surgical Procedure**
  - ○ The graft includes urethra, erectile tissue (corpus cavernosum and corpora spongiosum), penile skin, dorsal penile nerve, and groin lymph node basins.
  - ○ Graft pedicle is mainly based on the dorsal penile artery but can also include external pudendal artery and cavernosal artery.
  - ○ Recipient vessels include native dorsal artery, femoral artery, and deep inferior epigastric artery.
- **Outcomes**
  - ○ Four out of five penile transplants have been successful. The failed transplant was due to psychological concerns. Two of the successful cases have resulted in recovery of full urinary and sexual function.
  - ○ The hypervascular nature of erectile tissue may lead to increased risk of congestion, thrombosis, or hematomas.
  - ○ Epithelial lining of the urethra may undergo early rejection.
  - ○ Chronic rejection could present as erectile dysfunction.

ETHICAL CONSIDERATIONS

- **Historical Background**
  - ○ In the early days of VCA, the ethical debate was focused on the morality of these procedures.
  - ○ Over two decades since the first successful hand transplant, VCAs have proven to be feasible and successful, with clear benefits to patients.
  - ○ The ethical considerations are now focused on how to perform these procedures ethically.
- **Ethical Value of VCA**
  - ○ VCAs are life enhancing. Solid organ transplants are lifesaving.
  - ○ Some patients may experience "social death" if there are significant social and psychological consequences as a result of severe disfigurement.
  - ○ VCA can be considered lifesaving if it allows the individual to reintegrate back into society and regain self-identity.
- **Patient Selection**
  - ○ How should patients be selected for transplantation?
    - Currently no consensus on inclusion and exclusion criteria.
    - Providers must make judgment based on the patients' physical condition, comorbidities, potential benefit gained from VCA, motivation to successfully manage a VCA graft, and amount of social support available.
  - ○ How should mental health be assessed in the perioperative period?
    - Assessment of mental health in VCA candidates is not standardized.
    - The level of involvement and the use of assessment tools vary vastly among mental health providers.
    - Some centers consider self-inflicted gunshot wound an absolute contraindication. Yet these less-than-ideal patients may potentially benefit the most.

- How should biases be addressed in the selection process?
  - Institutions and providers might choose the "easier" patient while denying VCA to another patient who qualifies for the procedure but is at a higher risk for negative outcomes.
  - Negative outcomes could potentially lead to financial and reputational consequences for institutions and providers.
- **Informed Consent**
  - How can providers ensure that patients understand the full scope of the procedure and its potential complications?
    - In additional to information about the operation and its complications, patients must understand the need for intense therapy (especially for hand transplantation), importance of compliance to immunosuppression, and the consequence of noncompliance.
    - Patient advocates and support groups may be useful in assessing patients' understanding and motivation preoperatively as well as provide ongoing support and advocacy postoperatively.
- **Donation**
  - How can we inform the public about the benefits of VCA?
    - Studies show that there is less public awareness and greater hesitancy to donate associated with VCA compared to solid organ transplantation. Similarly, people also express less willingness to receive a VCA.
    - The public has many misconceptions about VCA, such as VCA is used for cosmetic reasons or the recipient will assume the identity of the donor.
  - How can we ensure proper consent to donate in VCA?
    - Individuals provide first-person consent when they register as an organ donor obtaining a driver's license under the Uniform Anatomical Gift Act (UAGA).
    - However, the UAGA and state/national registries do not provide any explicit information regarding VCAs. As a result, consent to VCA donation has required surrogate family consent to date.
- **Procurement**
  - How can we ensure that procurement of VCAs does not interfere with solid organ procurement?
    - Close coordination with all members of the solid organ team is important to optimize procurement.
  - How can we avoid disfigurement to the deceased donor?
    - Prosthesis for the donor have been used.
- **Quality of Life After Transplant**
  - How do we compare quality of life before and after transplant?
    - Very difficult to quantify success after VCA.
  - What are the implications if a VCA is rejected and necessitates graft removal?
    - Consider the implications of removing the face.

ECONOMIC CONSIDERATIONS

- **Cost of Disability**
  - This is an emerging area of research with respect to general reconstruction. Understanding the costs of specific disabilities is complicated by various factors specific to the defect and the patient characteristics.
  - How does the type of injury correspond with economic disability?
  - Does occupation of the recipient affect economic cost of transplantation (eg, farmer who lost a hand vs actor with facial defect from cancer)?
  - How should the economic burden of physical disfigurement be assessed?
- **Cost of VCA**
  - Total cost of VCA is related to procurement, surgical cost, anesthesia cost, immunosuppression, rehabilitation, complications, equipment, and personnel cost.

○ Analysis of the total cost of VCA should include comparing it to the cost of care associated with traditional reconstructive methods.
- **Funding for VCA**
  ○ Most VCA programs in the United States have been funded by research grants.
  ○ Insurance typically only pays for immunosuppression and routine postoperative care.
  ○ With the transition of VCA as an experimental treatment to standard of care, the way in which VCAs are funded is likely to change in the future.
  ○ Who should shoulder the costs associated with VCA? Should it depend on the type of allograft performed?
  ○ Should different economic costs of patient care be shouldered by separate institutions (eg, surgery vs immunosuppression vs complications vs rehabilitation)?
  ○ Who are the potential payers for this procedure (eg, patient, worker's compensation/government/Medicare/Medicaid, hospital, employer, private insurers, NIH, military)?

PEARLS

1. Performing VCAs requires a multidisciplinary team, including surgery, anesthesiology, transplantation medicine, pathology, radiology, nursing, occupation and physical therapy, psychology, social work, patient advocate, and organ procurement organizations.
2. The skin typically shows signs of acute rejection first. It manifests as erythematous macules and diffuse redness. Histologic analysis shows lymphocytic infiltrate consisting of T cells.
3. Induction immunosuppression typically uses antithymocyte antibody to deplete recipient T cells. Maintenance immunosuppression uses a triple therapy with tacrolimus, mycophenolate mofetil, and prednisone.
4. Prednisone is associated with hypertension, diabetes, dyslipidemia, and risk of malignancy.

QUESTIONS YOU WILL BE ASKED

1. What is the most immunogenic tissue for transplantation?
   Skin.
2. What is the difference between allotransplantation and autotransplantation?
   Allotransplantation involves transferring tissue from one individual to another. Autotransplantation involves transferring tissue from one location to a different location on the same individual.
3. What are factors to consider when deciding whether someone should undergo VCA?
   Age, current physical state, cause of disfigurement, comorbidities, impact of disfigurement on quality of life and function, candidacy for traditional reconstruction options, mental health history, social support, patient motivation, and ability to comply with maintaining a VCA.

Recommended Readings
1. Caplan AL, Parent B, Kahn J, et al. Emerging ethical challenges raised by the evolution of vascularized composite allotransplantation. *Transplantation*. 2019;103(6):1240-1246.
2. Cetrulo CL, Ng ZY, Winograd JM, et al. The advent of vascularized composite allotransplantation. *Clin Plast Surg*. 2017;44:425-429.
3. Mendenhall SD, Brown S, Ben-Amotz O, et al. Building a hand and upper extremity transplantation program: lessons learned from the first 20 years of vascularized composite allotransplantation. *Hand*. 2020;15(2):224-233.
4. Siemionow M. The past the present and the future of face transplantation. *Curr Opin Organ Transplant*. 2020;25:568-575.

5 Tissue Expansion

Christine S. Wang

OVERVIEW

- **Definition**: Placement of an artificial filling device that is gradually filled with saline or air, resulting in stretch of local soft tissue to increase surface area to reconstruct adjacent defect when primary closure is not possible.
- **Advantages**
  - Reconstruct "like with like" by using donor tissue that offers similar color, texture, thickness, and hair-bearing qualities.
  - Less donor site morbidity because the expanded tissue is closed primarily.
  - Robust angiogenic response within expanded local tissue reduces risk of tissue necrosis.
  - Versatile, reliable, repeatable, and can be applied to many regions of the body.
- **Disadvantages**
  - Significant time commitment with multiple operations and outpatient visits required
  - Temporary but significant contour deformity at the donor site that is often difficult to conceal
  - Complications associated with presence of foreign material (eg, infection, exposure, extrusion)

BIOLOGIC PROPERTIES OF SKIN

- **Physiology**
  - Layers of skin
    - Epidermis: stratum corneum, lucidum, granulosum, spinosum, basale
    - Dermis: papillary and reticular
- **Biomechanics**
  - **Creep:** the tendency of tissue to deform permanently under influence of stress; it can be an acute (mechanical) or chronic (biological) response to sustained stretch.
    - Acute/mechanical creep
      - Acute tissue elongation as collagen fibers align parallel to the vector force and adjacent tissue is recruited from surrounding skin laxity zones.
      - Water is displaced from the ground substance and elastic fibers microfragment.
    - Chronic/biological creep
      - Chronic tissue elongation due to new tissue regeneration.
      - Sustained tissue stretch leads to new tissue within expanded field by activation of collagenogenesis, angiogenesis, and epidermal proliferation.
  - **Stress relaxation**
    - Stress is defined as the average force per unit surface area within the tissue.
    - Strain is defined as the amount of tissue deformation that occurs in response to stress.
    - Stress relaxation refers to the gradual decline in stress over time at constant strain in biological tissues. Clinically, this is important because the acutely stretched tissue can relax before the next expansion, thereby preventing ischemia-related complications of the overlying soft tissue envelope.

---

*Denotes common in-service examination topics.

- Histology
  - Epidermis
    - *Increase in thickness through hyperkeratosis (stratum corneum thickens) and acanthosis (stratum spinosum thickens).
    - Increase in mitosis with narrowing of intracellular spaces.
    - Melanocyte activity increases, which can cause hyperpigmentation.
    - Epidermal thickening returns to baseline ~6 months after expansion process.
  - Dermis
    - *Overall decrease in thickness due to reticular dermis thinning, no change in papillary dermis.
    - Increased fibroblast and myofibroblasts numbers with thickened collagen bundles.
    - Degenerative changes to sweat glands and hair follicles.
    - Rupture of elastin producing striae.
    - Can have decreased appreciation of pain, temperature, pressure and light touch.
    - *Dermal thinning returns to baseline ~2 years after expansion.
  - Muscle
    - *Decrease in mass and thickness.
    - Disorganization of myofibrils and myofilament.
    - No loss of muscle function but injury has been reported during expansion process (eg, reduced brow elevation due to frontalis damage).
  - Fat
    - *Decrease in thickness, specifically subcutaneous fat.
    - Permanent fat loss (30%-50%) due to atrophic adipocytes being replaced by fibrosis.
  - Tissue expander capsule
    - Forms within days due to foreign body reaction composed of parallel-oriented fibroblasts intervening with a dense layer of collagen bundles.
    - Capsulotomy can be formed to increase tissue advancement at time of tissue expander removal.
    - Capsulectomy should be used judiciously to avoid interrupting vascular supply to random-pattern flaps.
  - Bone
    - Thinning of bone but no change in bone density.
  - Vascularity
    - Expanded skin is hypervascular secondary to angiogenesis.
    - Greatest density of blood vessels found at interface between the capsule and the expanded local tissue.
    - No abnormal cellular architecture has been demonstrated in expanded tissues.

PROCEDURAL CONSIDERATIONS

PRINCIPLES OF TISSUE EXPANDER PLACEMENT

- Fundamental Design
  - Surface
    - Smooth: more likely to move in the pocket
    - Textured: capsule able to grow into device, minimizing migration
  - Shape
    - Available in many standard shapes; can also be customized.
    - **Round expanders:** most commonly used in breast reconstruction. Results in ~25% of theoretical tissue gain.
    - **Rectangular expanders:** most commonly used in trunk and extremities. Results in ~40% of theoretical tissue gain.
    - **Crescent expanders:** useful in scalp reconstruction. Results in ~30% of theoretical tissue gain.

- **Anatomic expanders:** differentially expand the overlying soft tissue envelope to more accurately recreate the body part (ie, tear-drop–shaped expanders for breast reconstruction).
- **Custom expanders:** designed for irregularly shaped defects and may be more expensive.
  - ○ Filling port
    - Remote port: connected to tissue expander via silastic tubing and can be placed subcutaneously (more common) or externally for direct access.
    - Integrated port: located within the expander. There is risk of expander puncture.
    - Port often ferromagnetic and labeled as MRI-unsafe due to potential interaction with the magnetic field of the machine.

TECHNIQUE

- **Incision Placement**
  - ○ *Incisions are generally placed radially to the expander pocket, perpendicular to the direction of expansion to minimize tension on the incision during expansion process; undue tension placed on the incision during expansion can cause dehiscence and exposure of the expander. Do not place expanders across joints.
  - ○ Consider future reconstructive options when planning incision placement such that the incisions can easily be incorporated into planned flaps or the tissue to be resected.
  - ○ Donor tissue sites should be well vascularized and free of unstable scar without infection/contamination.
  - ○ Minimally invasive placement of tissue expanders can be performed with endoscopy to decrease incision length and has been shown to decrease complications, operative time and hospital stay.
- **Choice of Expander**
  - ○ **Use the largest expander possible** with a base diameter ~2-3 times that of the diameter of the soft tissue defect to be reconstructed.
  - ○ **If the expander contains a base plate or rigid backing,** this side should be placed along the floor of the pocket to guide the direction of expansion outward.
  - ○ **Multiple expanders are sometimes needed** to reconstruct a single defect, depending on the availability of donor tissue.
- **Pocket**
  - ○ The expander pocket can be developed in the subcutaneous, submuscular, or subgaleal (scalp) planes depending on the location of the soft tissue defect.
  - ○ The size of the expander pocket should be individually tailored to allow the expander to lie completely flat with minimal wrinkling.
  - ○ Excessive dissection should be limited to prevent expander migration postoperatively, and meticulous hemostasis is important to minimize hematoma formation.
- **Expansion Process**
  - ○ Insert a 23G butterfly needle or Huber (noncutting) needle into the filling port perpendicularly; bigger needles should be avoided because they can cause valve leak due to increased back pressure.
  - ○ At the time of expander placement, an initial volume is infused intraoperatively to gently fill the expander pocket to prevent seroma formation, and in the case of breast reconstruction patients, to maintain the shape of the overlying soft tissue envelope. If there is concern for overlying skin viability, intraoperative fill can be deferred.
  - ○ The expansion process usually begins 2-3 weeks postoperatively and continues on a weekly basis thereafter.
  - ○ Approximately 50-100 cc can be infused during each expansion, but regardless of the volume infused, the expander is filled until the patient expresses discomfort or the overlying skin blanches.
  - ○ The expansion process is complete based on surgeon preference when he/she deems there is enough donor tissue available to reconstruct the soft tissue defect;

however, this is often a difficult decision and additional "over" expansion is often recommended to ensure adequate soft tissue coverage.

o Typically wait a minimum of 8 weeks before removing expander for the patient's reconstructive procedure to allow for adequate tissue equlibration.

CLINICAL APPLICATIONS

• Indications for reconstruction generally include traumatic, congenital, oncologic, or burn defects. **See Table 5-1**

• **Flap Pre-expansion**
   o Pre-expansion of axial fasciocutaneous flaps facilitates coverage of larger soft tissue defects using expanded local tissue and simultaneously limits donor site morbidity by allowing primary closure.
   o Pre-expansion of myocutaneous flaps improves safe flap transfer due to a robust angiogenic response within the expanded local tissue resembling an incisional delay phenomenon.

COMPLICATIONS

• **Major**
   o **Cellulitis and periprosthetic infection**
      ▪ Requires early and aggressive treatment with intravenous antibiotics.
      ▪ If caught early, salvage of the expander may be possible with intravenous antibiotics alone; however, removal of the expander is often needed due to decreased clearance of bacteria from around the expander.
      ▪ If the infection becomes periprosthetic, removal of the expander is absolutely mandated.
      ▪ Port site infections can sometimes be managed by externalizing the remote filling port.
   o **Hematoma**
      ▪ Evacuation of the hematoma is necessary to prevent ischemia of the overlying skin flaps and bacterial superinfection.
      ▪ Removal of the expander is often not necessary.
   o **Expander exposure or extrusion**
      ▪ Requires removal of the expander if bacterial colonization is suspected.
      ▪ Most commonly due to inadequate pocket creation or poor overlying skin quality.
      ▪ Treat infection, if present.
   o **Expander deflation**
      ▪ Usually presents clinically as a "flat tire," and most often the result of iatrogenic puncture during insertion of the filling needle.
      ▪ Requires removal and replacement with a new expander.
   o **Skin-flap ischemia**
      ▪ Avoid aggressive dissection during expander placement to prevent devascularization of the overlying skin flaps.
      ▪ Avoid expanding too much during an individual session. If the overlying skin turns white, remove some fluid from the expander.
      ▪ Partial-thickness necrosis can usually be managed with local wound care.
      ▪ Full-thickness necrosis requires debridement of all devitalized tissue and reclosure to ensure adequate soft tissue coverage of the expander.
      ▪ Treat infection, if present.

• **Minor**
   o Incorrect valve placement or valve tissue expander flipping
   o Inadequate expansion
   o Pain during expansion
   o Temporary contour deformity at the donor site
   o Widening of surgical scars
   o Transient neuropraxia of both motor and sensory nerves

TABLE 5-1 Indications for Reconstruction

Area	Placement	Incisions	Closure	Caution	Other
Scalp/forehead	Subgaleal	Frontotemporal hairline; brow line; vertical midline; relaxed skin tension lines	Rotation-advancement	Temporal branch of facial nerve	50% of scalp can be reconstructed
Facial	Subcutaneous centrally; over parotidomasseteric fascia laterally	Preauricular hairline; relaxed skin tension lines	Local flap	Zygomatic and buccal branches of facial nerve; Stensen duct	
Auricular	Subcutaneous	Postauricular hairline	Thin, non-hair-bearing skin draped for primary closure		
Neck	Above platysma	Relaxed skin tension lines	Local flap; primary closure	Marginal mandibular and cervical branches of facial nerve	
Breast (Refer to Chapter 50: Breast Reconstruction)	Subcutaneous or subpectoral	Based on mastectomy incisions (periareolar, transverse, wise pattern)	Primary closure		Irradiated tissue with higher risk of complication
Abdominal wall	Subcutaneous; in between external and internal oblique muscles	Midline; paramedian	Primary closure with components separation and/or mesh		50% of abdominal wall can be reconstructed
Extremity	Over deep investing fascia of muscles	Relaxed skin tension lines; should not cross joints/impinge joint motion	Primary closure	Sensory nerves or superficial vessels	*Associated with higher complication rates especially in lower limb

PEARLS

1. Methylene blue can be used to color the contents of the expander to help identify the valve correctly when filling and to detect leakage more easily. However, there is a small percentage of patients with severe allergies to this dye.
2. Expanded local tissue can be re-expanded 3-6 months later.
3. The epidermis is the only layer of skin that increases in thickness during tissue expansion.
4. The base diameter of the expander should be approximately two to three times that of the diameter of the soft tissue defect to be reconstructed.
5. Approximately 50% of the scalp and abdominal wall can be reconstructed using tissue expansion.

QUESTIONS YOU WILL BE ASKED

1. Describe the phenomena of creep as it relates to tissue expansion.
   Creep describes the biological response of cells, which proliferate in response to continued mechanical stress.
2. Describe the histological changes seen with tissue expansion.
   Gap junctions become disrupted, epidermis thickens, and dermis becomes thinner.
3. Describe the contraindications to tissue expansion.
   No absolute contraindications, but irradiated bed, infection, extremities in children are all relative contraindications.
4. What is the effect of tissue expander on overlying skin?
   Blood flow increases, causing tissue expansion to mimic the delay phenomenon.

Recommended Readings
1. Austad ED, Pasyk KA, McClatchey KD, Cherry GW. Histomorphologic evaluation of guinea pig skin and soft tissue after controlled tissue expansion. *Plast Reconstr Surg.* 1982;70(6):704-710.
2. Dong C, Zhu M, Huang L, et al. Risk factors for tissue expander infection in scar reconstruction: a retrospective cohort study of 2374 consecutive cases. *Burns Trauma.* 2021;8:037.
3. Egeland BM, Cederna PS. A minimally invasive approach to the placement of tissue expanders. *Semin Plast Surg.* 2008;22(1):9-17. doi: 10.1055/s-2007-1019137. PMID: 20567683; PMCID: PMC2884855.
4. Huang X, Qu X, Li Q. Risk factors for complications of tissue expansion: a 20-year systematic review and meta-analysis. *Plast Reconstr Surg.* 2011;128(3):787-797.
5. Radovan C. Tissue expansion in soft-tissue reconstruction. *Plast Reconstr Surg.* 1984;74(4):482-492.

6 Fat Grafting

Amy L. Strong and Jaclyn T. Mauch

OVERVIEW

- **Background**
  - Early reports of fat grafting by Neuber, Czerny, and Hollander demonstrated the positive, natural appearing results achievable with fat grafting for facial and breast reconstruction.
  - Despite early successes, subsequent reports were met with varying levels of failure often associated with asymmetry caused by fat resorption.
  - In the early 1990s, Coleman proposed several refinement techniques focused on fat harvest, processing, and reinjection that increased the predictability of fat grafting outcomes.
  - Fat grafting is safe, abundant, readily available, and completely biocompatible, making it the preferred soft tissue filler for facial atrophy, breast asymmetry for aesthetic and reconstructive purposes, radiation damage, chronic ulceration, scleroderma, and burn injuries.
  - In general, "fat grafting" can be further broken down into its components
    - **Mature adipocytes** (85%-90% volume).
    - **Stromal vascular fracture (SVF):** (10%-15%) preadipocytes, fibroblasts, vascular smooth muscle cells, endothelial cells, resident monocytes/ macrophages, lymphocytes, and adipose-derived stem/stromal cells (ASCs).
    - **Adipose-derived stem/stromal cells (ASCs):** (3%-5%) regenerative cells that secrete cytokines and chemokines that improve engraftment of cells by reducing circulating immune cells, inhibiting melanocyte proliferation and melanin synthesis, and promoting cell turnover.
  - Fat grafting is further subdivided into the parcel size of the fat lobules and cell type with different indications for each (**Table 6-1**).
    - **Nanofats** is a misnomer as it does not contain adipocytes and is composed solely of SVF cells, ASCs, growth factors, and extracellular matrix
- **Indications**
  - Macrofat
    - Augmentation in any subcutaneous location with tissue atrophy
    - Facial rejuvenation, specifically malar region in the deep plane
    - Lipodystrophic syndromes and atrophic areas
    - Breast reconstruction
    - Breast augmentation
    - Scar revision
    - Coup de sabre and scleroderma
    - Hemifacial microsomia or progressive facial atrophy
  - Microfat: facial
    - Facial rejuvenation, in the nasolabial folds, lips, brows, lower lids, jaw line, blending of the lid-cheek junction
  - Nanofat: facial
    - Rejuvenation to improve collagen and elastin regeneration to improve skin texture and elasticity.
    - Inhibit melanin synthesis to improve skin pigmentation.

'Denotes common in-service examination topics.

TABLE 6-1 Fat Grafting Parcel Size

	Size	Harvesting	Target
Macrofat	2-2.5 mm in diameter	3-mm harvesting cannula	Body (ie, breast reconstruction, contour irregularities) and malar eminence fat grafting in the deep plane of the face
Microfat	1-2 mm in diameter	2.1- to 2.4-mm harvesting cannula	Facial fat grafting into the lid-cheek junction, lips, and nasolabial fold
Nanofat	400-600 μm diameter	Processed with filter devices from macrofat or microfat	Used to improve skin elasticity and hyperpigmentation

FAT GRAFTING TECHNIQUE

HARVESTING

- **Coleman technique**
  - Method used to harvest macrofat.
  - 3-mm incisions.
  - Blunt tip attached to 10-mL Luer-Lok syringe.
  - Cannula pushed through harvest site as surgeon uses manipulation to create gentle negative pressure by pulling back on plunger (ie, 1-2 cc with a 10-cc syringe).
  - Plunger removed and syringe placed in centrifuge for processing.
- Different providers have variable preferences/beliefs about the effect of amount of suction during harvest, length of canula, and size of collection.
- Harvest can be done with handheld syringe or suction-assisted liposuction. Compared with suction-assisted liposuction, handheld syringe lipoaspirates have higher adipocyte count and viability with the dry technique. No differences observed when the wet technique was employed.
- *Using a larger cannula size to harvest fat increases viability, whereas no differences were observed between multiperforated cannula vs single port cannula.
- **Donor site** with the highest efficacy is the abdomen and thighs.
- **Superwet or tumescent techniques** have not been shown to be detrimental on fat graft viability, as this excess fluid is generally removed during the processing step. Alternatively, tumescent fluid can be injected after harvesting for hemostasis and pain control.

PROCESSING

- Optimized to increase the number of viable adipocytes, SVF, and ASCs in fat grafting.
- **Coleman technique:** lipoaspirate is loaded into 10-mL syringes.
  - Adipose tissue centrifuged at 3000 rpm for 3 minutes (variable).
- **Centrifugation:** separates aspirate based on density.
  - Separated into the oil layer (top), adipose tissue, infranatant (bottom), which includes blood, water, aqueous solution, or tumescent.
  - Blood and tumescent fraction drained from the bottom layer and the oil is decanted and wicked with a cotton pledget for 3 minutes from the top layer.
  - High-density fat contains greater concentration of SVF cells and ASCs with greater graft take and regenerative potential, first 1-3 cc of processed fat in the bottom of the centrifuged syringe.
- **Telfa gauze rolling:** removes excess fluids from the adipocytes and cells. Results in large fat grafts with good structural integrity.
- **Sedimentation or gravity separation (ie, AquaVage, Red Head):** higher degree of resorption due to increase in fluid retained in the process lipoaspirate.

- **Revolve:** active filtration combined with washing and/or centrifugation; closed system; an inline fat-processing system in which lipoaspirate is harvested directly into a canister device rather than a drain bag.
- **Puregraft:** passive filtration combined with washing and/or centrifugation; closed system; fat is harvested directly into a bag and washed with LR.
- **LipiVage:** used for smaller volumes; a filtration system within the harvesting syringe, and the same syringe is used for harvesting, processing, and lipofilling

REINJECTION

- **Smaller gauge** used than when harvesting.
- **Blunt tip** allows less traumatic introduction (Coleman: 17-gauge cannula with a 1-mL syringe, injecting tiny amounts with each pass).
- **Fat should be placed with multiple passes** laying down single layer of fat and avoiding clumping.
- Each injection should be a new tunnel creating multiple levels in a three-dimensional manner.
- *Reinjection speed plays a role in survival: slower reinjection results in lower shear and higher cell viability.
- If clump injected, flatten with digital manipulation.
- Usually placed just under the dermis.
- Augmentation over mandible and malar region should be injected over periosteum to prevent nodule formation.
- **Possible methods to improve survival**
  - Greater exposure of each adipocyte to vasculature.
  - Diffuse infiltration with multiple passes.
  - Small amount of placement per pass.
  - Large surface area of contact between fat and surrounding tissue.
  - Pure fat.
  - *Graft soon after harvesting (ideally within 1-2 hours of harvest).
  - Once you feel large open space with each pass, it is likely a good indication to stop.
- **Three zones of healing** among the adipocytes located in a newly fat-grafted bed
  - Necrotic zone: innermost zone; no cells survive because of hypoxia
  - Regenerating zone: revascularization starts from the periphery toward the center
    - Most adipocytes in the regenerative and necrotic zones die within the first 24 hours.
  - Surviving zone: both adipocytes and ASCs survive; outermost zone

OTHER CONSIDERATIONS

- Special considerations for microfat grafting
  - Harvested either with a 2.1-mm cannula or macrofat processed with several passes through two Luer-Lok syringe with a 1.2- or 2.0-mm filter.
  - Can be injected more superficially given the smaller size.
  - Some surgeons inject subdermally to fill rhytids observed in the forehead, glabella, lips, and neck.
  - Also used to blend the lid-cheek junction.
- Special considerations for nanofat grafting
  - Processed from microfat through several passes through two Luer-Lok syringes with a 1.2 and 2.0 filter followed by a 400 or 600 μm emulsifier to remove any adipocytes.
  - Enriched for SVF, ASCs, extracellular matrix proteins, and growth factors.
  - Injected with a 27-gauge needle, microneedling, or dissolved in a topical cream.
  - Injections can be carried out intradermally or subdermally as there are no adipocytes and only SVF cells.

- **Graft survival and healing**
  - Patients can have considerable postoperative edema due to multiple passes with injection.
  - *In general, graft viability is 50%-80%. Survival rate decreases with infection, trauma, and hypoxia.
  - **Overcorrection** needed to optimize results and account for graft loss in the body but not in the face, as this is a challenging problem to correct.
  - **Final volume determined by:**
    - Interactions between multiple cell types, including ASCs, viable adipocytes, and necrotic adipocytes.
    - These cells stimulate maintenance of a set volume as determined by the original composite of tissue transferred into the wound bed.
  - For most patients included in studies examining the effect of fat grafting after thermal or radiation injury, an average of two treatments are needed.
  - Often the second fat transplantation occurs 3 months after the initial procedure.

SPECIFIC CLINICAL USES

- **Facial volume correction**
  - Inject macrofat into the deep malar fat pad with an 18-gauge blunt with 0.05 cc per pass.
  - Inject microfat into the upper lips and perinasal area with 16-gauge needle from stab incisions made on each side of oral commissure. Inject into vermilion of lip to roll out vermilion and give patient more red lip.
  - Periorbital rejuvenation: inject microfat along inferior orbital rim in the plane close to the bone. Can inject nanofat into the dermis over the lower eyelids.
  - Temporal rejuvenation: macrofat placed subcutaneously in the plane above the temporalis fascia.
- **Breast augmentation**
  - Generally appropriate for women who want a small enhancement (~1 cup size) and likely requires serial fat grafting to achieve the desired size.
  - Injection using 14-gauge Coleman side hole needle with multiple sites of injection along inframammary fold.
  - Fat injected subcutaneously and not directly into the breast tissue.
  - May lead to increased number of mammograms for cancer surveillance.
- **Breast reconstruction**
  - Fat grafting for primary reconstruction postmastectomy:
    - Pro: autologous reconstruction with no donor site morbidity.
    - Cons: limited by donor fat availability, only small breast volumes achievable (A/B cup), requires up to 6 procedures spaced at least 3 months apart to achieve desired breast size, radiation history tends to require more sessions.
    - Mean total graft volumes range from 600 to 750 cc, with ~200-300 cc per session.
    - Centrifugation most commonly used, with sedimentation also reported.
    - Recipient site expansion methods include internal expansion (internal expander deflated each session), external expansion (BRAVA), or none.
    - Previous radiation predicts increased complications, while mastectomy flap type does not.
    - Common complications include palpable lumps, ulceration necrosis, and fat necrosis.
  - Fat-augmented latissimus dorsi flap
  - The latissimus dorsi flap provides inadequate volume for breast reconstruction but can be augmented with fat injected intramuscularly with multiple passes to increase volume (eg, LIFT procedure).
  - Fat grafting occurs at the time of reconstruction with subsequent grafting for insufficient volumes.

○ Other uses
- Postlumpectomy deformity to improve contour.
- Augment autologous-based reconstruction or improve contour irregularities, such as softening the transition between the flap and chest wall or improving areas of fat necrosis.
- In implant-based reconstruction, fat grafting can create a more natural transition in the superior pole from the implant to the chest wall; it can also improve animation deformity.
- Tuberous breast deformity.
- Poland syndrome.
- Gluteal augmentation: injection should be in the subcutaneous tissue and never into the muscle as this can cause fat embolism/death.

○ Cancer outcomes: clinical studies show no increase in cancer recurrence when fat grafting is used in reconstruction.

COMPLICATIONS

- *Fat embolism secondary to intramuscular injection of fat for gluteal augmentation has resulted in death. Gluteal augmentation with fat grafting should be performed in the subcutaneous plane only, no intramuscular injections.
- *Glabellar injection can cause blindness via retinal artery occlusion or ophthalmic artery occlusion.
- Skin necrosis.
- Fat resorption and necrosis.
- Irregularities.
- Fat necrosis in breast cancer can lead to additional surveillance studies.
- Unknown risk in head and neck patients.

ADIPOSE-DERIVED STEM CELLS

- Can be isolated from adipose tissue harvested either by liposuction or by excision of tissue.
- **If harvested by liposuction,** adipose tissue settles into two layers.
  ○ **Supernatant or processed lipoaspirate (PLA) layer:** consists of the suctioned adipocytes as well as their surrounding endothelium and stroma.
  ○ **The bottom layer** or liposuction aspirate fluid: consists of injected saline, erythrocytes, and denser pieces of the PLA layer.
  ○ **ASCs can be harvested from both layers;** however, the yield of adherent ASCs is significantly higher in the adipocyte layer than in the liposuction aspirate fluid cells.
    - **Terms for adipose-derived "stem cells" (ASCs):** adipose-derived adult stem cells, adipose-derived adult stromal cells, adipose-derived stromal cells, adipose mesenchymal stem cells, lipoblast, pericyte, preadipocyte, and PLA cells.
    - **International Federation for Adipose Therapeutics and Science** reached a consensus: ASCs to describe plastic-adherent, multipotent cell population.
    - **Culturing of these cells** eventually results in the appearance of a relatively homogeneous population of mesodermal or MSCs (usually after two to three passages) after nonadherent cells from SVF are washed away.
    - **Beneficial impact of ASCs may be due to soluble factors** produced by ASCs rather than their differentiation capability toward different mature lineages.
    - **ASCs secrete** hepatocyte growth factor, vascular endothelial growth factor, transforming growth factor-β, insulinlike growth factor-1, basic fibroblast growth factor, granulocyte-macrophage colony-stimulating factor, tumor necrosis factor-α, interleukin-6, interleukin-7, interleukin-8, interleukin-11, adiponectin, angiotensin, and cathepsin D.
    - **ASCs are mesodermal and can differentiate into** adipogenic, osteogenic, chondrogenic, myogenic, cardiomyogenic, angiogenic, tenogenic, and odontogenic lineages.

PEARLS

1. When harvesting fat for grafting, the goal is to reduce sheer force on the adipocytes by using handheld syringe devices.
2. Graft soon after harvesting to increase cell viability.
3. Important to use many small passes or aliquots for laying fat down to improve vascularity to fat grafts and decrease fat necrosis.
4. Once recipient site for fat grafting feels like a large open space, probably it is best to stop grafting.
5. Rate of injection alters fat graft survival; faster injection speed increases fat resorption due to injury to the adipocytes.

QUESTIONS YOU WILL BE ASKED

1. What is the 6-month viability of fat grafting?
   Around 50%-80%.
2. Why is processing the lipoaspirate important?
   Reduces resorption and the unpredictability of fat grafting.
3. What is the most common complication after fat grafting?
   Resorption.
4. With fat grafting, why is it important for very small volumes to be injected with each pass?
   To promote maximal contact between graft and surrounding bed.

Recommended Readings
1. Coleman SR. Structural fat grafting: more than a permanent filler. *Plast Reconstr Surg.* 2006;118(3 Suppl):108S-120S.
2. Gir P, Brown SA, Oni G, Kashefi N, Mojallal A, Rohrich RJ. Fat grafting: evidence-based review on autologous fat harvesting, processing, reinjection, and storage. *Plast Reconstr Surg.* 2012;130(1):249-258.
3. Locke MB, de Chalain TM. Current practice in autologous fat transplantation: suggested clinical guidelines based on a review of recent literature. *Ann Plast Surg.* 2008;60(1):98-102.
4. Strong AL, Cederna PS, Rubin JP, Coleman SR, Levi B. The current state of fat grafting: a review of harvesting, processing, and injection techniques. *Plast Reconstr Surg.* 2015;136(4):897-912.

7 Benign and Malignant Skin and Soft Tissue Lesions

Naomi Briones

OVERVIEW

SKIN EMBRYOLOGY

- **Ectoderm:** epidermis, pilosebaceous glands, apocrine glands, eccrine sweat glands, nails
- **Mesoderm:** dermis, Langerhans cells, macrophages, mast cells, fibroblasts, blood vessels, lymph vessels, adipose cells
- **Neuroectoderm:** *melanocytes, nerves, specialized sensory receptors, Merkel cells

SKIN HISTOLOGY

- **Epidermis**
  - Made up of five layers (superficial to deep): stratum corneum, lucidum, granulosum, spinosum, basale
  - Keratinocytes: primary cell in epidermis
    - Starts in basal layer (stratum basale) and make their way to surface to become a dead cornified layer (stratum corneum)
  - Melanocytes: basal layer; protect against ultraviolet (UV) radiation
  - Merkel cells: mechanoreceptors
  - Langerhans cells: antigen-presenting cells in stratum spinosum
- **Dermis**
  - Made up of two layers (superficial to deep): papillary and reticular
  - Cell types: fibroblast, macrophage, and mast cell
  - Papillary dermis
    - Similar thickness to epidermis; intertwines with rete ridges of the epidermis
    - Type III collagen > type I
    - Site of collagenase activity, terminal networks of Meissner corpuscles and capillaries
  - Reticular dermis: majority of the dermal layer
    - Mostly type I collagen bundles with elastic fibers between
    - Contains hair roots, sebaceous and sweat glands, receptors, and blood vessels.
  - Tissue components
    - Collagen: provides tensile strength.
      - *Type I to type III—4:1 ratio in adult skin
      - Immature scar type I to type III—2:1 ratio in adult skin
    - Elastin
      - Interdigitates with collagen; composed of fibrillin protein
      - Important in skin recoil and decreases with aging
    - Ground substance
      - Noncellular component of extracellular matrix with fibers
      - Composed of glycosaminoglycans (hyaluronic acid and proteoglycans)

---

*Denotes common in-service examination topics.

BENIGN LESIONS

EPIDERMAL LESIONS

- **Epidermal nevus** (linear nevus)
  - Present at birth or early childhood
  - May be associated with developmental delays and other neurologic and MSK abnormalities
  - Clinical presentation: tan or brown warty papules in linear array
  - Anatomic location: trunk and extremities
  - Treatment: excision, laser therapy (CO_2), topical therapies less effective
- **Inflammatory linear verrucous epidermal nevus**
  - Present at birth or early childhood
  - Clinical presentation: erythematous, scaly papules in linear array, pruritic
  - Anatomic location: on one extremity along lines of Blaschko
  - Treatment: excision or laser therapy (pulsed dye laser)
- **Seborrheic keratosis**
  - Derived from basal layer of epidermis. Cystic inclusions of keratinous material
  - Present in middle age around fifth decade
  - Clinical presentation: waxy, tan to black, stuck-on papules
  - Anatomic location: anywhere except palms, soles, mucous membranes
  - Treatment: cryotherapy, curettage, excision
- **Actinic keratosis:** most common premalignant skin lesion
  - Rate of transformation to SCC ~0.6%-16% per year
  - Clinical presentation: erythematous, scaly papules; actinic cheilitis if on lips
  - Anatomic location: sunlight-exposed areas (scalp, ears, face, and hands)
  - Histologically characterized by dyskeratosis, atypia in basal layer of epidermis
  - Treatment: 5-fluorouracil (FDA approved), imiquimod 5% (Aldara), cryotherapy, photodynamic therapy
- **Verruca vulgaris**
  - Common wart: caused by human papillomavirus (HPV).
  - Clinical presentation: scaly, rough appearance often with thrombosed capillaries.
  - Anatomic location: variable. Lesions arise from stratum granulosum.
  - Treatment: cryotherapy, imiquimod, candida antigen, salicylic acid, or excision.
- **Cutaneous horn**
  - Clinical presentation: well-circumscribed cone with hyperkeratosis.
  - Most commonly arise from actinic keratosis; SCC present in up to 20% of lesions.
  - Anatomic location: sun-exposed areas.
  - Treatment: excisional biopsy with careful evaluation of lesion base.
- **Leukoplakia**
  - Associated with chronic inflammation/irritation (alcohol or tobacco).
  - *May degenerate into SCC.
  - Clinical presentation/anatomic location: mucosal lesion; cannot be wiped away.
  - Treatment: removal of irritant, biopsy may be warranted.
- **Keratoacanthoma**
  - *Rapid growth phase followed by spontaneous regression
  - Clinical presentation: firm, dome-shaped nodule
    - Prominent horn-filled central depression and keratin with thick epidermis
  - Difficult to distinguish from SCC
  - Treatment: simple excision; consider 5-fluorouracil if multiple lesions

MELANOCYTIC LESIONS

- **Nevus of Ota/nevus of Ito**
  - Found in patients with Asian ancestry
  - Clinical presentation: appears at birth as large, blue-gray patch

- - Anatomic location
    - Ota: areas innervated by first and second branches of trigeminal nerve
    - Ito: posterior shoulder and areas innervated by posterior supraclavicular and lateral cutaneous brachial nerves
  - Treatment: laser therapy (Q-switched ruby, alexandrite, Nd:YAG)
- **Nevus spilus**
  - Appears at birth
  - Clinical presentation: tan patch with speckled hyperpigmented macules and papules
  - Anatomic location: commonly on trunk and extremities
  - Treatment: observation, laser therapy (Q-switched ruby, Nd:YAG); simple excision
- **Spitz nevus** (benign juvenile melanoma)
  - Appears in childhood or early adulthood
  - Clinical presentation: pink to brown, dome-shaped, smooth papules
  - Anatomic location: commonly located on the head and neck
  - Treatment: excision with margins to decrease recurrence risk (range from 1-2 mm to 1-2 cm depending on concern for melanoma)
  - May be difficult to distinguish histologically from spitzoid melanoma
- **Junctional nevus**
  - Nests of melanocytes located at dermoepidermal junction
  - Appears in childhood or early adulthood
  - Clinical presentation: skin colored to brown, evenly pigmented macule with well-defined borders
  - Anatomic location: any site
  - Treatment: observation, simple excision
- **Compound nevus**
  - Contains both junctional and intradermal components
  - Appears in childhood or early adulthood
  - Clinical presentation: skin colored to dark-brown papule with regular borders
  - Anatomic location: any site
  - Treatment: observation, simple excision
- **Intradermal nevus**
  - Located entirely within the dermis
  - Appears in the second or third decade of life
  - Clinical presentation: appears as a flesh-colored or light tan papule
  - Anatomic location: face or neck
  - Treatment: observation, simple excision
- **Common blue nevus**
  - Appears during adolescence.
  - Clinical presentation: blue or blue-black <1 cm papule.
  - Anatomic location: hands, feet, face and scalp.
  - Treatment: observation, simple excision.
  - Cutaneous metastasis of malignant melanoma can resemble blue nevus.
- **Cellular blue nevus**
  - Appears after second decade of life
  - Clinical presentation: blue-black 1-3 cm papule
  - Anatomic location: buttocks or sacral region
  - Treatment: observation, simple excision
- **Atypical (dysplastic) nevus**
  - Patients with dysplastic nevi and a family history of melanoma in a first-degree relative are at a higher risk of melanoma, warranting regular skin examinations.
  - Appear after puberty.
  - Clinical presentation: atypical pigment, borders, size, asymmetric.
  - Anatomic location: anywhere.
  - Treatment: excision with margins to prevent recurrence.
    - Sunscreen and avoidance of sunburning/tanning

ADNEXAL TUMORS: SEBACEOUS GLANDS, HAIR FOLLICLES, APOCRINE, OR ECCRINE SWEAT GLANDS

- **Hair follicle tumors**: located in lower dermis and subcutaneous fat
  - **Pilomatrixoma** (calcifying epithelioma of Malherbe)
    - Typically seen in younger patients (<20 years old)
    - Clinical presentation: single, solid subdermal nodule
      - Positive tent sign—stretching of overlying skin yields angulated shape.
      - Difficult to distinguish from calcified masses or carcinoma.
      - Histopathology: epidermoid cells with basophilic and eosinophilic cells.
    - Anatomic location: head and upper trunk
    - Treatment: excision (up to 1-2 cm margins); up to 10% recurrence rate
  - **Trichofolliculoma** (hair follicle nevus)
    - Clinical presentation: <1 cm and skin colored
    - Anatomic location: on face with thin pale hairs
    - Treatment: observation, biopsy
  - **Trichoepithelioma**
    - Seen in patients after puberty
    - Clinical presentation: solitary pink or flesh-colored papule
    - May be difficult to distinguish clinically and histologically from BCC
    - Anatomic location: if multiple, symmetric distribution around face and eyes
    - Treatment: observation, laser, electrosurgical destruction
  - **Trichilemmoma**
    - Cowden syndrome (multiple hamartoma syndrome): suspect if patients have multiple such tumors.
    - Histopathology: glycogen-rich epithelial cells surrounded by sheaths of cells resembling hair follicles.
    - Clinical presentation: smooth skin-colored papules
    - Anatomic location: found on scalp or other hair-bearing regions
    - Treatment: laser therapy (CO_2), electrosurgical excision, or simple excision due to similar appearance with BCC and trichilemmal carcinoma
- **Eccrine tumors**
  - Cylindroma
    - Appears in early adulthood
    - Multiple may indicate AD Brooke-Spiegler syndrome or multiple cylindromatosis
    - Clinical presentation: solitary, firm, smooth pink nodules
    - Anatomic location: often located on scalp
    - Treatment: laser therapy (CO_2), electrodessication/curettage, or simple excision
  - **Eccrine poroma**
    - Clinical presentation: firm, popular, or nodular lesions surrounded by rim of hyperkeratosis; may appear pedunculated
    - Anatomic location: most commonly palms and soles of feet
    - Treatment: simple excision
  - **Syringoma**
    - Appears in early adulthood, more common in women and with Down syndrome
    - Clinical presentation: small yellow-pink papules. May be confused with xanthelasma or trichoepithelioma
    - Anatomic location: most commonly periocular region (eyelids, upper cheek) but may involve trunk, neck, or extremities
    - Treatment: laser (CO_2), electrodesiccation, snip/simple excision
  - **Eccrine spiradenoma**
    - Appears in young adults

- Clinical presentation: painful, slow-growing, blue-purple nodule
- Anatomic location: head, neck or trunk
- Treatment: simple excision if symptomatic; laser (CO_2) for smaller lesions
  - Eccrine hidrocystoma
    - Dilated and obstructed sweat ducts histologically
    - Clinical presentation: skin colored to blue translucent firm papules
    - Swell in heat/humidity; regress in cooler/dry climate
    - Anatomic location: temples, cheeks, periorbital area, forehead
    - Treatment: puncture to release pressure
- Sebaceous tumors
  - Nevus sebaceus (of Jadassohn)
    - Appears at birth or early childhood.
    - Most commonly develops secondary benign adnexal tumors, most common malignant lesion (~2.5% cases) that develops within is a BCC (~1% cases).
    - Clinical presentation: appears as yellow/orange, waxy, smooth plaques prior to puberty and rough, verrucous, orange plaques after puberty.
    - Anatomic location: most commonly found on scalp.
    - Treatment: observation, complete excision.
  - Sebaceous hyperplasia
    - Appears in middle-aged or older adults
    - Clinical presentation: appears as shiny, small umbilicated, yellow-white papules
    - Anatomic location: most common on face
    - Treatment: cryotherapy, electrodesiccation, or laser (pulsed dye, Er:YAG, CO_2), may be excised due to similar appearance with BCC
  - Sebaceous adenoma
    - Appears in middle age
    - *May be associated with Muir-Torre syndrome—an autosomal-dominant syndrome associated with multiple keratoacanthomas, marked increase in visceral neoplasm
    - Clinical presentation: smooth, yellow papules
    - Anatomic location: located primarily in head and neck
    - Treatment: simple excision
- Apocrine tumors
  - Apocrine cystadenoma (aka hidrocystoma)
    - Contains brown or blue tinged fluid
    - Clinical presentation: appears as a single translucent nodule
    - Anatomic location: most common on face
  - Chondroid syringoma
    - Histology: sweat gland (epithelial) and cartilaginous elements (mesenchymal)
    - Treatment: excisional biopsy
  - Syringocystadenoma papilliferum
    - Appears during childhood
    - Clinical presentation: may be associated with nevus sebaceus
    - Anatomic location: most commonly found on scalp
    - Treatment: excision; ablative laser

SMOOTH MUSCLE TUMOR

- Leiomyoma
  - Abnormal proliferation of smooth muscle.
  - May become painful on exposure to cold/pressure.
  - Clinical presentation: smooth, pink to red-brown papules or nodules.
  - Treatment: laser (CO_2), excisional biopsy.
  - Malignant degeneration to leiomyosarcoma is rare.

CYSTS

- **Epidermal inclusion cyst** (epidermoid cyst)
  - May be incorrectly called a sebaceous cyst; however, not sebaceous in origin.
  - Appears in adulthood.
  - Clinical presentation: fluctuant, flesh-colored, well-circumscribed nodules.
    - Dilated punctum may be visible; may express foul-smelling keratinous debris.
  - Anatomic location: commonly found on face, neck, and trunk.
  - Treatment: excision if uninfected; if infected, incision and drainage with interval excision.
- **Dermoid cyst**
  - Appears at birth or early childhood
  - Clinical presentation: firm, deep-seated nodules
  - *Anatomic location: most commonly found on supraorbital ridge, lateral brow, nasal midline
  - Treatment: excision
  - *Midline nasal mass differential diagnosis: dermoid cyst, glioma, meningocele/encephalocele
    - **CT or MRI prior to excision to determine intracranial extension**
- **Pilar (trichilemmal) cyst**
  - Appears in adulthood
  - Clinical presentation: smooth, mobile, keratin filled
  - Anatomic location: most commonly found on scalp
  - Treatment: excision if uninfected; if infected, incision and drainage with interval excision

FIBROUS LESIONS

- **Dermatofibroma**
  - Appears in adulthood
  - Clinical presentation: brown-red papule with dimple sign (sinks when squeezed)
  - Anatomic location: most common lower extremities
  - Treatment: intralesional corticosteroids, simple excision
- **Angiofibroma**
  - Clinical presentation: skin colored to pink firm papules
  - Anatomic location: most commonly on nose
  - Treatment: simple excision for cosmesis
  - May be associated with tuberous sclerosis if multiple
- **Lipoma**
  - Benign fatty tumor that may be present at any age
  - Clinical presentation: painless, soft, flesh-colored nodule
  - Anatomic location: commonly found on the trunk and extremities
  - Treatment: simple excision
- **Dermatofibrosarcoma protuberans**
  - Appears in middle age.
  - Clinical presentation: reddish-brown, firm, slow-growing nodular plaque.
  - Anatomic location: more commonly found on trunk, extremities.
  - *Treatment is radical excision (>3 cm margins) given locally aggressive behavior.
  - Local recurrence is common; however, metastasis is rare.
- **Neurofibroma**
  - Composed of Schwann cells and endoneurial fibroblasts.
  - May appear at any age.
  - Clinical presentation: soft, flesh-colored or pink nodules; button-hole sign (invaginate when compressed).
  - Anatomic location: more common on the trunk and extremities.
  - Treatment: observation, excision.
  - Multiple neurofibromas may be associated with neurofibromatosis type I or II.
    - *Type I—café au lait spots, Lisch nodules (iris hamartomas), and optic nerve glioma
    - Type II—bilateral acoustic neuroma

OTHER DISORDERS

- **Calciphylaxis**
  - Metastatic calcification of blood vessels and necrosis of surrounding tissue
  - Associated with renal failure; may appear at any age; more common in women
  - Clinical presentation: painful necrotic ulcerations; red-blue mottling of skin (livedo reticularis)
  - Anatomic location: fat-bearing locations on trunk and extremities
  - Treatment: pain control, correct underlying electrolytes, intravenous sodium thiosulfate, or excision (although relatively contraindicated as often results in progressive calcification)
- **Hidradenitis Suppurativa**
  - Clinical presentation: chronic inflammation of apocrine sweat glands, which can progress to chronic draining sinus tracts and abscesses
  - Anatomic location: most commonly the axillae, breasts, perineum, and buttocks.
  - Treatment: topical clindamycin, oral or IV antibiotics, biologics (TNF-alpha inhibitors), wide local excision and skin grafting, unroofing
- **Dystrophic Epidermolysis Bullosa**
  - Hereditary disease with bulla formation of skin/mucosa following minor trauma
  - May result in encasement of digits with scar tissue
  - Treatment: scar release/Z-plasty, topical steroids, avoidance of trauma
- **Cutis Laxa**
  - Defect in elastic fibers; wound healing unaffected.
  - Skin hangs loose from folds; premature aging.
  - Blepharoplasty and face lift can be beneficial.
- **Pseudoxanthoma Elasticum**
  - Affects elastic fibers and collagen; wound healing is normal.
  - Skin thickens and appears cobblestoned; later becomes wrinkled and lax.
- **Ehlers-Danlos Syndrome (Cutis Hyperelastica)**
  - Autosomal recessive or x-linked causing genetic defects in collagen.
  - Hyperextensible skin, severe joint laxity, delicate blood vessels.
  - *Wound healing is abnormal: approach surgery with caution.
- **Acne Vulgaris**
  - Appears in younger patients.
  - Clinical presentation: comedones, inflammatory papules, deep-seated cysts.
  - Anatomic location: face.
  - Treatment: topical retinoids, topical and oral antibiotics and oral isotretinoin (accutane). Isotretinoin—risk of birth defects; patients must have two forms of contraception. Avoid if planning aesthetic facial rejuvenation with lasers or peels.
- **Rosacea**
  - Clinical presentation
    - Facial flushing (increased vascularity), thickened skin erythema, telangiectasia
    - Acne rosacea (papules and pustules)
    - Rhinophyma—nasal skin becomes erythematous with telangiectatic changes
  - Anatomic location: affects forehead glabella, malar region, nose, chin
  - Treatment: oral antibiotics, retinoic acid, dermabrasion, cryotherapy, laser (CO_2), tangential excision (for rhinophyma)
  - Reconstruct with secondary contraction vs skin graft
- **Pyoderma Gangrenosum**
  - Clinical presentation: superficial abscesses with significant ulceration and skin necrosis.
  - Consult dermatology for biopsy to evaluate, although a diagnosis of exclusion.
  - Treatment: systemic corticosteroids, immunosuppressants.
  - Given pathergy, avoid surgery, debridement or skin grafts (can induce PG at donor sites).
  - *Associated with IBD—refer to gastroenterologist for endoscopy.

SKIN MALIGNANCIES

- **Generally grouped into three types**
  - **Basal cell carcinoma** (BCC) > **squamous cell carcinoma** (SCC) > **melanoma**.
  - The ratio of BCC to SCC to melanoma is ≈40:10:1.
  - Incidence of all three types is increasing; fortunately, the more common types (BCC and SCC) are far less aggressive than melanoma.
  - More than 20% of the U.S. population develops a skin cancer during their lifetime.
  - There are more skin cancers in the U.S. population than all other cancers combined.

BASAL CELL CARCINOMA

EPIDEMIOLOGY

- **Incidence**
  - BCC is the most common skin cancer, accounting for ≈80% of all skin cancers.
  - Roughly 3.6 million new cases per year in the United States.
- **Risk Factors**
  - UV exposure (eg, PUVA) or ionizing radiation, fair skin, chemical exposure (eg, arsenic), immunosuppression (transplant patients), nevus sebaceus
  - Syndromes associated with BCC
    - **Basal cell nevus syndrome (Gorlin syndrome)**
      - Autosomal-dominant inheritance
      - Palmoplantar cysts, early-onset BCCs, jaw cysts (odontogenic keratocysts), skeletal anomalies, medulloblastomas, fibromas (ovarian and cardiac)
    - **Xeroderma pigmentosum (XP):** patients have increased incidence of BCC, SCC, and malignant melanoma (see below in Melanoma section).
      - Autosomal recessive disorder affecting DNA repair
      - Treatment: avoidance of sunlight, isotretinoin, 5-fluorouracil, or excision

BCC DISEASE BIOLOGY AND CHARACTERISTICS

- Basal keratinocytes are the cell of origin, residing in the basal layer of the epidermis at the dermoepidermal junction.
- No universal clinical precursor lesion.
- BCC is most common in areas with high concentrations of pilosebaceous follicles and thus >90% are found on the head and neck.
- Metastasis is rare.
- Morbidity is caused by invasion of the tumor into underlying structures, including the sinuses, orbit, and brain. Typically, only a problem if neglected for many years.
- **Types of BCC**
  - **Nodular BCC**
    - The most common type, usually presenting as a single lesion consisting of pearly papules with telangiectasias, pruritus, and occasional bleeding.
    - Lesion breakdown over time leads to nodulo-ulcerative BCC ("rodent ulcer").
    - Histology demonstrates palisading nuclei.
  - **Superficial spreading BCC**
    - Slow-growing, erythematous, minimal induration, and located primarily on the trunk.
    - It is easily confused with other scaly, eczematous dermatoses.
    - Shallow lesions with horizontal growth pattern; can become invasive.
  - **Morpheaform (sclerosing, fibrosing) BCC**
    - Flat, scarlike, white to yellow to pink plaque with scale, erosion.
    - The true extent of the lesion is usually greater than the clinical appearance.
    - High incidence of recurrence or incomplete excision due to "fingerlike" extensions.
    - Margins of 1 cm or Mohs surgery is warranted.

- Pigmented BCC: similar to nodular BCC; easily confused with melanoma due to its deep pigmentation and nodularity.
- Adnexal BCC
  - Uncommon and found in older individuals.
  - Tumors arise from sweat glands, and although they exhibit slow growth, they are locally invasive, with a high incidence of local recurrence.

TREATMENT OF BCC

- **Standard Surgical Techniques:** ≈95% cure rate
  - **Wide local excision of BCC:** 3- to 5-mm margins
    - Frozen sections may be used to confirm negative margins intraoperatively. False negatives are common. Surgeon must have confidence in pathologist/laboratory.
  - **Mohs surgery:** sequential horizontal excision with immediate frozen section testing by dedicated Mohs dermatopathologist; ~99% cure rate for primary BCC.
    - *Indications include morpheaform BCC and/or lesions in aesthetically sensitive areas (nose, eyelid, lip, etc.).
    - Advantages are tissue preservation and confirmation of complete excision.
- **Field Therapies**
  - Curettage and electrodessication can be used for superficial, low-risk BCCs.
  - Cryotherapy, PDT, topical imiquimod, or fluorouracil if poor surgical candidate.
  - Radiation is effective but requires multiple visits. High cure rates (≈90%), but recurrence is relatively common many years (10-15) later.
- **Topical Pharmaceuticals**
  - **Imiquimod:** immune stimulant. FDA approved only for superficial BCCs, with cure rates between 80% and 90%. The 5% cream is applied 5 times per week for 6 weeks or longer.
  - **5-Fluorouracil (5-FU):** chemotherapy. FDA approved for superficial BCCs, with similar cure rates to imiquimod. Five percent liquid or ointment is rubbed onto the tumor 2 times per day for 3-6 weeks.
- **Adjuvant Radiation Therapy** (after surgery): useful for advanced, deeply invasive BCC
- **Metastatic Disease:** rare, can treat with SMO inhibitors (vismodegib or sonidegib)

SQUAMOUS CELL CARCINOMA

EPIDEMIOLOGY

- **Incidence**
  - Second most common skin cancer after BCC
  - Roughly 1.8 million new cases annually in the United States
- **Risk Factors**
  - UV exposure (eg, PUVA) or ionizing radiation, fair skin, chemical exposure (eg, arsenic), immunosuppression (transplant, HIV), viral infection (HPV, HSV), Marjolin ulcer: SCC arising in a chronic wound (ie, chronic burn scars and pressure sores) secondary to genetic changes caused by chronic inflammation
  - Syndromes: xeroderma pigmentosum, oculocutaneous albinism, dystrophic EB

SCC DISEASE BIOLOGY AND CHARACTERISTICS

- **Precursor Lesions**
  - **Actinic keratoses** (AKs, or solar keratoses)—risk of malignant transformation is ~10%.
    - Erythematous macules and papules with coarse, adherent scale.
    - Histologically resembles SCC *in situ* (premalignant).
  - **Bowen disease** (SCC *in situ*)
    - Exhibits full-thickness cytologic atypia of the keratinocytes.
    - Erythroplasia of Queyrat is SCC *in situ* of the glans penis.

- Leukoplakia: white patch on oral or other mucosa; malignant transformation in 15%.
- Keratoacanthoma: resembles SCC, rapid growth followed by involution.
- **Types of SCC**
  - **Verrucous carcinoma (well-differentiated SCC):** slow-growing; exophytic; less likely to metastasize; found on plantar feet, genitalia or in oral cavity.
  - **Ulcerative SCC:** grows rapidly and is locally invasive.
    - Ulcerative SCC has very aggressive growth characteristics, raised borders, and central ulceration.
    - Around <50% 5-year survival if spread to lymph nodes in the head and neck.
  - **Marjolin ulcer:** arises within chronic wound or scar (burn, ulcer or fistula tracks).

SCC TREATMENT OPTIONS

- **Standard Surgical Techniques:** 90%-95% cure rates; similar to BCC options
  - **Wide local excision of SCC: 4- to 6-mm margins are usually sufficient.** Frozen sections may be used to confirm negative margins intraoperatively.
    - If <2 cm, low grade and extends to dermis, 4-mm margin
    - If >2 cm, grade 2-4, high risk or extension into fat, 6-mm margin
  - **Mohs surgery:** sequential horizontal excision with frozen section testing. Highest cure rate for SCC: ~97%
    - Indications include recurrent, high-risk SCC, and/or lesions in aesthetically sensitive areas (nose, eyelid, lip, etc.).
    - Advantages are tissue preservation and confirmation of complete excision.
- **Field Therapies**
  - **Curettage, electrodessication, and cryotherapy** are less used SCC treatment than in BCC due to risk of missed deep tumor portions and scarring obscuring SCC recurrences.
  - **Radiation** is reserved for unresectable lesions or for the very elderly. Cure rates vary widely. Must consider cosmetic damage and long-term risks.
- **Management of Nodal Disease**
  - **SLN biopsy:** considered for high-risk SCC without palpable nodes (controversial).
  - **Aggressive resection** indicated for histologically positive (palpable) lymph nodes.
- **Adjuvant Radiation Therapy:** postexcision for high-risk cutaneous SCC or if positive nodes
- **Chemotherapy:** cisplatin alone or combined with 5-FU or EGFR inhibitors
- **Immunotherapies:** cemiplimab (PD-1 inhibitor) FDA approved for metastatic SCC

MELANOMA

EPIDEMIOLOGY

- **Incidence is increasing,** faster than any other cancer in Western world.
  - A total of 106 000 new cases diagnosed in the United States in 2021; annual increase ~3%-7%.
  - Less than 1% of all skin cancers, but cause majority of skin cancer-related deaths.
  - Prognosis of metastatic disease has doubled since 2004 given treatment advancements.
  - Five-year risk of developing a second melanoma following primary is 8%.
  - Median age of diagnosis is 65.
- **Risk Factors:** genetics, personal or family history of melanoma, **history of UV exposure** (both UVA and UVB), indoor tanning, blistering burns, fair skin (Fitzpatrick I and II) (**Table 7-1**) and red hair, large number nevi and/or lentigines, immunosuppression.
- **Race:** incidence is lower, but prognosis is worse for African-Americans, due to delayed diagnosis and/or worse disease subtype.

TABLE 7-1 Fitzpatrick Classification of Skin Type

Skin type	Unexposed areas	Tanning history
I	Pale/milky white	Always burn, never tan
II	Very light brown, freckles	Always burn, minimal tan
III	White to olive	Minimal burn, gradual tan
IV	Light brown	Minimal burn, tans well
V	Brown	Rarely burn, profuse tan
VI	Dark brown to black	Never burn, deep tan

Section I: General

- **Family History:** vast majority of melanomas are sporadic; however, some hereditary forms exist (see also Genetics section below).
  - **Familial atypical multiple mole and melanoma (FAMMM) syndrome:** patients have a first- or second-degree relative with malignant melanoma and typically have at least 50 melanocytic nevi. Mutations in CDKN2A/CDK4. Two or more cases of melanoma in first-degree relatives may indicate familial melanoma, autosomal-dominant transference with variable penetrance.
  - **Xeroderma pigmentosum** (XP)
    - Heterogeneous group of syndromes, mutations in various DNA repair genes.
    - UV-induced DNA damage leads to early death secondary to metastasis.
    - Typically presents in childhood with multiple BCCs, SCCs, and melanomas.
    - Restriction from sunlight exposure is mandatory, with aggressive surveillance/treatment of skin lesions.

MELANOMA DISEASE BIOLOGY AND CHARACTERISTICS

- **Precursor Lesions**
  - Melanoma is caused by multiple processes leading to malignant transformation of melanocytes.
  - **Congenital melanocytic nevi**
    - Malignant potential correlates with size.
    - Giant congenital nevi (>40-60 cm): confer an ~6% risk of melanoma; prophylactic excision (often serially) is recommended.
  - **Common acquired nevi**
    - Arise in childhood, adolescence and slowly regress in later years.
    - The greater the number of nevi, the greater the chance of melanoma.
  - **Dysplastic or atypical nevi**
    - Often appear in puberty in sun-exposed areas.
    - Thought to confer as high as 32× increased risk of melanoma.
  - **Melanoma *in situ*/atypical junctional melanocytic hyperplasia (AJMH)/lentigo maligna**
    - No penetration of atypical cells beyond epidermal junction.
    - May arise within dysplastic nevi.
    - Full excision with 0.5-1.0 cm margins (see Table 7-3).
- **Genetic Mechanisms**
  - *p16/CDKN2A* gene: tumor suppressor gene that is mutated or deleted in the majority of melanoma cell lines; mutations found in some familial melanomas.
  - *CDK4* gene: cell cycle regulator–like CDKN2A; plays a role in melanoma progression in a small proportion of familial and sporadic melanomas.
  - *MCR1*: strong association with *BRAF*-mutant melanomas.

- ○ *MIT4*: missense mutation associated with melanoma and renal cell cancer.
- ○ *BAP1*: AD mutation associated with mesothelioma, melanoma, and renal cell carcinoma.
- **Classification of Melanoma Types**
  - ○ **Superficial spreading melanoma**
    - ▪ Most common type, ~60%-70% cases; affects both genders equally.
    - ▪ Upper back in men and lower legs in women are most common sites.
    - ▪ Irregular borders with color variegation; regression commonly observed.
    - ▪ Radial growth phase early, vertical growth phase late.
  - ○ **Nodular melanoma**
    - ▪ Second most common: ~15%-30% cases.
    - ▪ Most aggressive type; tend to be diagnosed at advanced stage with poorer prognosis.
    - ▪ More common in men than in women; less clear association with sunlight exposure.
    - ▪ Typically blue-black, can ulcerate and develop rapidly.
    - ▪ Vertical growth phase is a hallmark feature; no radial growth.
  - ○ **Lentigo maligna melanoma (LMM)**
    - ▪ Approximately 10% of cutaneous melanomas.
    - ▪ Least aggressive type; ~5% progress to invasive melanoma.
    - ▪ Most clearly associated with sunlight/UV exposure.
    - ▪ Head, neck, and arms of elderly (sun-exposed areas).
    - ▪ Usually >3 cm in diameter; irregular, asymmetric with color variegation.
    - ▪ **Melanoma precursor lesion is lentigo maligna** (histologically equivalent to melanoma *in situ*, or AJMH): radial growth phase only. Transition to vertical growth phase marks development of LMM.
  - ○ **Acral lentiginous melanoma**
    - ▪ Around 2%-8% of melanomas in Caucasians, 35%-60% of melanomas in African-Americans, Hispanics, and Asians.
    - ▪ ***Presents in palms, soles, and beneath nail plate (subungual); most common site is great toe or thumb.**
    - ▪ Must distinguish from melanonychia, a benign, linear, pigmented streak in the nail, common in African and Asian populations. Due to the risk of melanoma, biopsy of suspect lesions should be performed.
    - ▪ Irregular pigmentation, large size (>3 cm) common.
    - ▪ Long radial growth phase, transition to vertical growth phase occurs with high risk of metastasis.
- **Noncutaneous Melanoma**
  - ○ **Mucosal melanoma**
    - ▪ Mucosal melanomas represent ~1% of melanomas, most commonly presenting within the genital tract, anorectal region, and head and neck mucosal surfaces.
    - ▪ Difficult to detect; typically advanced at the time of diagnosis with poor prognosis.
    - ▪ Excision is best for prognosis, but difficult given anatomy and growth patterns.
  - ○ **Ocular melanoma** (choroid ≫ ciliary body > iris)
    - ▪ Represent ~5% of melanomas (most commonly noncutaneous melanoma).
    - ▪ Interference with vision leads to earlier diagnosis.
    - ▪ Melanomas of iris are like cutaneous melanomas in genetics/behavior; melanomas of the posterior uvea act more like mucosal melanomas and have a worse prognosis.
    - ▪ The eye has no lymphatic drainage; therefore, no nodal metastasis is seen.
    - ▪ The liver is the main site of metastatic disease.
    - ▪ Treatment is by resection, radiation therapy, and enucleation.

- **Melanoma With an Unknown Primary**
  - ○ Represent 3% of melanomas; diagnosis of exclusion.
  - ○ Nodal metastases are the most common presentation.
  - ○ Prognosis similar to metastatic melanomas with a known primary.

DIAGNOSIS AND STAGING OF MELANOMA

- **Physical examination** is 75%-90% sensitive for diagnosing melanoma. Serial photograph monitoring and use of dermoscopy significantly enhance diagnostic sensitivity.
- **Common clinical features** of melanoma lesions (ABCDE)
  - ○ Asymmetry
  - ○ Border irregularity
  - ○ Color variation
  - ○ Diameter >5 mm
  - ○ Enlarging/evolving lesion
- **Diagnosis of primary melanoma** is made by histologic analysis of full-thickness biopsy specimens.
  - ○ **Full-thickness excisional biopsy** is preferred for lesions <1.5 cm in diameter. If possible, excise lesion with 1- to 3-mm margins. Partial thickness acceptable for face or acral sites.
  - ○ **Avoid shave biopsies,** since they forfeit the ability to stage the lesion based on thickness.
  - ○ **Incisional biopsy** is controversial; excisional biopsy preferred.
  - ○ **Permanent sectioning** is used to determine tumor thickness (Breslow depth).
  - ○ **Do not cauterize or freeze** the specimen: tissue destruction makes it impossible to evaluate thickness and margins.
  - ○ **Wide local excision** for tissue diagnosis can disrupt and decrease efficacy of future lymphatic mapping. Biopsy scars should be parallel to lymphatic drainage.
  - ○ **Orientation of biopsy** incisions should also consider definitive surgical therapy.
    - ▪ Longitudinal biopsies on extremities; transverse over joints to prevent contractures.
    - ▪ Place head and neck incisions along relaxed skin tension lines, keeping facial aesthetic units in mind.
- **Major Prognostic Factors:** Tumor thickness, Nodal status, and Metastases—TNM
  - ○ *Breslow depth (mm) is a more accurate and better prognostic indicator than Clark level (invasion through histologic skin layers) (see Table 7-2).
- **Other Significant Prognostic Factors**
  - ○ **Anatomic location:** trunk, head, and neck lesions generally carry worse prognosis than those on the extremities.
  - ○ **Sex:** for a given melanoma, women generally have a better prognosis if localized.
  - ○ **Ulceration** and increased **mitotic rate** are poor prognostic signs.
  - ○ **Lymph node involvement** or in-transit metastases are more significant than any other prognostic factors; for stage IV disease, visceral distant metastases have poorer prognosis.
- The American Joint Committee on Cancer has developed a staging system based on TNM classification.

TABLE 7-2 Melanoma Thickness Grading

Breslow depth (mm)	5-y survival (%)
≤0.5	97
>0.5 to ≤0.75	92
0.75 to ≤1.0	71

MELANOMA TREATMENT

- **Definitive Management of Melanoma**
  - ○ Wide local excision is the treatment of choice.
  - ○ Recommended surgical margins depend on tumor thickness (**Table 7-3**).
  - ○ Subungual melanoma requires amputation proximal to the DIPJ for fingers and proximal to IP joint for the thumb.
- **Management of Regional Lymph Nodes**
  - ○ **Elective lymph node dissection (ELND)** involves removal of clinically negative lymph nodes from the nodal basin. No prospective survival benefit seen except for a subgroup with 1- to 2-mm (intermediate thickness) melanomas.
  - ○ **Sentinel lymph node biopsy (SLNB)**
    - ▪ SLN hypothesis: tumor cells migrate to first node receiving lymphatic drainage from primary tumor; thus, excision of the sentinel node alone is adequate for nodal status.
    - ▪ Sentinel node(s) can be detected in >90%-95% of patients. **SLNB is widely considered the standard of care.** Dependent on Breslow thickness, ulceration, and presence of satellites (**Table 7-4**).
    - ▪ SLNB is performed in conjunction with WLE of the primary tumor. Lymphatic mapping is performed to determine the first lymph node that drains the primary tumor site (sentinel node).
    - ▪ On the day of or prior to surgery, preoperative nuclear imaging is performed with radiolabeled sulfur colloid solution (technetium-99) injected intradermally at the primary tumor. Lymphoscintigraphic imaging localizes the sentinel node basin(s) (some tumor sites can drain to multiple basins).
    - ▪ In the operating room, a lymphangiography dye (eg, methylene blue) can be injected intradermally at periphery of primary tumor site prior to excision.
      - ▫ Mark edges of the lesion before injection to avoid obscuration with dye.
      - ▫ Potential sentinel nodes will appear blue when exploring the nodal basin, giving secondary confirmation to localization of ^{99}Tc with gamma detection probe.
      - ▫ Dye injection may briefly interfere with pulse-oximeter readings; alert anesthesiologist at the time of injection.
      - ▫ Caution: risk of allergy or anaphylaxis with dye injection.
    - ▪ Following primary tumor excision, drapes, instruments, gowns, and gloves are changed and regional lymph nodes identified by lymphoscintigraphy are explored. Nodes demonstrating maximal counts with gamma detection probe are excised.
    - ▪ Histologic analysis of sentinel node with immunohistochemical staining identifies micrometastases. Permanent sections are required; frozen sections cannot reliably differentiate normal from neoplastic melanocytes.
- **Surveillance and Treatment of Melanoma Recurrence**
  - ○ **Asymptomatic patients** should be seen every 3-6 months with clinical lymph node exam (depending on pathological stage) for 2 years, then annually. All patients should be educated on and should receive thorough review of symptoms.

TABLE 7-3 Recommended Surgical Margins for Melanoma Excision

Melanoma thickness (mm)	Margin (cm)
In situ	0.5-1
≤1 mm (T1)	1
1-2 (T2)	1-2
>2 (T3-T4)	2

TABLE 7-4 Indication for Sentinel Lymph Node Biopsy for Melanoma

Breslow thickness	Ulceration	Satellites	SLNB recommendation
N/A	Absent/present	N/A	Not recommended
<0.8 mm	Absent	Not detected	Presence of adverse features? Absent → not recommended Present → discuss and consider
<0.8 mm	Present	Not detected	Discuss and consider
0.8-1.0 mm	Absent/present	Not detected	Discuss and consider
>1.0-2.0 mm	Absent	Not detected	Discuss and offer
>1.0-2.0 mm	Present	Not detected	Discuss and offer
>2.0-4.0 mm	Absent	Not detected	Discuss and offer
>2.0-4.0 mm	Present	Not detected	Discuss and offer
>4.0 mm	Absent	Not detected	Discuss and offer
>4.0 mm	Present	Not detected	Discuss and offer
≤4.0 mm	Absent/present	Microscopic	Discuss and offer
>4.0 mm	Absent/present	Microscopic	Discuss and offer

- ○ Imaging surveillance: CT of chest, abdomen, and pelvis considered for stage IIB and higher and regional nodal US every 4 months for positive SLNB without CLND; CLND does not offer survival benefit (MLST-2 trial). PET-CT for in-transit/satellite metastases.
- ○ Local recurrence: defined as regrowth within 2 cm of surgical scar; incidence 3%-5%; usually due to incomplete excision of primary or hematogenous dissemination. Resection is treatment of choice. Offered imaging, lymphatic mapping, and SLNB. Aggressive therapy warranted as local recurrences can indicate disseminated disease.
- ○ In-transit metastases: >2 cm from primary but not beyond regional nodal basin, presumed due to lymphatic spread. Imaging, SLNB, and systemic therapy typically warranted. Resection considered for limited disease.
- ○ Radiation therapy: can treat portions of unresectable metastases to brain or bone.
- ○ Cytokine therapy: interferon-α (IFN-α) and interleukin-2 (IL-2) produce tumor response, albeit transient. Little or no improvement in overall survival.
- ○ Immunotherapies: checkpoint inhibitors (nivolumab, pembrolizumab, ipilimumab) have largely replaced cytokine therapy and prolong life in nearly half of all patients.
- ○ Targeted therapy: melanomas that harbor BRAF mutations treated with BRAF inhibitors (dabrafenib, encorafenib, vemurafenib) or MEK inhibitors (trametinib, cobimetinib, binimetinib) or in combination and extend overall survival.
- ○ Chemotherapy: less effective than immunotherapy or targeted therapy, not used as initial treatment in advanced disease. Dacarbazine (DTIC), carmustine, cisplatin, and tamoxifen in combination are most frequently used.

LESS COMMON SKIN CANCERS

- • Merkel Cell Carcinoma (MCC)
  - ○ Rare, malignant neuroendocrine tumor arises from cells of neural crest origin in dermis.

- Incidence increasing; 2000 cases per year in the United States; 70% survival at 5 years.
- Risk factors include median age 75-80; UV exposure; fair skin; immunosuppression.
- Merkel cell polyomavirus implicated in 80% of MCC cases; positive prognostic factor.
- Pink to red-brown, firm, subcutaneous nodule; 50% involve the head and neck.
- Has very aggressive, radial spread, high local recurrence, regional, and systemic metastasis.
- Treatment: WLE with up to 3 cm margins; SLN biopsy with dissection in select patients.
- Advanced disease: adjuvant radiation, avelumab (PD-L1 inhibitor) and pembrolizumab (PD-1 inhibitor) are both FDA approved.
- **Microcystic Adnexal Carcinoma**
  - Slow-growing firm, flesh-colored to yellow nodule primarily on the head and neck.
  - Pathophysiology debated; favor dual follicular and eccrine differentiation.
  - Tumor is invasive and locally destructive; treat with Mohs or standard excision.
- **Sebaceous Gland Carcinoma**
  - Malignant tumor derived from adnexal epithelium of sebaceous glands.
  - Most are periocular; sebaceous gland carcinomas elsewhere are rare.
  - Yellowish to pink, slowly growing papulonodule on eyelid (resembles chalazion).

SOFT TISSUE SARCOMAS

EPIDEMIOLOGY

- Approximately 13 000 new cases diagnosed annually in the United States.
- Approximately 1% of all malignancies in adults and 15% of those in children.
- Approximately 50% are located on the extremities.
- Risk Factors
  - The majority of sarcomas have no clearly defined environmental or genetic etiology.
  - **Radiation exposure**
    - Associated with osteosarcomas and malignant fibrous histiocytomas.
    - Typically, there is a 10- to 20-year latency period after exposure.
    - Thorium dioxide (Thorotrast): contrast agent used in 1940-1950s for radiologic procedures; linked with a high incidence of hepatic angiosarcoma.
  - **Chemical exposure:** arsenic, vinyl chloride, and dioxin (found in Agent Orange).
  - **Genetic factors**
    - Type 1 neurofibromatosis: benign neurofibromas can undergo malignant change to malignant peripheral nerve sheath tumors
    - Mutation in *Rb1* tumor suppressor gene: retinoblastoma (sarcoma of the eye)
    - Mutation in *p53* tumor suppressor gene: Li-Fraumeni syndrome (variety of sarcomas)
  - **Lymphedema or chronic irritation**
    - Surgical procedures, radiation therapy, parasitic infection, idiopathic
    - 10- to 20-year latency for the development of lymphangiosarcoma
  - **Kaposi sarcoma:** strongly associated with HIV infection and HHV8

DIAGNOSIS

- Paucity of local symptoms often leads to advanced disease at diagnosis.
- Tumors grow along tissue planes; compress nearby normal tissue leading to pseudocapsule.
- Most commonly spread hematogenously depending on histology.
- **Extremity Sarcoma:** generally painless. Delay in diagnosis is common and patients are often erroneously treated for a hematoma or "pulled muscle."

o Suspicious findings include mass >5 cm, enlarging or symptomatic mass, mass present for >4 weeks, or recurrence after removal.

o MRI is the preferred imaging modality.

o Pulmonary metastases are the most common location for metastatic disease.

o Around 65% 5-year survival rate for all forms of soft tissue sarcoma.

• **Sarcoma of the Abdomen or Retroperitoneum**

o Can present with vague abdominal complaints (early satiety, pain, obstruction).

o Metastatic disease: most commonly to lungs.

o Palpable mass in 80% of patients at the time of presentation.

o Imaging: CT is the preferred diagnostic tool to evaluate primary site and rule out metastasis to lungs, liver, or peritoneum. MRI may be helpful for disease in pelvis.

o Biopsy: low threshold for percutaneous core needle biopsy if diagnosis in doubt.

CLASSIFICATION AND STAGING

• Subtypes are named for the cell of origin (**Table 7-5**). Undifferentiated pleomorphic sarcoma, liposarcoma, and leiomyosarcoma are the most common sarcomas in adults and rhabdomyosarcoma is the most common in children.

• Histologic type has little prognostic significance; histologic grade (including frequency of mitotic aures, cellular atypia, and presence or absence of tumor necrosis) is the best for prognosis and therapy.

• **Staging Criteria**

o **Histologic grade is the most important prognostic factor:** indicator of malignancy and distant metastases and death, but poor predictor of local recurrence.

o Tumor size: risk of local recurrence and distance metastases increase with tumor size.

o Nodal and distant metastases are associated with poor prognosis. Classified as stage III in retroperitoneum and stage IV on trunk and extremities.

• **Imaging**: various techniques used to define etiology and determine extent for surgical planning including X-ray, CT, MRI, and PET-CT.

SARCOMA MANAGEMENT

• **Extremities** (especially the thighs) are the most common sites for sarcoma.

o **Surgery**

▪ Complete resection while avoiding tumor plane violation is the mainstay of treatment.

▪ WLE is the standard of care, with **3- to 5-cm margins** of normal tissue proximally and distally. En bloc resection of uninvolved fascial plane with tumor is performed for control of the other margins.

▪ WLE is performed after excisional biopsy even if the margins are clear.

▪ Major neurovascular structures are generally preserved for low-grade lesions but are sacrificed and reconstructed as needed for high-grade tumors.

▪ There is no survival benefit of amputation compared to limb-sparing procedure.

TABLE 7-5 Tissue Classification of Soft Tissue Sarcomas

Tissue of origin	Benign soft tissue tumor	Malignant soft tissue tumor
Fat	Lipoma	Liposarcoma
Fibrous tissue	Fibroma	Fibrosarcoma
Smooth muscle	Leiomyoma	Leiomyosarcoma
Skeletal muscle	Rhabdomyoma	Rhabdomyosarcoma
Cartilage	Chondroma	Chondrosarcoma
Bone	Osteoma	Osteosarcoma
Blood vessel	Hemangioma	Angiosarcoma

○ **Radiation therapy** is not indicated for small (<5 cm) low-grade tumors due to excellent prognosis with WLE alone. It can be used as primary therapy for patients who cannot tolerate or refuse surgery; also useful as combination therapy for sarcomas up to 10 cm.
○ **Chemotherapy** is of undetermined benefit in soft tissue sarcoma.
• **Retroperitoneal and intra-abdominal sarcomas** have a uniformly poor prognosis. Excision with tumor-free margins is curative but difficult to achieve. Radiation is rarely used because surrounding organs cannot tolerate therapeutic doses.

PEARLS

1. Skin and soft tissue neoplasms are derived from a myriad of skin components and are the most common cancers of the body. Treatment depends on patient characteristics and outcome.
2. Changing, symptomatic skin lesions are suspicious for malignancy, warranting biopsy.
3. Perform full-thickness biopsies of pigmented lesions (ie, excisional) rather than shave biopsy or curettage so the depth of the lesion can be determined if it is a melanoma.
4. Excision is appropriate when definitive pathology and/or margins are required.
5. Design excisions as ellipses with sharp corners to facilitate closure and avoid if dog ears.

QUESTIONS YOU WILL BE ASKED

1. Should you undermine the wound arising from excision of a suspected malignant skin lesion to facilitate wound closure?
   No. It will permit the spread of malignancy.
2. A 35-year-old breast augmentation patient also mentions a 5-mm, nonhealing wound on the face that has been present for 2 months. What do you recommend?
   Immediate biopsy.
3. What is the risk of malignant transformation of an actinic keratosis, and what type of skin cancer can it progress to?
   Rates of AK progression to SCC are ~0.6 percent at 1 year and 2.6% at 4 years. Of SCCs, 75% considered invasive and the remainder were *in situ*.
4. What is the most common location of dermoid cysts?
   Periocular region.
5. What malignancy can Spitz nevi appear histologically similar to?
   Melanoma.

Recommended Readings
1. Apalla Z, Nashan D, Weller RB, et al. Skin cancer: epidemiology, disease burden, pathophysiology, diagnosis, and therapeutic approaches. *Dermatol Ther.* 2017;7:5-19.
2. Keung EZ, Gershenwald JE. The eighth edition American Joint Committee on Cancer (AJCC) melanoma staging system: implications for melanoma treatment and care. *Expert Rev Anticancer Ther.* 2018;18:775-784.
3. Lee EH, Nehal KS, Disa JJ. Benign and premalignant skin lesions. *Plast Reconstr Surg.* 2010;125:188e-198e.
4. Netscher DT, Leong M, Orengo I, et al. Cutaneous malignancies: melanoma and nonmelanoma types. *Plast Reconstr Surg.* 2011;127:37E.
5. Rogers-Vizena CR, Lalonde DH, Menick FJ, et al. Surgical treatment and reconstruction of nonmelanoma facial skin cancers. *Plast Reconstr Surg.* 2015;135:895e-908e.

8 Lymphedema and Vascular Anomalies

Geoffrey E. Hespe

LYMPHEDEMA

THE LYMPHATIC SYSTEM

- Structure
  - Made up of superficial (capillary) and deep (collecting) lymphatic vessel networks connecting to lymphoid organs, which direct lymph fluid in a unidirectional flow back to the venous system
    - Superficial lymphatics are open-ended, single-layer thick, valveless vessels, which absorb interstitial fluid and macromolecules.
    - Deep lymphatics contain valves and are surrounded by smooth muscle cells, which allow for propulsion of lymph fluid unidirectionally.
    - The thoracic duct is the main collecting lymphatic vessel for the majority of the body except the right upper extremity, right head and neck, and right hemithorax.
      - The terminal end of the thoracic duct can have varying anatomy and can anastomose to the internal jugular vein, left subclavian artery, or the junction of the two.
    - The right lymphatic duct drains the right upper extremity, right head and neck, and right hemithorax, and terminates typically at the junction of the right internal jugular and right subclavian veins.
  - Found in all tissues except cornea, retina and bone marrow
    - Ongoing research has recently identified lymphatics in bone, brain and spinal cord, tissues traditionally thought to be void of lymphatics
- Function
  - Collects and transports interstitial fluid back to the vascular system
  - Participates in the immune response by trafficking antigens and immune cells to lymphoid organs
  - Transports fats, lipids, and chylomicrons from the GI tract to the circulatory system

LYMPHEDEMA

- Definition: end-organ dysfunction of the lymphatic system that leads to stasis of protein-rich lymph fluid in the interstitium leading to edema, adipose deposition, and fibrosis.
- Most common cause of lymphedema in developing countries is from **filariasis**, a parasitic infection of *Wuchereria bancrofti*; in developed countries, it is secondary to cancer therapy.
- Affects ~250 million people worldwide.
  - Primary vs secondary
    - **Primary lymphedema:** developmental abnormality in lymphatic vessels with variable penetrance and severity of disease
      - **Congenital lymphedema (10%-25%):**
        - Usually present at birth
        - More commonly seen in females

---

*Denotes common in-service examination topics.

- Affects lower extremities > upper extremities; **typically** bilateral lower extremity lymphedema
- **Milroy disease** (hereditary lymphedema type I): ~2% of all congenital lymphedemas; sex-linked genetic mutation in vascular endothelial factor receptor-3 (VEGFR-3)
  - Results in malformation and agenesis of lymphatic vessels resulting in lymphedema, steatorrhea, and defective cell-mediated immune system
- □ Hereditary lymphedema type II (**lymphedema praecox, Meige disease;** 80%): typically **unilateral lower extremity** lymphedema due to fewer and small lymphatic vessels
  - Most common form of primary lymphedema
  - *Develops between birth and age 35; typically around puberty
  - More common in females 4:1
- □ **Lymphedema tarda** (<10%): lymphedema that develops after the age of 35 usually in lower extremities secondary to hypoplastic lymphatic vessels without valves
- **Secondary lymphedema:** result of damage and/or mechanical obstruction of lymphatic vessels
  - □ *Filariasis: most common cause of secondary lymphedema worldwide (120 million people worldwide)
    - Caused by parasitic roundworm *W bancrofti*, which obstructs lymphatic vessels
    - Typically affects the lower extremity or genitalia
    - Endemic to India, Indonesia, Bangladesh, and Nigeria
    - Treatment: ivermectin
  - □ Cancer treatment
    - Postmastectomy lymphedema
      - Affects ~4%-40% of women
      - Increased risk in patients who receive axillary lymph node dissection (ALND), receive radiation therapy, and/or are obese
      - Decreasing incidence due to increase in prevalence of sentinel lymph node dissection (approximately 5% risk)
      - Presents as persistent swelling, pain, and at increased risk of infection
- **Location**
  - ○ Lower extremities (90%)
  - ○ Upper extremities (10%)
    - Occurs in ~14%-49% of women after mastectomy with ALND
    - 8-10× increased risk of lymphedema in women after axillary node dissection and radiation
  - ○ Genitalia (<1%)
- **Pathophysiology**
  - ○ Remains poorly understood.
  - ○ Studies have demonstrated that it is likely due to fibrosis of lymphatic vessels secondary to chronic inflammation.
    - CD4+ T cells and macrophages have been shown to play a role in lymphedema.
  - ○ Leads to chronic lymphedema, which is characterized by soft tissue fibrosis and adipose tissue deposition secondary to chronic inflammation and sclerosis of lymphatic vessels.
- **Risk Factors**
  - ○ Obesity (>30 BMI; 3.6× increased risk)
  - ○ Radiation (2-4.5× increased risk)
  - ○ Infection
  - ○ Genetics

DIAGNOSIS

- **History and physical examination**
  - Family history of lymphedema
  - Comorbidities (eg, heart failure, venous stasis, renal dysfunction)
  - Recent surgery or trauma
  - Foreign travel: concern for *W bancrofti* infection (filariasis)
  - Malnutrition
  - Symptoms: limb swelling, extremity heaviness, skin tightness, skin infections
  - Examination
    - Nonpitting edema that usually affects hands/feet.
    - Usually not painful.
    - Minimal pigment change or ulceration.
    - Often unilateral (can measure limb circumference to document progression of disease).
    - Fluid protein content is 1-5 g/dL.
    - *Positive Stemmer sign: inability to grasp the skin of the second toe or finger due to thickening of the subcutaneous tissues.
- Limb circumference/volume changes: measure at standardized intervals between limbs, and a difference of 2 cm in circumference or volume difference of 200 mL is significant.
  - Prone to discrepency due to user variation in measurements
- Bioimpedance spectroscopy: noninvasive method used to measure fluid content of a limb by measuring electrical current transmission through tissues.
- **Lymphoscintigraphy (gold standard):** injection of radiolabeled colloid into distal effected limb to evaluate uptake at draining lymph node.
  - Sensitivity: 96%; specificity: 100%
- MR lymphangiography: uses gadolinium-based contrast agents injected into web spaces to help specifically visualize lymphatic vessels.
- CT/US: used to evaluate thickness of skin/subcutaneous tissues and appearance of fluid stasis and rule out other causes for limb asymmetry (eg, deep venous thrombosis, venous stasis).
- Indocyanine Green (ICG) Lymphography: ICG is injected into the interdigital webspaces and a near-infrared camera is used to visual lymphatic vessels.

DIFFERENTIAL DIAGNOSIS

- Venous insufficiency.
- Lipedema: excessive deposition of adipose tissue typically in the extremities sparing the hands and feet; affects females > males; can have a normal BMI.
- Obesity-induced lymphedema: bilateral lower extremity typically in patients with BMI > 40; mainstay treatment is weight loss.
- Myxedema: swelling of skin and soft tissue secondary to deposition of mucopolysaccharides in severe hypothyroidism.

STAGING

- Multiple classification schemes have been described:
  - International Society of Lymphology, Koshima, MD Anderson, Cheng Classification System (**Table 8-1**)

COMPLICATIONS

- Cellulitis
  - Can be severe so prompt antibiotic therapy is key
  - Patients with more than three episodes of cellulitis, consider prophylactic antibiotics
- Hyperkeratosis
- Lymphangiosarcoma: <1% incidence but biopsy any suspicious lesions in the setting of lymphedema
- Decreased patient quality of life

TABLE 8-1 Lymphedema Staging Classifications

| | | Staging system | | |
Stage	International Society of Lymphology	Koshima et al. Staging System for Lymphedema	M.D. Anderson Classification Based on ICG	Cheng Lymphedema Grading Scale
0	Subclinical lymphedema; may have complaint of extremity heaviness	Normal type: normal lymphatic vessels and function		Reversible with <10% arm circumference difference with partial occlusion on lymphoscintigraphy
1	Pitting edema due to accumulation of protein-rich fluid; completely resolves with elevation; no fibrosis	Ectasia type: increase in endolymph pressure leading to lymphatic vessel dilation	Numerous patent lymphatic vessels with minimal areas of dermal backflow	Mild symptoms with 10%-19% arm circumference difference with partial occlusion on lymphoscintigraphy
2	Nonpitting edema that does not respond to elevation; presence of fibrosis	Contraction type: thickening of the lymphatic vessel wall due to smooth muscle cell proliferation	Moderate patent lymphatic vessels with dermal backflow in a segmental distribution	Moderate symptoms with 20%-29% circumference difference with total occlusion on lymphoscintigraphy
3	Elephantiasis with significant fibrosis and skin changes (eg, hyperkeratosis)	Sclerosis type: narrowing of the lymphatic vessel due to fibrosis leading to inability to transport lymphatic fluid	Few patent lymphatic vessels with dermal backflow that is extensive and involves the entire arm	Severe symptoms with 30%-39% circumference difference with total occlusion on lymphoscintigraphy
4			No evidence of patent lymphatic vessels with extensive dermal backflow that now involves the entire arm and dorsum of the hand	Very severe symptoms with >40% circumference difference and total occlusion on lymphoscintigraphy

TREATMENT

- **Non-surgical Management**
  - ○ Elevation of the extremity and proper skin hygiene to decrease risk of infection
    - Use low pH solutions and water-based products to keep skin clean and daily moisturizers.
    - Avoid skin damage.
    - Treat any dermatologic conditions as they arise.
  - ○ **Complete decongestive therapy:** key component of lymphedema management
    - Multimodality approach overseen by certified lymphedema therapist
      - □ Involves education, skin care, manual lymphatic drainage, multilayered short stretch bandages, specialized exercises
      - □ Divided into two phases
        - Phase I: decongestion—employing the above components to achieve maximal volume reduction usually with daily therapy
        - Phase II: maintenance—continued manual lymphatic drainage, exercises, skin care, and compression to maintain improvement
      - □ Can result in reduction of extremity volume by 25%-60%
      - □ Need compression >20 mm Hg
  - ○ Intermittent pneumatic compression: inflatable device in which the extremity is placed in and is filled with air to compress the extremity
  - ○ Exercise: important component to increase muscle strength, increase lymph movement, and increase joint mobility
- **Surgical Management:** Physiologic vs Excisional
  - ○ Indications: loss of function, frequent infections, failure of conservative/nonsurgical management, significant psychological burden
    - **Physiologic**
      - □ **Lymphovenous bypass (LVB)/lymphovenous anastomosis (LVA)**
        - Employs principle that lymphatics drain interstitial fluid back to the venous system via the thoracic duct
        - Utilizes supermicrosurgery to anastomose functioning lymphatic vessels to adjacent venules
      - □ **Vascularized lymph node transfer**
        - Vascularized free tissue transfer of donor lymph nodes to lymphedematous extremity.
        - Possible mechanism of actions: transplanted lymph nodes act as sump pump collecting lymph and directing into the venous system or they may result in lymphangiogenesis and reestablishing new functional lymphatic vessels.
        - Lymph node donor sites: groin, thoracic, submental, supraclavicular, and omental.
        - Complications: donor site lymphedema.
    - **Excisional**
      - □ Charles procedure: removes entire skin and soft tissue with skin grafting to cover underlying muscle
        - Rarely used due to morbidity of procedure
      - □ Wedge resection
      - □ Staged subcutaneous excision ± skin grafting
        - First line for penile/scrotal lymphedema
      - □ Liposuction: useful for later stages of lymphedema where main component is adipose deposition

VASCULAR ANOMALIES

Classification: Mulliken and Glowacki described a histology-based classification system in 1982, which was most recently updated by the International Society for the Study of

Section I: General

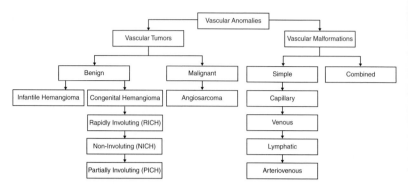

Figure 8-1 Flowchart of vascular anomalies.

Vascular Anomalies (ISSVA) in 2014 classifying vascular anomalies as **vascular tumors** and **vascular malformations (Fig. 8-1)**.

VASCULAR TUMORS

- **Infantile hemangioma (IH):** benign proliferation of endothelial cells, which is **present after birth**
  - Most common tumor of infancy
  - Incidence: 1:10 infants
    - 10% of White infants
    - 2% of Black infants
  - 3:1 female to male ratio
  - Most commonly found in the head and neck
  - Phases of growth: typically present within the first week of life followed by rapid postnatal growth switching to slow involution
    - Proliferative phase (0-12 months)
      - Rapid expansion of endothelial cells and pericytes (mostly during 6-8 months of age).
      - Vascular endothelial growth factor (VEGF) drives proliferation.
      - 80% of growth completed by 3 months.
    - Involuting phase (12 months to 10 years)
      - Progressive shrinking of lesion volume with deposition of fibrous tissue and degeneration of endothelial cells (continues to 5-10 years of age).
      - Mast cells downregulate endothelial cell turnover.
    - Involuted phase (>10 years)
      - Loose fibroadipose tissue replaces previous parenchymal tissue.
    - Dogma suggests 50% involution by age 5, 70% by age 7, and >90% by age 9; little data to support this, and likely involution starts earlier around 8-9 months with completion in most individuals by 3-5 years.
  - **Diagnosis**
    - *Primarily based on history and physical examination → lesions that are present after birth and enlarge during infancy.
    - Additional testing is not necessarily required, but MRI with contrast (gold standard) for evaluation especially if visceral hemangioma are suspected.
    - Ultrasound can be used to show shunting pattern of flow but can be difficult to distinguish hemangioma from arteriovenous malformation (AVM) due to both being high-flow lesions.

- **Congenital hemangioma**
  - **Rapidly involuting (RICH)**—similar histological appearance to IH except GLUT-1 negative; will typically involute by 1 year of age.
  - **Noninvoluting (NICH)**—similar histological appearance to IH except GLUT-1 negative; lesions grow in proportion to the child.
  - **Partially involuting (PICH)**—as the name suggests, these lesions begin as RICH but do not completely involute and become more like NICH.
- Other associated conditions with hemangiomas
  - **Spina bifida occulta**—associated with lumbar hemangioma.
  - **PHACES**—posterior fossa anomalies, hemangiomas, cardiac anomalies, eye abnormalities, sternal cleft.
  - **Kasabach-Merritt syndrome:** hemangioma + thrombocytopenia.
  - Platelet count <10 000, normal PT/PTT.
  - Diagnosis can be confirmed with MRI.
  - **von Hippel-Lindau disease:** retinal hemangiomas, hemangioblastomas of the cerebellum, visceral cysts, mental retardation.
  - **Cutaneous visceral hemangiomas:** Multiple hemangiomas (>5) should elicit concern for visceral hemangiomas.
    - Associated with: congestive heart failure, hepatomegaly (intrahepatic hemangiomas), anemia
- **Treatment**
  - **Observation** is appropriate in most cases.
    - Reassurance to parents is important.
    - Serial photographs to monitor progress.
  - Minor ulceration/bleeding can be treated with topical antibiotics ± hydrocolloid dressing to improve healing.
  - Indications for treatment
    - Bleeding/ulceration (5% cases): mostly seen in hemangiomas in the lip or anogenital areas.
    - Major ulceration, destruction, or distortion of surrounding structures, and/or obstruction of vital structures (10% cases). Most commonly occurs in the eyelid, nose, lip, and ear.
    - Eye/eyelid: Obstruction can cause deprivation amblyopia in as little as 1 week; hemangiomas can directly distort the cornea and damage vision.
    - Airway: Subglottic hemangioma can cause stridor/obstruction of the airway.
  - Nonsurgical management
    - *β-Blockers—has become the first-line treatment; effective at reducing bulk during the proliferative phase
      - Propranolol—2 mg/kg/d
      - Topical timolol—0.5% twice a day
      - Side effects: hypotension, bradycardia, hypoglycemia
        - Consider admitting patient for observation.
    - Systemic corticosteroids—historically used as first-line therapy but has fallen out of favor due to improved side effect profile of β-blockers
      - 2-3 mg/kg/d for 4-6 weeks.
      - Initial response visible after 7-10 days.
      - 85% of hemangiomas respond by regression or stabilization of growth after completion of corticosteroid therapy.
      - Side effects: **cushingoid facies**, myopathy, cardiomyopathy, premature thelarche, and hirsutism.
    - Intralesional steroid injection—alternative option with less systemic side effects
      - 1-2 mg/kg injected into the hemangioma at low pressure.
      - Care should be taken when injecting near the eye to avoid retinal artery occlusion.

- **Interferon α-2A**—alternative therapy when failed other options
  - Effective in Kasabach-Merritt syndrome.
  - 1-3 million units/m^2 injected subcutaneously daily.
  - Response seen over 6-10 months; 80% of patients demonstrate a response.
  - Side effects: fever on initiation (pretreat with acetaminophen), transaminitis, transient neutropenia, anemia, spastic diplegia (must stop immediately).
- **Vincristine**—alternative therapy when failed other options
  - >80% response rate
  - Given through central line
  - Side effects: peripheral neuropathy, sepsis, hair loss, central line complications (eg, infections, placement complications)
- **Laser therapy**—typically pulse dye lasers targeting oxyhemoglobin (585-595 nm)
  - Lightens the color of the hemangioma but does not reduce size or bulk
  - Only penetrates 0.75-1.2 mm into the dermis
  ○ **Surgical management**
  - Excision of the hemangioma
  - Indications
    - Infancy
      - Obstruction or deformation of a critical/vital structure (eg, eye, subglottic airway)
      - Bleeding/ulceration that is unresponsive to medical management
      - Easily excisable area with acceptable scar
    - Childhood (includes the above plus)
      - Excision of resultant scar from ulceration or residual fibroadipose tissue
      - Staged excision and reconstruction of large lesions
- Locally aggressive or borderline
  ○ Kaposiform hemangioepithelioma—result in **platelet consumption**; often have a lymphatic component; potential for malignant transformation
  ○ Retiform hemangioepithelioma—slow growing, low-grade vascular neoplasm that presents as singular nodule or plaque
  ○ Kaposi sarcoma—neoplasm associated with painless, purple raised, or flat lesions; associated with human herpesvirus 8
- Malignant
  ○ Angiosarcoma—typically solitary limb mass, locally recurrent

VASCULAR MALFORMATIONS

- Common features
  ○ *Vascular malformations are always present at birth, which helps distinguish from hemangiomas (are not seen at and grow after birth).
  ○ Lesions grow proportional to infant, and they do not involute.
  ○ 1:1 female:male ratio.
  ○ Vessels are inherently abnormal due to aberrant signaling pathways that determine apoptosis and proliferation pathways.
- **Diagnosis**
  ○ Clinical history and physical examination
  ○ Imaging
    - Doppler ultrasound: can differentiate high-flow vs low-flow lesions
    - **MRI with contrast:** gold standard for evaluation of vascular malformations; allows for differentiation between different forms of vascular malformations
    - Arteriography: invasive study; usually performed in conjunction with embolization

- Classification: simple vs combined
  - Simple
    - **Capillary malformation** → low-flow lesion
      - Appearance: dilated, thin-walled capillaries localized to the papillary and superficial reticular dermis.
      - Must be differentiated from other common macular stains of the face (eg, nevus flammeus).
      - The autonomic nervous system influences the development of this lesion, which is why it is often localized to distinct nerve distributions (eg, port-wine stains of the face associated with V1 nerve distribution).
      - Incidence: 0.3% of newborns. Most common location is on the face.
      - 3:1 female:male ratio.
      - **Treatment**
        - **Observation** is appropriate although important to note
          - Lesions do not regress.
          - Can progress to "cobblestone" appearance.
        - **Pulsed dye laser**
          - Typically requires multiple treatments.
          - 70%-80% of patients respond with decrease in pigmentation of the lesion.
          - More favorable results on the lateral face as compared to midface, trunk, and extremities.
        - **Surgical excision:** must be used for management of soft tissue/skeletal hypertrophy to address contour deformity
    - **Venous malformation** → low-flow lesion
      - **Appearance:** bluish, soft, compressible lesion, which swells on dependent positioning; cluster of thin-walled veins with smooth muscle surrounding, many veins lack valves.
        - Changes in hormone levels can cause enlargement.
      - **Must monitor for coagulopathy:** Always perform coagulation profile studies as patients can develop Disseminated intravascular coagulation.
      - **Treatment**
        - **Observation**
        - **Compression therapy**
          - Useful for pain and edema
          - Minimizes phlebothrombosis
        - **Sclerotherapy:** most effective if performed on small cutaneous lesions using ethanol
          - Side effects: blistering, full-thickness necrosis, neural deficits.
          - Make sure no important neural structures are nearby if using ethanol sclerotherapy.
        - **Surgical excision:** performed most commonly after sclerotherapy to improve cosmetic appearance or remove mass tissue to optimize function
    - **Lymphatic malformation** → low-flow lesion
      - **Appearance:** Anomalous lymphatic channels filled with lymphatic tissue, which may be clustered into vesicles.
        - Further classified as microcystic vs macrocystic
      - **Most common cause of macroglossia, macrocheilia in children.** Can also cause facial asymmetry, distortion of surrounding tissue, soft tissue/skeletal hypertrophy.
      - **Treatment**
        - **Observation**
          - Intralesional bleeding can be treated with NSAIDs for pain control and rest.
          - Antibiotics indicated for cellulitis/other infections.

- **Sclerotherapy** (mainstay treatment)
  - Lesion is instilled with ethanol, doxycycline, sodium tetradecyl sulfate.
  - Can be used effectively when macrocysts are present (large volumes of lymphatic fluid without small loculations as seen on US or MRI). Microcystic disease, in which many small loculations are present, is not readily amenable to sclerotherapy.
- **Surgical resection**
  - Direct excision can be effective but carries a high likelihood of significant complications.
  - Suction-assisted lipectomy has been used to debulk lesions.
  - Complications often include the following
    - Cellulitis
    - Hematoma
    - Persistent drainage
    - Recurrence of vesicular lesions
    - Need for skin graft depending on extent of excision
- **Arteriovenous malformation** → high-flow lesion
  - **Appearance:** abnormal connections between arteries and veins
    - Arteries have thick, fibromuscular veins with prominent elastic lamina and stroma.
    - Veins are "arterialized" and hyperplastic.
  - **Clinical features**
    - Intracranial AVMs are more common than extracranial AVMs.
    - **Always present at birth, but NOT always apparent.** Puberty and trauma can stimulate enlargement.
    - Schobinger stages of development
      - Stage 1 Quiescence—bluish discoloration and warmth of skin with AV shunting noted on Doppler examinations
      - Stage 2 Expansion—AVM begins to enlarge and demonstrates bruit, thrill, and pulsations
      - Stage 3 Destruction—begins to bleed, cause pain, and destroy surrounding tissue
      - Stage 4 Decompensation—persistent destruction to surrounding tissue with cardiac failure
  - **Associated syndromes**
    - Bannayan-Zonana syndrome: AVM + microcephaly + lipomas
    - Riley-Smith syndrome: AVM + microcephaly + pseudopapilledema
    - Osler-Weber-Rendu disease
      - Multiple cutaneous telangiectasias with visceral AVMs (most commonly in lungs, liver, brain)
      - Often presents as frequent nosebleeds
  - **Treatment**
    - **Observation:** used for small, clinically stable, asymptomatic lesions
    - **Embolization with surgical excision**
      - Used for stage 3-4 lesions.
      - Ligation/embolization of proximal feeding vessels must never be performed. Can cause recruitment of nearby vessels to exacerbate AVM.
      - Wide local excision is necessary to minimize recurrence rates.
      - Reconstruction with flaps is often necessary after excision.
- Malformations associated with other anomalies
  - **Klippel-Trenaunay syndrome:** capillary and/or lymphatic venous malformation (patchy port-wine stain on an extremity); skeletal and soft tissue hypertrophy (axial/transverse) of an extremity

- ○ **Parkes Weber syndrome:** capillary malformation + AVM with associated soft tissue/skeletal hypertrophy
- ○ **Servelle-Martorell syndrome:** similar to Klippel-Trenaunay syndrome with limb hypertrophy secondary to venous malformation, occasionally arterial, with skeletal hypoplasia
- ○ **Sturge-Weber syndrome**
  - ▪ Port-wine stain (capillary malformation) in V1/V2 distribution of the face
  - ▪ Leptomeningeal malformations
    - ▫ Seizures
    - ▫ Contralateral hemiplegia
    - ▫ Warrants MRI of the head
  - ▪ Developmental delay
  - ▪ Glaucoma and retinal detachment: screen using biannual fundoscopic and tonometry examinations for 1-3 years, then yearly examinations
- ○ **Maffucci syndrome:** enchondromatosis with multiple cutaneous hemangiomas
- ○ **Cobb syndrome:** capillary malformation localized to the trunk; associated with spinal AVM
- • **Combined:** involves more than two types of vascular malformation in one lesion

PEARLS

1. The lymphatic system is collects and transports fluid back to the venous system, transports antigens and immune cells and transports fat, lipids and chylomicrons from the GI tract.
2. Imaging with lymphoscintigraphy, MR lymphangiography and ICG lymphography are important to staging, monitoring and surgical planning.
3. Surgical success in management of lymphedema is dependent on patient selection; determining if the patient has edema, adipose deposition and/or functional lymphatics will aid in selection of a physiologic or excisional procedure.
4. Determining if the vascular anomaly was present at birth (eg vascular malformation) vs present after birth (eg hemangioma) is key to diagnosis.

QUESTIONS YOU WILL BE ASKED

1. What is the most common cause of secondary lymphedema in developing and developed countries?
   In the developing world, it is filariasis caused by *W bancrofti* (120 million cases). In the developed world, it is the result of cancer treatment, specially lymph node dissection.
2. What is the difference between the timing of presentation of hemangiomas vs vascular malformations?
   Vascular malformations are present at birth and continue to grow as the child ages. They do not involute. Infantile hemangiomas present after birth and continue to grow until approximately 1 year of age after which time they often begin to involute. The exception is congenital hemangiomas, which are present at birth.
3. What are the indications to perform operative intervention on a hemangioma?
   (1) Obstruction or deformation of critical structures such as the eye or airway.
   (2) Bleeding or ulceration that is unresponsive to pharmacologic management.
   (3) Easily excisable area with potential for an acceptable scar.
4. What nerve distribution do port-wine stains usually affect?
   V_1 and V_2 branches of cranial nerve V
5. Name the different syndromes associated with hemangiomas and vascular malformations along with associated signs.
   See sections on pages 7, 10 and 11.

Recommended Readings
1. Couto RA, Maclellan RA, Zurakowski D, Greene AK. Infantile hemangioma. *Plast Reconstr Surg.* 2012;130(3):619-624. doi:10.1097/PRS.0b013e31825dc129
2. Cox JA, Bartlett E, Lee EI. Vascular malformations: a review. *Semin Plast Surg.* 2014;28(2):58-63. doi:10.1055/s-0034-1376263
3. Kung T, Champaneria M, Maki J, Neligan P. Current concepts in the surgical management of lymphedema. *Plast Reconstr Surg.* 2017;139(4):1003e-1013e. doi:10.1097/PRS.0000000000003218
4. Rockson SG, Keeley V, Kilbreath S, Szuba A, Towers A. Cancer-associated secondary lymphoedema. *Nat Rev Dis Primers.* 2019;5(1):22. doi:10.1038/s41572-019-0072-5
5. Schaverien M, Coroneos C. Surgical treatment of lymphedema. *Plast Reconstr Surg.* 2019;144(3):738-758. doi:10.1097/PRS.0000000000005993

9 Lasers in Plastic Surgery

Naomi Briones

OVERVIEW

DEFINITIONS

- Laser is an acronym for light amplification by stimulated emission of radiation
- Light Characteristics
    - Monochromaticity: light emitted is of a well-defined wavelength.
    - Coherence: light waves are in phase temporally and spatially.
    - Collimation: light waves travel in parallel without spreading.
- There are four outcomes when laser light hits the skin
    - Reflection: character of target material's surface. No biological effect.
    - Absorption: light hits appropriate target (chromophore) and transforms to heat through tissue interaction.
    - Transmission: light passes through tissue unaltered.
    - Scattering: incoming beam is spread in all directions; limits depth of penetration.
- Lasers are selected based on indication and the target chromophore
    - Chromophores (eg, pigment, water, melanin, hemoglobin) absorb the light, and heat is produced to create the clinical effect.
        - If no heat is produced, no clinical effect. If excess heat is produced, scarring can result from thermal injury.
        - For example, darker skin has a greater amount of melanin and greater chromophore concentration. Therefore, it is more likely to generate heat and thermal damage with laser therapy compared with lighter skin tones.

PROPERTIES

- Key Parameters
    - Wavelength: laser dependent and determined by target chromophore.
    - Fluence (J/cm^2): amount of energy delivered per unit area.
    - Spot size: diameter of surface beam. Increase for deeper penetration.
    - Pulse width (duration): how long the tissue is exposed to the laser.
    - Cooling: extracts heat at skin surface and minimizes epidermal damage.
- Lasers can be delivered in several modes
    - Continuous mode: a constant, uninterrupted beam (eg, argon lasers).
    - Quasicontinuous: rapid succession of low-energy pulses; behaves like continuous mode (eg, 1064 nm ND:YAG)
    - Pulsed mode (Hz): single or train of pulses (eg, pulsed dye laser [PDL])
    - Q-switched mode: high-power, short-pulse duration (eg, Q-switched ruby)

LASER PHYSICS

- All lasers have four essential parts
    - A medium (gas, liquid, solid, semiconductor), through which energy excites atoms.
    - Power supply or a source of energy to excite the medium.
    - Mirrors for amplification.

---

*Denotes common in-service examination topics.

○ Delivery system to deliver light to the target.
- **Selective photothermolysis is the primary principle behind laser surgery**
  ○ Wavelength must penetrate to depth of skin target and correspond to absorption by chromophores within that target.
  ○ The time of laser exposure (pulse duration) is shorter or equal to thermal relaxation time (cooling time) of the chromophore.
    ▪ Thermal relaxation time (proportional to the square of the target diameter): time required for the heated tissue to lose half of its heat.
    ▪ If a pulse duration is longer than the thermal relaxation time, heat is not confined to target structure and can damage surrounding tissue.

LASER APPLICATIONS (TABLE 9-1)

- *The three main chromophores of the skin are water, hemoglobin, and melanin, and laser therapy is directed toward these targets (Fig. 9-1).

SKIN RESURFACING

- **Can improve fine to medium wrinkles** in patients with Fitzpatrick I or II skin (eg, perioral rhytids) due to skin contraction from synthesis and reorganization of new collagen and elastin.
  ○ Results in thermal injury to the skin with wound healing.
  ○ Reepithelialization occurs through proliferation of progenitor cells within hair follicles and sweat glands.
  ○ Increased dermal collagen synthesis for 3-6 months.
  ○ Reorganization of elastic fibers into a parallel and tight configuration.
- **Ablative vs nonablative lasers**
  ○ **Ablative:** removes dermis/epidermis, thermal injury induces wound healing response (eg, CO_2, Er:YAG)
  ○ **Nonablative:** heat underlying tissue to induce wound-healing response without trauma (eg, pulsed-dye, ND:YAG, alexandrite)
- **Contraindications**
  ○ **Relative:** smoking, previous resurfacing, diabetes, prior skin irradiation, active acne, hypertrophic scarring, skin hypersensitivity, vitiligo, and pigmentation disorders
  ○ **Absolute:** keloids, scleroderma, systemic lupus erythematosus, and isotretinoin use within the previous year
- **CO_2 laser:** ablative
  ○ Pulsed or continuous wave modes. Fractional setting decreases amount of thermal injury but still stimulates tissue regeneration.
  ○ Water absorbs energy, converting light to heat which vaporizes or ablates tissue. Effects are similar to a controlled partial-thickness burn.
  ○ Ablation threshold—the necessary amount of energy that achieves tissue vaporization. Ablation threshold for CO_2 laser is 5 J/cm^2.
  ○ Side effects: prolonged healing or erythema, scarring (infrequent), transient hyperpigmentation, risk of permanent hypopigmentation (infrequent), possible yeast, bacterial, viral infections, **HSV outbreak** (*can give valcyclovir PO for prophylaxis**), contact dermatitis.
  ○ Indications: photoaged skin, rhytids, acne scars, skin laxity, hypertrophic burn scars, some linear epidermal nevi, sebaceous hyperplasia, and seborrheic keratoses.
  ○ Relative contraindications: vitiligo, scleroderma, darker skin, unrealistic expectations.
  ○ Best candidate: Fitzpatrick type I or II skin.
  ○ Avoid using supplemental oxygen to prevent fires from CO_2 laser.
- **Erbium:yttrium-aluminum-garnet (Er:YAG):** ablative
  ○ Compared with the CO_2 laser, more passes are required for the same depth of penetration but with less thermal damage.

TABLE 9-1 Common Applications of Lasers in Plastic Surgery

Indication	Laser	Wavelength (nm)	Chromophore	Medium	Applications
Skin resurfacing	CO_2	10 600	Water	Gas	Rhytides, photodamage, acne scars, epidermal nevi, sebaceous hyperplasia, seborrheic keratoses, skin laxity
	Er:YAG	2940	Water	Solid	Rhytides, acne scars, skin laxity, photodamage
Vascular lesions	Pulsed dye	585-595	Oxyhemoglobin	Liquid (dye)	Capillary vascular malformations, hemangiomas, telangiectasias in rosacea, port-wine stains
	KTP	532	Hemoglobin, melanin	Solid	Pigmented lesions, vascular lesions including resistant port-wine stains
	Nd:YAG	1064	Oxyhemoglobin	Solid	Hemangiomas, venous malformations, telangiectasias, spider veins
Pigmented lesions	Q-switched Ruby	694	Pigment	Solid	Pigmented lesions, blue/black/green tattoo
	Q-switched alexandrite	755	Pigment	Solid	
	Nd:YAG	1064	Pigment	Solid	Pigmented lesions, blue/solar, lentigines, macules, black tattoos
	Frequency-doubled Nd:YAG	532	Pigment	Solid	Pigmented lesions, red/orange/yellow
Hair removal	Normal mode Ruby	694	Melanin	Solid	Hair removal
	Normal mode alexandrite	755	Melanin	Solid	Hair removal
	Normal Nd:YAG	1064	Melanin	Solid	Hair removal
	Diode	800-810	Melanin	Solid	Hair removal

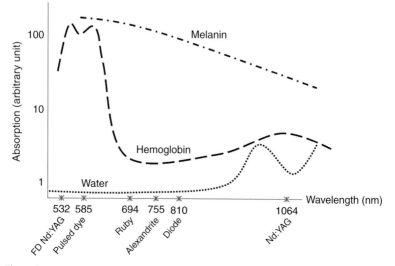

Figure 9-1 Wavelength depth of commonly used lasers. (Adapted from DiBernardo BE, Cacciarelli A. Cutaneous lasers. *Clin Plast Surg.* 2005;32:141-150, with permission from Elsevier.)

- ○ Ablation threshold for Er:YAG laser is 1.6 J/cm^2.
- ○ Side effects similar to CO_2.
- ○ Indications: rhytids, photodamage, acne scars, skin laxity.
- ○ Best candidate: Fitzpatrick type I or II skin.

VASCULAR LESIONS

- Indications: capillary malformations and hemangiomas are most common.
- Selective photothermolysis targets hemoglobin and oxyhemoglobin molecules in order to shrink or eliminate blood vessels.
- *Treatment of choice: IPL, 1064 nm Nd:YAG, 810 nm diode, 532 nm KTP, and 595 nm PDL.
- **Flashlamp pulsed dye laser**
    - ○ **Indications:** capillary vascular malformations, hemangiomas, telangiectasias, port-wine stains, recalcitrant verrucae.
    - ○ **Side effects:** erythema/purpura for 7-14 days, dyspigmentation.
    - ○ Usually requires several treatments for lightening of vascular lesions.
    - ○ Best results for port-wine stains depends on location and size.
        - ▪ Lesions on the face and neck respond better than those on the leg and hand.
        - ▪ Lesions on forehead and lateral face respond better than central face.
        - ▪ Chest, upper arm, and shoulder respond well.
        - ▪ Initial port-wine stain <20 cm^2 clear more than those larger than 20 cm^2.
- ND:YAG laser
    - ○ Indications: early stage hemangiomas, capillary vascular malformation, venous malformations, facial telangiectasias, spider veins
    - ○ Side effects: pain, redness, swelling, bruising, pigmentary changes
- **KTP (potassium-titanyl-phosphate) laser**
    - ○ Indications: epidermal pigmented lesions and vascular lesions. Similar response rates as PDL for some lesions, red tattoo-ink.
    - ○ Side effects: less purpura than PDL; scarring has been reported.
    - ○ Consider for resistant port-wine stains and large venous malformations.

PIGMENTED SKIN LESIONS

- Common lesions amenable to laser treatment: lentigines, ephelides, café au lait macules, thin seborrheic keratoses, nevus of Ota, nevus of Ito, blue nevi.
- May require multiple treatments, especially for café au lait macules, nevus of Ota/Ito.
- Diagnose melanocytic nevi before treating. Controversial as inadvertent treatment may slow the diagnosis of dysplasia or melanoma.
- Chromophore: melanin.
- *Q-switched lasers are now the treatment of choice for pigmented lesions.
  - Q-switched ruby laser: 694 nm
  - Q-switched alexandrite: 755 nm
  - Q-switched Nd:YAG: 1064 nm; use for patients with darker skin because of decreased risk of dyspigmentation
- Complications: pigmentary changes (hypopigmentation or hyperpigmentation), partial removal, infection, bleeding, textural changes, scarring (<5%).

TATTOO REMOVAL

- Lasers in Q-switched mode are used for tattoo removal.
- Chromophore: tattoo pigment.
- *Three types of lasers are currently used for tattoo removal.
  - Q-switched ruby (694 nm) and Q-switched alexandrite (755 nm)
  - Q-switched Nd:YAG (532 nm)
  - Q-switched Nd:YAG (1064 nm)
- Absorption peak of pigment must match wavelength of laser, which heats the tattoo particles within lysosomes, leading to cavitation and epidermal whitening.
- Multiple treatments are necessary with treatments separated by 5-10 weeks. Complete clearance may not be achieved.
- Tattoos exhibit "complementary matching" of laser with pigment (**Table 9-2**).
- Caution with cosmetic tattoos (eg, tattooed lip liner) due to oxidation of certain tattoo pigments (ie, ferric oxide and titanium oxide) leading to paradoxical darkening.
- Complications: pigmentary changes (hypopigmentation or hyperpigmentation), partial removal, infection, bleeding, textural changes, tattoo ink darkening, scarring (<5%).

TABLE 9-2 Tattoo Pigment Wavelength

Pigment	Wavelength
Blue green tattoos	400-450 nm and 505-560 nm
Yellow tattoos	410-510 nm
Orange tattoos	500-525 nm
Red tattoos	505-560 nm
Purple tattoos	550-640 nm
Blue tattoos	620-730 nm
Green tattoos	630-730 nm
Black and gray tattoos	600-800 nm

HAIR REMOVAL

- Numerous lasers targeting unwanted hair include diode laser, normal mode ruby, alexandrite, and normal Nd:YAG.
- Using lasers with longer pulse duration achieves two goals.
  - Epidermal melanosomes are not affected.
  - The light-absorbing melanized bulb and shaft diffuses heat to surrounding follicle.
- Higher fluences lead to better results but also more discomfort and complications.
- Requires multiple treatments. All lasers lead to hair reduction, not permanent removal.
- Cooling essential for safe reduction in darkly pigmented skin.
- Ideal patients have dark hair and fair skin. The treatment of light or white hairs remains a challenge due to lack of melanin target.

FRACTIONAL PHOTOTHERMOLYSIS

- Only a portion of the epidermis and dermis is treated with columns of energy to create targeted areas of thermal damage (microthermal treatment zones [MTZs]).
- The untreated areas are a reservoir of collagen and promote tissue regrowth.
- Allows for greater penetration with decreased risk of scarring.
- Pattern density: number of MTZs within the treatment area.
  - Greater number of MTZs yields a greater surface of the skin treated at each pass.
- **Energy**: depth of MTZ penetration into the dermis.
- **Nonablative fractional devices**
  - Lasers: erbium-glass laser (1540 nm); Nd:YAG (1320 nm); diode (1450 nm)
  - Indications: skin resurfacing, acne, striae, scarring, melisma, burn scars
  - Can be performed under topical anesthetic
  - Mild erythema and swelling, dry skin, flaking, superficial scratches, pruritus, pigmentary changes, and acneiform eruptions
  - Risk of herpes simplex virus and varicella zoster virus reactivation (use valacyclovir for prophylaxis as indicated)
- **Ablative fractional devices**
  - Ablative CO_2 or erbium lasers.
  - Fine rhytids, dyspigmentation, skin laxity.
  - Can be performed under topical anesthetic with nerve block.
  - May result in prolonged erythema, hypopigmentation, and scarring, although the risks are less compared with fully ablative therapy.

LASER SAFETY

- **Signs**
  - Signs on room door should have information about laser, its wavelength, and energy.
  - A pair of appropriate eyewear placed on the door outside the room.
- **Eye Protection**
  - CO_2 and Er:YAG lasers can injure cornea.
  - PDL and ruby lasers can injure retina.
  - Special glasses that match the emission spectrum of a laser must be worn by laser operator and all other personnel in the room.
  - Manufacturer of protective eyewear has the wavelengths of light for which protection is provided printed on goggles.
  - Patient can wear
    - Metal corneal eye shields if laser will be used around orbits.
    - Burnished stainless steel eye cups.

- **Fire Risk**
  - ◦ Prep solution should be nonflammable (avoid chlorhexidine or alcohol).
  - ◦ Surround the area to be treated with wet towels.
- ***Laser Plume**
  - ◦ Ablative lasers create a plume, which may contain bacteria (coagulase negative *Staphylococcus*, *Corynebacterium*, *Neisseria*, and HPV).
  - ◦ Laser operator and personnel should wear surgical masks.
  - ◦ Use a smoke evacuator ~1-2 cm from laser smoke plume source.

Section I: General

PEARLS

1. Vascular lesions are most effectively treated using PDLs (585-595 nm).
2. Tattoos can be effectively treated with Q-switched lasers, and the appropriate wavelength depends on the color and depth of the pigment.
3. Fractional technologies are increasingly popular for skin rejuvenation and resurfacing, and only treat a portion of the skin surface. These techniques can potentially minimize patient side effects and complications.

QUESTIONS YOU WILL BE ASKED

1. Know the chromophores of each laser. Know for each clinical application, what are the lasers of choice?
2. What medication(s) should patients with history of HSV undergoing cutaneous laser resurfacing receive as prophylaxis?
   Valacyclovir.
3. Which skin types are at greatest risk for side effects or complications following laser therapy?
   Fitzpatrick IV and above.

Recommended Readings
1. Alam M, Warycha M. Complications of lasers and light treatments. *Dermatol Ther*. 2011;24:571-580.
2. Azadgoli B, Baker RY. Laser applications in surgery. *Ann Transl Med*. 2016;4:452.
3. Chuang J, Barnes C, Wong BJ. Overview of facial plastic surgery and current developments. *Surg J*. 2016;2:e17-e28.
4. Khalkhal E, Rezaei-Tavirani M, Zali MR, et al. The evaluation of laser application in surgery: a review article. *J Lasers Med Sci*. 2019;10:S104.
5. Nelson AA, Lask GP. Principles and practice of cutaneous laser and light therapy. *Clin Plast Surg*. 2011;38:427-436.

10 Burns

Emily Barrett

OVERVIEW OF THERMAL BURN INJURY

PATHOPHYSIOLOGY OF BURN INJURY

- Coagulation of protein due to intense heat
- Release of local inflammatory mediators
- Change in blood flow due to vasoconstriction and thrombosis
- Tissue edema

SYSTEMIC EFFECTS

- Loss of skin's barrier function leads to fluid loss and massive fluid shifts.
- Injured tissues release vasoactive mediators with secondary interstitial edema, hypoproteinemia, fluid shifts, and organ dysfunction.
- Bacterial translocation.
- Immune Function: hypermetabolic state
    - *Initial response: decreased cardiac output, decreased metabolic rate.
    - 24-48 hour after injury: increased cardiac output (2 times normal), increased metabolic rate (2 times normal).
    - Hypothalamic function altered: increased glucagon/cortisol/catecholamines.
    - GI barrier function breaks down, leads to bacterial translocation.
    - Nutritional needs dramatically increase (2-3 times normal).
    - Overall catabolic state.
    - Strategies to alter the hypermetabolic state have included antipyretics, β-adrenergic blockade, and NSAIDs.

INITIAL BURN EVALUATION AND MANAGEMENT

BURN INJURY SEVERITY

- **Calculating total body surface area (TBSA) burned and presence of inhalation injury are the most important.**
- Depth of burn can be affected by mechanism, temperature, duration of contact, and thickness of skin.
- Patient comorbidities and age are other important factors.
- Patients may have coexisting traumatic injury (motor vehicle accidents, explosions, etc.).
- Patients should always be treated initially via Acute Trauma Life Support (ATLS) guidelines.
- **TBSA can be estimated by the "Rule of Nines" (Fig. 10-1)**
    - The Rule of Nines is altered for children and infants whose heads are larger and extremities smaller than adult patients.
    - The size of a patient's palm is a reasonable estimate of 1% of TBSA.

---

*Denotes common in-service examination topics.

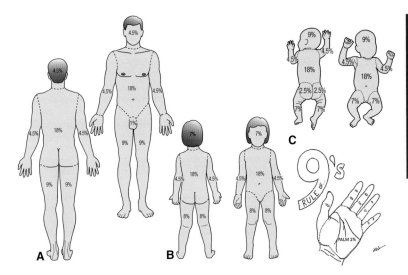

Figure 10-1 A-C. Percent total body surface area burn as estimated by location in adults (**A**), children (**B**), and infants (**C**). ("Rule of Nines"). (Modified from Dimick JB, ed. *Mulholland & Greenfield's Surgery.* 7th ed. Wolters Kluwer; 2022. Figure 12.2.)

DEPTH OF BURN

- **Superficial Burns (First Degree)**
  - Involve the epidermis.
  - **Symptoms similar to a bad sunburn** and include hyperemia, blanching skin, and tenderness to palpation.
  - **Blisters are not present.**
- **Partial-Thickness Burns (Second Degree)**
  - **Involve the dermis** and are categorized into superficial partial-thickness and deep partial-thickness burns. This distinction is the most important, as it will determine the need for excision and grafting vs dressings and observation.
  - **Superficial partial thickness.**
    - **Painful**
    - Papillary dermis involved without involvement of skin appendages.
    - Raw surfaces are deeper red and tender to palpation.
    - Blisters (either intact or ruptured) will be present.
    - *Blanches with pressure.
    - If the dermal appendages are intact, then healing without skin grafting is possible.
  - **Deep partial thickness**
    - Reticular dermis involved with skin appendages
    - No capillary refill
    - White
    - *Decreased to absent sensation
- **Full-Thickness Burns (Third Degree)** result in destruction of the epidermal and dermal layers
  - Burns extend into the subcutaneous tissues, muscle, or bone.
  - **Skin is white and nonblanching** or, in deeper burns, dry and leathery in appearance. No sensation is present. If a burn is painful, it is not full thickness (sensory nerves are preserved).
  - Will not heal on its own and will require excision and coverage.

INHALATION INJURY

- Occurs in ~10% of burn patients.
- **History** often includes fire in an **enclosed space** such as a basement.
- **Physical Examination**: singed nasal hairs, facial burns, carbonaceous sputum, and/or hoarseness
  - Agitation or shortness of breath may be caused by hypoxia.
  - Fluorescein eye examination is mandatory for patients with facial burns to rule out corneal abrasions.
- *Definitive diagnosis is made by direct airway examination using nasopharyngeal scope or fiberoptic bronchoscopy.
  - Early intubation for airway protection is mandatory.
  - Intubation becomes much harder when the airway swells.
  - Extubation criteria: passed spontaneous breathing trial (with a cuff leak), reasonable fluid balance, able to protect airway and manage secretions, CXR assessed for remaining edema/pneumonia, no OR planned in next 24 hours.
  - BiPAP will likely not be an option due to facial burns, but heated high flow through a nasal cannula is an alternative.
- **Inhalation injury can be graded according to the Abbreviated Injury Score (AIS) on bronchoscopy**
  - Grade 0 (no injury)—absence of carbonaceous deposits, erythema, edema, bronchorrhea, or obstruction
  - Grade 1 (mild injury)—minor or patchy areas of erythema or carbonaceous deposits in the proximal or distal bronchi
  - Grade 2 (moderate injury)—moderate degree of erythema, carbonaceous deposits, bronchorrhea, or bronchial obstruction
  - Grade 3 (severe injury)—severe inflammation with friability, copious carbonaceous deposits, bronchorrhea, or obstruction
  - Grade 4 (massive injury)—evidence of mucosal sloughing, necrosis, endoluminal obliteration
- **HAM Treatment for Intubated Patients With Suspected or Known Inhalation Injury**
  - Nebulized heparin 100 000 IU/3 mL NS, Nebulized albuterol 2.5 mg, Nebulized Mucomyst (*N*-acetylcysteine) 3 mL of 20% solution
  - Therapy to continue for 7 days or until patient is extubated
- Systemic Toxicity
  - **Carbon monoxide (CO) poisoning**
    - Should be suspected in any patient who was in an enclosed space fire.
    - Occurs because CO has 200 times affinity for hemoglobin compared to O_2.
    - CO will shift oxygen disassociation curve to the left and create tissue hypoxia.
    - Physical examination demonstrates cherry red color of mucous membranes, altered level of consciousness, and agitation.
    - Pulse oximetry may be normal (cannot distinguish between CO and O_2).
    - Treatment is 100% oxygen because CO half-life is 4 hours on room air vs 1 hour on 100% FiO_2.
  - Cyanide toxicity
    - Hydrogen cyanide is released during combustion of synthetic polymers.
    - Should be suspected in any patient who was in an enclosed space fire, is unconscious, or has a lactic acidosis (lactate >4).
    - Interferes with oxygen transfer in mitochondria, which results in tissue anoxia.
    - Pulse oximetry is unreliable because oxygen uptake and carrying capacity are normal.
    - Patients should be treated if in enclosed space fire exposure within the past 6 hours and any of the following: hypotension with SBP < 90, almond odor, or GCS ≤ 9.
    - *Treatment is Cyanokit (hydroxocobalamin 5 g IV). Will turn the urine dark pink and will cause wound exudate to develop pink hue. No need to repeat dose.

CRITERIA FOR TRANSFER TO BURN CENTER

- Partial- or full-thickness burns >10% TBSA
- Burns involve the face, hands, feet, genitalia, perineum, or major joints
- Electrical or chemical burns
- Inhalation injuries
- Children in hospitals not equipped to treat pediatric patients
- Patients with significant comorbid medical conditions
- Trauma patients where the burn injury poses the greatest risk of morbidity or mortality
- Patients with burns who require social, emotional, and rehabilitative services

FLUID RESUSCITATION

- *The Parkland formula is widely used to estimate fluid requirements in the first 24 hours
  - *First 24-hour requirement = 4 cc × %TBSA × weight in kilograms
    - For fluid resuscitation, only partial- and full-thickness burns count toward TBSA; do not include superficial degree burns.
    - Lactated Ringer solution should be used as its composition is closest to extracellular fluid.
    - Do not resuscitate with colloids (though some studies show patients with low albumin might benefit).
  - *Administer half of the above volume during the first 8 hours (calculated from the time of injury, not the time of hospital admission), and the other half over the next 16 hours.
  - Pediatric patients
    - Add maintenance fluid with D5 lactated Ringer solution.
    - Infants and children have limited stores of glycogen in liver, which can quickly lead to hypoglycemia.
  - *The adequacy of resuscitation is best judged by hourly urine output (0.5 mL/kg/h in adults or 1 mL/kg/h in children).
  - Also important to follow trend of base deficit, lactate and pH. These should continue to go down with adequate resuscitation.
  - Swan Ganz Catheter or bedside ultrasound (IVC filling and cardiac contractility) can also be used to assess fluid status.
- *Jackson burn model describes the distinct areas within every burn wound (Fig. 10-2)
  - Zone of coagulation
    - Tissue is severely damaged and will not recover.
    - Treatment: excision and grafting.
  - Zone of stasis
    - Tissue is inflamed with impaired vasculature.
    - Tissue may recover with appropriate resuscitation.
    - Surrounds zone of coagulation.
    - Treatment: aggressive resuscitation.
  - Zone of hyperemia
    - Tissue has intense vasodilation with increased blood flow and should recover.
    - Treatment: aggressive resuscitation.
- Fluid resuscitation should be assessed on an hourly basis
  - Fluids should be regularly adjusted to maintain adequate urine output as both under- and over-resuscitation have severe consequences. Keep in mind that urine output might lag early in the resuscitation and it is important to avoid giving too much fluid to just increase urine if other parameters continue to improve.
  - Jackson zone of stasis can potentially be salvageable with judicious fluid resuscitation. Under- or over-resuscitation may result in additional tissue loss.
  - Over-resuscitation can predispose to:
    - Pulmonary edema with prolonged ventilator requirements.
    - Increased tissue edema with subsequent need for escharotomy.

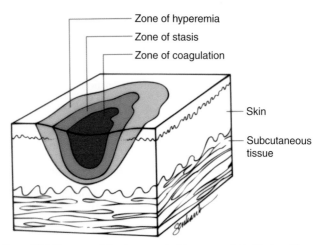

Figure 10-2 Recommended escharotomy incisions are marked with *dotted lines.*

CIRCUMFERENTIAL BURNS AND ESCHAROTOMY (FIG. 10-3)

- **Circumferential Burns**
  - Can produce a tight, inelastic contraction with limited ability for expansion of tissues.
  - As tissue edema develops during resuscitation, supraphysiologic pressures can develop with subsequent tissue ischemia and necrosis.
- **Burned Extremities**
  - Physical signs are often obscured by the burn injury or tissue edema. However, physical examination remains your best clinical diagnostic tool.
  - Doppler examination is unreliable in estimating tissue perfusion.
- **Burned Chest:** circumferential burns can cause difficulty in ventilation with high peak pulmonary pressures.
- **Burned Abdomen**
  - Circumferential burns can create an abdominal compartment syndrome.
  - Bladder pressure is a good estimate of intra-abdominal pressure and can be measured via the Foley catheter.
- **Escharotomy** is an incision of burned skin to relieve constriction.
  - When designing escharotomy incisions, remember that all burned skin will eventually be excised, so standard rules (eg, not making an incision perpendicular to a joint) do not apply.
  - **Electrocautery incision** is the method of choice and can be performed at the bedside, as the burned skin is anesthetic.
    - Need to connect unburned skin to unburned skin.
    - Burn eschar will "pop" when the constriction is released and a gap between edges of burned tissues will be created.
    - Healthy, viable tissue (usually fat) should be present at the wound base.
  - **Arms and legs**
    - Can be decompressed with axially oriented medial and lateral incisions.
    - Digital escharotomies are not typically needed.
  - **Chest and upper abdomen**
    - Can be decompressed with bilateral midaxillary releases.
    - These can be connected with one or multiple horizontal incision to form an "H."

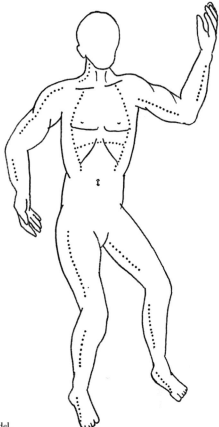

Figure 10-3 Jackson burn model.

BURN WOUND CARE

- **All blisters and nonviable tissue should be débrided at the bedside. Wounds should be dressed with a topical antimicrobial agent.**
  - ○ **Silvadene** (1% silver sulfadiazine) has broad coverage for gram-negative and positive bacteria.
    - ▪ Wound penetration is moderate.
    - ▪ Can damage the cornea so use near the eyes is contraindicated.
    - ▪ *Can cause neutropenia so white blood cell count should be followed.
    - ▪ Avoid in patients with sulfa allergy.
  - ○ **Sulfamylon** (10% mafenide acetate) has broad coverage for gram-positive bacteria and gram negative including coverage of pseudomonas and is bacteriostatic.
    - ▪ Wound and eschar penetration is excellent.
    - ▪ Sulfamylon is the topic agent of choice for **exposed cartilage** of the ear or nose.
    - ▪ *Sulfamylon is a carbonic anhydrase inhibitor and can cause hyperchloremic acidosis, particularly when used in large burns.
    - ▪ Avoid use in burns >20% TBSA.
  - ○ **Silver nitrate** (0.5% solution) has broad-spectrum coverage with coverage of *Staphylococcus* and *Pseudomonas*.
    - ▪ Silver nitrate solution does not penetrate eschar well.

- Silver nitrate solution will discolor the adjacent skin and surrounding dressings and bedding to a black color.
- *Silver nitrate can cause hyponatremia. Sodium level should be followed.
- Cost effective.

○ **Acticoat** is a silver-impregnated dressing that is available in sheets. Moisture activates the silver ions, which act as a topical antimicrobial agent.
  - Sheets can be placed over clean burn wounds and moistened with normal saline several times per day. Dressings can be changed every 3-5 days.
  - Acticoat is available in glove form, which is ideal for clean, partial-thickness burns of the hand.
  - Will also discolor the skin to a darker color from silver.

○ **Bacitracin zinc ointment** can provide coverage for gram-positive organisms.
  - Bacitracin penetrates burn eschar.
  - Commonly used for facial burns.
  - Bacitracin is safe for use around the eye.

○ **Xeroform** is a sterile, fine mesh gauze impregnated with 3% Bismuth and petroleum.
  - Sheets are nonadherent to wound sites and helps maintain a moist wound environment.
  - Used for superficial and partial thickness burns, as well as fragile STSGs.
  - Provides little antimicrobial coverage. Frequently used with bacitracin.
  - Preferred due to easy up-keep and flexible changing schedule.

NUTRITIONAL SUPPLEMENTATION

- **A hypermetabolic response is common to all large burns**
  ○ The metabolic rate is proportional to the size of the burn, up to 60% TBSA, and remains constant thereafter.
  ○ This response begins soon after injury, reaching a plateau by the end of the first week.
  ○ Most burns >30% TBSA require intensive nutritional support until wound healing is complete.
  ○ *Curreri formula for caloric requirements: 24 hour caloric requirement = (25 kcal × kg body weight) + (40 kcal × %TBSA).
  ○ Protein requirements: 2.5-3 g/kg/d are recommended. In children, requirements are 3-4 g/kg/d.
- **Intestinal feeding should be performed early**
  ○ Initial feeds can be performed using a nasogastric tube.
  ○ If feeds are administered to the stomach, feeding should be held 6 hours prior to the OR.
  ○ A postpyloric Dobhoff tube is appropriate for long-term feeding. Postpyloric feeds can be continued in the perioperative period.
- Weekly nutrition labs, prealbumin levels are drawn to monitor nutrition status.
- Early involvement of a registered dietician is imperative.

SURGICAL MANAGEMENT OF BURN WOUNDS

- **Initial débridement of blisters** should be performed at the bedside prior to initial wound dressing.
- **Formal débridement and grafting** in the operating room is performed after adequate resuscitation and when the patient is hemodynamically stable
  ○ Early débridement can prevent burn wound infection; the first débridement is often within 2-4 days of injury to allow for tissue injury to declare itself.
  ○ For large burns, sequential débridement and grafting is appropriate.
  ○ Ideally, all burn wounds would be grafted by 3 weeks to prevent hypertrophic scar formation; however, in very large burns, it is important to perform early escharotomies to remove the large bioburden of dead tissue.
- **Tangential excision** allows sequential excision of thin layers of nonviable tissue until bleeding, healthy tissue is reached.

○ At débridement, the most important distinction is between superficial and deep partial-thickness burns.
  - *Superficial partial-thickness injuries will heal on their own without grafting.
  - *Deep partial-thickness burns require skin grafting.
○ Delayed grafting can be performed if inadequate donor skin is present. Cover wounds first with cadaveric allograft or a nonbiologic dressing to protect against fluid losses and burn wound infection (see below).
- **Grafting Techniques (See Chapter 2: Grafts)**
  ○ **Split-thickness grafts**
    - Usually 12-14/1000th of an inch.
    - Thinner grafts preserve donor site for reharvesting and have higher take rates but are more prone to secondary contraction.
  ○ **Meshing is typically performed at a 1:1.5 ratio** to increase surface area and for fluid to escape from beneath the graft.
    - Higher mesh ratios (eg, 1:2, 1:3, or 1:4) can be used but prolong healing.
    - Even if using a meshed graft, the less you need to spread out the graft, the better the graft appearance will be in the future and the less likely it will break down.
  ○ **Unmeshed sheet grafts are typically used on cosmetic or functional areas,** such as the face, breast, and hands.
- Graft failure can occur for many reasons
  ○ Inadequate wound débridement prior to graft application is the primary cause.
  ○ Infection: Quantitative cultures showing more than 10^5 cells will result in graft loss.
  ○ Fluid collection beneath the graft, including hematoma (most common) or seroma.
  ○ Shear force to graft from inadequate immobilization and compression.
  ○ Poor nutrition or overall physiologic status.

COVERAGE OPTIONS

Coverage option	Properties	Advantages	Disadvantages
Autograft	A patient's own skin and is the preferred grafting material when available	Single-stage reconstruction and reliable take on a clean, vascularized wound bed	Creation of a second partial-thickness donor site
Allograft	A skin graft taken from a cadaver	Limitless quantities when autograft is sparse Can temporarily revascularize and dermal elements may incorporate Allows coverage of burn wounds to minimize fluid loss and burn wound infection	Cost Potential for disease transmission Will eventually reject
Xenograft	A tissue graft between species (eg, porcine)	Limitless quantities when autograft is sparse Allows coverage of burn wounds to minimize fluid loss and burn wound infection Good for patients with painful superficial partial-thickness burns that will likely not require grafting	Predictable slough at ~7 d because the graft cannot obtain blood supply Potential for disease transmission exists

(continued)

Coverage option	Properties	Advantages	Disadvantages
Integra	A bilaminate bovine collagen construct that provides a decellularized matrix to be populated by patient's own cells	Ability to cover over nonvascularized surfaces such as bone without periosteum or tendon without paratenon Will provide a vascularized wound bed in 3-4 wk for grafting Allows usage of thin (6-8/1000th of an inch) skin graft to conserve donor site	High incidence of infection Need for a second operation for skin grafting Need for thin autograft harvest at second surgery
Cultured epithelial autograft cells	A patient's own skin cells that are expanded in cell culture prior to grafting	Expansion of available autograft in patients with large surface area burns (>80%)	3-4 wk lag time before cells are ready for grafting Creation of a thin, unstable coverage with no dermal elements High cost Squamous cell cancer has been reported in patients treated with these grafts

BURNS OF THE FACE, EYES, AND EARS

- The central face has deeper skin appendages and excellent blood supply, resulting in a greater healing capacity.
- **Assessed Using the Subunit Principle:** when >50% of a subunit requires grafting, excision and grafting of the entire subunit optimizes aesthetic outcome
  - Use unmeshed sheet grafts, applied by aesthetic units.
  - Thicker grafts (16-20/1000th of an inch) are preferable on the face.
  - Facial grafting should be performed <2 weeks from the time of injury to decrease scarring.
- **Eyes:** lid edema usually protects the eyes in the early stages. Patients are at risk of corneal exposure and corneal abrasion as edema subsides.
  - Ophthalmology consult and fluorescent staining often indicated to assess for corneal abrasions.
  - Eye lubrication and/or temporary tarsorrhaphy may be required.
  - Definitive surgical correction to address anterior, middle, and posterior lamella.
  - Goals
    - Restore the lid to the proper functional position.
    - Covering the inferior margin of the corneoscleral limbus in neutral gaze.
- **Ears:** ear skin is very thin and exposed cartilage is common.
  - *Twice-daily sulfamylon is the best wound dressing for exposed cartilage.
  - Avoid any external pressure to the ear.
  - Suppurative chondritis requires urgent débridement.
  - If no cartilage exposure is present, split-thickness skin grafting and a bolster are appropriate.
  - Small amounts of exposed cartilage may be débrided to allow primary wound closure.
  - Large amounts of exposed cartilage necessitate vascularized coverage prior to grafting. An ipsilateral temporal-parietal fascia flap is ideal.

BURNS OF THE HANDS AND FEET

- Have a low threshold for early escharotomies of severely burned extremities.
- Superficial extremity burns are treated with elevation, topical antimicrobials, and passive ROM for each joint BID.
- *Burned hands should be splinted in the intrinsic plus position with the thumb maximally abducted.
- Important to get occupational therapy on board early to help with splinting and ROM.
- If prolonged hospitalization and severe burns with exposed tendon, should consider K-wire hand in intrinsic plus.
- Deep partial- and full-thickness burns
  - Early excision and sheet grafting are preferred, particularly on the dorsum of the hand and fingers.
  - After 5 days of immobilization, ROM exercises should be restarted.
- Exposed tendon may require local tissue rearrangement vs flap coverage vs integra placement.
- Palmar skin is thick and only 20% of palmar burns ultimately require resurfacing. A conservative approach is recommended to preserve thick fascial attachments.
- May need to perform z-plasties or local tissue rearrangements if contractions develop (See Chapter 11: Burn Reconstruction).
- Burns of the feet are managed similarly to hand burns.

GENITAL BURNS

- Place burned foreskin into its normal position to prevent paraphimosis.
- Topical antibiotic therapy may be instituted for several weeks as needed. Any remaining open wounds should then be sheet grafted.
- Early consultation with an experienced urologist is recommended. The Foley catheter may be removed at their discretion.

OPHTHALMOLOGIC INJURY

- Important to consult ophthalmology if concern for elevated intraocular pressures
- Important to keep eyes well lubricated and consider tarsorrhaphy

ELECTRICAL INJURY

- Electrical injuries represent <5% of burn injuries admitted to major burn centers.
- The typical patient is a young male; often work related.
- Total body surface area (TBSA) is not necessarily associated with prognosis and does not quantify damage to deep tissues.

MECHANISM OF INJURY

- Pathophysiology of electrical burn is based on the following
  - Type of current: low frequency alternative current (AC) results in muscle contraction where the person cannot let go of the electrical source usually resulting in worse injury; direct current (DC) usually causes a single shock.
  - Voltage: low voltage is <1000 V and high voltage is >1000 V.
  - *Resistance: tissue resistance in decreasing order = bone, fat, tendon, skin, muscle, vessel, nerve. (Bone heats to a high temperature and burns surrounding structures.)
- Thermal: can generate temperatures over 100 degrees.
- Electroporation: electrical force drives water into lipid membrane and causes cell rupture.

- Assessment of entry and exit wounds not always useful but should be evaluated.
- Difficult to determine type and severity of damage between entrance and exit.

SYSTEMIC EFFECTS

- All must be considered prior to determination of a management plan.
- Current flows through tissue can cause burns at entrance/exit wounds and burns to deep tissue.
  - Current will preferentially travel along low-resistance pathways.
  - Nerves and blood vessels have low resistance. Bone has high resistance.
  - Current will pass through soft tissue, contact high-resistance bone, and travel along bone until it exits to the ground.
- Vascular Injury to Nutrient Arteries
  - Damage to intima and media
  - Thrombosis
- Cardiac Effects
  - Arrhythmia—EKG monitor for at least 24 hours
  - Coronary artery spasm
  - Myocardial injury and infarction
- Gastrointestinal (GI) Effects
  - Injury to solid organs
  - Acute bowel perforation
  - Delayed bowel perforation
  - Gallstones after myoglobinuria
- Genitourinary (GU) Effects
  - Rhabdomyolysis with elevated CK levels, hyperkalemia, hyperphosphatemia, and myoglobinuria
- Electrical arcs have incredibly high temperatures and can cause flash burns.
- Electricity can ignite clothing or structures with secondary flame burns.

INITIAL MONITORING

- Based on ATLS guidelines (ABCDE)
- **Airway Maintenance:** C-collar until c-spine cleared
- **Breathing and Ventilation**—100% oxygen
- **Circulation and Cardiac status**
  - Cardiac monitor
  - Two large-bore IV catheters
  - Assess peripheral perfusion
  - ECG
  - 24-hour monitor if
    - Ectopy or dysrhythmia present
    - Loss of consciousness
    - Cardiac arrest
    - Abnormal rate or rhythm
- **Disability, Neurological Deficit, and Gross Deformity**
  - Assess level of consciousness.
  - Note any neurological deficit.
  - Note any gross deformity.
- **Exposure and Environmental Control**
  - Stop the burning process and remove clothes.
  - Avoid hypothermia.
- **Renal Function Analysis and Urine Myoglobin**

FLUID RESUSCITATION

- **TBSA provides an inadequate estimation of burn severity**
- Unlike thermal injury, electrical injury often occurs deep to the skin and is not visible. Thus, standard fluid resuscitation models (Parkland formula) may underestimate fluid resuscitation needs.
- **The Parkland formula** can be used to provide a minimum volume estimate. If no urine pigmentation is present, the minimum acceptable urine output is 0.5 mL/kg/h.
- **Pigmented urine can be caused from myoglobin** (secondary to rhabdomyolysis) and/or free hemoglobin (from damaged RBCs)
  - For myoglobinuria, the urine dipstick will be positive for blood. However, microscopy will not demonstrate RBCs.
  - *The goal urine output for rhabdomyolysis and myoglobinuria is 2 mL/kg/h or about 75-100 cc/h.
    - Insufficient volume resuscitation can predispose to myoglobin-induced acute tubular necrosis.
    - In addition to adequate fluid resuscitation, myoglobin excretion can be promoted using mannitol (12.5 g/h osmotic diuresis) and/or urine alkalinization with 50 mEq/L of bicarbonate.
    - Follow urine myoglobin levels every 6 hours until a downward trend is seen.

COMPARTMENT SYNDROME CAN OCCUR AFTER HIGH-VOLTAGE INJURY TO AN EXTREMITY

- Current travels along bone, which has high resistance.
- The bone serves as a conductor and "cooks" adjacent tissue from deep to superficial.
- *In the upper extremity, flexor digitorum profundus and flexor pollicis longus will be most severely affected (closest to bone).
- Overaggressive fluid resuscitation can worsen tissue edema, resulting in increased tissue pressures, and exacerbating raised compartment pressures typically occurs within 48 hours of injury.
- **Compartment Syndrome**
  - Clinical concern for raised compartment pressures mandates an evaluation of compartment pressures or a trip to the operating room.
  - The 6 "P" signs/symptoms include pain out of proportion, paresthesia, pallor, paralysis, pulselessness, and poikilothermia.
  - Raised compartment pressures can be used as an adjunct to clinical diagnosis, or when the patient is unable to participate in clinical examination
    - *Absolute pressure ≥30 mm Hg.
    - Pressure within 20 mm Hg of the diastolic blood pressure is also diagnostic of compartment syndrome.
  - Compartment pressures can be measured using a Stryker intracompartmental pressure monitor or an arterial line pressure transducer.
- **Upper extremity compartment syndrome** is managed with surgical release of the volar and extensor compartments, the mobile wad, carpal tunnel, Guyon canal, and nine compartments of the hand.
- **Lower extremity compartment syndrome** managed with fasciotomies of the anterior, lateral, superficial posterior, and deep posterior compartments.

CHEMICAL BURNS

GENERAL APPROACH TO CHEMICAL BURNS

- Protect yourself with personal protective equipment: always consider that the chemicals are still present and must be neutralized or temporized.
- Clothing that is saturated with chemical should be removed. Any powders that are present on the skin should be brushed off.
- With few exceptions (see below), all chemical burns should be copiously irrigated with water. This dilutes but does not neutralize the chemical and cools the burning area.
- Neutralization of a chemical burn is generally contraindicated because neutralization may generate heat and cause further burn injury.
- Water irrigation is contraindicated or ineffective in several scenarios
  - Contraindicated with elemental sodium, potassium, and lithium as this will precipitate an explosion.
  - Dry lime should be brushed off, not irrigated.
  - *Phenol is water insoluble and should be wiped from the skin with 30% polyethylene glycol–soaked sponges.

TYPES OF CHEMICAL BURNS (TABLE 10-1)

- **Alkali mechanism** of injury is via liquefaction necrosis and protein denaturation
  - Oven, toilet and drain cleaners, fertilizer, wet cement.
  - Alkali injury will extend deeper into tissues until the source is removed or diluted.
- **Acids** damage tissue via coagulation necrosis and protein precipitation
  - Acid injury is typically self-limited and confined to the region of exposure.
  - Acids are commonly found in household cleaners and rust removers.

TABLE 10-1 Chemical Burns

Acid burns	Mechanism	Appearance	Texture
Sulfuric Nitric HCl TCA Phenol	Exothermic reaction, cellular dehydration, protein precipitation	Gray, yellow, brown, or black depending on duration of exposure	Soft to leathery eschar depending on duration of exposure
Hydrofluoric	Same as in other acids plus liquefaction and decalcification	Erythema with central necrosis	Painful, leathery eschar
Alkali burns			
KOH NaOH Lime	Exothermic reaction, hygroscopic cellular dehydration with saponification of fat and protein precipitation	Erythema with bullae	Painful "soapy" slick eschar
Ammonia	As with other bases, plus laryngeal and pulmonary edema	Gray, yellow, brown, or black, often very deep	Soft to leathery depending on duration of exposure
Phosphorous	Thermal effect, melts at body temperature, ignites at 34 °C, acid effect of H_2PO_4	Gray or blue green, glows in the dark	Depressed, leathery eschar

- **Organic compounds** cause damage via multiple mechanisms
  - Phenol and petroleum
    - Cutaneous damage due to fat solvent action (cell membrane solvent action)
    - Systematic absorption with toxic effects on the liver and kidneys
- When in doubt about the type of burn, check the label on the can or bottle. Your local poison control office may be a helpful resource.

SPECIFIC TYPES OF CHEMICAL BURNS

- **Hydrofluoric acid (HF)** is a potent and corrosive acid commonly used as a rust remover, in glass etching, and to clean semiconductors
  - HF is a weak acid but the fluoride ion is toxic.
  - HF can cause severe pain and local necrosis.
  - Acid exposure is treated with copious water irrigation.
  - *Fluoride ion can be neutralized with topical calcium gel (1 amp calcium gluconate in 100 g lubricating jelly).
  - If symptoms persist, can consider intra-arterial calcium infusion (10 mL calcium gluconate diluted in 80 mL of saline, infused over 4 hours) and/or subeschar injection of dilute (10%) calcium gluconate solution.
  - *Fluoride ion can bind free serum calcium. Make sure to check the serum calcium and replace with IV calcium as needed.
- **Phenol** is commonly used in disinfectants and chemical solvents
  - Phenol is an acidic alcohol with poor water solubility.
  - Phenol causes protein disruption and denaturation that results in coagulation necrosis.
  - Phenol is associated with cardiac arrhythmia and liver toxicity: cardiac and liver function should be monitored.
  - Phenol is cleared by the kidneys.
  - Phenol causes demyelination and has a local anesthetic effect. Thus, pain is not a reliable indicator of injury.
  - *Treatment of phenol exposure includes copious water irrigation and cleansing with 30% polyethylene glycol or ethyl alcohol.
  - EKG is required.
- **Tar** is used in the paving and roofing industry as a durable, waterproof coating
  - Tar can be heated to 260 °C (~500 °F) prior to application. In addition to thermal injury, tar solidifies as it cools and will become enmeshed with hair and skin.
  - Tar should be cooled with copious water irrigation to stop the burning process.
  - Tar removers promote micelle formation to break the tar-skin bond.
    - A sterile surfactant mixture (De-Solv-it or Shur-Clens) allows tar to be wiped away in real time.
    - Wet dressings using polysorbate (Tween 80) or neomycin cream for 6 hours prior to tar removal can also be effective.
- **White phosphorus** is used in the manufacture of military explosives, fireworks, and methamphetamine
  - White phosphorous explosions will deposit chemical particles on the skin.
  - These particles will smoke when exposed to air.
  - Obvious particles should be brushed off. The skin should be irrigated with a 1%-3% copper sulfate solution.
  - Copper sulfate stains the particles black for identification.
  - Copper sulfate will also prevent ignition when particles are submerged in water.
  - After copper sulfate irrigation, the exposed area should be placed in a water bath and the white phosphorous should be removed.
- **Anhydrous ammonia** is an alkali used in fertilizer
  - Skin exposure is treated with irrigation and local wound care.
  - Anhydrous ammonia exposure is associated with rapid airway edema, pulmonary edema, and pneumonia: consider early intubation for airway protection.

- **Methamphetamine**
  - Tachycardia (greater than expected with a similar size burn)
  - Hyperthermia
  - Agitated
  - Paranoid

INJURY TO EYES

- Prolonged irrigation with Morgan lenses.
- Eyelids may need to be forced open due to edema or spasm.
- Utilize topical ophthalmic analgesic.
- Consult an ophthalmologist.
- Electrical injuries can cause late cataracts, therefore, good to get a baseline.
- Can cause increase in intra-ocular pressures.
- Can get corneal abrasions if corneas not protected and/or lubricated.

FROSTBITE

PATHOPHYSIOLOGY

- Heat loss can occur via four distinct mechanisms
  - Evaporation: direct absorption of body heat by water (sweat)
  - Conduction: direct loss of heat via contact with colder object
  - Convection: heat loss via movement of current/airflow
  - Radiation: direct loss of body heat to air
- **Patients at highest risk for frostbite** have decreased awareness of cold, loss of instinct to seek shelter, loss of shivering reflex, and/or cutaneous vasodilation. An easy way to remember these risk factors is the "I's" of frostbite (from Mohr, 2009).
  - Intoxicated (alcohol or other drugs)
  - Incompetent (patients with mental illness or dementia)
  - Infirm (elderly patients ± falls)
  - Insensate (extremity neuropathy)
  - Inducted (increased risk in wartime)
  - Inexperienced (those new to cold climates)
  - Indigent (homeless)

SPECTRUM OF COLD INJURY (TABLE 10-2)

- The spectrum of cold injury relates to:
  - How rapidly the body part is cooled.
  - Presence or absence of ice crystals in the tissue.
    - Rapid freezing causes intracellular ice crystallization, leading to architectural damage and cell death.
    - Slow freezing causes extracellular ice crystallization, leading to intracellular dehydration from osmotic fluid shift out of cells.
  - Frostnip is a mild, reversible cold injury with skin pallor, pain, and local numbness.
  - Pernio or chilblains is a more severe cold injury from repeat exposures to near-freezing temperatures. This presents as violaceous nodules and plaques with local pain and pruritus on repeat cold exposure.

TABLE 10-2 The Spectrum of Cold Injury

Rate of cooling	No ice crystals in tissue	Ice crystals in tissue
Fast	Frostnip	Flash-freeze injury
Slow	Pernio/chilblains	Frostbite

o Flash freezing occurs when tissue is rapidly cooled, resulting in ice crystal formation. An example of this would be licking a metal pole in winter.

PATHOPHYSIOLOGY AND STAGING

- Frostbite occurs in response to slow rate of cooling with ice crystal formation in tissue.
- Ice crystal formation occurs when tissue temperature reaches 28 °F.
- Concentrated solutes draw fluid out of cells and ice crystals subsequently cause cell membrane puncture.
- Intravascular ice crystals cause direct vascular damage and indirect vascular sludging.
- With rewarming, tissue thaws from blood vessels outward.
- Freeze-induced endothelial damage allows capillary leak that allows extravasation of polymorphonuclear leukocytes and mast cells. This results in inflammation, edema, and microvascular stasis and occlusion.
- Blisters will form at 6-24 hours when extravasated fluid collects beneath detached epidermal sheet. If dermal vascular plexus is disrupted, hemorrhagic blisters will be present.
- Stages of Frostbite
  o **First degree:** hyperemia, intact sensation, no blisters on rewarming, no tissue loss expected
  o **Second degree** with blisters containing clear or milky fluid, local edema, no tissue loss expected
  o **Third degree** with hemorrhagic blisters, edematous tissue, shooting or throbbing pain, and likely tissue loss
  o **Fourth degree** with mottled or cyanotic skin, hemorrhagic blisters, and frozen deeper structures. Mummification occurs over several weeks.

TREATMENTS AND OUTCOMES

- General treatment considerations
  o **Do not rewarm if any chance of refreezing exists.**
  o **Multiple freeze-thaw cycles** causes multiplicative, not additive, damage to the affected tissues.
  o **Intact blisters should be left alone.** Débride ruptured blisters and apply bacitracin ointment or silvadene.
  o **Beware of the afterdrop phenomenon** during rewarming
  o Afterdrop occurs when central rewarming results in peripheral vasodilation.
  o This returns cold blood from the extremities to central circulation and can result in systemic hypothermia.
- *Initial Frostbite Treatment
  o Rapid rewarming of affected area in 104 °F-108 °F water bath, not radiant heat
  o Ibuprofen 400-600 mg PO QID
  o Antibiotic prophylaxis to cover Staph, Strep, Pseudomonas
  o Pentoxifylline 400 mg PO TID
  o Elevation of limb with splinting to decrease movement
  o No smoking, caffeine, or chocolate
  o Tetanus prophylaxis
  o Three-phase bone scan may identify "at-risk" tissue
- **Acute Interventions**
  o For stable patients with severe frostbite, rapid extrication to a center with interventional radiology capabilities within 12 hours is indicated.
    ▪ Arterial catheterization can identify and treat vasospasm and microvascular thrombosis with tPA or heparin.
    ▪ Reversal of local microvascular thrombosis may restore perfusion before irreversible necrosis and ischemia occur.

- Several studies have shown significant decrease in amputation and tissue loss with this aggressive protocol.
  ○ Early regional sympathectomy of an affected extremity is controversial.

PROGNOSIS

- Tissue necrosis may be superficial with underlying viable tissue.
- Complete demarcation usually takes several weeks. Therefore, amputation should not be considered until complete tissue loss is established.
- Cold intolerance and an increased susceptibility to cold injury are likely in the affected part or extremity.

STEVENS-JOHNSON SYNDROME AND TOXIC EPIDERMAL NECROLYSIS

ETIOLOGY

- **Both Stevens-Johnson syndrome (SJS) and toxic epidermal necrolysis (TEN)** have widespread necrosis of the superficial portion of the epidermis.
- *SJS/TEN is commonly associated with sulfonamides, trimethoprim-sulfamethoxazole, oxicam NSAIDs, chlormezanone, and carbamazepine. However, a single offending drug is identified in <50% of cases.
  ○ Antibiotic-associated SJS/TEN presents ~7 days after drug is first taken.
  ○ Anticonvulsant-associated SJS/TES can present up to 2 months after drug is first taken.
- TEN can also be caused by staphylococcal infections in immunocompromised patients.

CLASSIFICATION

- **SJS:** total involvement <10% TBSA. Widespread erythematous or purpuric macules or flat atypical targets are present.
- **Overlap SJS-TEN:** total cutaneous involvement of 10%-30% TBSA. Widespread purpuric macules or flat atypical targets are present.
- **TEN with spots:** total cutaneous involvement of >30% TBSA. Widespread purpuric macules or flat atypical targets are present.
- **TEN without spots:** total cutaneous involvement >10% TBSA. Large epidermal sheets present. No purpuric macules or targets.

PRESENTATION

- Initial symptoms can be a 2- to 3-day prodrome of nonspecific findings like fevers, headaches, and chills.
- Symptoms of mucosal irritation like conjunctivitis, dysuria, and/or dysphagia may be present. These symptoms are followed by mucosal and cutaneous lesions.
- Mucosal irritation, typically at two or more sites. Involved sites may include vaginal, urinary, respiratory, gastrointestinal, oral, and/or conjunctival.
- Skin lesions are diffusely present
  ○ Lesions are typically erythematous macules with purple, possibly necrotic centers.
  ○ Nikolsky sign is typically positive (rubbing the skin causes exfoliation of outermost layers and/or a new blister to form).
- Differential diagnosis of acute, diffuse blistering includes staphylococcal scalded skin syndrome, pemphigus vulgaris, pemphigus foliaceus, paraneoplastic pemphigus, bullous pemphigoid, acute graft vs host disease, and linear IgA dermatosis.
- Diagnosis of SJS/TEN is largely clinical and can be confirmed by skin biopsy and histology.

TREATMENT

- **Discontinue all potentially offending drugs.**
- Transfer to a burn ICU for fluid/electrolyte monitoring, dressing changes, and temperature regulation is recommended.
- Débride flaccid bullae. Initial wound care with dressing changes until extent of skin loss is known.
- Empiric systemic antibiotics have been associated with increased mortality and are not indicated.
- Consider hemodialysis to remove potentially offending drugs with long half-lives.
- Early ophthalmology consultation. Over 50% of SJS/TEN patients can develop symblepharon or entropion.
- Can involve other consultant services (pulmonary, urology, OB/GYN, gastroenterology) as needed.
- Administration of steroids and IVIG is controversial. TEN is known to overexpress FAS, which promotes apoptosis of keratinocytes by binding to the FAS/CD95 receptor. IVIG blocks the CD95 receptor and has been efficacious in small series of TEN patients.

OUTCOMES

SJS has a mortality of between 1% and 5%. TENS has a mortality of up to 44%.

PEARLS

1. The Parkland formula is only a guide to approximate fluid replacement. Real-time monitoring of urine output (0.5 cc/kg/h adults, 1 cc/kg/h in children) is the most important indicator of adequate resuscitation.
2. Be wary of inhalation injury and have a low threshold for early endotracheal intubation.
3. Wounds that are not closed by 3 weeks (through healing on their own or skin grafting) are at high risk for hypertrophic scar formation.
4. Electrical injury can cause harm via multiple mechanisms, including cutaneous burns from arc or clothing fire, deep tissue burns from current flow along bones, concomitant traumatic injury, and cardiac arrhythmia.
5. Compartment syndrome is treated with decompressive fasciotomy.
6. The most important immediate frostbite intervention is rapid rewarming in a 104 °F-108 °F water bath.

QUESTIONS YOU WILL BE ASKED

1. How does a skin graft survive?
   a. *Initially the graft survives by imbibition or diffusion of nutrients from the surrounding serum (first 48 hours).
   b. Inosculation (days 2-3) connections forming between vessels in the skin graft and from the recipient site.
   c. Revascularization, with new blood vessel ingrowth into the graft (days 5-7).
2. How should we deal with exposed ear cartilage?
   a. Sulfamylon is the preferred topical wound dressing because it has good cartilage penetration.
   b. Small amounts of exposed cartilage can be resected with primary closure.
   c. Large amounts may require temporal-parietal flap closure with skin grafting.
3. What factors cause a skin graft to fail?
   a. Shear forces
   b. Infection or inadequate débridement
   c. Fluid collection beneath the graft (hematoma most common, seroma)
   d. Poor nutrition

4. How is compartment syndrome diagnosed and treated?
   a. Compartment syndrome is a clinical diagnosis, typically made using the 6 "P's" (see above). Measurement of intracompartmental pressures is a useful adjunct when clinical diagnosis is unclear or the patient is unresponsive. Compartment syndrome requires compartment release of the affected areas, typically the fore-arm and/or hand.
   b. *Diagnosis: absolute pressure ≥30 mm Hg or pressure within 20 mm Hg of the diastolic blood pressure is also diagnostic of compartment syndrome.
5. Which is worse: acid burns or alkali burns?
   Alkali. Alkali burns will continue to extend deeper into tissues until the source is removed or diluted. Acid injury is typically limited to the exposed area.
6. Who is at risk for frostbite?
   Any patient with cutaneous dilation, decreased awareness of their surroundings, or loss of instinct to seek shelter.

THINGS TO DRAW

1. Draw basic schematic of percent burn percentage per body part (**Fig. 10-1**).
2. Draw incision lines for escharotomy (**Fig. 10-3**).

Recommended Readings
1. Arnoldo B, Klein M, Gibran NS. Practice guidelines for the management of electrical injuries. *J Burn Care Res*. 2006;27(4):439-447.
2. Bruen KJ, Ballard JR, Morris SE, Cochran A, Edelman LS, Saffle JR. Reduction of the incidence of amputation in frostbite injury with thrombolytic therapy. *Arch Surg*. 2007;142(6):546-551. discussion 551–553
3. Friedstat JS, Klein MB. Acute management of facial burns. *Clin Plast Surg*. 2009;36(4):653-660.
4. Gerull R, Nelle M, Schaible T. Toxic epidermal necrolysis and Stevens-Johnson syndrome: a review. *Crit Care Med*. 2011;39(6):1521-1532.
5. Hazin R, Ibrahimi OA, Hazin MI, Kimyai-Asadi A. Stevens- Johnson syndrome: pathogenesis, diagnosis, and management. *Ann Med*. 2008;40(2):129-138.
6. Klein MB, Moore ML, Costa B, Engrav LH. Primer on the management of face burns at the University of Washington. *J Burn Care Rehabil*. 2005;26(1):2-6.
7. Mohr WJ, Jenabzadeh K, Ahrenholz DH. Cold injury. *Hand Clin*. 2009;25(4):481-496.
8. Palao R, Monge I, Ruiz M, Barret JP. Chemical burns: pathophysiology and treatment. *Burns*. 2010;36(3):295-304.
9. Schulz JT, Sheridan RL, Ryan CM, MacKool B, Tompkins RG. A 10-year experience with toxic epidermal necrolysis. *J Burn Care Rehabil*. 2000;21(3):199-204.
10. Sterling J, Gibran NS, Klein MB. Acute management of hand burns. *Hand Clin*. 2009;25(4):453-459.

11 Burn Reconstruction

Megan Lane and Ayana K. Cole-Price

OVERVIEW

TECHNIQUES IN ACUTE BURN CARE THAT CAN DECREASE LONG-TERM RECONSTRUCTIVE NEEDS

- Please **see Chapter 10: Burns** for appropriate resuscitation of thermal injuries.
- Fasciotomies, entrapment release, and repair of any ocular injuries are critical in the acute burn period.
- Use sheet grafts when possible and full-thickness grafts for the hands and face with attention to the aesthetic units of the face.
- Initiate early motion and pressure garments as soon as possible.
- Apply splints with hands in intrinsic plus and joints in extension to prevent flexion contracture.
- For patients with eyelid burns, tarsorrhaphy in the first weeks following burn can be helpful in preventing exposure keratopathy.
- Exposed cartilage and severe microstomia require urgent reconstruction in the subacute period.

MAJOR RECONSTRUCTIVE CHALLENGES FOLLOWING BURN INJURIES

- Burn Contractures
  - Tight, shortened scars from tissue deficit.
  - Can form across joint creating limitation of movement.
  - Can involve more than skin: causes shortening and fibrosis of underlying muscle, fascia, and joints.
  - More common on flexor surface because flexors are stronger and flexed position is position of comfort.
  - Assessment of contracture should include description of functional limitation, presence of joint involvement, quality of scarred skin, condition, and availability of surrounding tissue.
  - Nonoperative treatments include occupational therapy and pressure garments.
  - Pressure garments thought to reduce hypertrophic scarring and contractures by reorienting collagen fibers and reduce fiber thickness.
- Scar Deformity
  - Risk factors: wound closure, infection, Fitzpatrick scale
  - Characteristics of problematic scars: poor pliability, hypertrophic scarring, tissue loss, uneven surface, pigment change, fragility, chronic open wounds
  - Have high suspicion for malignancy Marjolin's ulcer in chronic wounds, which have been persistent for years

---

*Denotes common in-service examination topics.

- Pigment and Hair Loss
  - **Pigment**
    - Hyperpigmentation and hypopigmentation can develop at the burn site or the donor site.
    - Topical treatment options: hydroquinones and retinoids can be used for hyperpigmentation.
    - Lasers additionally useful. Pulsed dye can be utilized for red scars and fractionated CO_2 laser can soften thick scars.
  - **Hair Loss**
    - Can occur in grafted region or in region of deep burn without grafting.
    - Small areas addressed with excision and tissue rearrangement, large areas with tissue expansion.
    - Micrografts can be used for eyebrows and moustache region.
    - Excess hair from thick grafting can be treated with laser (Alexandrite or Nd:YAG) or electrolysis.
- Timing for Reconstructive Surgery
  - Urgent Reconstructive Surgeries
    - Severe microstomia
    - Exposed cartilage
    - Release of vital structures (eg, eyelid, exposed cornea)
- Semi-elective Procedures (Should Be Done Within First Few Months to 1 Year)
  - Release of joint limited by range of motion
  - Progressive deformities
- Elective Procedures (Should Be Done After 1 Year to Allow Scars to Mature)
  - Aesthetics
  - Hypertrophic scars

SURGICAL TECHNIQUES

CONTRACTURE RELEASE

- Linear incision through scar overlying point of maximum tightness, oriented perpendicular to line of contracture.
- Incise skin and then keep area on tension and carefully push with scalpel.
- If contracture persists, may need to release underlying fascia, muscle, tendon, or joint.
- Commonly paired with local tissue rearrangement.

LOCAL TISSUE REARRANGEMENTS (SEE CHAPTER 4)

- For example, the standard Z-plasty (**Fig. 11-1**).
- Like contracture release, the central limb of Z-plasty is perpendicular to the area of scar being released.
- Prior to inset, assess the transposition of the Z. If the Z does not transpose, deepen the Z-plasty.
- Jumping man and series of Z-plasties are commonly used within burn reconstruction, particularly in web spaces or in joint contractures.

GRAFTS

- Please see **Chapter 2: Grafts** for more details
- In general, defects lead to loss of skin and thus skin graft is common technique used to address this.

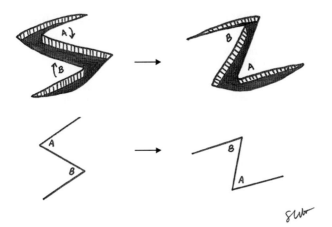

Figure 11-1 Z-plasty.

- Please see the débridement and grafting section of the acute burn chapter for acute débridement and grafting.
- For reconstruction, if using split-thickness skin graft (STSG), should use a thicker setting (0.012-0.020 in). Useful for forehead, upper eyelids, or closure of peripheral areas.
- Full-thickness skin graft (FTSG): consists of entire dermis, therefore, less remodeling and secondary contracture.
  - Preferred over STSG for face, hand, and joint surfaces

DERMAL SUBSTITUTES

- Used prior to skin (autograft) grafting to prepare wound bed
- Cadaveric skin (homograft)
- Skin substitutes derived from porcine or bovine (xenograft)
- Integra (Life Sciences): collagen-glycosaminoglycan biodegradable matrix covered by semipermeable silicone. Secured to burn in a similar way to skin graft
  - *Provides temporary coverage and allows for thinner STSG to be used (0.005-0.008 in)
  - May graft onto granulated surface in ~21 days if using traditional dressing and 10 days if using a wound vac
  - Disadvantage: expensive

FLAPS

- Local
  - Flaps can be utilized if there is noninjured local tissue
  - Groin or intercostal flaps also possible in severe hand burn
- Free Flaps
  - Thin free flap options such as fascia only with skin graft or fasciocutaneous free flaps
  - Common flaps: anterolateral thigh, scapular/parascapular, radial forearm (see Chapter 4: Vascularized Composite Allotransplantation)

TISSUE EXPANSION (SEE CHAPTER 5 FOR FURTHER DETAILS)

- Produces additional tissue with similar appearance to recipient site.
- Expanded tissue has improved vascularity.
- Especially helpful for burn alopecia.
- Expander base dimensions should be planned preoperatively.
- When first placing expander, it is important to make sure that the expander is not folded. The pocket must not be made too large in order to prevent unwanted changes in position of the expander.
- Create small tract distal from expander for filling port and use remote port in a different pocket than expander.

NONSURGICAL OPTIONS

- Laser therapy can improve the thickness and color of scar.
- Common laser therapy used in burn care: pulsed dye (for persistent scar erythema), fractionated CO_2 (for scar thickness), alexandrite (for hair removal from flaps and full-thickness grafts).
- **See Chapter 9: Lasers in Plastic Surgery** for full discussion of available laser therapies.
- Continued occupational and physical therapy is essential for reconstructive success.

CONSIDERATIONS FOR SPECIFIC ANATOMIC AREAS

FACIAL BURNS

- Ideally graft by facial subunit with use of FTSG
- If not possible, graft smaller subunits with FTSG and larger units with thick STSG
- For extensive, disfiguring burns, can also consider facial transplantation or other complex free flap–based reconstruction

MOUTH

- Reconstruction should focus on maintain oral competence and prevent microstomia
- **Commissure**
    - ○ The commissure should form an acute angle at a vertical line dropped from the medial limbus in repose. Burn contractures can blunt the oral commissure.
    - ○ Successful splinting may counteract, or prevent, the natural tendency for a mild to moderate perioral burn
    - ○ Commisureplasty techniques to correct microstomia
        - ■ Buccal mucosal advancement flap-following burn excision and contracture release at the oral commissure, mucosal flaps are developed and advanced into the defect (typically in V to Y fashion).
        - ■ Myomucosal advancement flap-contracture is released and the orbicularis oris muscle is incised and advanced laterally toward the commissure. A vermillion flap is additionally elevated and advanced laterally. The mucosa of the oral vestibule is elevated and advanced to cover remaining exposed orbicularis.
        - ■ Staged lip reconstruction (Estelander, Karapandzic flaps, **see Chapter 26: Lip and Cheek Reconstruction**)
- **Upper Lip**
    - ○ Three subunits: two lateral lip elements and the philtrum.
    - ○ Philtrum can be recreated using skin graft or philtral shaped cartilage graft.
    - ○ The columella can be lengthened with "fork flaps" from the upper lip.
    - ○ Important to preserve and realign white roll where possible.
    - ○ May also use staged lip reconstruction techniques.

- **Lower Lip**
  - Can place scars in labiomental creases.
  - Maintain soft tissue of pogonion for chin prominence.
  - Severe neck contracture can cause lip eversion.

EYEBROW

- If contralateral brow unaffected, create template from this side
- May use micrografts or hair-bearing FTSG
- Additionally can utilize vascularized island flap based on superficial temporal artery
- Tattoo

EYELID

- Reconstructive challenges: corneal exposure, ectropion (from internal or external contracture), and canthal contracture
- Tarsorraphy may be helpful in the first few weeks to prevent corneal exposure and keratitis
- **Ectropion:** caused by inadequate tissue; therefore, in addition to release, the surgeon will need to replace tissue, often with a FTSG.
  - Extrinsic contracture: need to release scar and provide additional tissue to prevent recurrence.
  - Release 2 mm from the ciliary margin, extending 15 mm beyond the medial and lateral canthi.
  - FTSG form contralateral side for upper lid and from retroauricular region for lower lid.
  - Dissect the orbicularis oculi muscle free from all scar tissue, re-drape the muscle over the entire eyelid as a sling, and secure it laterally to the orbital rim and medially to the nasal sidewall.
- **Intrinsic Contracture**
  - Requires addressing all lamellae
  - Upper lid: if ipsilateral lower lid is intact: Hughes or Cutler-Beard flaps
  - Lower lid: Mustarde cheek advancement with deep anchoring. If no local tissue is available, pedicled temporoparietal fascia flap.
    - Subperiosteal mid-face lift can be performed to reduce tension of the lower eyelid
  - Medial: Z-plasties, V-M plasties, or double opposing Z-plasties
  - Lateral: local transposition flap, lateral canthoplasty, or lateral canthotomy
  - Middle lamella: palatal mucosal graft for support

NOSE

- Layers to consider: skin, cartilage, and mucosa
- Consider nine aesthetic nasal subunits: dorsum, tip, columella, sidewalls (×2), soft triangles (×2), ala (×2)
- Dermabrasion followed by STSG or FTSG in an aesthetic unit
- Total or subtotal reconstruction: forehead flap
- Cartilage defects: conchal or septal cartilages

EAR

- **Small helical rim defects:** Antia-Buch advancement flap.
- **Larger helical rim defects:** Davis conchal transposition flap
  - Elevation of a composite flap of skin and cartilage from the concha, pedicled at the crus helix, is transferred to the upper third of ear. The donor site is closed with a skin graft.
- Extensive defects: a temporoparietal fascial flap is used to cover a cartilage framework.

- An osseointegrated prosthesis is an excellent option for total ear loss with significant burn scar on surrounding tissue.

NECK AND CHIN

- *Neck contractures are the most common complication of burn injury
- Key components: range of motion and oral competence
- Release scar contracture down to platysma or subplatysmal followed by coverage with large FTSG or thick STSG followed by aggressive range of motion 5 days after having patient in neck brace
- Can use multiple tissue expanders in infraclavicular region
- Can also use thin free flaps to resurface neck contractures
- Postoperative management: compression garments for 6-18 months and a neck brace to keep neck extended to prevent recurrence

SCALP

- Small defects: advancement or rotation flaps with donor site closed or covered with skin graft
- Moderate: tissue expansion with expander placed in subgaleal plane (deep to frontalis)
- Extensive: omentum or latissimus dorsi flap

BREAST

- Key deformities: tight skin envelope, asymmetry, nipple-areola complex malformations
- Tissue expansion or autogenous reconstruction: TRAM or latissimus dorsi if tissue uninjured
- Can do contralateral reduction to aid in symmetry
- *Prepubescent breast burns—important to release contracture to allow for development of breast

AXILLA

- Regions: anterior axillary fold, mid-axillary line, and posterior axillary line
- Common because difficult to maintain ideal position (shoulder should be at 90°-120° abduction and 15°-20° flexion) in acute phase of burn
- Three Grades of Axillary Contractures
  - Type I: both the anterior and posterior axillary folds are involved leaving the normal skin in the hair bearing central part. A web is formed during abduction.
  - Type II: the inner portion of the upper arm and the adjacent trunk as well as one axillary fold are involved.
  - Type III: the upper arm and the lateral aspect of the trunk and completely included in one mass of scar.
- Types I and II: contracture sequential release and thick STSGs or FTSGs
- Type III: local and distant flaps, including parascapular and latissimus flaps
- Must pay attention to where hair-bearing regions are transposed
- May need release pectoralis major or latissimus dorsi muscles
- Intraoperative OT range of motion including shoulder
- Postoperative OT and splinting necessary to prevent recurrence

ELBOW (TABLE 11-1)

- Results from scarring along antecubital fossa or dorsal forearm and upper arm
- No bone exposed: FTSG or thick unmeshed STSG
- May need to perform tendon lengthening of the biceps tendon
- Bone exposed: local fasciocutaneous flap—reverse radial forearm or propeller flap
- Bone exposed and no local tissue available: free fascia only or thin fasciocutaneous flap

TABLE 11-1 Classification of Elbow Burn Contracture Severity and Commonly Used Reconstructive Options

Severity of antecubital contracture	Problem	Reconstructive options
Mild	Superficial linear scar bands that span the antecubital fossa Scarring does not involve the deeper layers	Local tissue rearrangement (simple or serial Z-plasty or V-Y-plasty) Full-thickness or thick split-thickness skin grafting
Moderate	Wide areas of scar over the antecubital fossa requiring excision that may result in need for soft tissue coverage of exposed vital structures Patients may require ulnar nerve decompression	Small local perforator flaps Local fascial or fasciocutaneous flaps: Radial artery Ulnar artery Posterior interosseous artery
Severe	Burn scarring that involves deeper structures, such as fascia, muscle, and joint capsule Elbow range of motion is significantly reduced and function is severely limited Requires release of each scarred component Patients routinely require ulnar nerve decompression Heterotopic ossification is common	Lateral arm Medial arm Local muscle: Flexor carpi ulnaris Brachioradialis Regional pedicled: Latissimus dorsi Serratus anterior Free tissue: Anterolateral thigh Gracilis Rectus abdominis Contralateral radial forearm flap Free-style perforator flap

From Kung TA, Jebson PJ, Cederna PS. An individualized approach to severe elbow burn contractures. *Plast Reconstr Surg.* 2012;129(4):663e–673e. doi:10.1097/PRS.0b013e3182450c0c

HAND

- Prevention of hand contracture is key. Patients should be splinted in intrinsic plus (MC flexed at 70°-90°, wrist 20°-30°, IP joints in full extension and thumb kept abducted and slightly opposed) in acute phase of burn.
- Unchecked burn hand contracture: wrist flexion, MCP joint hyperextension, PIP flexion, boutonniere deformities of digit, and thumb adduction contracture
- **Flexion Deformities**
  - Isolated scar bands volarly or excision of scar and FTSG
  - Small defects after release: local skin flaps
  - If joint affected: release of volar plate, joint capsule, and collateral ligaments
- **Boutonniere deformity (see Chapter 38: Tendon Injuries and Tendonitis)**
- **MCP Hyperextension**
  - Requires contracture release and grafting
  - If scar released and not sufficient gain in flexion, may need dorsal capsulotomy
- **Palmar Contractures**
  - Avoid excision of palmar skin
  - FTSG to resurface small defects, though may need dorsal neurocutaneous island flap for large defects
- **Web Space Contractures**
  - Postburn syndactyly is the most common secondary deformity and usually involves dorsal skin of web space

- Treatment options: Y-V advancement, Z-plasty, jumping man
- Thumb most difficult and often best treated by jumping man
- **Burn Syndactyly**
  - Unlike congenital syndactyly, there is not enough laxity or surrounding tissue for reconstruction. Usually requires release and FTSG
  - Thumb reconstruction includes web space deepening, pollicization, and toe thumb transfer

PERINEUM

- Perineal webs result from burn to genitalia and perineum and deep burns to proximal thigh, interfering with hygiene and ambulation
- Early scar release and grafting important in severe deformities
- Labia and scrotum: release of webbing and skin grafting
- Complete reconstruction utilizes the techniques of gender-affirming surgery

FOOT

- Based on the complexity, depth, and severity of the contracture, a classification system was developed to describe each toe burn scar contracture as mild, moderate, or severe (**Table 11-2**).
- Mild: superficial tissues only. Treatment: scar excision or rearranging the local tissue, that is, with a Z-plasty burn scar release.
- Moderate: soft tissue deficits. Treatment: scar excision and resurfacing with skin grafts. Sometimes require ancillary procedures, such as closed capsulotomy of the metatarsal phalangeal or interphalangeal joints.
- Severe: involvement of deeper structures, including tendons, ligaments, and joint capsules. Treatment: multiple procedures, including skin grafting, possible free flaps for adequate soft tissue coverage, tendon lengthening, open capsulotomy, tenotomy, and pin fixation.

HETEROTOPIC OSSIFICATION

- Formation of extraskeletal bone.
- Risk of heterotopic ossification increases with percent body surface area burned and more common in blast injuries.
- Thought to be caused by trauma-induced activation of local mesenchymal cells or endothelial to mesenchymal transition of local endothelial cells.
- Current diagnosis strategies inadequate and include X-ray and CT.
- Possible prophylaxis includes NSAIDs, specifically indomethacin.
- Treatment includes radical resection of osseous tissue and contracture release.

TABLE 11-2 Decision Tree for Foot Burns

	Scarring limited to superficial tissues	Mild contracture	Scar excision Local tissue rearrangement
Extent of burn	Significant soft tissue deficits	Moderate contracture	Scar excision Skin grafts Occasional closed capsulotomy
	Significant involvement of deeper structures (tendon, joints)	Severe contracture	Skin grafts Tendon lengthening Open capsulotomy Pin fixation

PEARLS

1. Acute burn care plays a critical role in decreasing secondary burn reconstruction needs.
2. Adequate splinting in the acute setting as well as following elective burn reconstruction is critical to reconstructive success.
3. Full-thickness skin grafts are preferred in the face and hands.
4. Burned lid ectropion should to address the internal, middle, and outer lamella.
5. Burn scar finger syndactyly often has a greater tissue deficit than congenital syndactyly and almost always requires a skin graft.
6. Burned breast reconstruction in children requires release of the cutaneous scar restricting the breast bud to allow breast growth.

QUESTIONS YOU WILL BE ASKED

1. What angle should you set up the limbs of a Z-plasty?
   In general, between 60° and 70°.
2. What are you gaining by doing a Z-plasty?
   Gaining length at the expense of width.
3. What flap is ideal to improve a web space contracture of the thumb?
   Jumping man flap.
4. What is heterotopic ossification?
   Formation of extraskeletal bone. It is most common in large total surface area burns and blast injuries.

THINGS TO DRAW

1. Z-plasty and serial Z-plasty including where to place and how it rearranges tissues
2. Jumping man flap

Recommended Readings
1. Klein MB. Burn reconstruction. *Phys Med Rehabil Clin N Am.* 2011;22(2):311-325. vi–vii
2. Klein MB, Donelan MB, Spence RJ. Reconstructive surgery. *J Burn Care Res.* 2007;28(4):602-606.
3. Klein MB, Moore ML, Costa B, Engrav LH. Primer on the management of face burns at the University of Washington. *J Burn Care Rehabil.* 2005;26(1):2-6.
4. Orgill DP, Ogawa R. Current methods of burn reconstruction. *Plastic and Reconstructive Surgery.* 2013;131(5):827e-836e.
5. Parsel S, Winters R. Commissuroplasty. *Operative Techniques in Otolaryngology.* 2020;33:33-37.
6. Ranganathan K, Wong VC, Krebsbach PH, Wang SC, Cederna PS, Levi B. Fat grafting for thermal injury: current state and future directions. *J Burn Care Res.* 2013;34(2):219-226.
7. Wainwright DJ. Burn reconstruction: the problems, the techniques, and the applications. *Clin Plast Surg.* 2009;36(4):687-700.

12

Preoperative Cardiopulmonary Risk Stratification and Prophylaxis

Kory LaPree

PULMONARY

AIRWAY

- **Mallampati Scores (Fig. 12-1)**: a high Mallampati score (either 3 or 4) is associated with more difficult mask ventilation and intubation.
  - Class I: full visibility of tonsils, uvula, and soft palate.
  - Class II: visibility of hard and soft palates, upper portions of tonsils, and uvula.
  - Class III: soft and hard palates, as well as base of uvula, are visible.
  - Class IV: hard palate is the only visible structure.
- **The LEMON method of airway assessment** is a useful screening tool. Patients who meet multiple LEMON criteria should be referred for preoperative anesthesia consultation.
  - **L** = Look externally (for beard/mustache, facial trauma, macroglossia, micrognathia)
  - **E** = Evaluate the 3-3-2 rule
    - Mouth opening <3 finger breadths (the patient's fingers) with normal dentition quality
    - Hyoid-mentum distance <3 finger breadths
    - Thyroid cartilage-hyoid bone <2 finger breadths
  - **M** = Mallampati score of 3 or 4
  - **O** = Obstruction (from large tonsils, peritonsillar abscess, trauma, macroglossia)
  - **N** = Neck mobility (cervical extension and flexion)
- Other patients to refer to preoperative anesthesia for airway issues include
  - Patients with a history of difficult airway.
  - Patients with other barriers to intubation (such as a halo).
  - Consider patients with known obstructive sleep apnea or supermorbid obesity if in combination with any LEMON criteria from above.

CARDIOVASCULAR

RISK STRATIFICATION AND PROPHYLAXIS FOR ENDOCARDITIS

- In general, invasive procedures performed through surgically scrubbed skin are not likely to produce clinically relevant bacteremia.
- Patients that require prophylactic antimicrobial therapy based on 2017 AHA/ACC guidelines (high risk only).
  - Dental procedure that involves the manipulation of gingival tissue, periapical region of teeth, or perforation of the oral mucosa.
  - Urologic surgery if the urinary mucosa is pierced in the setting of active urinary tract infection or colonization.

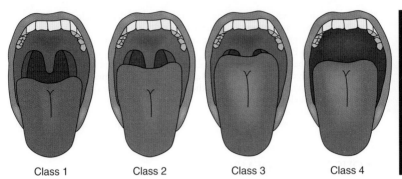

| Class 1 | Class 2 | Class 3 | Class 4 |

Figure 12-1 Mallampati classification.

- **High-Risk Categories**
  - Prosthetic cardiac valves
  - Patients with implanted prosthetic material, such as annuloplasty rings and artificial chordae tendineae
  - Patients with a history of infectious endocarditis
  - Patients with a history of unrepaired cyanotic congenital heart disease, including patients with a repair, but with a residual shunt or valvular regurgitation
  - Patients with a history of cardiac transplantation who have a regurgitant valvular lesion due to a structurally abnormal valve

AMERICAN HEART ASSOCIATION GUIDELINES FOR PERIOPERATIVE β-BLOCKADE

- Revised Cardiac Risk Index (RCRI): tool used by AHA/ACC to estimate patient's risk for perioperative cardiac complications (2 or more = high-risk patient)
  - Creatinine >2.0 mg/dL
  - Heart failure
  - Insulin-dependent diabetes mellitus
  - Intrathoracic, intra-abdominal, or suprainguinal vascular surgery
  - History of CVA or TIA
  - Ischemic heart disease
- **Preoperative Evaluation**
  - *If the patient is already on a β-blocker for a cardiovascular indication (angina, arrhythmia, hypertension), plan to continue this medication in the perioperative period.
  - Consider starting higher risk patients on β-blockade at least 1 week prior to surgery or refer them back to their primary care provider to address this issue.
  - The initiation of beta-adrenergic blockade within 1 day of elective noncardiac surgery has been associated with a decreased risk of myocardial infarction. Although NOT recommended because of the elevated risks of clinically significant hypotension, bradycardia, stroke, and death based on POISE trial of 2008.
  - Higher-risk patients also include
    - Vascular surgery patients with coronary artery disease
    - Vascular surgery patients with multiple cardiac risk factors listed above in the RCRI
    - Patients with cardiac ischemia present on preoperative testing
    - Patients having high-risk procedures such as intrathoracic, aortic, or major transplant (heart, lung, or liver) for cardiac events

- o The utility of β-blockade is unknown for lower-risk patients, including
  - Patients undergoing low- or intermediate-risk surgery
  - Vascular surgery patients without known coronary artery disease
- **Electrocardiogram Preoperative**
  - o According to the 2014 guidelines, it is reasonable to perform a preoperative ECG in patients with coronary heart disease, significant arrhythmia, peripheral arterial disease, cerebrovascular disease, or other significant structural heart disease who are undergoing elevated-risk surgery.
- **Postoperative Management**
  - o Continue β-blockers in patients receiving them preoperatively for cardiovascular indications.
  - o Watch for hypotension and bradycardia.

VENOUS THROMBOEMBOLISM

- **Venous thromboembolism (VTE) includes deep venous thrombosis and pulmonary embolism**
  - o Major source of morbidity and mortality among hospitalized patients.
  - o Considered potentially preventable through use of sequential compression devices (SCDs) and, in some cases, chemoprophylaxis like heparin or low molecular weight heparin.
- **VTE risk stratification and prophylaxis for inpatient surgery**
  - o 2005 Caprini Risk Assessment Model (**Table 12-1**) has been validated to predict 60-day VTE risk in plastic surgery patients.
  - o If NO chemoprophylaxis is given, expected 60-day VTE rates include
    - Caprini scores of 3-4 = 0.6%
    - Caprini scores of 5-6 = 1.3%
    - Caprini scores of 7-8= 2.7%
    - Caprini scores of >8 = 11.3%
  - o For inpatients with Caprini scores of >7, weight-based prophylactic dose enoxaparin given during the inpatient stay can decrease observed 60-day VTE rate by 50%.
    - When started 6-8 hours after surgery, a 0.7% increased rate of reoperative hematoma can be expected.
    - This can be balanced against the risk reduction for potentially fatal VTE events.
  - o Unless a contraindication is present, all patients should have SCDs while in the hospital.
- **VTE risk stratification and prophylaxis for outpatient surgery (Table 12-2)**
  - o Outpatient surgery is generally considered to be low risk for VTE.
  - o Recent risk stratification models have shown that a distinct, high-risk subgroup exists within the generally low-risk outpatient surgery population.
  - o The risk stratification model shown below can predict 30-day VTE risk and identify both low- and high-risk patients.
  - o No data are available for VTE prevention among outpatients.
    - The role of chemoprophylaxis remains unknown.
    - Unless a contraindication is present, all patients having surgery under general anesthesia or IV sedation should have SCDs placed.

ANESTHETIC CONSIDERATIONS

PECTORAL BLOCKS

- Pectoralis nerve (PECS) block is a fascial plane block that provides analgesia to the upper anterior chest wall, most indicated for analgesia for breast surgery post-op. They are an alternative to and more efficacious than paravertebral blocks for breast surgery, as well as better pain scores and less opioid use overall in post-op periods.

- ○ *PECS I block lateral pectoral nerve from C5 to C7 that runs between pec major and minor and medial pectoral nerve from C8 to T1 that runs deep to pec minor. Useful for breast expanders, subpectoral prosthesis.
- ○ *PECS II block anterior and lateral divisions of the thoracic intercostal nerves T2-T6, which run between intercostal muscles and provides analgesia along long thoracic nerve (C5-C7) to the serratus anterior muscle and thoracodorsal (C6-C8) to latissimus dorsi muscle. Useful for extensive breast surgery/mastectomy involving pec major and minor, serratus anterior muscle, and the axilla.

LOCAL ANESTHETIC SYSTEMIC TOXICITY

- **Signs/symptoms:** prodromal symptoms of perioral numbness/paresthesia's/tinnitus, dizziness/confusion, tremors followed by central nervous system seizures/loss of consciousness followed by respiratory depression/cardiovascular collapse
- *Treatment for adult over 70 kg: lipid emulsion 20% 100 mL over 2 minutes followed by 250 mL over 20 minutes (repeat bolus/infusion if unstable).
- LAST ACLS use less epi (<1 mcg/kg) and avoid local anesthesia, calcium channel blockers/β-blockers, and vasopressin.
- **Bupivacaine (Marcaine) toxic dose limit is 2.5 mg/kg.**
  - ○ Bupivacaine 0.25% allows for mL used to match the weight (kg) of patient
    - ■ A patient that weighs 70 kg may receive up to 70 mL of bupivacaine
  - ○ Bupivacaine 0.50% allow for ½ mL used to be half the weight of patient
    - ■ A patient that weighs 70 kg may receive up to 35 mL of bupivacaine
  - ○ Always confirm toxic doses with anesthesiologist before injecting large amounts
- Other local anesthetic toxic doses
  - ○ Lidocaine: 4.5 mg/kg
  - ○ Lidocaine with epinephrine: 7 mg/kg
  - ○ Ropivacaine/tetracaine: 3 mg/kg
  - ○ Chlorprocaine: 12 mg/kg

MALIGNANT HYPERTHERMIA

- **Malignant Hyperthermia**
  - ○ Life-threatening reaction to certain anesthetic agents, including volatile anesthetics and succinylcholine.
  - ○ Uncontrolled increase in skeletal muscle metabolism due to mutation in ryanodine receptor inherited in an autosomal-dominant fashion.
  - ○ The disorder exhausts oxygen and leads to rapid increase in carbon dioxide overcoming the body's ability to excrete.
  - ○ *Initial signs can be an increase in end-tidal carbon dioxide, masseter muscle rigidity, and tachycardia/arrhythmia with temperature increase as a late sign.
  - ○ Left unchecked, circulatory collapse and death will occur.
  - ○ *Appropriate treatment includes discontinuation of offending agent, IV dantrolene 2.5 mg/kg, and cooling treatment (ice-filled sponges, gastric lavage, cold wound irrigation) in addition to cardiovascular support.
  - ○ Monitor ABG/electrolytes, I/O balance, core temp, CVP, and CK in ICU for 24 hours.
  - ○ Patients with a personal or family history of malignant hyperthermia should be referred to anesthesia preoperatively.

TABLE 12-1 The 2005 Caprini Risk Assessment Model

Choose all that apply

Each Risk Factor Represents 1 Point

☐ Age 41-60 y
☐ Minor surgery planned
☐ History of prior major surgery (<1 mo)
☐ Varicose veins
☐ History of inflammatory bowel disease
☐ Swollen legs (current)
☐ Obesity (BMI > 25)
☐ Acute myocardial infarction
☐ Congestive heart failure (<1 mo)
☐ Sepsis (<1 mo)
☐ Serious lung disease including pneumonia (<1 mo)
☐ Abnormal pulmonary function (COPD)
☐ Medical patient currently at bed rest

Other risk factors _____

Each Risk Factor Represents 2 Points

☐ Age 60-74 y
☐ Arthroscopic surgery
☐ Malignancy (present or previous)
☐ Major surgery (>45 min)
☐ Laparoscopic surgery (>45 min)
☐ Patient confined to bed (>72 h)
☐ Immobilizing plaster cast (<1 mo)
☐ Central venous access

Each Risk Factor Represents 3 Points

☐ Age over 75 y
☐ History of DVT/PE
☐ **Family history of thrombosis***
☐ Positive factor V Leiden
☐ Positive prothrombin 20210A
☐ Elevated serum homocysteine
☐ Positive lupus anticoagulant
☐ Elevated anticardiolipin antibodies
☐ Heparin-induced thrombocytopenia (HIT)
☐ Other congenital or acquired thrombophilia If yes:

Type _____

*Most frequently missed risk factor

Each Risk Factor Represents 5 Points

☐ Elective major lower extremity arthroplasty
☐ Hip, pelvis, or leg fracture (<1 mo)
☐ Stroke (<1 mo)
☐ Multiple trauma (<1 mo)
☐ Acute spinal cord injury (paralysis) (<1 mo)

For Women Only (Each Represents 5 Points)

☐ Oral contraceptives or hormone replacement therapy
☐ Pregnancy or postpartum (<1 mo)
☐ History of unexplained stillborn infant, recurrent spontaneous abortion (≥3), and premature birth with toxemia or growth-restricted infant

<u>**Total Risk Factor Score**</u> ☐

From Pannucci CJ, Dreszer G, Wachtman CF, et al. Postoperative enoxaparin prevents symptomatic venous thromboembolism in high-risk plastic surgery patients. *Plast Reconstr Surg.* 2011;128(5):1093-1103. PMID: 22030491.

TABLE 12-2 Weighted Risk Stratification Tool for 30-Day VTE Events After Outpatient Surgery

Two-point factors	Three-point factors	Five-point factors
☐ Age 40-59 ☐ OR time ≥120 min ☐ BMI ≥ 40	☐ Age ≥60	☐ Active cancer
Six-point factors	**Eight-point factors**	**Ten-point factors**
☐ Arthroscopic surgery	☐ Current pregnancy	☐ Sapheno-femoral junction surgery
Eleven-point factors		
☐ Non-GSV venous surgery	**TOTAL SCORE** _____	

Total score	30-day VTE rate	Risk level
0-2	<0.1%	Low
3-5	0.1%-0.3%	Moderate
6-10	0.3%-0.5%	High
≥11	Up to 1.2%	Highest

Reprinted from Caprini JA. Thrombosis risk assessment as a guide to quality patient care. *Dis Mon.* 2005;51 (2-3):70-78. PMID: 15900257, with permission from Elsevier.

PEARLS

1. "First do no harm." Assess each surgical candidate for their perioperative risk and treat/prophylaxis accordingly. Anesthetic, endocarditis, cardiac, and VTE risks should be specifically considered.
2. The most overlooked risk factor for VTE is a positive family history.
3. Consider a PECS II block for extensive breast surgery/mastectomies to improve patient's postoperative recovery.
4. Lipid emulsion 20% is used emergently for patients with local anesthetic systemic toxicity.
5. IV dantrolene 2.5 mg/kg is used emergently for patients with malignant hyperthermia.

QUESTIONS YOU WILL BE ASKED

1. Which patient characteristics increase the risk for VTE?
   Many factors are known to increase risk for perioperative VTE. Major factors include cancer, central venous catheters, and a personal or family history of VTE.
2. What options exist for prophylaxis against perioperative VTE?
   The most important decision-making tool for prophylaxis is appropriate risk stratification. Once risk has been quantified, appropriate prophylaxis may include SCDs, early ambulation, and/or chemoprophylaxis. Risk factor modification is also important in the preoperative setting.
3. What is the appropriate treatment for patients suspected of having malignant hyperthermia?
   Appropriate treatment for malignant hyperthermia includes removing the offending agent, administration of dantrolene, and cardiovascular support as necessary.

Recommended Readings

1. Caprini JA. Thrombosis risk assessment as a guide to quality patient care. *Dis Mon.* 2005; 51(2-3):70-78.
2. Dajani AS, Taubert KA, Wilson W, et al. Prevention of bacterial endocarditis. Recommendations by the American Heart Association. *Circulation.* 1997;96(1):358-366.
3. Fleisher LA, Fleischmann KE, Auerbach AD, et al. 2014 ACC/AHA guideline on perioperative cardiovascular evaluation and management of patients undergoing noncardiac surgery: a report of the American College of Cardiology/American Heart Association Task Force on Practice Guidelines. *Circulation.* 2014;130(24):e278-e333.
4. Nishimura RA, Otto CM, Bonow RO, et al. 2017 AHA/ACC focused update of the 2014 AHA/ACC Guideline for the management of patients with valvular heart disease: a report of the American College of Cardiology/American Heart Association Task Force on Clinical Practice Guidelines. *Circulation.* 2017;135(25):e1159-e1195.
5. Pannucci CJ, Dreszer G, Wachtman CF, et al. Postoperative enoxaparin prevents symptomatic venous thromboembolism in high-risk plastic surgery patients. *Plast Reconstr Surg.* 2011;128(5):1093-1103.
6. Pannucci CJ, Fleming KI, Bertolaccini C, et al. Optimal dosing of prophylactic enoxaparin after surgical procedures: results of the double-blind, randomized, controlled, fixed or variable enoxaparin (FIVE) trial. *Plast Reconstr Surg.* 2021;147(4):947-958.

13 Cleft Lip

Gina N. Sacks

OVERVIEW

- Cleft lip (CL) and cleft lip/palate (CLP) are the same entity along a morphologic continuum (**Fig. 13-1**).
  - Variable extent of clefting of the primary palate occurs (**Fig. 13-1**) in CL, including: upper lip, nasal floor (or nostril sill), alveolus, and hard palate (anterior to incisive foramen).
  - May involve the secondary palate (posterior to incisive foramen), and this combination is termed "cleft lip and palate."

EPIDEMIOLOGY

- Incidence of CL with or without cleft palate
  - Caucasian ancestry: 1:1000 live births
  - Asian ancestry: 1:500 live births
  - African ancestry: 1:2000 live births
- Demographics
  - Male:female = 2:1
  - Left:right:bilateral = 6:3:1
- *Risk of clefting in subsequent children
  - *If one child or one parent has CLP, there is a 4% chance of subsequent clefting in successive pregnancies
  - *If two children have CLP: 9%
  - *If one child and one parent both have CLP: 17%

ETIOLOGY

- Most cases are sporadic, multifactorial, and no genetic cause is identified
- Risk factors
  - Fetal exposure to substances including phenytoin, EtOH, steroids, phenobarbital, diazepam, and isotretinoin
  - Maternal smoking
  - Maternal diabetes
  - Parental age, especially advanced paternal age
  - Family history of clefting (see above)
- CLP is syndromic in <15% of cases
  - **Van der Woude syndrome**
    - Most common syndrome associated with CL
    - **Autosomal dominant,** with variable penetrance. Due to mutations in *IRF6* gene
    - **Associated with lip pits** (accessory salivary glands)
    - May also have hypodontia (absent second molar), syndactyly, abnormal genitalia, and popliteal pterygia
  - Waardenburg syndrome (sensorineural hearing loss, iris pigment abnormality, hair hypopigmentation, and lateral displacement of medial canthi)

---

*Denotes common in-service examination topics.

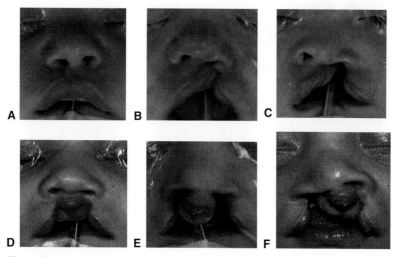

Figure 13-1 The spectrum of cleft lip. A. Microform unilateral cleft lip. **B.** Incomplete unilateral cleft lip. **C.** Complete unilateral cleft lip. **D.** Incomplete bilateral cleft lip. **E.** Complete bilateral cleft lip with "flyaway" premaxilla. **F.** Right complete cleft and left incomplete cleft lip. (From Chung KC. *Grabb and Smith's Plastic Surgery*. 8th ed. Wolters Kluwer; 2020. Figure 25.5.)

- ○ Trisomy 21 (Down syndrome)
- ○ Trisomy 13 (Patau syndrome)
- ○ Trisomy 18 (Edward syndrome)

EMBRYOLOGY/PATHOPHYSIOLOGY

- ***Cleft lip is caused by interrupted mesenchymal migration and failure of fusion between the medial nasal process and maxillary prominence**
  - ○ Neural crest cells are responsible for fusion of facial prominences.
- Critical developmental period: 4-6 weeks
  - ○ Medial nasal processes fuse with maxillary prominences to form philtrum and primary palate (failure causes CL).
  - ○ Maxillary prominences become the lateral upper lip and maxilla and secondary palate.
  - ○ The two lateral palatine shelves that initially lie in a vertical plane adjacent to the tongue move into horizontal plane and fuse at midline along with the primary palate (failure causes CP).
  - ○ Nasal septum forms from fusion of medial nasal prominences and grow downward to join the fused palatal shelf.

CLASSIFICATIONS

- Unilateral vs bilateral
  - ○ **Unilateral CL (Fig. 13-1A-C):** divided into greater segment and lesser segment
    - ▪ Lesser segment collapse, with medial and posterior displacement
  - ○ **Bilateral CL (Fig. 13-1D-F)**
    - ▪ Central prolabium and premaxilla
    - ▪ May have "flyaway" premaxilla **(Fig. 13-1E)** and collapsed bilateral lesser segments

- Variable severity per side (**Fig. 13-1F**)
- More likely to be complete, wide clefts
- Severity/extent (**Fig. 13-1**)
  - **Microform CL** ("forme fruste" or "minor cleft lip"; **Fig. 13-1A**)
    - Vermilion notching, scarlike line or depression, lip shortening
    - ± Nasal deformity, usually mild
    - Surgery may or may not be indicated based on severity
  - **Incomplete CL** (**Fig. 13-1B**)
    - Intact nasal sill (termed "Simonart band"—skin bridge that contains no muscle)
    - Intact alveolar ridge
  - **Complete CL** (**Fig. 13-1C**)
    - Clefting of the lip, nostril sill, and alveolus
    - Wider than incomplete clefts with greater cleft nasal deformity
  - **Complete CLP**
    - CL deformity is same as above
    - Includes CP (posterior to incisive foramen)

RELEVANT LIP ANATOMY

- **Normal lip anatomy** (see Chapter 26: Lip and Cheek Reconstruction, Fig. 26-1)
  - Central philtrum demarcated laterally by philtral columns and inferiorly by Cupid's bow and tubercle
  - Above the junction of vermilion-cutaneous border is mucocutaneous ridge ("white roll")
  - Within red vermilion, noticeable junction demarcating dry and wet vermilion ("wet-dry border")
  - Vertical height of upper lip = peak of Cupid's bow to nasal sill
    - Newborn—10 mm
    - 3 months—13 mm
    - Adult—17 mm
- **Musculature**
  - Orbicularis oris—primary muscle of lip, has two well-defined components (CN VII)
    - Deep (internal)
      - Fibers circumferentially from modiolus to modiolus
      - Functions as the primary sphincter for feeding
    - Superficial (external)
      - Fibers run obliquely, decussate in the midline, and insert into the skin lateral to the opposite philtral groove forming the philtral columns.
      - Philtral dimple is depressed centrally because no muscle fibers directly insert into the dermis in the midline.
      - Provides subtle shades of expression and precise movements of lip for speech.
    - Pars marginalis—portion of orbicularis along the vermilion forming the tubercle of the lip with eversion of the muscle
  - Levator labii superioris
    - Fibers arise from medial aspect of infraorbital rim, insert near vermilion-cutaneous junction helping to define the lower philtral column and peak of Cupid's bow.
    - Functions to elevate the upper lip.
- **Blood supply**
  - Superior labial arteries, bilaterally; columellar branch centrally
    - Branches of bilateral facial arteries
- **Sensory innervation**: upper lip, maxillary division of trigeminal nerve (CN V_2)
- **Motor innervation**: zygomatic and buccal branches of the facial nerve (CN VII)

CLEFT ANATOMY

- **Unilateral CL**
  - ○ Muscles
    - ▪ Pathological insertion of orbicularis oris
      - □ Runs parallel along the edge of cleft and inserts on alar base (cleft side), base of columella (noncleft side)
      - □ Responsible for nasal distortion and widening of cleft with smiling
      - □ In incomplete cleft lips, some superficial orbicularis fibers may traverse superior lip across the cleft
    - ▪ Hypoplasia and disorientation of pars marginalis associated with disappearance of vermilion-cutaneous ridge (white roll) at cleft margin
  - ○ **Vertical lip height is decreased on noncleft side**
  - ○ Nasal abnormalities (**Fig. 13-2**)
    - ▪ Hypoplastic, flattened alar dome on the affected side
    - ▪ Lack of upper lateral cartilage overlap of lower lateral cartilage
    - ▪ Subluxed lower lateral cartilage with alar base displaced cephalad and posteriorly
    - ▪ Hypoplastic bony foundation (maxilla)
    - ▪ Caudal septum is pulled toward the noncleft side by aberrant insertion of orbicularis oris
    - ▪ Flattening of the nasal bones
    - ▪ Shortened columella
- **Bilateral CL**
  - ○ Two lateral components (lesser segments) of lip-alveolus-palate with an intervening prolabium and premaxilla that varies in its degree of protrusion (mild vs "flyaway")
    - ▪ Total absence of orbicularis muscle in prolabial segment results in the absence of philtral dimple/columns/white ridge and median tubercle
    - ▪ Aberrant dry and wet vermilion on prolabial segment
    - ▪ Absence of normal labial-gingival sulcus in premaxillary segment
  - ○ Absence of Cupid's bow
  - ○ Nasal abnormalities
    - ▪ Widened alar bases, with laterally flared alar domes and malpositioned cartilages
    - ▪ Shortened columella
    - ▪ Obtuse nasolabial angle

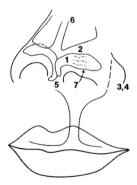

Figure 13-2 **The cleft nasal deformity.** The lower lateral cartilage on the cleft side is abnormally shaped and improperly positioned. Numbers *1* and *7*, hypoplastic, flattened alar dome on the affected side; *2*, lack of upper lateral cartilage overlap of lower lateral cartilage; *3*, subluxed lower lateral cartilage with alar base displaced cephalad and posteriorly; *4*, hypoplastic bony foundation (maxilla); *5*, the caudal septum is pulled toward the non-cleft side; and *6*, flattening of the nasal bones.

EVALUATION

- Often diagnosed prenatally on ultrasound
- Evaluate for associated anomalies (especially with isolated CP)
- Consultations
  - Genetics
  - Social work
  - Feeding/nutrition
    - Monitor for appropriate weight gain
    - May require Haberman bottle or cross-cut nipple to reduce the work of feeding, especially with CP
  - Otolaryngology
    - Eustachian tube dysfunction (**see Chapter 14: Cleft Palate**) often requires myringotomy tubes.
    - Repeat otitis media affects hearing and speech development.

MANAGEMENT

EARLY INTERVENTIONS

- Preoperative molding may be used to bring cleft segments together to minimize tension during repair
  - Taping
    - Applied across both segments of the lip
    - Requires compliant and reliable parents
  - Nasoalveolar molding (NAM)
    - Custom fabricated oral appliance with nasal stents adjusted weekly
    - Positions nasal cartilages and alveolar processes to facilitate closure
    - **Lengthens deficient columella**
    - Takes advantage of increased plasticity of neonatal cartilage
  - Active presurgical infant orthopedics
    - Orthodontic appliance (Latham device) rigidly fixed to palatal segments
    - Parents adjust daily to bring alveolar segments into alignment
    - Removed at the time of definitive lip repair
  - Lip adhesion: suturing cleft margins together
    - Incisions should be made in region that will be discarded at subsequent operation (mark key landmarks)
    - Goal: turn a complete CL into an incomplete CL
    - Definitive lip repair performed several weeks to months later

TIMING OF REPAIR

- 3 months of age, generally accepted
- "Rule of Tens" (historical criteria) for suitability for surgery
  - 10 weeks old
  - 10 lb
  - Hemoglobin 10 mg/dL
- May delay in syndromic patients with systemic concerns

GOALS OF REPAIR

- Goals of unilateral repair
  - Lengthen medial lip element
  - Reconstitute orbicularis oris
  - Restore Cupid's bow, aligning white roll and wet-dry vermilion
  - Correct nasal deformity (primary rhinoplasty)
    - Upright caudal septum
    - Narrow alar base on the cleft side

- Establish convexity of lower lateral cartilage on the cleft side
- May use nasal conformers to maintain shape
  ○ Goals for bilateral repair
    - Reconstitute orbicularis oris across premaxilla
    - Achieve proper prolabial size and shape
      □ ~10 mm height
      □ ~3 mm from midline to each Cupid's bow peak
    - Formation of median tubercle from lateral lip vermillion-mucosa (see "Techniques" later)
    - Correct nasal deformity (primary rhinoplasty)
      □ Narrowing alar base is key difference in emphasis from unilateral technique.
      □ Nasal conformers also used.
    - Symmetry

KEY LANDMARKS (FIG. 13-3)

- Alar bases (ie, *subalare*: alar insertion point onto upper lip)
- Columellar base midpoint
- Commissure bilaterally
- White roll
  ○ At the peak of Cupid's bow on non-CL
  ○ At the trough of Cupid's bow (tubercle) on non-CL
  ○ Additional mark equidistant from the trough to the peak on medial cleft element
    - Define peak of Cupid's bow for CL segment
    - Peaks are ~3 mm from the trough on each side
- *Noordhoff point: vanishing point of white roll on the CL segment
  ○ Most critical and difficult point to identify
  ○ Should correspond to region of thickest vermillion and robust white roll
  ○ In bilateral cases, this is marked on each cleft segment

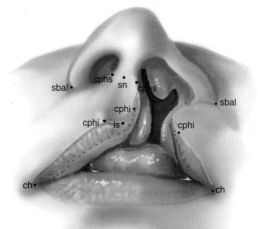

Figure 13-3 Key landmarks in a cleft lip. sbal, subalare; sn, subnasale; cphs, crista philtra superior; cphi, crista philtra inferior (aka Cupid's bow peak), ls, labiale superius; ch, cheilion. (From Chung KC, Disa JJ, Gosain A, Lee G, Mehara B, Thorne CH, van Aalst J. *Operative Techniques in Plastic Surgery.* Wolters Kluwer; 2020. Tech Figure 8.3.1A.)

SURGICAL TECHNIQUES

UNILATERAL CL REPAIR

- Multiple variations of techniques that have evolved over time
- Most are Z-plasty–based reconstructions
- **Straight-line repair (Rose-Thompson):** excision of cleft margin and primary straight-line closure
    - Incorporates Z-plasty to establish normal vertical height of the lip
- **Quadrangular flap (Le Mesurier):** uses a back-cut above Cupid's bow and a laterally based inferior rectangular flap to fill in the rotational defect of the medial lip element
- **Triangular flap (Randall-Tennison, Trauner, and Skoog):** incorporates Z-plasty to restore vertical height
    - May result in excess vertical length
    - Places scar in the center of lip with oblique portion crossing philtrum
- **Rotation advancement: most common type of repair**
    - *Millard: see (Fig. 13-4) for step by step details
        - Incorporates the Z-plasty superiorly
        - "Cut-as-you-go" technique
        - Medial lip rotated downward
        - **C-flap** (*"c" is for columella*): C-flap back-cut is variable and is determined intraoperatively
            - Rotated to create the nasal sill or used to lengthen the columella (more common)
        - **L-flap:** Nasal lining is repaired with L-flap from mucosal portion of lateral segment (*"l" is for lining*)
            - This is required because the cleft ala is posteriorly displaced (**Fig. 13-2**).
            - When ala advanced forward to desired position, mucosal defect must be filled to prevent contraction.
            - May also be filled with turbinate flap.
        - **M-flap:** Gingivolabial sulcus is augmented with M-flap from mucosal portion of medial segment (*"m" is for mucosa*).
        - Scar follows the line of philtral column and preserves Cupid's bow.
        - Orbicularis oris muscle repair is important to restore dynamic lip function.
            - Muscle fibers are inappropriately inserted into the alar base and columella.
            - Must be completely disinserted and repaired in a transverse position.
        - Primary rhinoplasty
            - Diffuse undermining of alar cartilage
            - Transnasal suture techniques to secure desired position
            - May use nasal conformers to maintain shape
        - Common pitfall: inadequate rotation and inadequately corrected vertical lip height on noncleft side; "whistle deformity"
    - **Mohler repair**
        - Similar to Millard but the back-cut is moved from the medial lip element to the columella
            - Allows for scar to simulate the unaffected philtral column
        - End result appears more like an asymmetric Z-plasty repair than rotation advancement
    - **Fisher repair** (anatomic subunit, Fisher DM; *Plast Reconstr Surg.* 2005) (**Fig. 13-5**)
        - Markings are similar to Millard but closure lines are placed along anatomic subunits
        - Stresses the importance of complete leveling of the Cupid's bow
            a = greater lip height
            b = lesser lip height

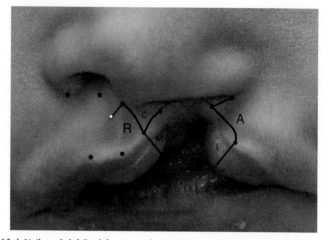

Figure 13-4 Unilateral cleft lip deformity, with preoperative markings for (Millard) repair. For clarity, descriptive anatomy is used in place of numbers. First mark the peak of Cupid's bow on the noncleft side. Then mark the nadir of Cupid's bow. Extrapolate the proposed peak of Cupid's bow in the cleft equidistant from the nadir of Cupid's bow. Next, mark the wet-dry junction on the noncleft side. Then mark the superior point of the philtral column on the noncleft side: this is the height of the normal philtral column that you must achieve on the cleft side. You also need to establish the normal width of the nostril floor. To do this, mark the midpoint of the columellar base and subalare. This distance must equal the distance between subalare on the cleft side and your midline columellar base mark. The defect in the nasal floor will need to be closed to close this distance. At the junction of the nasal floor and the lip skin, mark off a proposed "wedge excision" (two marks here) that will achieve this. Noordhoff's point: the point at which the white roll begins to fade and where the vermillion begins to thin toward the cleft must now be marked. In the Millard repair, the incision is made through the vermillion to the new Cupid's bow peak and then up toward the columellar midpoint. A back-cut via "cut-as-you-go" is then made toward the open circle. This releases the lip, thereby lengthening the noncleft side. Care must be taken to avoid crossing the noncleft philtral column. On the cleft side, the incision is carried through the vermillion and Nordhoff point, to the superior-medial most point on the cleft lip, then back laterally toward subalare along the skin/nostril sill junction. Nasal dissection for primary rhinoplasty is then performed through these incisions. Once the muscle is dissected free of the skin and mucosa, and disinserted from its abnormal attachments, it can be reapproximated transversely in the midline. The mucosa is also closed in a separate layer, using the M-flap, and then the L-flap is used for nasal lining. The C-flap rotates toward the columella for inset, and closure of the lip commences with the white roll. A, advancement flap; R, rotation flap.

- c = difference between "a" and "b"
- A white roll triangular flap (a "Nordhoff triangle" or "c") is used to achieve Cupid's bow symmetry
- The equation: $a - b - 1 \text{ mm} = c$
  □ Accounts for 1 mm lengthening effect
  □ "Rose-Thompson" effect: lip repair via closure as an ellipse will "automatically" lengthen the incision
- Vermilion height is equalized by using a similar triangle as a vermilion flap

BILATERAL CL REPAIR—MILLARD (FIG. 13-6)

- Prolabium is used to create the philtrum only
  ○ Prolabial white roll and vermillion are discarded; the remaining prolabial mucosa is rolled inward to reconstruct the central gingivolabial sulcus

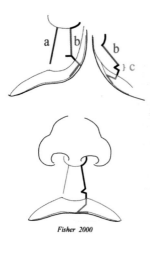

Figure 13-5 Unilateral cleft lip Fisher repair. The height of the greater lip segment is measured from white roll to the apex of philtral column "a." The height of the lesser lip segment is similarly measured "b." The difference between "a" and "b" is made up with a triangle from the cleft lip element "c." Because of the Rose-Thomson effect, 1 mm is subtracted from triangle "c." Noordhoff point is marked on the cleft side. From the proposed location of the philtral column apex on the cleft side, the length "b" is marked with a compass so that it coincides with Nordhoff point and the triangle "c." A back-cut is made beneath "a" to admit the triangle "c." A similar triangle may be required in the vermillion to augment the thickness of the vermillion on the medial aspect of the cleft.

Fisher 2000

- Prolabial vermillion lacks minor salivary glands→using this tissue results in dry, chapped, keratotic "patch"
- Prolabial vermillion previously used in Manchester repair (of historical interest)
- Tip: make width of philtral flap near columella 1-2 mm narrower than inferior portion near white roll to allow for subsequent widening
- Cupid's bow and tubercle reconstructed from lateral lip segments, which are advanced medially beneath the elevated philtral flap
- Alar cinch suture to reposition alar bases
- Common pitfall(s)
  - Inadequate columellar length
  - Poor projection of tubercle
  - May have significant widening of the prolabium

POSTOPERATIVE CARE

GENERAL CONSIDERATIONS
- Early postoperative airway monitoring is required.
- Nerve blocks may be used to help with postoperative pain control.
- Arm restraints are often used but have not been shown to affect complication rates.

COMPLICATIONS
- Early: airway obstruction, hematoma, infection, dehiscence
- Late
  - Hypertrophic scars: consider massage, silicone sheeting, and/or steroid injections
  - **Short scar/lip**
    - May be amenable to the addition of Z-plasty
    - Likely requires complete revision
  - Deficient tubercle
    - Most commonly encountered following bilateral repair
    - If deficiency is minor, can consider dermal or frat graft
    - If deficiency is larger, will likely require Abbe flap
      - Lip sharing procedure from the lower lip
      - Usually performed after maxillary growth or Le Fort I advancement

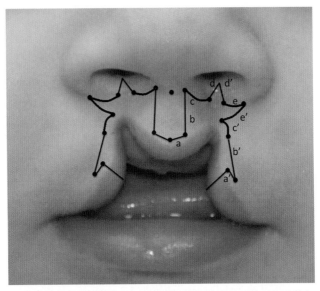

Figure 13-6 Bilateral cleft lip deformity, with preoperative markings. The most inferior point on the prolabium is marked; this will become the trough of the Cupid's bow. The proposed peaks of the Cupid's bow are marked ~3 mm lateral, on each side, to this point. The center of the columellar-labial junction is also marked, and 2 mm lateral to this, on each side, a mark is also made. Draw a neck-tie that connects these dots. On the lateral lip elements, Nordhoff points are defined and marked above the white roll. About 3 mm lateral to these points, a mark is made that will allow (a) and (a') to coincide upon closure. Mark subalare bilaterally. The height of the philtrum (b) is transferred to each lateral lip element (b'). Line (c) is marked extending into the nasal floor and (c') is made to equal length. A similar concept to the unilateral repair is applied to the nasal floor in the bilateral repair, in that a wedge must be taken from the floor to narrow it. This corresponds to (f) and (f'). The prolabial skin inside of the original markings is discarded and the mucosa is used for lining. Lines (e) and (e') are made to close the distance in vertical lip height to subalare. The lateral lip elements rotate downward, forming the tubercle in the midline.

SECONDARY RHINOPLASTY

- May be performed at any age, but commonly at skeletal maturity
- Open approach requires creative use of preexisting incision or judicious planning of transcolumellar incisions
- Requires stable bony foundation for the base of nasal pyramid (ie, previously suitable alveolar bone grafting to address maxillary deficiency)
- Must address poor tip projection and abnormal alar position
- Columella and caudal septum may require repositioning to the cleft side and suturing to the ANS
- Requires addition of anatomic and nonanatomic cartilage grafts
- Alar contour grafts
  - Onlay tip grafts
  - L-strut grafts
  - Severe septal deviation may require aggressive submucous resection of ethmoid in addition to septal cartilage (used for grafts)
- Spreader grafts often needed for airway patency at internal nasal valve (see **Chapter 60: Rhinoplasty**)

QUESTIONS YOU WILL BE ASKED

1. Describe basic CLP epidemiology
   a. Asians>Whites>Blacks
   b. Left:right:bilateral; 6:3:1
2. What are key timepoints and events in CLP embryology?
   a. 4-7 weeks, critical period
   b. Cleft lip: failure of fusion medial nasal process and maxillary prominence
   c. Cleft palate: failure of fusion palatal shelves
3. What is most common CLP syndrome and what are the findings?
   a. Van der Woude
   b. Autosomal dominant with lip pits and CLP
4. What is pathologic anatomy of cleft nasal ala?
   a. Posterior and superior displacement
   b. Loss of convexity of lower lateral cartilage
5. What is primary goal of unilateral CL repair?
   a. Increase the height of medial CL segment
   b. Restore continuity of orbicularis
   c. Reposition alar base(s)

Recommended Readings

1. Fisher DM. Unilateral cleft lip repair: an anatomical subunit approximation technique. *Plast Reconstr Surg.* 2005;116(1):61-71.
2. Millard DR Jr. Complete unilateral clefts of the lip. *Plast Reconstr Surg Transplant Bull.* 1960;25:595-605.
3. Millard DR Jr. Refinements in rotation-advancement cleft lip technique. *Plast Reconstr Surg.* 1964;33:26-38.
4. Mulliken JB. Primary repair of bilateral cleft lip and nasal deformity. *Plast Reconstr Surg.* 2001;108(1):181-194.

14 Cleft Palate

Katelyn G. Makar

OVERVIEW

EPIDEMIOLOGY

- **Isolated cleft palate (CP)** must be differentiated from cleft lip and palate
- **CP**
  - 1 in 700 born with orofacial cleft
  - 6 in 10 000 born with isolated CP
  - No ethnic variation in isolated CP
- **Syndromes and major congenital malformations more common with isolated CP**
  - **DiGeorge syndrome**
    - Most common
    - Cardiac defects
    - Chromosome 22q deletion
  - **Stickler syndrome**
    - Autosomal dominant
    - Mutation in type 2 collagen
- **Cleft lip and palate (see Chapter 13: Cleft Lip for further information)**
  - The vast majority of cleft lips arise spontaneously and are not inherited
  - Ethnic variation in incidence
  - Asians (1 in 500)
  - Whites (1 in 1000)
  - Blacks (1 in 2000)
    - Syndromic conditions less common (eg, Van der Woude syndrome)
    - Predominantly sporadic
    - Always involves the primary palate, with variable involvement of the secondary palate

NORMAL PALATE ANATOMY

- **Hard Palate (Bony Palate; Fig. 14-1)**
  - **Primary palate**
    - Anterior to incisive foramen
      - Nasopalatine nerve
      - Sphenopalatine artery
    - Forms by fusion of median palatine processes (4-7 weeks' gestation) and fuses with developing secondary palate
      - Failure of fusion on one side results in unilateral cleft lip and alveolus
      - Failure of fusion on both sides results in bilateral cleft lip and alveolus
  - **Secondary palate**
    - Posterior to incisive foramen
    - Forms by fusion of lateral palatal shelves of maxillary prominences (8-12 weeks' gestation)
    - Contains the greater palatine foramen
      - Greater palatine nerve and artery (vascular supply for mucoperiosteal flaps)

---

*Denotes common in-service examination topics.

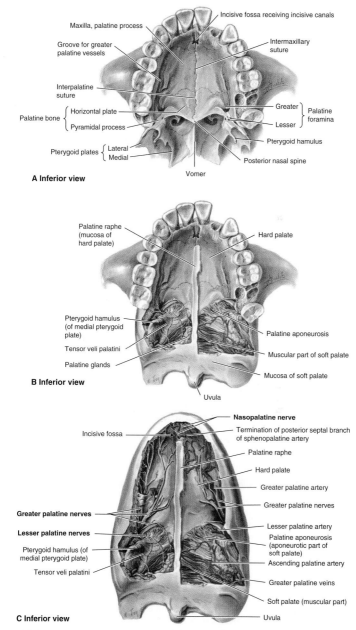

Figure 14-1 Anatomy of the hard palate. A. Normal palatal anatomy with all soft tissue removed. **B.** Palatal anatomy with anterior (hard) palate soft tissue removed. **C.** Palatal anatomy with soft tissue intact, depicting neurovascular supply to palatal muscles and to mucosa. (From Dalley AF II, Agur AMR. *Moore's Clinically Oriented Anatomy*. 9th ed. Wolters Kluwer; 2023. Figures 8.86 and 8.87B.)

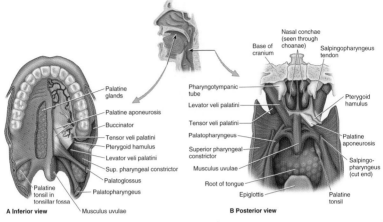

Figure 14-2 Normal palate muscle anatomy. Views of the palatal muscles and their interaction with the pharyngeal constrictors as shown from (**A**) inferior and (**B**) posterior views. (From Dalley AF II, Agur AMR. *Moore's Clinically Oriented Anatomy.* 9th ed. Wolters Kluwer; 2023. Figure 8.88.)

- **Soft Palate (Velum; Fig. 14-2):** mucosa and muscles involved in velopharyngeal (VP) closure (with corresponding innervation)
  - **Levator veli palatini (LVP, CN X)**
    - Lifts velum against posterior pharynx
    - Function: key muscle involved in VP closure
    - Normally oriented transversely across velum to decussate with contralateral muscle in midline, but in CP it is oriented longitudinally and inserts on posterior hard palate
  - **Tensor veli palatini** (CN V)
    - Travels around the hamulus (sphenoid bone)
    - Tendon often divided in repair to further release LVP (intravelar veloplasty [IVV])
    - Function: open eustachian tube
  - **Palatoglossus** (CN X)
    - Originates from the tongue, passes through anterior tonsillar pillar, and inserts on anterior velum
    - Function: velar depression and glossal elevation
  - **Palatopharyngeus** (CN X)
    - Originates from posterior pharynx, passes through posterior tonsillar pillar, and inserts on velum
    - Function: velar depression and retrodisplacement, medialization of pharyngeal walls
    - Used for dynamic sphincter pharyngoplasty
  - **Musculus uvulae** (CN X)
    - Originates from posterior nasal spine
    - Inserts into the base of the uvula (uvula is mostly devoid of muscle)
    - Function: works with LVP to elevate and extend velum
  - **Superior pharyngeal constrictor** (CN X)
    - Broad muscle that encloses naso- and upper oropharynx
    - Originates from pterygomandibular ligament and medial pterygoid plate
    - Inserts into posterior midline at pharyngeal ligament

- Function: medial/sphincteric movement of lateral pharyngeal wall
- Works with palatopharyngeus to form Passavant ridge
- **Vascular Supply**
  - Greater palatine arteries are primary blood supply for palatal mucosa
    - Pedicle for most mucoperiosteal flaps for hard palate closure
    - Located in posterolateral hard palate
  - Lesser palatine arteries: supplies soft palate
    - Sphenopalatine artery
    - Ascending pharyngeal artery of external carotid
    - Ascending palatine branch of facial artery
- **Innervation**
  - Hard palate: greater palatine (CN V) and nasopalatine nerves (CN V)
  - Soft palate: lesser palatine nerve (CN V)

CP ANATOMY AND CLASSIFICATION

- **Variable Severity**
  - **Bifid uvula only**
  - **Submucous CP:** intact mucosa with aberrant musculature, only requires repair if patient demonstrates velopharyngeal insufficiency (VPI)
    - Bifid uvula
    - Hard palate notch (palpable on exam)
    - Zona pellucida: pale midline mucosa
  - **Soft palate cleft only (Veau type I)**
  - **Cleft of soft palate and bony palate up to incisive foramen** (soft and hard palate, Veau type II)
  - **Complete cleft** (a component of cleft lip and CP)
    - Primary and secondary palate
      - If unilateral complete, **Veau III**
      - If bilateral complete, **Veau IV**
- **Anomalous Insertion of Tensor and LVP**
  - Eustachian tube dysfunction and decreased middle ear drainage
    - Recurrent otitis media leading to hearing loss
    - Myringotomy tubes
      - Placed in 95% of CP patients
      - Often at time of CP repair
  - *LVP muscles abnormally oriented in anteroposterior direction instead of transverse direction, inserting onto posterior margin of hard palate

PALATAL EMBRYOLOGY

- **Primary Palate (4-7 Weeks)**
  - Lip, alveolus, nostril sill, and hard palate anterior to incisive foramen.
  - Medial and lateral nasal prominences of frontonasal process migrate and fuse to form median palatine process.
  - Median palatine process forms from fusion of bilateral median nasal prominences and becomes premaxilla.
- **Secondary Palate (8-12 Weeks)**
  - Includes hard palate posterior to incisive foramen and soft palate.
  - Bilateral palatine shelves develop from medial maxillary process.
  - Lateral palatine shelves hang vertically then lift horizontally.
    - Right lateral palatal process becomes horizontal before left, which may explain higher incidence of left-sided clefts.
    - Fusion takes 1 week longer in females, which may explain increased incidence in females.
  - Fusion starts at incisive foramen and moves posteriorly. When interrupted, CP results.

ETIOLOGY
- **Genetics**
    - CP: usually sporadic unless associated with a syndrome
    - CLP: polygenic, usually sporadic
- **Environment**
    - Smoking: inconclusive but many studies have implicated its role
    - Teratogens: alcohol, isotretinoin, topiramate increase risk
    - Obesity
    - Folic acid supplementation may be protective
- **Robin Sequence**
    - Micrognathia leads to glossoptosis, which may cause CP
        - Lateral palatine processes may be unable to fuse due to glossoptosis, causing CP
    - **Clinical triad of micrognathia, glossoptosis, and airway obstruction** (do not have to have a CP to be diagnosed with Robin sequence)
        - Conservative measures: prone positioning and nasopharyngeal airway
        - Sleep study
        - Laryngoscopy to assess if other levels of airway obstruction exist (tracheomalacia, bronchomalacia)
        - Consider mandibular distraction if single-level obstruction at tongue base

INITIAL EVALUATION
- **Feeding and Weight Gain**
    - Haberman or cross-cut nipple required due to poor oral suction.
    - Palate repair is often performed at age 1 year but may be delayed if the patient has multiple comorbidities or if language is delayed.
- **Examination**
    - Use penlight and tongue depressor.
        - Crying infant is easier to examine.
        - Place child supine and upside-down on parent's lap.
        - Look for bifid uvula.
        - Vomer will be visible above palate in cases of bilateral CLP (**Fig. 14-3A**).

MANAGEMENT

GOALS
- **Closure of Cleft**
    - Separate oral and nasal cavities.
    - Prevent nasal regurgitation of oral contents.
- **Normalization of Speech**
    - Requires competent VP mechanism
        - Operative goals: close cleft, reposition LVP, increase length
    - Prevent maladaptive compensatory misarticulations
        - Perform repair by 1 year of age
        - Timing of speech milestone (first words)
            - Prelinguistic testing may indicate need for earlier surgery
- **Hearing**
    - Recurrent otitis media commonly occurs in patients with CP
        - Eustachian tube dysfunction: abnormal LVP insertion impairs "milking" action, which leads to poor venting of middle ear
        - Permanent impairment results with recurrent infection
    - Myringotomy tubes often placed at time of CP repair
        - Some surgeons advocate for tensor tenopexy during palatoplasty to improve eustachian tube function postoperatively
        - Restoration of velar anatomy improves eustachian tube function

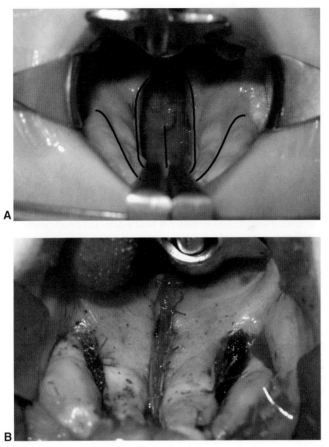

Figure 14-3 Von Langenbeck palatoplasty. A. Preoperative appearance of bilateral cleft palate, surgeons view. Incisions are planned along the cleft margins and in the vomerine mucosa (midline). Lateral relaxing incisions are also shown. The *dotted lines* anteriorly would be incised to convert this bipedicled technique to a unipedicled island flap (Bardach) repair. In the soft palate, a straight-line repair (IVV) is planned. **B.** Appearance of palate after closure of oral mucosa, muscle, and nasal mucosa. Cellulose material has been placed into the lateral defects for hemostasis. (Photos courtesy of Dr. Craig Birgfeld.)

- **Maintenance of Facial Growth**
  - *Palate repair in early childhood may adversely affect maxillary growth, but this drawback is outweighed by the improvements in speech achieved by early correction.
  - Early soft palate and delayed hard palate repair has been advocated (controversial two-stage approach) by some European cleft centers to maximize midfacial growth.
    - Variable speech outcomes.
    - Nearly 90% of U.S. surgeons perform single-stage repair.
  - *Around 25% of patients will require orthognathic surgery in adolescence (Le Fort I advancement; see **Chapter 18: Orthognathic Surgery**) for midface hypoplasia and class III malocclusion.

REPAIR TECHNIQUES

- In CLP (Veau III or IV), both the primary and secondary palates require repair
  - The entire hard palate mucoperiosteum must be elevated for oral sided closure
  - Nasal mucosa elevated off bony cleft margins to provide two-layer closure
  - Vomer flaps utilized for nasal layer closure
  - Soft palate dissection allows for nasal, oral, and muscle repair
- In isolated CP, only the secondary palate requires repair
  - Veau I—soft palate repair only with closure of nasal, muscle, and oral layers
  - Veau II—soft palate repair and posterior hard palate repair that may require lateral relaxing incisions or bipedicled mucoperiosteal flaps if cleft is wide
- Soft Palate Repair Techniques
  - Straight-line repair with intravelar veloplasty (IVV) (Fig. 14-3)
    - IVV first described by Kriens in 1967
    - Useful in wide clefts
    - Three-layered closure (nasal mucosa, muscle, oral mucosa)
    - Correct aberrant insertion of LVP from hard palate and rotate posteriorly into transverse orientation IVV: complete LVP dissection from nasal and oral mucosa, disinsertion from posterior hard palate, and muscle repair in the midline
    - Adverse sequelae: potential for short palate and subsequent VPI
  - Furlow palatoplasty or double-opposing Z-plasty (Fig. 14-4)
    - Opposing Z-plasty flaps for *both* oral and nasal closure
      - Posteriorly based oral myomucosal flap is on the patient's left
        - Conventional technique
        - Remember: easier for right-handed surgeon to elevate the left-sided myomucosal triangle first
      - Posteriorly based nasal myomucosal flap is on the patient's right
    - Rotation of triangles will "automatically" bring LVP muscles into anatomic alignment (recall: anomalous LVP insertion)
    - Lengthens soft palate
    - Offsets the nasal and oral suture lines (decreasing risk for fistulas)
    - Adverse sequelae: sacrifice of width in order to gain length; may not be possible in wide clefts (consider IVV)
- Hard Palate Repair Techniques
  - Von Langenbeck repair (Fig. 14-3)
    - Bipedicled mucoperiosteal flaps
      - Anterior pedicle: blood supply via sphenopalatine a.
      - Posterior pedicle: blood supply via greater palatine a.
    - Parallel incisions are made along cleft margin.
    - Lateral relaxing incisions along lingual side of alveolus left open to heal secondarily.
    - Nasal and oral mucosal flaps are mobilized to midline and sutured in two layers.
    - Adverse sequelae: potential for maxillary growth restriction; high tension repair, which may lead to dehiscence.
  - V-Y pushback (Veau-Wardill-Kilner)
    - Unipedicled flaps
    - V-Y advancement of mucoperiosteal flaps
    - Lengthens palate for speech
    - Adverse sequelae: significant potential for maxillary growth restriction
  - Two-flap palatoplasty (Bardach repair)
    - Requires elevation of entire palatal mucosa: island flap based on greater palatine a.
    - May be used in wide cases of isolated CP to gain extra mucosa for closure

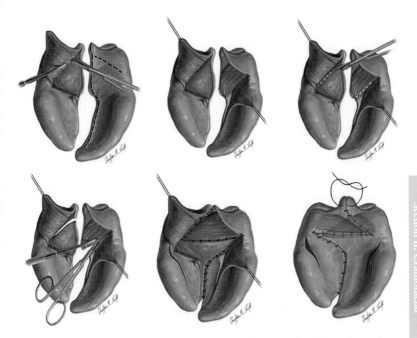

Figure 14-4 Furlow double-opposing Z-plasty. The procedure is not that different from primary cleft palate repair. _Above, left_: the posteriorly based oral musculomucosal flap is elevated first. The clefted levator muscle is detached from its hard palate attachment and nasal mucosa. When the lateral extent of the dissection nears the hamulus, the levator as a distinct muscle bundle coming into the flap. _Above, center_: The lateral limb incision is made from the base of the uvula to just lateral to the hamulus. As the flap is elevated, care is taken to separate the mucosa from the underlying muscle. The plane should be deepened to the back of the hard palate and carefully detached from it, without damaging the greater palatine vessels. _Above, right_: The anteriorly based nasal mucosal flap is incised from the base of the uvula to the superior constrictor. _Below, left_: The posteriorly based nasal musculomucosal flap is created by incising the nasal mucosa 3 to 4 mm from the posterior edge of the hard palate toward the eustachian orifice for ~1 cm. With the tip of the flap pulled transversely, the levator muscle is released carefully from the new free margin of the nasal mucosal incision, and the lateral limb incision is extended until the tip of the flap will reach the end of the contralateral nasal mucosal flap lateral limb incision. This brings the distal end of the levator muscle against the contralateral superior constrictor and immediately under the contralateral levator. _Below, center_: Flaps are then inset, beginning with the nasal musculomucosal flap, bringing the tip of the levator muscle to the contralateral superior constrictor. _Below, right_: The tip of the oral musculomucosal flap is positioned at the point along the lateral limb incision over the contralateral levator muscle belly, just posterior to the hamulus, orienting the levator transversely to complete the overlapping levator sling. (Reprinted with permission from Naran S, Ford M, Losee JE. What's new in cleft palate and velopharyngeal dysfunction management? *Plast Reconstr Surg.* 2017;139(6):1343e-1355e. Figure 4.)

- ▪ Most common repair in Veau III and IV
- ▪ Adverse sequelae: anterior areas heal secondarily causing maxillary growth restriction
- **Additional Maneuvers for Wide Clefts**
  - ○ Infracture of the hamulus can bring lateral elements toward midline
  - ○ Osteotomy of greater palatine foramen for increased pedicle length

○ The periosteal sheath around pedicle can be released with meticulous dissection to gain additional pedicle length

ADJUNCTIVE TECHNIQUES

- **Buccal Fat Pad Flaps**
  - ○ Used to cover raw surfaces of hard palate laterally to minimize scarring and secondary growth restriction or to fill in dead space at areas of high tension (hard-soft palate junction) to decrease risk of fistula
  - ○ Small incision made just lateral to maxillary tuberosity
  - ○ Fat "teased" from buccal space with gentle spreading motion
  - ○ Can be spread to cover surprisingly large surface area
  - ○ Will mucosalize secondarily
- **Vomer Flaps**
  - ○ Based superiorly
  - ○ Used for nasal mucosal closure anteriorly in all Veau III/IV repairs
- **Facial Artery Myomucosal Flap**
  - ○ Intraoral mucosal flap based on facial artery.
  - ○ Often used to repair palatal fistulae secondarily
- **Gingivoperiosteoplasty**
  - ○ Can obviate the need for secondary bone grafting during mixed dentition
  - ○ May be indicated at time of lip repair to close alveolar segments
  - ○ Only feasible if greater and lesser segments are within ~1 mm of each other
    - Performed frequently at cleft centers that utilize nasoalveolar molding or Latham devices

POTENTIAL COMPLICATIONS OF CP REPAIR

- **Acute Airway Obstruction**
  - ○ Bleeding/aspiration/laryngospasm.
  - ○ Tongue swelling due to reperfusion injury from Dingman mouth gag.
  - ○ Reintubation in immediate perioperative period is ~1%.
  - ○ Some patients require ICU admission for closer monitoring.
  - ○ Place tongue stitch and nasopharyngeal airway postoperatively.
  - ○ Pulse oximetry overnight.
- **Dehiscence of Palatal Flaps**
  - ○ Undue tension
  - ○ Poor flap vascularity
  - ○ Poor tissue handling
- **Palatal Fistula**
  - ○ Reported rates range from 5% to 50%.
  - ○ More common in Veau III/IV than Veau I/II.
  - ○ *Hard/soft palate junction is the most common location.
  - ○ Requires repair if causes nasal regurgitation of food or hypernasality.
- **Midfacial Growth Restriction**
  - ○ Intrinsic midface growth problems are present in children with CP or CLP.
  - ○ Scarring/secondary healing from palate repair exacerbates maxillary growth restriction.
  - ○ May be reduced by avoiding secondary intention healing.
    - Limit undermining when possible.
    - Use buccal fat pad flaps to close lateral open areas.
  - ○ Timing of palate repair: as late as possible to allow maximal growth, but before the emergence of speech.
- **Hyponasality:** much less common than VPI; related to overaggressive closure of velopharynx
- **VPI** (Please see **Chapter 15: Velopharyngeal Insufficiency** for details)

- ○ **Incomplete closure of velum**
  - ▪ Air escape through nasopharynx
  - ▪ Hypernasal speech
  - ▪ Secondary to inadequate palatal length or poor muscle function
- ○ 20% incidence following palatoplasty
- ○ **Patient develops maladaptive compensatory substitutions** of abnormal for normal sounds in order to be understood
  - ▪ Pharyngeal fricatives
  - ▪ Glottal stops
- ○ Treatment
  - ▪ **Obturator** (prosthesis) to fill areas of tissue deficit
  - ▪ **Posterior pharyngeal flap** (PPF)
    - □ Static, nonphysiologic technique
    - □ Myomucosal flap from posterior pharynx
      - ▪ Mucosa and superior pharyngeal constrictor m.
      - ▪ Superiorly based and sutured to soft palate
    - □ Appears as a tissue "bridge" with two lateral ports
    - □ Requires the patient to have movement of lateral walls
  - ▪ **Dynamic Sphincter Pharyngoplasty (DSP)**
    - □ Dynamic technique
    - □ *Superiorly based myomucosal flaps from posterior tonsillar pillar flaps (palatopharyngeus m.)
    - □ Crossed and overlapped (to variable degrees) in midline
    - □ Indicated with absent or minimal medial excursion of lateral walls
    - □ Appears as a single port
  - ▪ **Buccal myomucosal flaps**
    - □ Myomucosal flaps elevated intraorally from buccal mucosa
    - □ Soft palate released from hard palate
    - □ Flaps used to fill subsequent defect, with one providing nasal closure and the other providing oral closure
    - □ Decreased risk of sleep apnea compared with PPF and DSP
  - ▪ **Posterior pharyngeal fat grafting** (PPFG)
    - □ Hand-assisted liposuction
    - □ Injection into submucosa of posterior pharyngeal wall to narrow distance to velum
    - □ Usually indicated in very small defects identified on nasendoscopy (0.5-1 cm^2)
- • **Obstructive sleep apnea (OSA)**
  - ○ Increasingly diagnosed in CP population
  - ○ More likely following secondary speech operations: PPF, DSP, and PPFG

PEARLS

1. Be prepared to place the Dingman mouth gag and mark the incisions on the palate. All residents should attempt this, no matter what PGY level.
2. At the University of Michigan, we place the Furlow incisions more posteriorly in the soft palate in order to increase mobilization and allows the surgeon to take advantage of the laxity of the buccal mucosa, rather than the immobile hard palate mucosa. We still dissect the entire muscle off the posterior hard palate, such that the myomucosal flaps have a "tongue" of muscle that extends beyond the mucosal flap tips.
3. In very wide clefts, you may need to consider a straight-line repair as opposed to a Furlow palatoplasty. The Furlow technique gains length at the expense of width (as do all Z plasties), and if your cleft is extremely wide, you may not have the freedom to sacrifice width.

4. Tag your oral Furlow flaps with a Vicryl and "hang" the Vicryl on the Dingman. This keeps the flaps out of your way as you incise the nasal flaps and helps keep you oriented when it is time to close.
5. As you close the nasal mucosa, keep your knots on the nasal side. This helps prevent irritation and inflammation between your layers as the sutures dissolve and also prevents pooling of mucus at the suture line within the nose.

QUESTIONS YOU WILL BE ASKED

1. What is the effect of palatoplasty on maxillary growth?
   It causes maxillary growth restriction.
2. What is the most common location for a palatal fistula?
   At the junction of hard and soft palates.
3. What is the blood supply to the hard and soft palate?
   Hard palate: greater palatine artery. Soft palate: lesser palatine artery, ascending pharyngeal artery, and ascending palatine branch of facial artery.
4. What muscle is being reoriented and repaired?
   Levator palatini.

THINGS TO DRAW

Draw out a Furlow palatoplasty. See Figure 14-4.

Recommended Readings
1. Fisher DM, Sommerlad BC. Cleft lip, cleft palate, and velopharyngeal insufficiency. *Plast Reconstr Surg.* 2011;128(4):342e-360e.
2. Furlow LT Jr. Cleft palate repair by double opposing Z-plasty. *Plast Reconstr Surg.* 1986;78(6):724-738.
3. Liau JY, Sadove AM, van Aalst JA. An evidence-based approach to cleft palate repair. *Plast Reconstr Surg.* 2010;126(6):2216-2221.
4. Smith DM, Losee JE. Cleft palate repair. *Clin Plast Surg.* 2014;41(2):189-210.
5. Woo AS. Evidence-based medicine: cleft palate. *Plast Reconstr Surg.* 2017;139(1):191e-203e.

15 Velopharyngeal Insufficiency

Alexandra O. Luby

OVERVIEW

- Children born with cleft lip and palate are at a high risk for developing disorders of speech, language, resonance, and voice. This can be due to abnormalities in dentition or occlusion, hearing loss, upper airway obstruction, or velopharyngeal insufficiency.
- The primary goal of cleft palate repair: structural and functional restoration of the palate to allow for normal speech. Yet, ~20%-30% of children with repaired palate develop velopharyngeal dysfunction.
- **Velopharyngeal Dysfunction (VPD):** inability of the velum (soft palate) to completely close the nasal cavity during production of oral sounds
- **Velopharyngeal Insufficiency (VPI):** anatomic or structural abnormality (ie, tissue deficit) that prevents complete velopharyngeal closure, resulting in a persistent connection between the nasal and oral cavities
  - Most common type of VPD.
  - Results in hypernasal speech, increased nasal resonance, nasal air emission.
  - Often develop some degree of velopharyngeal mislearning in attempt to compensate
    - Compensatory misarticulations: due to incorrect articulation due to abnormal structure
    - Examples: glottal stops, pharyngeal fricatives
  - Can dramatically impact overall speech intelligibility and negatively impact quality of life including social interactions.
  - Most common cause of VPI: cleft palate. In repaired cleft palates, VPI is most often due to inadequate velar length, levator veli palatini (LVP) dysfunction, and scarring of the velum.
  - Other causes: submucous cleft palate, iatrogenic VPI due to adenoidectomy or uvulopalatopharyngoplasty (UP3), palatopharyngeal imbalance as in 22q11.2 deletion.

VELOPHARYNGEAL ANATOMY AND PHYSIOLOGY OF SPEECH PRODUCTION

- Velopharyngeal Sphincter (**Fig. 15-1**)
  - Comprised of the soft palate anteriorly, lateral pharyngeal walls, posterior pharyngeal wall
    - Muscles: LVP, tensor veli palatini, palatoglossus, palatopharyngeus, muscularis uvulae, superior constrictor muscles
  - Function: allows closure of the VP port to separate nasal and oral cavities
  - Important for coordinated speech and swallow
  - Regulates air flow between nasal and oral cavities and prevents regurgitation of food/drink
  - Physiology of VP closure: LVP contracts and pulls the velum posteriorly and superiorly, while the lateral pharyngeal walls move medially, and posterior pharyngeal wall moves anteriorly

*Denotes common in-service examination topics.

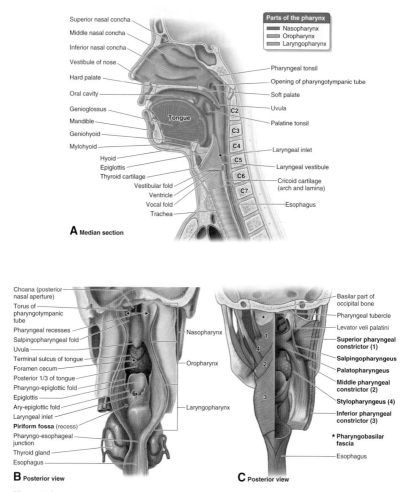

Figure 15-1 Pharyngeal anatomy. Nasopharynx, oropharynx, and laryngopharynx. **A.** Parts of pharynx. **B.** Anterior wall of pharynx. The posterior wall has been incised along the midline and spread apart. **C.** Muscles. The posterior wall of the pharynx has been incised in the midline and reflected laterally, and the mucous membrane has been removed from the right side. (Based on Tank PW, Gest TR. *Lippincott Williams & Wilkins Atlas of Anatomy.* 2008:305, plate 7.10. In: Agur AMR, Dalley AF II. *Moore's Essential Clinical Anatomy.* Wolters Kluwer; 2020. Figure 9.22.)

- **Sound Production**
  - VP closure with adequate seal is important to be able to direct air to the oral cavity with enough pressure to produce certain sounds.
  - Oral sound production: palate must close off the nasal cavity and so that all air is directed through the mouth.
    - Essentially all consonants except m, n, ng (p, b, t, s, d, k, g, f, v, z, etc.) and vowel sounds
    - Enough oral pressure is required to produce oral plosives ("p" sound), fricatives ("s" sound), and affricatives ("ch" sound)

- o Nasal sound production: palate remains open to allow air through the nose (m, n, ng).
- o During spontaneous, connected speech, the palate must move quickly to coordinate air movement through the air and nose to produce appropriate sounds.
- **Resonance**
  - o Balance of sound energy as it travels through the vocal cords, oral cavity, and nasal cavity.
  - o Augmenting the size and shape of these cavities augments the sound.
  - o Types of resonance
    - ▪ Hypernasality: occurs when too much sound is transmitted through the nasal cavity during speech
      - ▫ Presents as nasalization of voiced consonants
      - ▫ Examples: m for b, n for d
      - ▫ Note: patients with oronasal fistulas will often have hypernasal speech but this is a separate etiology from VPI
    - ▪ Hyponasality: occurs when obstruction in the nasopharynx or nasal cavity prevents sound from resonating in the nasal cavity
    - ▪ Mixed resonance: occurs when there is hypernasality on oral consonants and hyponasality on nasal consonants

PREOPERATIVE EVALUATION

- **Patient History**
  - o Past medical history: history of cleft palate, submucous cleft, any syndromes including 22q11 deletion syndrome, neurologic disorders
  - o Past surgical history: adenoidectomy, tonsillectomy, prior palate repair
  - o Feeding/swallowing history
  - o Airway history, history of snoring or obstructive sleep apnea (OSA) diagnosis
  - o Developmental history (including motor, speech, language, learning)
  - o Otologic history: previous hearing assessment, history of recurrent ear infections
  - o Speech: previous or current speech therapy, current speech concerns from parents, patient, teachers
- **Subjective Speech Assessment**
  - o Evaluate speech intelligibility, resonance, articulation, and nasal air escape.
  - o Many ways to assess speech: single word articulation tests, syllable repetition, sentence repetition, counting, spontaneous connected speech.
    - ▪ Examples of short sentences to assess hypernasality
      - ▫ "Do it today for dad," "puppy pulls a rope," "buy baby a bib," "sissy sees the sky," "zip up the zipper"
    - ▪ Counting: have the child count from 60 to 70 ("s")
  - o Facial grimace during speech: grimace constricts the nasal passage to decrease nasal air escape.
  - o Evaluate for air escape: hold a mirror under nose and look at nasal air flow during speech.
  - o Evaluate resonance
    - ▪ Nasal occlusion test: pinch nose to occlude the nares, and have child say phrase without nasal constants (eg, "buy baby a bib")
      - ▫ In normal resonance, should be no change
      - ▫ In hypernasality, resonance will be improved with nasal occlusion
- Formal perceptual speech evaluation by a licensed speech language pathologist
  - o Remains the gold standard for diagnosis of VPI
  - o Perceptual analysis can be used to predict VP gap size
- **Physical Exam**
  - o Palate
    - ▪ Assess size, shape, elevation, movement
    - ▪ Assess for any oronasal fistulas

- If no history of cleft palate, assess for signs of submucous cleft: notching of hard palate, bivid uvula, zona pellucida secondary to levator diastasis
  - Tonsils, uvula, dentition, occlusion, relationship of the tip of the tongue to the alveolar ridge
  - Intranasal exam: assess nasal mucosa, turbinates, and nasal septum
- **Further Diagnostics**
  - Nasometry
    - Method of measuring nasal air emission and calculating nasalance—the ratio between nasal and oral sound emission through a computer-based instrument
    - Produces a quantitative value that can be compared with age normative values
    - Does not characterize VP gap (size, location, closure pattern)
  - Nasoendoscopy
    - Nasal endoscopy allows direct visual observation of the velopharyngeal mechanism during phonation
    - Determines the degree and pattern of VP closure, size of VP gap, position and function of the LVP, length and movement of the soft palate, movement of lateral and posterior pharyngeal walls
    - Best procedure to visualize VP movement and closure during speech to formulate patient specific treatment plans, especially for surgical planning
    - VP closure patterns in VPI
      - Coronal closure: posterior pharyngeal wall and palate
      - Sagittal closure: lateral pharyngeal walls
      - Circular closure: symmetric
  - Video fluoroscopy
    - Two-dimensional view of the velopharynx movement during speech through a series of x-rays
    - Provides less information than nasoendoscopy but better tolerated than nasoendoscopy
  - CTA or MRA
    - Not routine but should be considered in the preoperative work-up of patients with 22q11.2 deletion syndrome as they often have aberrant anatomy of internal carotid with medial displacement

TREATMENT

- **Nonsurgical**
  - Speech therapy
    - Key component of treatment of VPI
    - Can be used to correct compensatory misarticulations after surgery
  - Prosthetics
    - Obturator to fill area of tissue deficit to allow for VP closure
    - Custom prosthetic appliance made by prosthodontist
    - Important for patients who are not surgical candidates or as a temporary solution for those awaiting surgery
- Speech Surgery
  - Type of surgery is based on formal perceptual speech analysis, VP closure characteristics (VP gap size, closure pattern, location), and surgeon preference.
  - Ideally speech surgery should be done around 5 years of age.
- **Palatal Lengthening Techniques**
  - **Double opposing Z-palatoplasty**
    - Indications: small VP gaps with sagittal closure pattern and sagittally oriented LVP; either in unrepaired or in previously repaired palate with minimal muscle repositioning
    - Repositions LVP transversely, improves palatal motion, lengthens palate (**see Chapter 14: Cleft Palate**)

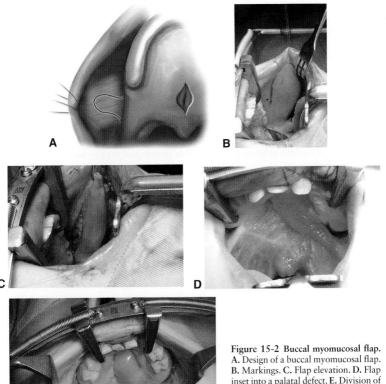

Figure 15-2 Buccal myomucosal flap. A. Design of a buccal myomucosal flap. **B.** Markings. **C.** Flap elevation. **D.** Flap inset into a palatal defect. **E.** Division of base of flap. (From Pearson GD. Palatal fistula. In: Chung KC, ed. *Operative Techniques in Plastic Surgery*. Wolters Kluwer; 2020:2696-2705. Tech Figure 8.13.3.)

- ○ Buccal myomucosal flap (**Fig. 15-2**)
  - ▪ Indications: small to moderate central VP gaps
  - ▪ Buccinator myomucosal flaps are raised from the bilateral cheeks
    - □ Buccal mucosa and buccinator m.
    - □ Transposed and advanced lengthens the soft palate
- • **Pharyngeal Augmentation Techniques**
  - ○ Posterior pharyngeal flap
    - ▪ *Indications: moderate to large VP gap but with good lateral wall motion
    - ▪ Static, nonphysiologic technique
    - ▪ Myomucosal flap from posterior pharynx
      - □ Mucosa and superior pharyngeal constrictor m.
      - □ Superiorly based and sutured to posterior soft palate
    - ▪ Creates a tissue "bridge" between palate and posterior pharyngeal wall with two lateral ports for nasal airflow, which are occluded by the lateral pharyngeal walls during VP closure
  - ○ Sphincter pharyngoplasty
    - ▪ *Indications: restricted or absent lateral pharyngeal wall movement
    - ▪ Dynamic, physiologic technique

- Superiorly based myomucosal flaps from the posterior tonsillar pillars
  □ Mucosa and palatopharyngeus m.
  □ Flaps are transposed and overlapped in midline of posterior pharyngeal wall
- Creates a single, central VP port
○ **Posterior pharyngeal wall augmentation**
  - Indications: small, central VP gaps or to augment other techniques with small gap.
  - Can be used to augment the posterior pharyngeal wall.
  - Historically, many different materials used for augmentation, but fat is most common.
  - Hand assisted liposuction on available donor site, usually abdomen or flank.
  - Inject fat into submucosa of posterior pharyngeal wall to narrow distance to velum.

COMPLICATIONS

- Acute Airway Obstruction
- Obstructive Sleep Apnea
  ○ Up to 35% of patients who have posterior pharyngeal flap can develop OSA in the early postoperative period.
  ○ Estimated 9% of patients with posterior pharyngeal flap will need revision for OSA.
- Persistent Velopharyngeal Insufficiency: normal in the early postoperative period, will need to continue with speech therapy initially but should gradually improve in time
- Hyponasality: can be caused by excessive narrowing of the VP port, minimizing air movement

QUESTIONS YOU WILL BE ASKED

1. What defines the velopharyngeal port?
   Velum, lateral pharyngeal walls, posterior pharyngeal wall.
2. What must a patient have in order to be considered for a posterior pharyngeal flap for VPI?
   Good lateral wall movement.
3. What muscle is included in the sphincter pharyngoplasty?
   Palatopharyngeus.

Recommended Readings
1. Gart MS, Gosain AK. Surgical management of velopharyngeal insufficiency. *Clin Plast Surg.* 2014;41(2):253-270.
2. Goudy SL, Tollefson TT. Complete cleft care: cleft and velopharyngeal insufficiency treatment in children. In: Hiscock TY, Owen Zurhellen J, eds. *Speech/Resonance Evaluation.* Thieme; 2015.

16 Craniosynostosis and Craniofacial Syndromes

Alexandra O. Luby

CRANIOFACIAL EMBRYOLOGY AND DEVELOPMENT

- Skeletal tissues of the head and face derive from mesenchyme and cranial neural crest cells.
- Bone (Fig. 16-1)
  - Skull development starts at 23-26 days of gestation.
    - **Neurocranium:** develops into calvarium
    - Membranous neurocranium: precursor to the cranial vault
      - Paired frontal, parietal, squamosal temporal, and superior occipital bones
      - *Bone formation through intramembranous ossification (direct ossification of mesenchyme)
    - Cartilaginous neurocranium: precursor to the skull base
      - Sphenoid, ethmoid, mastoid, petrous portion of temporal bone, and inferior occipital bones.
      - *Bones develop through endochondral ossification (ossification of cartilaginous precursor).
  - Viscerocranium: precursor to the bones of the facial skeleton.
    - **Neural crest cells of the first pharyngeal arch (Meckel cartilage)** gives rise to the following:
      - **Maxillary process** (dorsal portion of first pharyngeal arch) forms premaxilla, maxilla, zygoma, and squamous temporal bone.
      - **Mandibular process** (ventral portion of first pharyngeal arch) forms the mandible, malleus, and incus.
    - *Second pharyngeal arch (Reichert cartilage) gives rise to stapes, styloid process of the temporal bone and lesser horn and superior body of the hyoid bone.
    - Bone formation through intramembranous ossification.
- Cranial Sutures
  - Fibrous joints between calvarial bones
  - Metopic, sagittal, coronal, lambdoid, and squamosal sutures (Fig. 16-1)
    - Adjacent osteogenic fronts, interposed mesenchymal tissue, and underlying dura
    - Allow for head expansion during development and deformational changes (ie, passage through birth canal)
      - *Primary stimulus for skull growth is brain growth.
      - Brain is 25% of adult size at birth, 50% at 6 months, and 75% at 1 year.
      - Full adult volume by ~2.5 years.
  - Fontanelles (infantile "soft spots") are the confluence of two or more cranial sutures
    - Anterior fontanelle (bregma): Closes around 2 years of age
    - Posterior fontanelle (lambda): Closes around 2 months of age
  - Suture fusion sequence
    - Metopic: 3-9 months (only suture to obliterate during childhood)
    - Sagittal: 20-22 years
    - Coronal: 23-24 years
    - Lambdoid: 26 years

---

*Denotes common in-service examination topics.

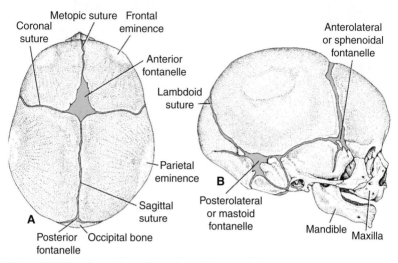

Figure 16-1 Major bones, fontanelles, and cranial sutures of the newborn skull as seen from (**A**) superior and (**B**) lateral views. (From Digestive System. In: Sadler TW. *Langman's Medical Embryology*. 15th ed. Wolters Kluwer; 2024:232-258. Figure 10.5.)

- **Sinus Development**
  - Maxillary and sphenoid: begins at 3 months gestation, complete during childhood
  - Ethmoid: begins at 5 months gestation, complete during childhood
  - Frontal: begins at 5 years old, complete during adolescence; the only one to begin development postnatally

CRANIOSYNOSTOSIS

OVERVIEW

- Premature fusion of the cranial sutures
- *Virchow Law
  - Growth restriction occurs perpendicular to the affected suture.
  - Compensatory skull growth occurs parallel to the affected suture.
- **Nonsyndromic (Primary) Craniosynostosis**
  - Isolated suture fusion without associated abnormalities
  - Largely sporadic pattern of occurrence (incidence 0.6 in 1000 live births)
- **Syndromic Craniosynostosis**
  - Heterogeneous group of disorders marked by premature suture fusion
  - Associated dysmorphic features and congenital abnormalities
  - Genetic heritability patterns (eg, autosomal dominant, a. recessive, and X-linked)
  - Linked to specific gene mutations in some cases (see below)
- **Secondary Craniosynostosis:** premature suture fusion due to other disease processes
  - Hyperthyroidism
  - Idiopathic hypercalcemia
  - Rickets
  - Microcephaly
  - Mucopolysaccharidoses

- ○ Hematologic disorders (thalassemia, polycythemia vera, and sickle cell)
- ○ Iatrogenic (eg, after shunt placement for hydrocephalus)
- **Diagnosis, Workup, and Consultations**
  - ○ History
    - ▪ Abnormal head contour
    - ▪ Sleep disturbances
    - ▪ Regression or failure to meet developmental milestones
  - ○ **Physical exam**
    - ▪ Palpable ridge along synostotic sutures
    - ▪ Lack of movement along sutures with palpation
    - ▪ May have dysmorphic facial features or facial asymmetry
    - ▪ Abnormal head circumference when compared with age-predicted norms
    - ▪ Poorly defined, absent or bulging fontanelles
  - ○ **Evaluate for elevated intracranial pressure (ICP)**
    - ▪ Approximately 10% of single suture synostosis and 40% of patients with multisuture synostosis have elevated ICP.
    - ▪ Irritability, growth impairment, inconsolability, vomiting, bulging fontanelles.
    - ▪ Fundoscopic examination for papilledema.
    - ▪ Requisite neurosurgical consultation in all confirmed patients.
  - ○ **Imaging: CT scan**
    - ▪ Routinely used in diagnosis.
    - ▪ Three-dimensional reformatting for preoperative planning.
    - ▪ Evidence of elevated ICP may be manifested as hydrocephalus or Lückenschädel ("copper beaten") skull.
  - ○ **Genetics evaluation.**
  - ○ **Neuropsychological evaluation** to determine baseline cognitive functioning.
  - ○ **Speech and audiology assessment** should be performed to ensure ongoing language acquisition during development.

NONSYNDROMIC CRANIOSYNOSTOSIS

- **Metopic Synostosis—Deformity: Trigonocephaly**
  - ○ Relatively uncommon: <10% of craniosynostosis
  - ○ Keel-shaped skull with pointed forehead, frontal bossing, bitemporal narrowing, hypotelorism, and recessed superior orbital rims
- **Sagittal Synostosis—Deformity: Scaphocephaly** (Dolichocephaly)
  - ○ *Most common: >50% of craniosynostoses
  - ○ Male predominance: 4:1 male/female ratio
  - ○ Sporadic with 2% genetic predisposition
  - ○ Associated findings: increased AP length of skull, "boatlike" appearance, decreased biparietal width, and frontal and occipital bossing
- **Unilateral Coronal (Unicoronal) Synostosis—Deformity: Anterior Plagiocephaly**
  - ○ Second most common: 20% of craniosynostosis
  - ○ Ipsilateral frontal bone flattening, contralateral frontal bossing, shortened AP dimension on affected side, anterior displacement of ipsilateral ear, and deviation of nasal tip to contralateral side
  - ○ *Harlequin eye deformity
    - ▪ Lack of ipsilateral descent of greater wing of sphenoid during development
    - ▪ **Pathognomonic for unicoronal synostosis**
- **Bilateral Coronal (Bicoronal) Synostosis—Deformity—Brachycephaly**
  - ○ *Most commonly associated with syndromic craniosynostosis (such as Crouzon and Apert syndromes)
  - ○ Frontal bossing, vertical elongation of frontal bones, widening of anterior cranial base, shortened AP skull dimension, occipital flattening, shallow orbits, and hypertelorism

- **Lambdoid Synostosis—Deformity: Posterior Plagiocephaly**
  - Least common: <3% of craniosynostosis
  - May be unilateral or bilateral
  - Flattening of ipsilateral occiput, posterior/inferior displacement of ipsilateral ear, and contralateral occipitoparietal bossing
- **Multiple Suture Synostosis**
  - Usually occurs as a feature of syndromic craniosynostosis.
  - Dysmorphic features depend on the pattern of involved sutures.
  - **Pansynostosis:** fusion of all cranial sutures.
    - **Nonsyndromic pansynostosis**
      - Inadequate volume expansion secondary to impaired brain growth.
      - Skull is normocephalic in contour but microcephalic in volume.
    - **Syndromic pansynostosis**
      - Normal brain growth, which is constrained by the fusion of all sutures
      - Kleeblattschädel deformity: clover leaf skull
        - Ballooning of cranial vertex and squamosal sutures.
        - Immediate surgical decompression at birth to avert neurologic compromise.
        - May require cerebrospinal fluid (CSF) shunt.
        - C-spine must be evaluated for additional abnormalities.

DEFORMATIONAL PLAGIOCEPHALY (POSITIONAL HEAD DEFORMITY, OR POSITIONAL PLAGIOCEPHALY)

- Results from external pressure applied to the pliable fetal or infant skull
- **Must be differentiated from lambdoid or coronal synostosis (Fig. 16-2)**
- **Causes:**
  - Supine sleeping position, which is recommended to decrease the risk of sudden infant death syndrome. This is the most common cause of positional plagiocephaly.
  - *In utero* compression.
  - Vertebral abnormalities.

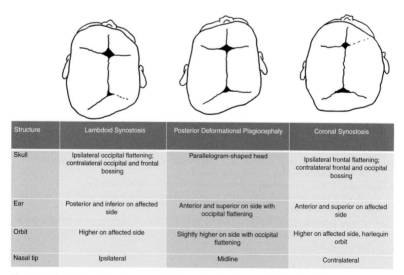

Structure	Lambdoid Synostosis	Posterior Deformational Plagiocephaly	Coronal Synostosis
Skull	Ipsilateral occipital flattening; contralateral occipital and frontal bossing	Parallelogram-shaped head	Ipsilateral frontal flattening; contralateral frontal and occipital bossing
Ear	Posterior and inferior on affected side	Anterior and superior on side with occipital flattening	Anterior and superior on affected side
Orbit	Higher on affected side	Slightly higher on side with occipital flattening	Higher on affected side, harlequin orbit
Nasal tip	Ipsilateral	Midline	Contralateral

Figure 16-2 Distinguishing features of deformational and synostotic plagiocephaly.

- ○ Congenital muscular torticollis (often occurs with deformational plagiocephaly).
- ○ Ocular torticollis: visual field deficits causing preferential head positioning.
- • **Treatment Specific to the Underlying Cause**
  - ○ **Supervised prone positioning** ("tummy time"), physical therapy, stretching and possible muscle release for torticollis, head and neck rotation while feeding, encouraging looking to affected side by positioning infant
  - ○ **Shaping helmets**
    - ▪ Fitted to widest skull dimension.
    - ▪ Compensatory growth occurs due to external forces applied by helmet.
    - ▪ Must be worn for >23 hours per day, for 2-3 months or longer.
    - ▪ Less effective after 18 months of age; early helmeting is much more effective.
    - ▪ Multiple helmet fittings required as cranial contour improves.

SYNDROMIC CRANIOSYNOSTOSIS

- • **Apert Syndrome (Fig. 16-3A)**
  - ○ Genetics
    - ▪ Autosomal dominant inheritance but vast majority of cases represent sporadic mutations
    - ▪ *FGFR2 mutation (chromosome 10)
  - ○ Craniofacial features
    - ▪ Bicoronal craniosynostosis, turribrachycephaly (short AP skull dimension, wide transverse dimension, and increased vertical excess of skull), orbital hypertelorism, proptosis, midface hypoplasia with class III malocclusion, "parrot beak" nose, high-arched palate, occasional cleft palate, and acne
    - ▪ Elevated ICP common
  - ○ *Extremities: severe complex syndactyly of hands and feet in which most or all digits are fused, including phalanges; all interphalangeal joints of fingers are stiff; lack PIP joints; also often have stiffness affecting elbow and shoulder joints; 4-5 metacarpal synostosis; and radial clinodactyly of the thumb
  - ○ Mental status: variable
- • **Crouzon Syndrome (Fig. 16-3B)**
  - ○ Genetics
    - ▪ Autosomal dominant
    - ▪ *FGFR2* mutation
  - ○ Craniofacial features
    - ▪ Coronal and lambdoidal synostosis, turribrachycephaly, exorbitism/proptosis leading to exposure keratitis, midface hypoplasia, class III malocclusion
    - ▪ Features less severe than Apert
    - ▪ Conductive hearing loss due to cranial base abnormalities
  - ○ Extremities: normal
  - ○ Mental status: variable
- • **Saethre-Chotzen Syndrome**
  - ○ Genetics
    - ▪ Autosomal dominant
    - ▪ *TWIST-1 mutation
  - ○ Craniofacial features: asymmetric coronal synostosis, shallow orbits, telecanthus, ptosis of eyelids, midface hypoplasia, deviated nasal septum, low hairline
  - ○ Extremities: partial syndactyly
  - ○ Mental status: usually normal
- • **Pfeiffer Syndrome**
  - ○ Genetics
    - ▪ Autosomal dominant
    - ▪ *FGFR1*, *FGFR2*, *FGFR3* mutations
  - ○ Craniofacial features: turribrachycephaly, coronal and/or sagittal synostosis, shallow orbits, hypertelorism, downslanting palpebral fissures, and midface hypoplasia
  - ○ *Extremities: broad thumbs and great toes, partial syndactyly of digits 2 and 3
  - ○ Mental status: variable

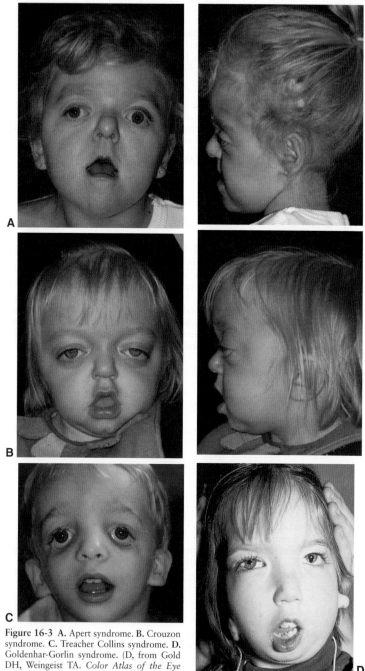

Figure 16-3 A. Apert syndrome. B. Crouzon syndrome. C. Treacher Collins syndrome. D. Goldenhar-Gorlin syndrome. (D, from Gold DH, Weingeist TA. *Color Atlas of the Eye in Systemic Disease*. Lippincott Williams & Wilkins; 2001. Figure 122.1.)

- **Jackson-Weiss syndrome**
  - Genetics
    - Autosomal dominant
    - *FGFR2* mutation
  - Craniofacial features: highly variable, may appear similar to other syndromes
  - Extremities: broad great toes or syndactyly of toes
- **Carpenter Syndrome**
  - Genetics
    - Autosomal recessive (most syndromic craniosynostosis are AD)
    - **RAB23* mutation
  - Craniofacial features: variable suture synostosis, flat nasal bridge, low set ears, abnormal globe, and canthi
  - Extremities: brachydactyly, syndactyly of hands and feet, and short stature
  - Mental status: impaired
- **Boston-Type Craniosynostosis**
  - Genetics
    - Autosomal dominant
    - *MSX2* mutation
  - Craniofacial features: craniosynostosis, soft palate cleft
  - Extremities: short first metatarsal head, triphalangeal thumb

FUNCTIONAL SEQUELAE OF CRANIOSYNOSTOSIS

- **Central Nervous System**
  - Varying degrees of cognitive impairment
  - Possible elevations in ICP (neurosurgical consultation is requisite in all patients)
- **Ocular**
  - Exorbitism may lead to exposure keratitis and visual compromise.
  - Strabismus.
  - Bony orbit and ocular abnormalities may lead to deprivation amblyopia.
- **Airway**
  - Midface hypoplasia may result in varying degrees of airway compromise: from obstructive sleep apnea to critical airway stenosis.
  - Tracheostomy may be required.
  - Monobloc or Le Fort III advancement may also be required.
- **Abnormal Speech and Hearing**

TREATMENT

- **Multidisciplinary team** includes plastic surgeon, neurosurgeon, otolaryngologist, pediatrician, oral surgeon, orthodontist, pediatric dentist, ophthalmologist, geneticist, child neuropsychologist, speech therapist, social worker, dietician, and nurses.
- **Preoperative Considerations**
  - Parents should be engaged in operative plan of care.
  - Preoperative hematocrit with type and cross (~80% perioperative transfusion).
  - Two large-bore peripheral intravenous lines, urinary catheter, and arterial line.
  - ICU bed for 24-48 hours postoperatively.
  - Perioperative antibiotics.
  - Perioperative steroids may be used to decrease swelling.
  - Prone vs supine positioning depending on involved suture(s) and surgeon preference.
    - Special head rest may be necessary.
    - Modified prone positioning.
      - Greater exposure
  - Preoperative cervical spine films required.
  - Ophthalmic ointment and corneal shields.
  - Anesthetic considerations.
    - Warming device to maintain normothermia
    - Hypotensive anesthesia

- Cell-saver devices for directed autotransfusion
- Antifibrinolytics (Amicar) and erythropoietin to mitigate bleeding risk
- **Operative Interventions**
  - Timing: 3 months to 1 year of age (earlier if evidence of elevated ICP).
  - Earlier operation: patient maintains capacity for dural-induced ossification of small cranial defects.
    - Intraoperative tranexamic Acid (TXA) has been show to decrease blood loss and need for transfusion
- **Postoperative Care**
  - ICU monitoring for 24-48 hours.
  - Neurologic checks every 1-2 hours.
  - Serial hematocrits to evaluate ongoing bleeding.
  - Electrolyte abnormalities (especially Na^+) due to disruption of hypothalamic-pituitary axis.
    - SIADH (syndrome of inappropriate antidiuretic hormone): low serum sodium, treat with fluid restriction, salt tabs, or increased sodium in IV fluids.
    - Diabetes insipidus: high serum sodium and increased urine output. Treat with fluid resuscitation due to the risk of dehydration.
  - ICP monitoring (only in select cases).
  - Postoperative fever is very common; postoperative infection is rare.
  - Other complications: venous air embolism, dural lacerations, CSF leak, visual changes, seizures, meningitis, and death.

CRANIOFACIAL (TESSIER) CLEFTS

- **Etiology**
  - Lack of fusion of facial processes
  - Lack of migration of mesoderm
  - Possible amniotic banding
- **General Considerations**
  - Incidence: 1:100 000 births
  - *Tessier classification (Fig. 16-4)
  - "Oculocentric"
    - Cranial clefts extend superiorly from the lid margin.
    - Facial clefts extend inferiorly from the lid margin.
    - Corresponding cranial and facial clefts sum to 14 (eg, 0 and 14, 1 and 13, and 6 and 8).
    - **Tessier 7 cleft**
      - Most common of all craniofacial clefts
      - *Findings: ipsilateral microtia and macrostomia
    - Clefts 0-3: oral-nasal, clefts 4-6: oral-ocular, clefts 7-9 lateral facial.
- Soft tissue abnormalities predict the underlying bony clefts (eg, irregular hairline and lid margins).
- Clefts may involve globe (coloboma) and extraocular muscles.

BRANCHIAL ARCH SYNDROMES AND HEMIFACIAL MICROSOMIA

- Heterogeneous group of syndromes involving Tessier clefts 6, 7, and 8
- Includes Treacher Collins-Franceschetti complex, Goldenhar syndrome, and hemifacial (craniofacial) microsomia
- **Etiology**
  - Vascular insults during embryogenesis (ie, stapedial artery thrombosis)
  - Teratogens: thalidomide and retinoic acid
  - Maternal diabetes

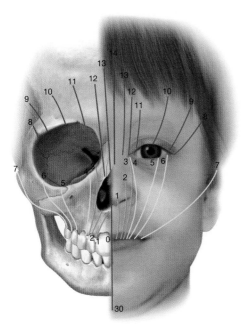

Figure 16-4 Tessier classification of craniofacial clefts. (From Goldstein JA, Losee JE. Craniofacial Clefts and Orbital Hypertelorism. In: Chung KC, ed. *Grabb and Smith's Plastic Surgery*. 8th ed. Wolters Kluwer; 2020:301-311. Figure 32.1.)

Section II: Craniofacial

TREACHER COLLINS-FRANCESCHETTI COMPLEX
(Mandibulofacial Dysostosis, Fig. 16-3C)

- **Genetics**
  - Autosomal dominant
  - *TCOF1* mutation (chromosome 5)
  - *Craniofacial features: features are bilateral and symmetrical, Tessier clefts 6-8, with hypoplasia of body and arch of zygoma, mandibular hypoplasia, retrusion of chin, prominent facial convexity, hypoplastic lower eyelids with coloboma (congenital cleft of eyelid), absence of medial lower eyelashes, and downslanting palpebral fissures, and upper eyelids show tissue redundancy and pseudoptosis
- **Associated Abnormalities**
  - Microtia and middle ear anomalies result in conductive hearing loss.
  - Cleft palate.
  - Abnormalities of hairline.
  - Airway compromise.
    - Decreased pharyngeal diameter secondary to mandibular hypoplasia
    - May necessitate early airway intervention
- **Mental Status:** normal intelligence

HEMIFACIAL (CRANIOFACIAL) MICROSOMIA

- Abnormal development in derivatives of the first and second branchial arches
- **Genetics**
  - Largely sporadic, occasional familial clustering
  - Incidence: 1 in 4000-5000 live births

- ○ Male predominance
- ○ Bilateral involvement in 10%-15% of cases
- **Craniofacial Features**
  - ○ Variable hypoplasia of the skeleton and overlying soft tissues. Three structures most commonly affected: mandible, maxilla, and auricle.
  - ○ Mandible is always involved to a degree. Deformity ranges from mild hypoplasia to complete absence of the ramus, condyle, or temporal mandibular joint.
  - ○ Maxillary hypoplasia, upward occlusal cant on affected side, cross bite, open bite, and macrostomia. "C" deformity on frontal facial view.
  - ○ Orbital dystopia and upper lid colobomas.
  - ○ Facial muscle atrophy and weakness.
  - ○ Cranial nerve abnormalities are frequent—the most common is facial paralysis due to agenesis of facial nerve (CN7).
  - ○ External ear abnormalities with variable middle and inner ear anomalies.
- **Mental Status:** mental deficiency in 10% of cases
- **Classification Systems:**
  - ○ Several classification systems have been proposed.
  - ○ OMENS+: Orbital dystopia, Mandibular hypoplasia, Ear abnormalities, Nerve involvement, Soft tissue deficit, +extra-craniofacial manifestations. Characterizes an individual's manifestations, but does not guide treatment.
  - ○ Pruzansky-Kaban: classification based on the severity of mandibular hypoplasia and TMJ derangement, usually determined by 3D CT. Can be used to guide treatment (**Table 16-1**).
- **Treatment**
  - ○ Treatment depends on patient's phenotype and needs.
  - ○ Mild cases may not require treatment.
  - ○ Mandibular distraction osteogenesis during early adolescence ± reconstruction.
  - ○ Le Fort osteotomy, bilateral split osteotomy of mandible, and genioplasty may be required in skeletally mature patients.
  - ○ External ear reconstruction.
  - ○ Audiologic evaluation and treatment for hearing loss.

TABLE 16-1 Pruzansky-Kaban Classifications of Hemifacial Microsomia and Associated Treatments

Pruzansky-Kaban type	Description	Treatment
Type I	Hypoplastic temporomandibular joint (TMJ), but normal mandibular and TMJ shape	Orthodontia ± orthognathic surgery
Type IIa	Hypoplastic mandibular ramus, condyle, and TMJ with abnormal shape but TMJ articulation maintained	Mandibular distraction
Type IIb	Hypoplastic mandibular ramus with abnormal shape and location, lacking articulation with temporal bone	Mandibular distraction OR nonvascularized bone graft of ramus and condyle
Type III	Absent mandibular ramus, condyle, and TMJ (with or without adequate mandibular body bone stock)	Nonvascularized bone graft (ie, costochondral or iliac crest) OR if inadequate mandibular body bone stock, free fibula

GOLDENHAR-GORLIN SYNDROME
(Oculoauriculovertebral Dysplasia; Fig. 16-3D)

- **Genetics:** majority of cases are sporadic.
- **Craniofacial Features**
  - Within the spectrum of hemifacial microsomia but more severe
  - Prominent frontal bossing, low hairline, mandibular and maxillary hypoplasia, facial muscle weakness, epibulbar dermoids (ocular dermoid tumors), preauricular skin tags and ear pits, conductive hearing loss, and vertebral abnormalities
- **Treatment:** similar to hemifacial microsomia

QUESTIONS YOU WILL BE ASKED

1. What is Virchow law.
   Growth restriction occurs perpendicular to the affected suture, whereas compensatory skull growth occurs parallel to the affected suture.
2. What is the difference between synostotic and deformational plagiocephaly.
   Deformational plagiocephaly results from external pressure applied to the pliable fetal or infant skull vs craniosynostosis, which is due to premature fusion of cranial sutures and resultant compensatory growth according to properties of Virchow law.
3. What is the most common craniofacial cleft.
   Tessier cleft 7 resulting in ipsilateral microtia and macrostomia.
4. Describe the characteristic findings in syndromic craniosynostosis.
   See Section Syndromic Synostosis and **Figure 16-3**.

Recommended Readings
1. Czerwinski M, Hopper RA, Gruss J, Fearon JA. Major morbidity and mortality rates in craniofacial surgery: an analysis of 8101 major procedures. *Plast Reconstr Surg.* 2010;126(1):181-186.
2. Czerwinski M, Kolar JC, Fearon JA. Complex craniosynostosis. *Plast Reconstr Surg.* 2011;128(4):955-961.
3. Fearon JA, Ruotolo RA, Kolar JC. Single sutural craniosynostoses: surgical outcomes and long-term growth. *Plast Reconstr Surg.* 2009;123(2):635-642.
4. Kaban LB, Padwa BL, Mulliken JB. Surgical correction of mandibular hypoplasia in hemifacial microsomia: the case for treatment in early childhood. *J Oral Maxillofac Surg.* 1998;56(5):628-638. doi:10.1016/s0278-2391(98)90465-7
5. Oh AK, Wong J, Ohta E, Rogers GF, Deutsch CK, Mulliken JB. Facial asymmetry in unilateral coronal synostosis: long-term results after fronto-orbital advancement. *Plast Reconstr Surg.* 2008;121(2):545-562.
6. Smartt JM Jr, Reid RR, Singh DJ, Bartlett SP. True lambdoid craniosynostosis: long-term results of surgical and conservative therapy. *Plast Reconstr Surg.* 2007;120(4):993-1003.
7. Tessier P, Kawamoto H, Posnick J, Raulo Y, Tulasne JF, Wolfe SA. Taking calvarial grafts, either split in situ or splitting of the parietal bone flap ex vivo—tools and techniques: V. A 9650-case experience in craniofacial and maxillofacial surgery. *Plast Reconstr Surg.* 2005;116(5 Suppl):54S-71S; discussion 92S-94S.
8. Warren SM, Proctor MR, Bartlett SP, et al. Parameters of care for craniosynostosis: craniofacial and neurologic surgery perspectives. *Plast Reconstr Surg.* 2012;129(3):731-737.

Section II: Craniofacial

17 Reconstruction of Congenital Ear Deformities

Chien-Wei Wang

EXTERNAL EAR EMBRYOLOGY AND ANATOMY

- **Embryology of the External Ear**
  - Auricle
    - Hillocks of His: six condensations of mesoderm that develop into the auricle (**Fig. 17-1**)
      - □ Contribution from both 1st (mandibular) and 2nd (hyoid) brachial arches
        - *1-3 anterior (1st brachial arch): tragus, root of the helix, and helix.
        - *4-6 posterior (2nd branchial arch): antitragus, antihelix, and lobule. Lobule is the last to develop.
    - Development time frame: begins at 6-8 weeks and is fully formed by 4 months.
    - The auricle forms in the lower neck and migrates cranially during mandibular development. Arrested growth results in low-set ears.
  - External auditory canal (EAC)
    - Canalization of the meatal plug: ectodermal cells (1st brachial cleft) degenerate at 28 weeks to form the EAC
      - □ Failure to canalize leads to congenital aural atresia or stenosis.
    - Sigmoid shaped and ~2.5 cm in length and 1 cm in diameter
      - □ Outer one-third: fibrocartilaginous
      - □ Inner two-thirds: bony
  - Tympanic membrane (ear drum)
    - Development: thin membrane formed from invagination and meeting of the 1st brachial cleft (groove) with the 1st branchial pouch
    - Three layers: outer epithelial layer (ectoderm), middle fibrous layer (mesoderm), and inner mucosal layer (endoderm)
    - Two parts: pars flaccida (small, triangular, flaccid) and pars tensa (large, oval-shaped, tense)
    - Separates external ear from middle ear
- **Surface Topographic Landmarks (Fig. 17-1)**
- **Anatomy**
  - Blood supply
    - Arterial supply from branches of external carotid artery (**Fig. 17-2A**)
      - □ *Posterior auricular artery: dominant blood supply to both the anterior (through perforating branches) and posterior surfaces of the ear
      - □ Superficial temporal artery: supplies the anterior surface of the ear and forms numerous interconnections with the posterior auricular artery, allowing ear replantation based solely on either arterial network
      - □ Occipital artery: supplies the posterior surface of the ear (minor contributor) and the retroauricular skin
    - Venous drainage: follows the feeding arteries and empties into the retromandibular vein (external jugular system)
  - Sensory innervation (**Fig. 17-2B**)
    - Great auricular nerve (C2, C3)

---

*Denotes common in-service examination topics.

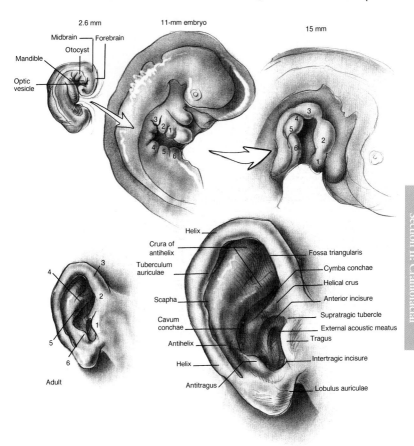

Figure 17-1 The auricle is formed from six auricular hillocks, three each from branchial arches I and II. Surface anatomy of the auricle (*bottom right*). (From Johnson J. *Bailey's Head and Neck Surgery.* 5th ed. Wolters Kluwer; 2014. Figure 146.1.)

- □ Innervates: lower half of both anterior and posterior surfaces of the ear
- □ Landmarks
  - Erb point (6.5 cm below the tragus at the posterior border of the SCM)
  - Runs posterior and parallel to the external jugular vein
- Auriculotemporal nerve (V3)
  - □ Innervates the upper half of the anterior surface of the ear and the anterior portion of the EAC
  - □ Landmarks: ascends with the superficial temporal vessels
- Lesser occipital nerve (C2)
  - □ Innervates: upper half of the posterior surface of the ear
  - □ Landmarks: Erb point and ascends along the posterior border of sternocleidomastoid muscle
- Auricular branch of the vagus nerve (X, Arnold nerve)
  - □ Innervates: the concha and the posterior portion of the EAC

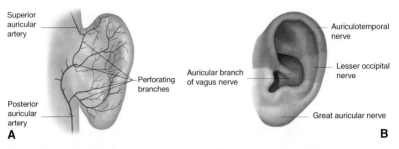

Figure 17-2 A. Arterial anatomy of the posterior ear. (The right ear is shown.) The posterior auricular artery anastomoses with the superficial temporal artery via the superior auricular artery. (From Hanasono M. Postauricular flap for ear reconstruction. In: Chung KC, Disa JJ, Gosain A, eds. *Operative Techniques in Plastic Surgery*. Wolters Kluwer; 2020:1133-1137. Figure 3.30.1B.) **B.** The auriculotemporal nerve innervates the superior aspect of the external ear, the lesser occipital nerve is responsible for the mid posterior external ear, and the great auricular nerve innervates the inferior aspect of the ear. (From McNabb JW, O'Connor F. *A Practical Guide to Joint & Soft Tissue Injection*. Wolters Kluwer; 2022. Figure 7.12A.)

- □ *A ring block will not provide adequate anesthesia to the concha; direct local infiltration is required
  - External auditory canal receives sensory innervation from cranial nerves V, VII, IX, and X
  - ○ Lymphatic drainage
    - Parallels embryologic development
    - The tragus, root of helix, and superior helix (1st branchial arch) → parotid nodes
    - The antitragus, antihelix, and lobule (2nd branchial arch) → cervical nodes
  - ○ Vestigial musculature
    - Intrinsic muscles: helicis major and minor, tragicus, antitragicus, and the transverse and oblique auricular muscles
    - Extrinsic muscles: anterior, posterior, and superior auricular muscles
- Clinical Measurements of the Normal Ear
  - ○ Growth
    - Approximately 85% of ear growth is achieved by the age of 3
    - Ear width reaches full size by the age of 10, while ear height continues to grow into adulthood
    - *Near-adult size is routinely considered between the ages of 6 and 7
  - ○ Location
    - The ear is located roughly 6 cm, or a single ear-length, posterior to the lateral orbital rim.
    - The superior aspect of the helix is at the level of the lateral brow.
    - The inferior aspect of the lobule is at the level of the nasal ala.
    - On frontal view, the helical rim is slightly lateral to the antihelical fold.
  - ○ Measurements
    - Normal auricular angles
      - □ The long axis of the ear is inclined posteriorly 20°.
      - □ **Auriculocephalic angle:** the angle formed between the midpoint of the lateral helix and the mastoid bone (normally between 20° and 30°).
      - □ **Conchoscaphal angle:** the angle formed between the scapha and the concha (normally <90°).
      - □ **Conchomastoid angle:** the angle formed between the concha and the mastoid (normally about 90°).

- Normal auricular projections
  - □ Upper third: 10-12 mm
  - □ Middle third: 16-18 mm
  - □ Lower third: 20-22 mm

RECONSTRUCTION OF CONGENITAL EAR DEFORMITIES

- **Microtia**
  - ○ **Epidemiology**
    - Incidence: 1 in 6000 births.
    - Prevalence: higher in Hispanics, Asians, and Native Americans.
    - Male to female ratio is 2:1.
    - ***Right/left/bilateral ratio of 6:3:1.**
    - Etiology: poorly understood
      - □ Most cases are isolated and sporadic.
      - □ Proposed causes: ischemia (eg, acute vascular obstruction), drugs (eg, thalidomide, isotretinoin, retinoic acid), and infection (eg, rubella).
    - Commonly associated syndromes: **hemifacial microsomia, Goldenhar syndrome, and Treacher-Collins syndrome.**
    - Based on embryologic development, the inner ear is often spared, but defects of the external auditory canal and middle ear are common.
      - □ Hearing loss is predominantly due to atresia or stenosis of the external auditory canal but can result from the absence or structural abnormalities of the ossicular chain.
      - □ Conductive component (80%) is more prevalent than a sensorineural component (20%).
  - ○ **Classification**
    - Many classification systems have been proposed, but they are rarely clinically useful.
    - Marx classification: based on severity of the microtia deformity.
    - Nagata classification: most commonly used; based on vestigial structures present
      - □ **Lobular type:** microtic ears have a remnant ear and lobule but lack a concha, acoustic meatus, and tragus (correspond to **grade III**).
      - □ **Conchal type:** microtic ears possess some degree of a lobule, concha, acoustic meatus, and tragus (correspond to **grade II**).
      - □ **Small conchal type:** microtic ears contain the remnant ear and lobule with a small indentation for a concha.
      - □ **Anotia:** absence of auricular tissue (correspond to **grade IV**).
  - ○ **Timing of repair**
    - ***General rule of thumb: delayed until ear reaches near-adult size for optimal result**
      - □ Usually around age of 6-7
      - □ Wait until the patient (not the parents) requests surgery
        - Self-awareness of the ear deformity
        - Ability to participate postoperative care and comply with restrictions
    - Different techniques have different age requirements for optimal reconstructive outcomes
      - □ Brent technique: performed at the **age of 6** (ear maturity)
      - □ Nagata technique: performed at the **age of 10** when patient's chest circumference **is at least 60 cm** at the level of xiphoid process (need of additional cartilage for tragal reconstruction)
    - If there is presence of conductive hearing loss, coordination of operative care with an otolaryngologist is paramount

- □ Unilateral microtia with normal contralateral hearing: bone-anchored hearing aids (BAHAs) and middle ear reconstruction are not routinely required.
- □ *If contralateral conductive hearing loss is present: BAHA placement should be deferred until completion of ear reconstruction to avoid compromising the vascularity of the skin envelope.
- ○ **Surgical management of microtia**
  - **Brent technique (four stages) (Fig. 17-3)**
    - □ Stage 1: a cartilaginous ear framework is carved from the synchondrosis of the contralateral sixth through eighth ribs, which is then inserted into a subcutaneous pocket beneath the retroauricular skin.
    - □ Stage 2: lobular transposition is performed.
    - □ Stage 3: elevation of the ear framework, creation of the retroauricular sulcus, and coverage of the posterior reconstructed ear with a full-thickness skin graft.
    - □ Stage 4: conchal excavation and tragal reconstruction.
  - **Nagata technique (two stages)**
    - □ Stage 1: a cartilaginous ear framework is carved from the synchondrosis of the ipsilateral sixth through ninth ribs, which is then inserted into a subcutaneous pocket beneath the retroauricular skin. Lobular transposition and tragal reconstruction are both performed during this initial stage.
    - □ Stage 2: elevation of the ear framework, creation of the retroauricular sulcus, and coverage of the posterior reconstructed ear with a tunneled temporoparietal fascial flap (TPFF) and split-thickness skin graft.
  - **Alloplastic framework**
    - □ Options
      - Silicone elastomer (Silastic, Cronin)
        - High complication rate and failure rate
        - Silicone is walled off by the host and prone to extrusion and scar tissue formation
      - Porous polyethylene (Medpor, Reinisch)
        - Porous structure allows tissue ingrowth
        - Superior and safer result than silicone
    - □ Major advantage is no donor site morbidity, but higher rates of infection and extrusion compared to autogenous reconstruction.
    - □ Coverage with a TPFF decreases the complication rate.
  - **Ear prosthesis**
    - □ Indications: failed autogenous reconstruction, paucity of local tissue, radiation, burn, trauma, cancer, and in the elderly.
    - □ Previously considered a poor option because adhesives are required for the prosthesis to "stick" to the patient's head.
    - □ With the advent of osseointegrated titanium implants, ear prostheses are now more practical and widely used.
    - □ Requires meticulous daily hygiene to prevent the skin-abutment interfaces from becoming inflamed/infected.
- ○ **Postoperative care**
  - Closed-suction drainage system to avoid pressure dressings, which may cause skin necrosis
  - Close monitor for hematoma or infection
- ○ **Complications**
  - Skin necrosis
    - □ Causes: tight pressure dressings or raise too thin of a flap when creating subcutaneous pocket

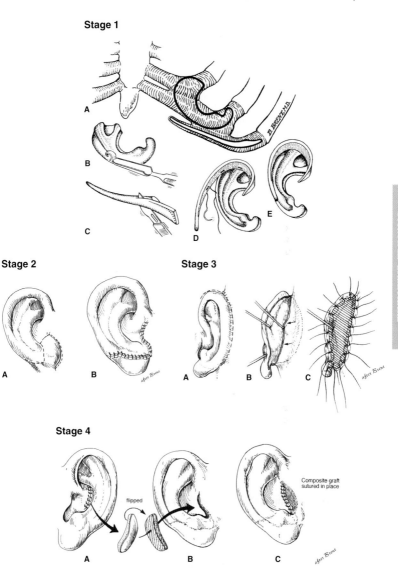

Stage 1

Stage 2

Stage 3

Stage 4

Composite graft sutured in place

flipped

Figure 17-3 Brent technique for microtia reconstruction. Stage 1: A-E. The base plate of the framework and the helix and the crura are carved from autologous costal cartilage grafts. The framework is implanted subcutaneously. **Stage 2: A, B.** The lobule is created by transposing a flap from the microtia remnant or adjacent skin. **Stage 3: A-C.** The ear is elevated and then a skin graft is placed on its posterior surface to increase lateral projection from the head. **Stage 4: A-C.** The tragus is reconstructed using a contralateral composite conchal cartilage graft, which is then secured to the previously placed framework. (From Thorne CH, ed. *Grabb and Smith's Plastic Surgery.* 7th ed. Lippincott Williams & Wilkins; 2014. Figures 27.9-27.12.)

- Management:
  - Partial-thickness necrosis: conservative management with local wound care
  - Full-thickness necrosis: excisional débridement and local flap coverage
- Infection
  - Early recognition and treatment are the mainstay of therapy.
  - **Superficial infections can sometimes be managed nonoperatively with antibiotics alone.**
  - **Deep infections (ie, gross purulence or suppurative chondritis) require irrigation of the subcutaneous pocket, drain placement, and removal of the ear framework.**
- Hematoma
  - **Classically presents as sudden onset unilateral ear pain.**
  - Treatment is immediate clot evacuation.
- Hypertrophic scarring
  - Commonly occurs at the chest wall donor site
  - Design incisions that will not interfere with future breast growth
- Hair growth
  - Commonly occurs in patients with a low temporal hairline.
  - Our preferred treatment is preoperative laser hair ablation.
- Pneumothorax
  - Can be evacuated using a red rubber Robinson catheter.
  - Rarely requires placement of a thoracostomy tube.
  - Chest plain film is obtained in recovery and on the first postoperative morning.
- Chest wall deformity
  - Usually more noticeable in thinner patients and when more donor rib cartilage is harvested.
  - Cartilage may regenerate if the perichondrium is left intact.
- Resorption of cartilage graft
  - Usually due to infection or a tight, restrictive skin envelope.
  - If severe, may require regrafting.
  - Most cartilage grafts retain their size and shape or grow slightly larger over time.
- **Prominent Ear (Fig. 17-4)**
  - **Epidemiology**
    - Affects ~5% of the general population
    - Most likely hereditary but can be associated with fragile X syndrome
  - **Anatomic causes**
    - Underdeveloped antihelical fold
      - *Most common cause of prominent ear
      - Definition: conchoscaphal angle more than 90°
      - Results in prominence of the upper third of the ear
    - Conchal hypertrophy
      - Definition: excess conchal cartilage (more than 1.5 cm deep)
      - Results in prominence of the middle third of the ear
    - Protruding lobule
      - Least common cause of the prominent ear
      - Results in prominence of the lower third of the ear
  - ***In newborns less than 6 weeks of age, ear molding can be performed to help reshape the deformed ear**
    - **Circulating maternal estrogens lend malleability to the ear cartilage.**
    - Soft putty is shaped into a custom mold that can be adjusted as the newborn grows (worn for several weeks to months).

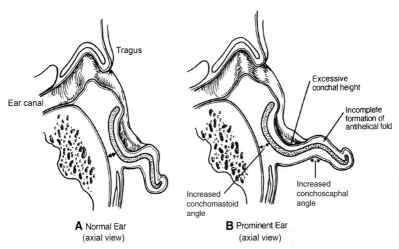

Figure 17-4 Comparison of normal and prominent ear anatomy. (From Thorne CH, ed. *Grabb and Smith's Plastic Surgery*. 7th ed. Lippincott Williams & Wilkins; 2014. Figure 49.1.)

○ **Surgical management of the prominent ear**
  ▪ Timing: 6-7 years of age (similar to microtia); when patient can participate in the decision for surgery and comply with postoperative restrictions
  ▪ The type of otoplasty performed will depend on the anatomic abnormality present; often more than one technique is required
  ▪ **Cartilage-scoring techniques**
    □ Gibson and Davis law: cartilage bends away from the scored surface due to the release of intrinsic stresses
    □ **Stenström:** anterior scoring via an anterior approach
    □ **Chongchet:** anterior scoring via a posterior approach
  ▪ **Cartilage-suturing techniques**
    □ *Conchoscaphal (Mustardé) sutures: recreate the antihelical fold using permanent mattress sutures, thereby reducing upper-third prominence.
    □ *Conchomastoid (Furnas) sutures: reduce the auriculocephalic angle, and consequently middle-third prominence, using permanent mattress sutures.
  ▪ **Cartilage-incising or -excising techniques**
    □ A powerful tool in patients with stiffer ear cartilage or those with very severe deformities, but the major drawbacks are palpable step-offs and an overly chiseled appearance
    □ **Converse-Wood-Smith:** recreates the antihelical fold by first incising the cartilage and then placing permanent mattress sutures
    □ **Luckett:** similar to Converse-Wood-Smith, except that a crescent-shaped piece of skin and cartilage is excised
  ▪ **Lobule repositioning**
    □ Correction of upper- and middle-third prominences may reveal or accentuate prominence in the lower third of the ear.
    □ **Webster:** repositions the helical tail next to the concha but is often ineffective because the helical tail does not extend into the lobule.
    □ Other techniques involve either fusiform, wedge, or fishtail excisions on the posterior surface of the lobule, and then suturing the fibrofatty tissue of the lobule to either the concha or mastoid periosteum.

- ○ Postoperative care
  - ▪ Avoid any trauma to the ears.
  - ▪ Head-band protocol: wear head band for protection of ears at all times for 3-4 weeks. Afterward, wear the headband at bedtime and when engaging in physical activities for 3 months.
- ○ Complications
  - ▪ Recurrence
    - ▫ More common in patients with stiffer ear cartilage.
    - ▫ **Early recurrence is most likely due to suture pull-through or suture breakage.**
  - ▪ Asymmetry and contour irregularity
    - ▫ More common with cartilage-incising or -excising techniques.
    - ▫ **Telephone deformity:** relative upper- and lower-third prominences of the ear caused by either overcorrection of the middle third or undercorrection of the upper and lower thirds.
    - ▫ **Hidden helix:** the helix is unable to be seen on frontal view due to overcorrection of the upper and middle thirds.
  - ▪ Infection
    - ▫ Superficial infections can sometimes be managed nonoperatively with antibiotics alone.
    - ▫ If not recognized early, suppurative chondritis may develop leading to cartilage loss and residual deformity.
    - ▫ Spit sutures can be irritating and should be removed.
  - ▪ Hematoma
    - ▫ Classically presents as sudden onset unilateral ear pain.
    - ▫ Treatment is immediate clot evacuation.
  - ▪ Keloids
    - ▫ More common in dark-skinned patients.
    - ▫ Treat initially with pressure earrings and steroid injections.
    - ▫ In severe cases, surgical excision and postoperative radiotherapy may be required.
- • **Other Congenital Ear Deformities**
  - ○ **Cryptotia (Fig. 17-5A)**
    - ▪ Definition: adherence of the superior helix to the temporal skin with absence of the superior auriculocephalic sulcus
    - ▪ Surgical correction: release of the superior helix from the temporal skin and creation of a new superior auriculocephalic sulcus using skin grafts or local flaps
  - ○ **Stahl ear (Fig. 17-5B)**
    - ▪ Definition: an abnormal third crus that arises from the antihelix and extends horizontally to the helical rim
      - ▫ The superior crus is often hypoplastic or absent.
      - ▫ The scapha is malformed, while the concha is normal.
    - ▪ Surgical correction: wedge excision of the third crus with helical advancement
  - ○ **Constricted ear (Fig. 17-5C)**
    - ▪ Definition: an inadequate circumference of the helical rim causing the superior helix to fold over the scapha
      - ▫ Also known as a cup ear or lop ear deformity
    - ▪ Surgical correction: detaching the superior helix from the scapha and reattaching it at the proper position and angle

PEARLS

1. Patients with oropharyngeal cancer may complain of referred otalgia via Arnold's nerve.
2. A ring block will not provide adequate anesthesia to the concha; direct local infiltration is required.

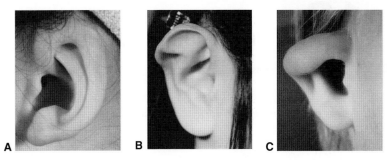

A   **B**   **C**

Figure 17-5 Congenital ear deformities. A. Cryptotia. **B.** Stahl ear. **C.** Constricted ear. (From Thorne CH, ed. *Grabb and Smith's Plastic Surgery.* 7th ed. Lippincott Williams & Wilkins; 2014. Figure 49.4.)

3. Children with microtia or prominent ears are usually operated on between the ages of 6 and 7 when ear growth is nearly complete and when they are able to participate in postoperative care and restrictions.
4. In newborns <6 weeks of age, ear molding can be performed to help reshape many deformed ears due to circulating maternal estrogens lending malleability to the ear cartilage.

QUESTIONS YOU WILL BE ASKED

1. What is the most common complication of otoplasty?
   Recurrence.
2. What is the blood supply to the anterior surface of the ear?
   Perforating branches of the postauricular artery. Superficial temporal artery only supplies the triangular fossa.
3. What suture technique is most commonly used to correct prominent ear and how is it placed?
   Mustardé suture: horizontal mattress sutures placed between the scapha cartilage and the conchal cartilage to recreate the antihelical fold.
4. What are the causes of prominent ear?
   Underdeveloped antihelical fold (most common), conchal hypertrophy, and protruding lobule.

THINGS TO DRAW

Draw the surface anatomy of the ear.

Recommended Readings
1. Beahm EK, Walton RL. Auricular reconstruction for microtia: part I. Anatomy, embryology, and clinical evaluation. *Plast Reconstr Surg.* 2002;109(7):2473-2482. doi:10.1097/00006534-200206000-00046
2. Brent B. Auricular repair with autogenous rib cartilage grafts: two decades of experience with 600 cases. *Plast Reconstr Surg.* 1992;90(3):355-374; discussion 375-376.
3. Janis JE, Rohrich RJ, Gutowski KA. Otoplasty. *Plast Reconstr Surg.* 2005;115(4):60e-72e.
4. Thorne CH, Wilkes G. Ear deformities, otoplasty, and ear reconstruction. *Plast Reconstr Surg.* 2012;129(4):701e-716e. doi:10.1097/PRS.0b013e3182450d9f
5. Walton RL, Beahm EK. Auricular reconstruction for microtia: part II. Surgical techniques. *Plast Reconstr Surg.* 2002;110(1):234-387. doi:10.1097/00006534-200207000-00041

18 Orthognathic Surgery

Hossein E. Jazayeri

There is no excellent beauty that hath not some strangeness in the proportions.
—Francis Bacon

OVERVIEW

- From Greek—Ortho: "straight" or "correct" + Gnath: "jaw."
- Goals of treatment include restoration of form and function.
  - Proper occlusion for mastication.
  - Ideal facial proportions with harmonious maxillomandibular relationship.

DENTITION

- **Pediatric:** primary or deciduous teeth
  - **Eruption sequence** (months)
    - *Incisors: 6 months; first teeth
    - First molars: 12 months
    - Canines: 16 months
    - Second molars: 20 months
  - **Nomenclature for the 20 primary teeth**
    - Letter system: A-P
    - Mnemonic: **All Just Kids Teeth (Fig. 18-1B)**
      - A, right maxillary second molar
      - J, left maxillary second molar
      - K, left mandibular second molar
      - T, right mandibular second molar
- **Mixed Dentition:** when both primary and secondary teeth are present; age 6-9 years
- **Adult:** secondary, permanent
  - **Eruption sequence** (years)
    - *First molars: 6-7; first adult teeth
    - Incisors: 6-9
    - Canines: 9-10
    - First premolars: 10-12
    - Second premolars: 11-12
    - Second molars: 11-13
    - Third molars: 17-21; "wisdom" teeth
  - **Numbering (international standard): 1-32 (Fig. 18-1A)**
    - 1, right maxillary third molar
    - 17, left mandibular third molar

DENTAL ANATOMY

- **Crown:** above the gingiva
- **Root:** within the bone
- **Cusp:** protruding portion of occlusal surface
- **Groove:** intruding portion of occlusal surface

---

*Denotes common in-service examination topics.

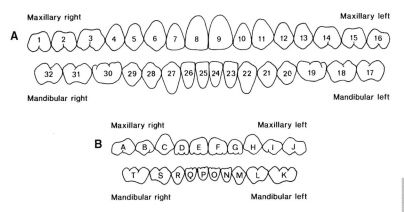

Figure 18-1 Permanent teeth numbering (**A**) and primary teeth numbering (**B**). (From Wilkins EM. *Clinical Practice of the Dental Hygienist.* 12th ed. Wolters Kluwer; 2017. Figure 9.1.)

TERMINOLOGY

- **Mesial:** toward midline (eg, incisors are mesial to molars).
- **Distal:** away from midline.
- **Buccal:** toward the cheek.
- **Lingual:** toward the tongue.
- **Overbite:** vertical relationship of the maxillary and mandibular tooth apices.
- **Overjet:** horizontal relationship of the maxillary and mandibular tooth apices.
- **Proclination:** angulation of apex toward the lips.
- **Retroclination:** angulation of apex toward the tongue.
- **Apertognathia:** open bite, negative overbite.
- **Incisal show:** amount of vertical show of maxillary central incisor in repose.
- **Centric occlusion:** maximal intercuspation of teeth.
- **Centric relation:** mandibular condyles fully seated in glenoid fossae.
- **Open bite:** part of the dentition does not occlude (can be anywhere).
- **Deep bite:** a pronounced overbite.
- **Crossbite:** can be buccal, neutral (normal), or lingual. Often caused by tilting of the maxillary teeth. Crossbite can occur in either anterior or posterior dentition.

ANGLE CLASSIFICATION (EDWARD HARTLEY ANGLE, "FATHER OF MODERN ORTHODONTICS")

- *Angle Classification: based on the relationship between the buccal groove of the mandibular first molar and the mesiobuccal cusp of the maxillary first molar (Fig. 18-2)
- **Class I:** mesial buccal cusp of maxillary first molar in buccal grove of mandibular first molar
- **Class II:** mesial buccal cusp of maxillary first molar is mesial to buccal grove of mandibular first molar
  - Division 1: maxillary incisors are proclined with an overjet beyond the normal 2-4 mm range
  - Division 2: retroclination of maxillary incisors
- **Class III:** mesial buccal cusp of maxillary first molar is distal to buccal grove of mandibular first molar

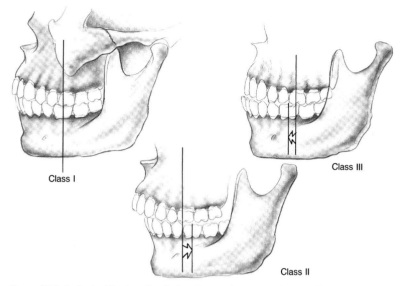

Figure 18-2 Angle classification of occlusion. (From Johnson J. *Bailey's Head and Neck Surgery.* 5th ed. Wolters Kluwer; 2014. Figure 80.2.)

ORTHOGNATHIC SURGERY EVALUATION

HISTORY AND PHYSICAL EXAMINATION

- **Close Coordination With Orthodontist**
- **Complete Medical and Dental History**
  - Functional concerns: obstructive sleep apnea (OSA), temporomandibular joint disease (TMD), cleft lip, cleft palate, craniofacial syndromes (hemifacial microsomia, Treacher-Collins, Pierre-Robin sequence)
  - Aesthetic concerns: maxillary/mandibular protrusion, maxillary/mandibular retrotrusion, facial profile discrepancies, retruded/protruded chin
- **Oral Exam**
  - **Occlusion:** number of dental contacts; angle classification
    - Curve of Spee: AP curvature of occlusal plane
    - Curve of Wilson: lateral curvature of occlusal plane
  - **Midline:** coincidence (alignment) of maxillary and mandibular central incisors
  - **Cant:** discrepancy of occlusal plane from horizontal
  - *Ideal incisal show: 2-4 mm in women; 0-2 mm in men
  - **Restorations** and overall dental health (wear of dentition, chips/cracks)
  - **TMJ:** MIO, protrusion, laterotrusion, presence of crepitus, clicking, subluxation, pain
- **Aesthetic Evaluation**
  - Neoclassical canon
    - Measure horizontal thirds and vertical fifths
    - Assess nose-lip-chin relationship
  - Determine facial symmetry
  - Determine facial profile (straight, convex, concave)

RADIOGRAPHIC (CEPHALOMETRIC) EVALUATION

- **PA and Lateral Cephalogram** ± Orthopantomogram (Panorex)
- **Determine Convexity/Concavity**

- **Facial Divergence**
  - ○ Anteriorly divergent: soft tissue pogonion anterior to glabella
  - ○ Posteriorly divergent: soft tissue pogonion posterior to glabella
- ***Key Anatomic Points on Lateral Cephalogram)**
  - ○ Sella: midpoint of the sella turcica of sphenoid bone
  - ○ Nasion: most concave point on the nasal bone
  - ○ A point: most concave point on the maxilla
  - ○ B point: most concave point on the mandible
  - ○ Pogonion: most forward projecting point on anterior surface of the chin
  - ○ Gonion: the lowest, posterior and lateral point of the mandibular angle
  - ○ Gnathion: the midpoint between the pogonion and menton
  - ○ Menton: the lowest point on the mandibular symphysis
  - ○ **Normative angle values** (differ based on race/ethnicity, sex)
    - ▪ Stella, Nasion, A point (SNA) = 82
    - ▪ Stella, Nasion, B point (SNB) = 80

DIAGNOSES AND GENERAL MANAGEMENT

- **Treatment Planning**
  - ○ **Expansion of the soft tissue envelope** with anterior skeletal movement is generally preferred to the opposite
    - ▪ Anterior movements produce a more youthful, rather than aged, appearance
    - ▪ Consider but "ignore" normative angles
  - ○ **"Decompensate" occlusion**
    - ▪ Orthodontic correction of proclined/retroclined teeth in preparation for postoperative occlusion
    - ▪ Worsens preoperative occlusion
  - ○ **Virtual surgery can be helpful in preoperative planning**
    - ▪ Two-dimensional software (eg, Dolphin).
    - ▪ Cone-beam CT or fan CT obtained, and virtual model of the skull is generated.
      - ▫ The mandible is defined to prepare the virtual osteotomies.
      - ▫ The planned osteotomies are defined using the software.
      - ▫ The maxilla can be manipulated in any plane.
      - ▫ A virtual intermediate splint can be designed and printed using CAD/CAM technology.
      - ▫ Distal segment of the mandible is manipulated to the desired occlusion after which a final splint can be designed and printed.
      - ▫ May determine soft tissue response to skeletal movement
      - ▫ Estimates postoperative SNA/SNB angles.
      - ▫ Three-dimensional treatment planning is also used (eg, Medical Modeling).
  - ○ **Casts, model surgery, and occlusal splints**
    - ▪ Dental impressions followed by plaster casts
    - ▪ Casts enable determination of maximal intercuspation: centric occlusion
    - ▪ Casts facilitate fabrication of occlusal splint to guide positioning following osteotomy
      - ▫ For "two-piece" Le Fort I cases (ie, maxillary arch must be widened with sagittal osteotomy), a splint is required to maintain desired palatal width
      - ▫ For "two-jaw" or "double-jaw" cases (ie, maxillary and mandibular osteotomies), two splints are required: intermediate and final
    - ▪ In "double-jaw" cases, facebow transfer is required to establish the relationship of the maxilla to the skull base
      - ▫ Bite registration needed to then relate mandibular cast to maxillary cast on articulator

□ Maxillary cast osteotomy (model surgery) performed on articulator to fashion intermediate splint
□ Final splint fabricated on separate models mounted on Galetti articulator
○ **Arch bars or braces with brackets required**

GENERAL MANAGEMENT CONSIDERATIONS

- *Vertical Maxillary Excess
  ○ **Examination findings**
    ▪ Long face/"gummy smile" with excess gingival show
    ▪ Greater than 4-mm incisor show
    ▪ Mentalis strain
    ▪ Flattened midface
    ▪ Class II malocclusion most common but can have any occlusion
    ▪ SNA and SNB are decreased; ANB increased
  ○ **Etiology:** open-mouthed breathing-nasal airway obstruction, myotonic dystrophy, adenoid hypertrophy, and familial
  ○ **Treatment:** Le Fort I impaction, possible mandibular advancement. With maxillary impaction, mandible will autorotate into occlusion with maxillary dentition
    ▪ This will improve SNB angle without mandibular osteotomy
    ▪ Concomitant genioplasty sometimes needed to correct relative chin retrusion or midline menton discrepancy
- **Vertical Maxillary Deficiency**
  ○ **Examination findings**
    ▪ Short face: see very little maxillary dentition in repose and with smiling
    ▪ No incisor show
    ▪ Aged, edentulous appearance, prominent chin with jowling
    ▪ **Class II malocclusion**
    ▪ **Increased SNA and SNB angles**
  ○ **Treatment:** downfracture Le Fort I with bone grafting, possible mandibular advancement
  ○ **Orthodontics:** curve of Spee (vertical wave in occlusal plane) is corrected postsurgically
- **Maxillary Retrusion/Midface Hypoplasia**
  ○ **Examination findings**
    ▪ Flat or dish face
    ▪ Depressed nasal tip and wide alar base
    ▪ Negative overjet
    ▪ Short upper lip
    ▪ **Class III malocclusion**
    ▪ **Decreased SNA;** normal to larger SNB; negative ANB
  ○ **Etiology:** often history of cleft lip ± palate, CPAP (continuous positive airway pressure) during childhood
  ○ **Treatment:** maxillary advancement
    ▪ High-winged Le Fort I
      □ Improves malar position with one operation
      □ Obviates need for implants or bone grafts
    ▪ Le Fort I via distraction osteogenesis
      □ Used in large advancements (>10 mm)
      □ Requires halo mounted to cranium during initiation, activation, and consolidation phases
      □ Unable to precisely establish final occlusion
    ▪ *Le Fort I advancement changes the nasal appearance
      □ Widened alar base
      □ Increased tip projection
      □ Increased nasolabial angled
      □ Narrowing of upper lip show (smaller vermillion)

- Soft tissue of upper lip moves 0.5-0.9 compared with the bone
- **Retrognathia**
  - **Examination findings**
    - Decreased mandibular projection
    - Obtuse cervicomental angle, redundant submental soft tissue
    - May have excessive eversion of lower lip
    - Positive overjet
    - **Class II** malocclusion
    - **Decreased SNB angle**
  - Orthodontic presurgical management seeks to eliminate crowding (limits the amount by which the mandible can be advanced)
  - **Etiology:** may have history of Pierre-Robin sequence
  - **Treatment:** bilateral sagittal split osteotomy (BSSO), possible genioplasty
- **Prognathia**
  - **Examination findings**
    - Prominence mandible with apparent midface retrusion
    - Mandibular over-rotation
    - Negative overjet
    - **Class III** malocclusion
    - **Increased SNB angle**
  - **Treatment**
    - Consider maxillary advancement only
    - Setback mandible only in severe cases
      □ BSSO
      □ Intraoral vertical ramus osteotomy (IVRO)
        ■ If setback is >10 mm
        ■ Requires postoperative maxillomandibular fixation (MMF)
- **Obstructive sleep apnea (OSA)**
  - **With severe OSA** not amenable to CPAP, "bi-max" advancement, also known as maxillomandibular advancement (MMA), is considered.
  - **Advancement of maxillomandibular skeleton** improves airway patency and relieves upper airway obstruction.

OPERATIVE TECHNIQUES

- **Anesthetic Considerations**
  - Hypotensive anesthesia
  - Reverse Trendelenburg positioning (head up) reduces bleeding intraoperatively
- **Le Fort I osteotomy (Fig. 18-3)**
  - Upper buccal sulcus incision.
  - Leave 2- to 3-mm cuff of tissue on gingiva for closure.
  - Avoid parotid papilla.
  - Identify infraorbital nerve in midpupillary line.
  - Dissect along buttresses in subperiosteal plane.
  - Elevate mucosa from nasal floor, septum, and sidewalls.
  - **Buttress osteotomies**
    - Nasomaxillary: reciprocating saw from piriform aperture medial to lateral in horizontal plane.
    - Zygomaticomaxillary: reciprocating saw directed from lateral to medial in horizontal plane.
    - Pterygomaxillary: curved osteotome behind maxillary tuberosity into pterygomaxillary fissure.
    - Nasal septum divided using double-ball, guarded osteotome.
    - Check lip-tooth relationship with acrylic splint in place.
    - Plate fixation at piriform ± maxillary buttress.

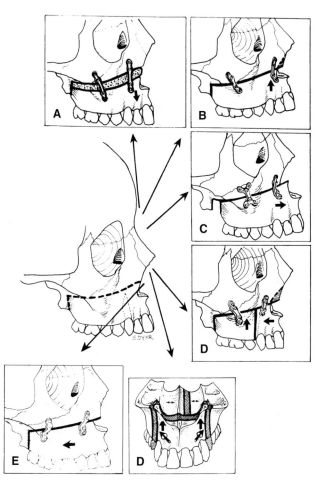

Figure 18-3 Versatility of the Le Fort I osteotomy. The Le Fort osteotomy can be varied to position portions of the maxilla in various ways. **A.** Inferior displacement (with bone graft) to increase vertical length. **B.** Impaction to reduce maxillary height. **C.** Anterior movement of the maxilla is possible. **D.** The surgeon may adjust the width of the maxilla as needed. **E.** Posterior movement of the maxilla is possible as well. (From Thorne CH, ed. *Grabb and Smith's Plastic Surgery.* 7th ed. Lippincott Williams & Wilkins; 2014. Figure 25.5.)

- V-Y vestibular closure: prevent nasal widening, thinning of upper lip, and commissure downturn.
- Check occlusion and revise hardware if incorrect.
- **Bilateral Sagittal Split Osteotomy (BSSO) (Fig. 18-4)**
    - Requires removal of third molars ~6 months preoperatively.
    - Intraoral incision over ascending ramus and external oblique ridge.
    - Subperiosteal dissection on medial surface of ramus
        - Above the level of occlusal plane at lingula
        - Point where inferior alveolar nerve enters the mandible

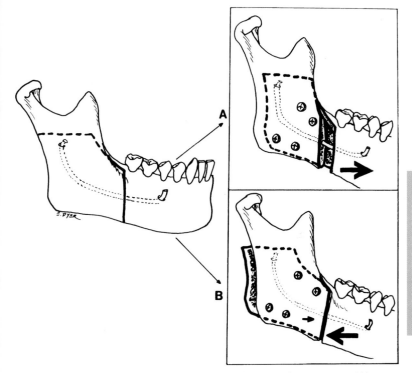

Figure 18-4 The sagittal split osteotomy. It may be used to move the anterior mandible into a more anterior position (**A**) or, more rarely, into a more posterior position (**B**). (From Thorne CH, ed. *Grabb and Smith's Plastic Surgery*. 7th ed. Lippincott Williams & Wilkins; 2014. Figure 25.4.)

- ○ Step-wise osteotomy in sagittal plane.
- ○ Segments mandible into three segments
  - ▪ Proximal (two segments, bilateral): contains ramus and condyle
  - ▪ Distal (one segment, central): contains body, both branches of inferior alveolar nerve
- ○ Acrylic splint guides the distal segment into occlusion.
- ○ Transbuccal trocar is used to assist in bicortical screw fixation of both mandibular segments.
- ○ Seat condyles in glenoid fossa (centric relation) during fixation.
- ○ Check occlusion on release of MMF and revise hardware if incorrect.
- **Intraoral Vertical Ramus Osteotomy (IVRO)**
  - ○ Intraoral incision over ascending ramus and external oblique ridge
  - ○ Subperiosteal dissection on lateral surface of ramus
    - ▪ Posterior to entrance of inferior alveolar nerve
    - ▪ Splits mandible in coronal plane between condyle and coronoid (sigmoid notch)
    - ▪ Internal maxillary artery traverses this bony interval
  - ○ Less favored technique of mandibular osteotomy
  - ○ Used when large mandibular setback is required (ie, class III malocclusion)
  - ○ No osseous fixation employed; requires MMF postoperatively

- **Genioplasty**
  - Lower buccal sulcus incision.
  - Leave the cuff of mucosa and mentalis muscle for two-layer closure.
  - Subperiosteal dissection centrally and along inferior mandibular border to reveal mental nerves
    - Located between first and second premolars
    - *May course ~2 mm beneath the mental foramen before exiting
  - Transverse osteotomy with sagittal saw.
  - Measured step plates may be used to achieve fixation at desired location.
- **"Double-Jaw" Surgery**
  - Le Fort I
  - BSSO or IVRO
  - Performed in series, beginning with Le Fort I osteotomy
  - Intermediate and final occlusal splints used to establish occlusion

POSTOPERATIVE CONSIDERATIONS

POSTOPERATIVE CARE

- **Use of Elastic Bands**
  - Temporary elastics used to secure desired occlusion during fixation
  - Often removed prior to extubation
  - May be left in place as "guiding elastics"
    - Class II elastics
      - Used to "correct" a class II malocclusion
      - Vector from anterior maxilla to posterior mandible
    - Class III elastics
      - Used to "correct" a class III malocclusion
      - Vector from anterior mandible to posterior maxilla
- **MMF**
  - Used in cases of suboptimal fixation or in large/unstable skeletal movements
  - May be kept in place for several months
  - Wire cutters required at bedside in cases of airway compromise and/or emesis
- Steroid (fluocinolone) cream used for labial swelling
- Peridex mouth rinses
- Soft diet
- Elevate head of bed and employ cool compresses

COMPLICATIONS

- **Relapse**
  - **Surgical:** loss of plate fixation (malunion).
  - **Dental:** persistent malocclusion; requires appropriate decompensation—MMF not performed appropriately with bimaxillary surgery or elastics not used postoperatively for maintenance of occlusion may lead to relapse and need for reoperation.
  - **Condylar**
    - Resorption of bone at condyle (progressive condylar resorption)
    - Related to residual apertognathia and unfavorable TMJ dynamics
    - TMJ displacement may require reduction
  - Soft tissue: recoil forces from "Moss functional matrix"
- ***Paresthesia**
  - Risk of inferior alveolar nerve injury in BSSO is 10%.
  - About 90% of patients have temporary postoperative symptoms.
  - Temporary paresthesia may last anywhere from 2 to 12 months postoperatively.
- **Infection:** may require abscess drainage but not removal of hardware in most cases

- ○ Acute versus chronic: <6 weeks or >6 weeks
- ○ Penicillin prophylaxis commonly used but postoperative infection still possible
- **Hemorrhage**
  - ○ **Le Fort osteotomy may damage internal maxillary artery** branches and pterygoid venous plexus during pterygomaxillary disjunction
    - Maintain subperiosteal dissection.
    - Ensure osteotome placement in pterygopalatine fossa.
  - ○ **Use hypotensive anesthesia** (SBP ~ 80 mm Hg) and reverse Trendelenburg position
- **Ischemia**
  - ○ **Rare occurrence** in Le Fort I advancement, presents as dusky, violaceous mucosal appearance—may also be compounded by risk factors such as history of radiation, chemotherapy, smoking, hematologic conditions, diabetes, trauma, and any other condition that may weaken wound healing capabilities.
  - ○ **More common in**
    - Large anterior movements
    - Cases of cleft lip and palate, and/or
    - Two-piece movements with osseous discontinuity
  - ○ **Blood supply to Le Fort I segment**
    - Interruption of descending palatine a. after osteotomy
    - Maintained on ascending palatine branch of facial a.
    - Anterior branch of ascending pharyngeal a., through mucosal attachments (soft tissue pedicle)
- **Blindness** may also occur—extremely rare
  - ○ Adverse damage to the optic nerve with osteotomy extending to the sphenoid bone leading to neuropathy and blindness
  - ○ Hypotensive anesthesia—transient ischemia

QUESTIONS YOU WILL BE ASKED

1. Describe the location of the mental and infraorbital nerves
   a. Mental n.: between first and second mandibular premolars
   b. Infraorbital n.: ~1 cm below rim in midpupillary line
2. Describe the course of the inferior alveolar nerve within the mandible.
   The nerve enters mandibular foramen at lingula on medial surface of ramus. The nerve enters from medial to lateral cortex distally. Finally, it curves below mental foramen prior to exiting.
3. Describe the characteristic nasolabial changes following Le Fort I advancement.
   Alar widening, increased tip projection, vertical lip shortening
4. What are the differences between centric occlusion and centric relation.
   a. Centric occlusion: maximal intercuspation of the teeth in wear facets
   b. Centric relation: normal resting relationship of mandibular condyle in glenoid fossa
   c. CO-CR shift
      i. Sacrifice of centric relation in order to obtain occlusion and increase mandibular projection
      ii. Common in class III malocclusion

Recommended Readings
1. Legan HL, Burstone CJ. Soft tissue cephalometric analysis for orthognathic surgery. *J Oral Surg.* 1980;38(10):744-751.
2. Panula K, Finne K, Oikarinen K. Incidence of complications and problems related to orthognathic surgery: a review of 655 patients. *J Oral Maxillofac Surg.* 2001;59(10):1128-1136. discussion 1137.
3. Proffit WR, Turvey TA, Phillips C. Orthognathic surgery: a hierarchy of stability. *Int J Adult Orthodon Orthognath Surg.* 1996;11(3):191-204.

19 Facial Palsy

Alisa Yamasaki

OVERVIEW

FACIAL NERVE ANATOMY AND FUNCTION

- The Facial Nerve Contains Motor and Sensory Nerve Fibers
  - Special visceral efferent
    - Motor control of muscles derived from the second branchial arch
    - Includes muscles of facial expression, posterior belly of digastric, stylohyoid, intrinsic muscles of auricle (posterior auricular nerve), and stapedius (nerve to stapedius)
  - General visceral efferent
    - Provides preganglionic parasympathetic secretomotor innervation
    - Sublingual and submandibular glands (chorda tympani)
    - Lacrimal, nasal, and palatine glands (greater superficial petrosal nerve)
  - Special visceral sensory afferent
    - Transmits taste from anterior 2/3 of tongue and hard/soft palate (chorda tympani)
  - General somatic sensory afferent
    - Transmits sensation from external auditory meatus, auricle, and retroauricular area (posterior auricular nerve)
  - General visceral afferent
    - Transmits feelings of pain from nasal cavity, sinuses, and soft palate (greater superficial petrosal nerve)
    - Very small component of facial nerve function
- **Intratemporal Facial Nerve**
  - Intracranial facial nerve and nervus intermedius travel in the cerebellopontine angle.
  - Enters the temporal bone with the vestibulocochlear nerve via the internal auditory canal and exits at the stylomastoid foramen.
  - Divided into the meatal (canalicular), labyrinthine, tympanic (horizontal), and mastoid (vertical) segments.
    - Labyrinthine segment is the narrowest and shortest segment, most susceptible to injury (eg, temporal bone trauma, infection) and vascular compromise.
- **Extratemporal Facial Nerve**
  - Begins at the stylomastoid foramen and branches into the posterior auricular nerve, stylohyoid branch, and digastric branch prior to innervating the facial mimetic muscles (**Fig. 19-1**).
  - *Three anatomic landmarks are commonly used to identify the main trunk of the facial nerve as it exits the stylomastoid foramen.
    - **Tragal pointer:** located 1 cm anterior, inferior, and deep to the tragal cartilage.
    - **Tympanomastoid suture:** located 6-8 mm deep to the inferior edge of the suture line.
    - **Posterior digastric muscle attachment to the digastric ridge:** delineates depth of facial nerve.

---

*Denotes common in-service examination topics.

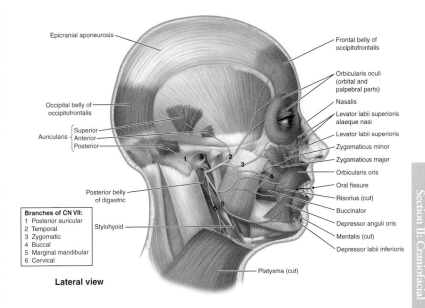

Lateral view

Branches of CN VII:
1 Posterior auricular
2 Temporal
3 Zygomatic
4 Buccal
5 Marginal mandibular
6 Cervical

Figure 19-1 Facial nerve anatomy and facial musculature. (From Dalley AF II, Agur AM, eds. *Moore's Clinically Oriented Anatomy.* 9th ed. Wolters Kluwer; 2023. Figure 10.11B.)

- A small branch off the occipital artery is often encountered just lateral to the nerve; thus, brisk bleeding is usually an indicator that the nerve is nearby.
- In children, the facial nerve runs more lateral and superficial.
- Main trunk divides into upper and lower divisions at the **pes anserinus** and divides the parotid gland into superficial and deep lobes.
    - Upper division: temporal, zygomatic, and buccal branches
    - Lower division: buccal, marginal mandibular, and cervical branches
- **Anatomic Pearls for Extratemporal Facial Nerve Branches**
    - Temporal (frontal) branch
        - *Lies superficial to the superficial layer of the deep temporal fascia and deep to the temporoparietal fascia that is continuous with SMAS
        - *Pitanguy's line: line drawn from 0.5 cm below the tragus to 1.5 cm above the lateral brow, approximating the course of the frontal branch
        - Especially prone to **symptomatic** injury due to its location and lack of redundancy (ie, it does not arborize)
    - Zygomatic branch
        - Crosses the zygomatic arch along the middle 1/3
        - **Zuker point**: midpoint of line drawn from helical root to oral commissure, approximating zygomatic/buccal branch that innervates the zygomaticus major
    - Buccal branch
        - Lies deep to the SMAS where it arborizes and forms extensive interconnections
        - *Most common facial nerve injury during rhytidectomy, but rarely symptomatic due to its redundancy
    - Marginal mandibular branch
        - Lies deep to the platysma muscle.

- ***Runs along inferior border of the mandible (80%) or 1-2 cm below it (20%) prior to its intersection with the facial vessels.**
- After crossing the facial vessels, it remains above the border of the mandible.
- Similar to the temporal branch, it is especially prone to **symptomatic** injury due to its lack of redundancy.
  - Cervical branch
    - Located ~1 cm below the half-way point of a line between the mentum and mastoid process (ie, below mandibular angle)
- **Muscles of Facial Expression (Fig. 19-1 and Table 19-1)**
  - Four layers of facial musculature, from superficial to deep:
    - Depressor anguli oris, zygomaticus minor, orbicularis oculi
    - Depressor labii inferioris, risorius, platysma, zygomaticus major, levator labii superioris alaeque nasi
    - Orbicularis oris, levator labii superioris
    - Mentalis, levator anguli oris, buccinator
  - *All muscles are innervated on their deep surface except for the buccinator, levator anguli oris, and mentalis

TABLE 19-1 Muscles of Facial Expression

Branch	Muscle	Function
Temporal	Corrugator supercilii	Brow depression and medialization
	Frontalis	Brow elevation
	Procerus	Brow depression
Temporal/zygomatic	Orbicularis oculi	Eyelid closure
Zygomatic/buccal	Zygomaticus major	Oral commissure elevation and lateralization (primary smile actuator)
Buccal	Buccinator	Cheek compression
	Depressor septi nasi	Nasal tip depression
	Levator labii superioris	Upper lip elevation
	Levator labii superioris alaeque nasi	Upper lip elevation and nostril dilation
	Levator anguli oris	Oral commissure elevation
	Nasalis	Transverse head: nostril dilation Alar head: nostril compression
	Orbicularis oris	Mouth closure and lip pursing
	Risorius	Oral commissure lateralization (secondary smile actuator)
	Zygomaticus minor	Upper lip elevation
Buccal/marginal mandibular	Depressor anguli oris	Oral commissure depression
Marginal mandibular	Depressor labii inferioris	Lower lip depression
	Mentalis	Chin elevation (soft tissue)
Cervical	Platysma	Oral commissure depression

ETIOLOGIES OF FACIAL PALSY

- Facial paralysis can result from a lesion anywhere along the length of the facial nerve
  - **Intracranial etiologies:** compressive masses tend to have an insidious onset, while acute vascular obstruction can cause sudden-onset facial paralysis
    - **Neoplastic:** cerebellopontine tumor (eg, vestibular schwannoma, meningioma), facial nerve schwannoma
    - **Traumatic:** penetrating trauma, shear injury
    - **Infectious:** encephalitis, meningitis, cerebral abscess
    - **Vascular:** aneurysm, stroke, vasculitis, intracerebral hemorrhage
    - **Neurodegenerative:** amyotrophic lateral sclerosis, multiple sclerosis
    - **Iatrogenic:** tumor extirpation
    - **Congenital:** Möbius syndrome, Goldenhar syndrome, hemifacial microsomia
      - *Möbius syndrome is the most common cause of bilateral facial palsy
      - Can also involve other cranial nerves (eg, abducens) as well as chest wall and limb abnormalities
      - *Patients typically present with a motionless face and inability to abduct the eyes
  - **Intratemporal etiologies:** injury often caused by swelling and/or compression of the nerve within the facial canal
    - **Neoplastic:** cholesteatoma, facial nerve schwannoma
    - **Traumatic:** temporal bone fracture
      - Classified as either longitudinal (80%; parallel to long axis of petrous pyramid) or transverse (20%); or otic capsule sparing vs otic capsule involving
      - Higher risk of facial paralysis with transverse and otic capsule-involving fractures
    - **Infectious:** otitis media/mastoiditis, Lyme disease, HSV, HIV, mononucleosis, syphilis, **Ramsay-Hunt syndrome ("herpes zoster oticus")**
      - Ramsay-Hunt is characterized by unilateral facial paralysis, otalgia, and a painful vesicular rash in the external auditory canal.
        - Oral corticosteroids and antivirals recommended within 72 hours of onset.
    - **Vascular:** cavernous hemangioma
    - **Iatrogenic:** Tumor extirpation, otologic surgery (eg, mastoidectomy, tympanoplasty, external auditory canal exostosis removal)
    - **Systemic:** Guillain-Barré, sarcoidosis, diabetes, Melkersson-Rosenthal syndrome (MRS)
      - MRS is characterized by recurrent facial paralysis, painless orofacial edema/granulomatous inflammation of the lips (granulomatous cheilitis), and a fissured tongue (lingua plicata)
        - Associated with uveitis, diverticulitis, ulcerative colitis, and Crohn disease
        - Treat with oral corticosteroids/immunosuppressants
    - **Toxins:** lead poisoning, carbon monoxide
    - **Idiopathic:** Bell palsy
      - *Most common cause of unilateral facial paralysis in adults.
      - Diagnosis of exclusion thought to involve a viral-induced inflammatory process leading to nerve edema and compression.
      - Defined by acute onset <72 hours, treat with oral corticosteroids and antivirals within 72 hours of onset.
      - Higher incidence in pregnant and diabetic patients.
      - Hyperacusis, age > 60, diabetes mellitus, hypertension, and severe radicular pain are poor prognostic factors.
      - Most patients (85%) experience some recovery within 3 weeks and complete recovery by 3-4 months.
      - Facial nerve decompression is controversial.

- Extratemporal etiologies
  - **Neoplastic:** parotid tumor, metastatic skin cancer, facial nerve schwannoma
  - **Traumatic:** penetrating trauma, birth trauma
    - *Exploration must be performed <72 hours of injury (prior to Wallerian degeneration) so that distal ends can be identified by electrical stimulation
    - *General "rule of thumb" is that facial nerve exploration is not warranted for distal injury (ie, medial to the lateral canthus)
    - Birth trauma typically involves neuropraxia that is managed conservatively
  - **Infectious:** parotitis
  - **Iatrogenic:** tumor extirpation, facial surgery (eg, parotidectomy), TMJ surgery
  - **Congenital:** congenital unilateral lower lip paralysis (CULLP)
    - Caused by hypoplasia or absence of the lower lip depressors
    - Typically presents with deviation of the lower lip toward the unaffected side (eg, when crying)
- **Bilateral facial paralysis** is not as common as unilateral facial paralysis but causes include Möbius syndrome, Lyme disease, toxins, and systemic infection (eg, HIV)

EVALUATION OF FACIAL PALSY

- **Assess Facial Nerve Prognosis and Muscle Viability**
  - **Onset and severity of symptoms:** gradual onset (eg, neoplastic, neurodegenerative, systemic) vs acute onset (eg, traumatic, vascular, infectious, iatrogenic, idiopathic), partial vs complete palsy, facial zones involved
  - **Determine potential etiologies** (see Etiologies of facial palsy section)
  - **Duration of symptoms:** determine viability of the affected facial musculature—muscle may be reinnervated 18-24 months following denervation
  - **Prognosis:** Determine likelihood of spontaneous recovery based on facial nerve status (ie, intact or not), signs of any clinical recovery 6-12 months after onset
- **Neuromuscular Examination**
  - Ask for a baseline photo of the patient; subtle facial asymmetries may exist prior to diagnosis of facial paralysis
  - **Assess for type of facial palsy**
    - Central vs peripheral etiology
      - Upper motor neuron lesion: contralateral facial paralysis that is forehead sparing
      - Lower motor neuron lesion: ipsilateral total facial paralysis
    - Flaccid paralysis vs partial palsy vs synkinesis
      - Flaccid paralysis: no facial movement on affected side
      - Partial palsy: weakness from decreased neural input/muscular atrophy
      - Synkinesis: postparalytic phenomenon thought to be caused by aberrant facial nerve regeneration, results in involuntary facial movements with volitional facial activation (eg, eye closure with smile)
  - **Flaccid facial palsy exam**
    - Smooth forehead with absence of wrinkles
    - Brow ptosis
    - Lagophthalmos—check for protective **Bell phenomenon** (superior rotation of globe with attempt at eye closure)
    - C-shaped nasal deformity with tip and philtral deviation away from paralyzed side, lack of nostril dilation during inspiration
    - Effacement of the nasolabial fold
    - Down-turned oral commissure, inability to smile or expose lower dentition
    - **Lower lip of paralyzed side can be more elevated due to lip depressor paralysis**
    - Inability to whistle or puff out cheeks

- **Partial facial palsy exam:** decreased facial movements due to intrinsic weakness, can also involve synkinesis
- **Synkinetic facial palsy exam**
  - Activation of non-native facial muscles on affected side
  - Smile asymmetry, oral commissure malposition, and oral incompetence due to tethering from simultaneous activation of antagonist muscles
  - Associated with significant facial and neck tightness
- Other physical findings include xerophthalmia (greater superficial petrosal nerve), hyperacusis (nerve to stapedius), dysgeusia (chorda tympani nerve), and gustatory lacrimation ("crocodile tears"; hyperlacrimation during salivation caused by "miswiring" of general visceral efferent fibers to the lacrimal gland instead of the salivary glands)

- **Facial Nerve Grading Systems**
  - **House-Brackmann scale:** one of the most common classification schemes—I (normal) to VI (complete facial paralysis), III signifies complete eyelid closure
    - Evaluates gross appearance and motion at the forehead, eye, and mouth
    - Limitations include its generalized assessment of facial nerve function, inability to detect small changes in facial nerve recovery, and lack of metrics for synkinesis
  - **Sunnybrook facial grading system:** measures zonal symmetry at rest and with voluntary motion, includes assessment of synkinesis
  - **eFACE:** electronic assessment that uses a visual analog scale to rate static, dynamic, and synkinetic function and zonal symmetry as well as overall facial disfigurement; scored from 0 to 100 (0 = severe asymmetry/palsy, 100 = normal symmetry/function) with −100 to 100 used for bidirectional parameters (eg, −100 = ptotic, 0 = normal, 100 = hyperelevated)

- **Electrodiagnostic Studies:** assist with prognostication and decision between surgical intervention vs observation
  - Normal side of the face is used as a control (ie, less useful in bilateral cases)
  - Perform >72 hours after symptom onset (ie, after Wallerian degeneration has occurred) to ensure accurate result
  - **Electroneurography (ENoG)**
    - Compares differences in compound muscle action potentials between normal vs affected side after transcutaneous stimulation of facial nerve
    - >90% axonal degeneration representing a poorer prognosis
    - Most predictive test for facial nerve recovery
  - **Electromyography (EMG)**
    - Performed 2-3 weeks after symptom onset—at rest, with needle insertion, and with voluntary muscle contraction
    - Fibrillation potentials: muscle denervation
    - Polyphasic potentials: muscle reinnervation
  - **Nerve excitability test (NET)**
    - Transcutaneous stimulation over the stylomastoid foramen until contraction of the paralyzed side is visualized
    - Difference >3.5 mA with the normal side is significant
    - Easy to perform, but highly subjective and examiner dependent
  - **Maximal stimulation test (MST)** is similar to the NET, except maximal current is used

- **Additional Workup**
  - In cases of trauma, use computed tomography to assess for temporal bone fractures
  - An audiogram should be obtained in all patients and, if abnormal, the next step is magnetic resonance imaging and referral to an otolaryngologist
  - For lagophthalmos—monitor for keratoconjunctivitis, corneal ulceration

TREATMENT OF FACIAL PALSY

NONSURGICAL MANAGEMENT

- **Acute Management**
  - ○ **Oral corticosteroids ± antivirals** treat edema/compression of the nerve, depending on etiology.
  - ○ For Bell palsy, begin treatment within 72 hours of symptom onset.
  - ○ **Eye care:** corneal ulceration and potential blindness can result if corneal sensation is impaired and eyes are not adequate protected.
    - ▪ Artificial tears for lubrication
    - ▪ Eyelid taping during sleep for corneal protection
    - ▪ Eye patches, moisture chambers, and scleral lenses can reduce evaporative losses
    - ▪ Eyelid weight to facilitate eye closure in paralytic lagophthalmos
- **Long-term Management**
  - ○ **Facial physical therapy**
    - ▪ Facial neuromuscular retraining for incomplete recovery and postoperative training
    - ▪ Can include EMG and mirror biofeedback
  - ○ **Botulinum toxin**
    - ▪ Targeted chemodenervation of muscle groups on both the normal and affected side to achieve facial balance
    - ▪ Commonly used to treat synkinesis and blepharospasm
  - ○ **Facial fillers** can be used as an adjunct to correct facial volume asymmetry
  - ○ Determine candidacy for surgical options

SURGICAL MANAGEMENT

- **Type of facial palsy, likelihood of spontaneous recovery, and viability of facial muscles** dictate surgical options—muscle remains viable for 18-24 months after denervation
  - ○ Flaccid facial palsy or weakness
    - ▪ Possible recovery: close observation for 9-12 months
    - ▪ No possible recovery with *viable* facial muscles: nerve transfer ± static procedures
    - ▪ No possible recovery with *nonviable* facial muscles: muscle transfer ± static procedures
  - ○ **Synkinesis:** selective neurectomy of nerve branches triggering undesired muscle activation
- **Static vs Dynamic Procedures**
  - ○ **Static procedures** re-establish resting facial symmetry and improve functional deficits but do not restore symmetry in facial movement
    - ▪ Brow lift for brow ptosis
    - ▪ Periocular procedures for paralytic lagophthalmos: platinum eyelid weight, palpebral spring, lower eyelid tightening (eg, lateral tarsal strip, tarsoconjunctival flap; refer to **Chapter 23: Eyelid Reconstruction**)
    - ▪ Suture suspension/static slings (eg, tensor fascia lata, palmaris longis, acellular dermis) to resuspend the nasal valve, nasolabial fold, and oral commissure
    - ▪ Lip depressor resection (eg, DLI, DAO) for smile asymmetry
    - ▪ Platysmectomy for cervical synkinesis
    - ▪ Asymmetric rhytidectomy to correct asymmetric facial soft tissue ptosis
  - ○ **Dynamic facial reanimation** restores facial movement, particularly for smile mechanism
    - ▪ **Volitional reanimation:** must consciously move face (eg, masseteric nerve transfer)
    - ▪ **Spontaneous reanimation:** occurs spontaneously (eg, cross-facial nerve graft)

- **Nerve Repair and Nerve Transfer**
  - **Primary nerve repair and/or nerve grafting** is favored when possible.
    - Repair must be tension-free—interposition grafts should be used if tension encountered in primary repair.
    - Incidence of synkinesis is increased with nerve grafting due to the presence of two coaptations instead of one with primary repair.
  - Nerve transfer is used if ipsilateral facial nerve is not viable.
    - **Cross-facial nerve graft (CFNG)**
      - Indicated when proximal ipsilateral nerve stump is unavailable for grafting but distal stump is present and facial muscles are viable for reinnervation.
      - A donor nerve graft (eg, sural nerve) guides regenerating nerve fibers from a redundant facial nerve branch on the normal side to a distal nerve stump on the paralyzed side—potential for spontaneous animation.
      - Nerve growth is monitored by an advancing Tinel sign.
      - Can be less predictable in older patients.
    - **Nerve transfers:** V to VII (masseteric), partial XII to VII
      - Powerful due to a greater number of nerve fibers being transferred compared to CFNG but does not provide spontaneous animation.
      - XII to VII uses 30%-40% of XII to avoid ipsilateral tongue atrophy and synkinesis.
      - Historically also performed with XI and phrenic nerves but no longer used due to significant donor site morbidity.
    - **Babysitter procedure**
      - Used for intermediate duration facial palsy (6-18 months) to prevent muscle atrophy and fibrosis while waiting for CFNG reinnervation.
      - CFNG is combined with a minihypoglossal transfer—XII "babysits" facial muscles until the regenerating nerve fibers arrive from the CFNG.
- **Muscle Transfers**
  - **Regional muscle:** temporalis muscle tendon transfer
    - Orthodromic transfer of the temporalis muscle (ie, no muscle inversion) with coronoidectomy, secured to oral commissure/lips using fascia lata strips
    - Can also tunnel temporalis under zygoma and transfer tendon to oral commissure with coronoid still attached (lengthening myoplasty technique)
    - Pro: single stage procedure with immediate movement
    - Con: not spontaneous, fixed oral commissure insertion with minimal control over smile vector/shape, degree of oral commissure excursion is variable
  - **Free muscle: gracilis free flap (Fig. 19-2)**
    - Obturator nerve and adductor artery/vein.
    - Powered by ipsilateral masseteric nerve and/or CFNG.
    - CFNG is performed during the first stage and muscle is transferred 9-12 months later during the second stage.
    - Pro: spontaneous activation can be achieved, ability to customize smile vector with reliable oral commissure excursion.
    - Con: requires microvascular expertise, time (performed 6-9 months after CFNG, monitor for movement 1-3 years postop), can create unwanted midfacial bulk.

PEARLS

1. Facial palsy includes a spectrum of facial motor disorders ranging from partial palsy to complete flaccid paralysis to postparalytic synkinesis.
2. Synkinesis refers to the involuntary contraction of facial muscles during volitional movement of other facial muscles, leading to facial asymmetry and/or decreased facial movement due to simultaneous contraction of antagonistic muscle groups.
3. Bell palsy is the most common cause of unilateral facial paralysis in adults (diagnosis of exclusion) and should be treated with oral corticosteroids and antivirals within 72 hours of symptom onset.

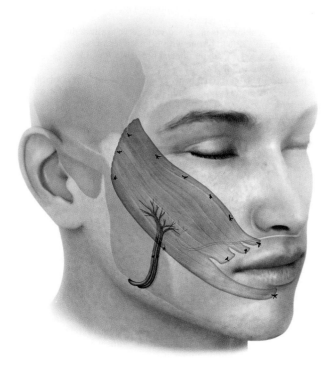

Figure 19-2 Free microneurovascular gracilis muscle transfer.

4. Facial muscles may remain viable for 18-24 months after denervation.
5. Surgical management of facial palsy depends on the degree and type of facial palsy (eg, flaccid vs synkinetic), potential for spontaneous recovery, and viability of facial muscles.

QUESTIONS YOU WILL BE ASKED

1. What three anatomic landmarks help identify the facial nerve as it exits the stylomastoid foramen?
   Tragal pointer (lies 1 cm anterior, inferior, and deep), tympanomastoid suture (lies 6-8 mm deep), and posterior belly of the digastric muscle (defines plane of facial nerve).
2. Describe how to find the temporal branch of the facial nerve.
   Follows the course of Pitanguy line, which is drawn from 0.5 cm below the tragus to 1.5 cm above the lateral brow.
3. What structures are continuous with the SMAS?
   Superficial temporal fascia (temporoparietal fascia) and platysma.
4. What nerves are commonly used to reinnervate paralyzed facial muscles?
   Contralateral VII, masseteric branch of V, and XII.

THINGS TO DRAW

Draw the course of the extratemporal facial nerve.

Recommended Readings
1. Azizzadeh B, Hjelm N. Modified selective neurectomy: a new paradigm in the management of facial palsy with synkinesis. *Facial Plast Surg Clin North Am.* 2021;29(3):453-457.
2. Garcia RM, Hadlock TA, Klebuc MJ, Simpson RL, Zenn MR, Marcus JR. Contemporary solutions for the treatment of facial nerve paralysis. *Plast Reconstr Surg.* 2015;135(6): 1025e-1046e.
3. Jowett N, Hadlock TA. A contemporary approach to facial reanimation. *JAMA Facial Plast Surg.* 2015;17(4):293-300.
4. Kim L, Byrne PJ. Controversies in contemporary facial reanimation. *Facial Plast Surg Clin North Am.* 2016;24(3):275-297.
5. Terzis JK, Konofaos P. Nerve transfers in facial palsy. *Facial Plast Surg.* 2008;24(2):177-193.

20 Facial Trauma

Chien-Wei Wang

PATIENT EVALUATION

- **History**
    - Mechanism of injury determines the degree of force
        - Interpersonal violence (usually low energy)
        - Motor vehicle accident (usually higher energy)
    - History of prior facial trauma/surgery
    - Time of injury
    - Loss of consciousness
    - Subjective complaints: diplopia, blindness, hearing loss, malocclusion, otorrhea and rhinorrhea
    - Environmental considerations: chemical exposure
    - Past medical/surgical history, medications, smoking, and drug abuse
- **Physical Exam**
    - **Trauma patients: ABCs** (airway, breathing, circulation) must be the first priority
        - Most facial trauma patients need clinical and radiographic cervical spine (c-spine) evaluation and management.
        - *Over 10% of facial trauma patients have associated c-spine injury.
    - **Control hemorrhage**—most hemorrhage can be controlled with pressure.
        - *Internal maxillary artery is the most common source of life-threatening hemorrhage associated with facial trauma.
        - Management: **secure airway** → posterior nasal packing.
        - Stable patient: consider angiography and embolization via interventional radiology.
        - Unstable patient: surgical ligation of external carotid artery.
    - Adequate lighting, irrigation, and suction are required.
    - Inspection: lacerations, abrasions, burns, edema, symmetry, septal hematoma, ruptured tympanic membrane, otorrhea and dental occlusion.
    - Palpation:
        - Skull, orbital rims, zygomatic arches, maxilla, and mandible
        - Assess for symmetry, step-offs, crepitus, and pain
    - **Complete cranial nerve exam** (prior to administration of local anesthetic) with emphasis on (**Table 20-1**).
        - Sensation: light touch in three divisions of CN V—ophthalmic, maxillary, and mandibular
        - Motor: test all CN VII branches (temporal, zygomatic, buccal, marginal mandibular, and cervical) and look for asymmetry
    - Eyes
        - Test visual acuity with pocket card
        - Pupillary response to light
        - Swinging flashlight test to rule out afferent papillary defect (optic nerve injury)
        - Diplopia (horizontal versus vertical)
        - Extraocular movements

---

*Denotes common in-service examination topics.

TABLE 20-1 Cranial Nerves and Their Foramina

Number	Name	Foramen
I	Olfactory	Cribriform plate
II	Optic	Optic foramen
III	Oculomotor	Superior orbital fissure
IV	Trochlear	Superior orbital fissure
V	Trigeminal: ophthalmic division (V1) Trigeminal: maxillary division (V2) Trigeminal: mandibular division (V3)	Superior orbital fissure Foramen rotundum Foramen ovale
VI	Abducens	Superior orbital fissure
VII	Facial	Internal acoustic meatus and stylomastoid foramen
VIII	Auditory	Internal acoustic meatus
IX	Glossopharyngeal	Jugular foramen
X	Vagus	Jugular foramen
XI	Accessory	Jugular foramen
XII	Hypoglossal	Hypoglossal canal

- □ *Perform forced duction to rule out muscle entrapment if intubated/sedated and periorbital fractures present
- □ Steps for forced duction test
  - ▪ Place 2 drops of tetracaine into the eyes. Patient may need additional anxiolytics.
  - ▪ Grasp the sclera (away from cornea) with fine forceps and move the globe into upward/downward/lateral gaze positions to test for entrapment of extraocular muscles.
  - ▪ When in doubt, perform forced duction on the normal side for comparison.
- ▪ Hyphema or globe injury
- ▪ Enophthalmos
- ▪ Eyelid position
- ▪ Medial canthal tendon stability (vs telecanthus)
- ○ Ears
  - ▪ Inspect external ear on all surfaces for lacerations, perichondral hematoma.
  - ▪ Observe for Battle sign: bruising of mastoid process indicative of skull base fracture.
  - ▪ Otoscopy: hemotympanum, cerebrospinal fluid (CSF) leak, perforation of tympanic membrane.
  - ▪ **Hematoma on external ear must be evacuated and bolstered to prevent reaccumulation.**
- ○ Nose
  - ▪ Assess contour and stability of nasal bones.
  - ▪ Use nasal speculum for intranasal exam: assess for lacerations, nasal obstruction, **rule out septal hematoma (can lead to septal necrosis if untreated)**

- ▫ Septal hematoma can be drained via small incision. After incision and drainage, nasal packing or nasal stent should be placed to prevent reaccumulation.
  - ○ Midface, cheek
    - ▪ *Lacerations should be examined for proximity to Stenson (parotid) duct (runs in middle third of a line drawn from oral commissure to tragus).
    - ▪ To assess integrity of the duct:
      - ▫ Cannulating the intraoral papilla at level of maxillary second molar with a lacrimal probe or small gauze IV catheter.
      - ▫ Instill propofol or half-strength hydrogen peroxide solution to see if any white solution or bubbling in the wound, which indicates ductal injury.
      - ▫ Any injury must be repaired or stented.
    - ▪ Look for malar flattening and downsloping of palpebral fissure (ZMC fractures).
    - ▪ Assess for midface mobility while stabilizing the skull (Le Fort fractures)
  - ○ Mandible, oral cavity, occlusion
    - ▪ Assess occlusion
      - ▫ Ask patient "Does your bite feel normal?"
      - ▫ Inspect wear facets of teeth—these will intercuspate if occlusion is normal. This is very useful in unresponsive patients.
      - ▫ Anterior or posterior open bite, cross bite.
    - ▪ Document loose/missing/broken teeth
      - ▫ Dentistry consult
    - ▪ Inspect oral lining for lacerations or ecchymosis.
    - ▪ Measure incisal opening distance.
    - ▪ Submucosal hematoma may indicate mandible fracture.
    - ▪ Palpate temporomandibular joint (TMJ) in external auditory canal with opening and closing of mouth.
    - ▪ Note oral hygiene and any carious teeth that may serve as source of infection.
- • Diagnostic Studies
  - ○ *Maxillofacial CT is the gold standard to evaluate for facial fractures (isolated nasal bone fractures do not require imaging. It is a clinical diagnosis)
    - ▪ Coronal views
      - ▫ Accurate assessment of nasal bones
      - ▫ Orbital walls and potential herniation of contents into maxillary sinus
    - ▪ Three-dimensional reformats are useful in planning complex panfacial fracture reconstruction.
    - ▪ Herald findings of fracture
      - ▫ Osseous deformity
      - ▫ Sinus opacification
      - ▫ Pneumocephalus or soft tissue air/edema
  - ○ Panorex may be sufficient in cases of mandible fracture (this requires a patient to sit up in the panoramic radiograph device and therefore cannot be done in unresponsive patients).
  - ○ Consider plain films, three views, to evaluate for missing mandibular segments (eg, gunshot wounds); also useful when Panorex not available.

FACIAL SOFT TISSUE INJURIES

FACIAL FIELD BLOCKS

Facial field blocks are useful for providing anesthesia in awake patients and usually take about 1-2 cc of local anesthetics for each nerve block (Fig. 20-1)
- • Supraorbital, Supratrochlear, and Infratrochlear Nerves
  - ○ Innervates: forehead/anterior scalp/upper eyelid/glabella.

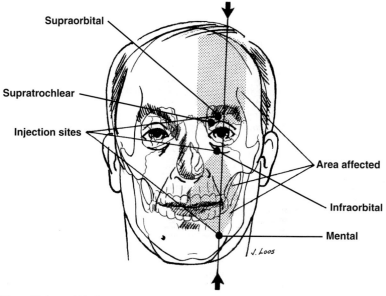

Figure 20-1 Facial blocks.

    ○ Insert needle in midpupillary line at supraorbital rim (just lateral to the mid brow), advance medially to capture supratrochlear nerve.
- **Infraorbital Nerve**
    ○ Innervates: lateral nose/upper lip/lower eyelid/medial cheek.
    ○ Transoral: insert needle into superior buccal sulcus above the canine tooth root at midpupillary line 6-10 mm below the infraorbital rim.
    ○ Transcutaneous: insert needle into a few millimeters lateral to the alar groove at the superior part of the nasolabial groove and advance to 6-10 mm below the infraorbital rim at midpupillary line.
        ■ With transcutaneous approach, operator can often feel the needle entering the foramen.
- **Zygomaticotemporal/Zygomaticofacial Nerves**
    ○ Innervates: temporal and lateral orbital regions/lateral cheek over the zygoma.
    ○ ZT block: insert needle from above just 1 cm behind the lateral orbital rim at the level just below the zygomaticofrontal suture. Insert along the bony wall to 1 cm below the lateral canthus and inject on the way out.
    ○ ZF block: always done after ZT block. Inject a dime-sized of injectate just at the junction of lateral and inferior orbit rims.
- **Dorsal Nasal Nerve**
    ○ Innervates: cartilaginous dorsum and tip.
    ○ Palpate nasal bone with thumb and index finger. Nerve exits ~6-10 mm from the middle line on both sides. Around 1-2 cc injectate is sufficient for each side.
- **Mental Nerve**
    ○ Innervates: lower lip/chin
    ○ *Insert needle into inferior buccal sulcus at **mandibular second premolar**
- **Cervical Plexus, Great Auricular, Transverse Cervical Nerves**
    ○ Innervates: posterior auricle/mandibular angle/anterior neck

- o *Both great auricular and transverse cervical nerves emerge at Erb point
  - ▪ 7 cm inferior to tragus
  - ▪ Posterior border of sternocleidomastoid (SCM) muscle
- o Mark patient's SCM when flexed, locate midpoint from clavicle to mastoid for injection
- **Auriculotemporal, Great Auricular, Lesser Occipital, Arnold Nerve**
  - o Ear "ring block."
  - o Begin with needle at junction of lobule and cheek and proceed with four injections circumferentially.
  - o Avoid superficial temporal artery.
  - o *Separate injection in external auditory canal for Arnold nerve (auricular branch of the vagus nerve, CN X).

LACERATION REPAIR

- **General Principles**
  - o The face has a robust vascular supply; avoid excessive debridement.
  - o Repair in layers under minimal tension.
  - o Copious irrigation with normal saline and betadine, remove foreign bodies.
  - o Deep dermis: 5-0 interrupted buried absorbable sutures (eg, Vicryl and Monocryl).
  - o Skin: 5-0 or 6-0 interrupted or running permanent suture (eg, nylon and Prolene).
  - o In young children, skin closure may be performed with 6-0 fast absorbing gut or 7-0 chromic gut to eliminate the need for suture removal.
  - o Nonabsorbable sutures are removed in 5-7 days; delayed removal will result in suture track marks.
  - o Avoid undermining and/or local tissue rearrangement.
    - ▪ Partial avulsions: tissue present on small pedicles will usually survive.
- **Scalp**
  - o Close with surgical staples or running locking absorbable suture (eg, chromic gut).
  - o Avulsions are indication for microvascular replantation.
    - ▪ Scalp can tolerate 12-18 hours cold ischemia time.
    - ▪ Superficial temporal or occipital vessels can serve as recipient vessels during scalp replantation.
- **Eyebrows**
  - o Direction of hair growth helpful in realigning wound edges
  - o Inspect within the wound for occult fracture
  - o Avoid cautery: cicatricial alopecia
  - o *Temporal branch of facial nerve: Pitanguy line
    - ▪ 0.5 cm inferior to tragus to 1.5 cm superior to lateral margin of eyebrow
    - ▪ **Deep surface of superficial temporal fascia** (ie, temporal parietal fascia) with superficial temporal artery
  - o Advance lateral brow if necessary to close, medial brow position more aesthetically important
- **Eyelids**
  - o Conjunctiva meets the skin at gray line on lid margin.
  - o Ptosis on exam may indicate levator injury.
  - o **Rounding and mobility of medial canthus may indicate nasoorbitoethmoid (NOE) fracture** (telecanthus) (normal intercanthal distance 32 mm).
  - o Epiphora (excessive tearing) indicates possible lacrimal canalicular injury.
  - o Repair techniques
    - ▪ Repair conjunctiva only if large defect present (eg, 5-0 fast absorbing chromic)
    - ▪ Repair tarsal plate (eg, 5-0 Vicryl)

- Repair lid margin with vertical mattress at gray line using polyfilament (eg, 6-0 Vicryl)
  - Eversion of closure prevents notching of lid margin
  - Avoids corneal abrasion from monofilament suture
  - May be removed in 5-7 days
- Keep all suture tails long, tied into an inferior suture knot away from globe
- **Lacrimal System Injury**
  - Canaliculus courses 2 mm perpendicular to lid margin then heads medially to lacrimal sac and nasolacrimal apparatus
  - *Drains into nose at inferior meatus
  - Laceration to medial third of eyelid ⇒ suspect canaliculus injury
    - Exploration: after dilating the punctum, place lacrimal probe in punctum and pass it into canaliculus, look for probe within the wound.
    - Place silastic lacrimal stent; "Crawford tubes" (±suture repair of duct)
      - Stents should exit from inferior nasal meatus. They should be tie and cut short.
    - Stent remains in place for 2-3 months.
    - Dacryocystorhinostomy may be necessary if cannulation is impossible with resulting epiphora.
    - *Jones I and II tests may be used clinically.
      - Jones I test: performed by instilling fluorescein into the conjunctival fornices and passing a cotton-tip into the inferior meatus to recover the dye. This is done at 2 and 5 minutes after instilling fluorescein.
      - Jones II test: performed after an unsuccessful Jones I test. Remaining of the fluorescein is injected into the punctum (after dilating) with a 23-gauge catheter. Failure to see dye at inferior meatus indicates negative test and possible lacrimal injury or obstruction.
- **Cheek**
  - **Stenson duct** penetrates buccinator to enter oral cavity opposite second molar; travels with buccal branches of facial nerve.
    - Probe intraoral papilla with 22G angiocath peripheral venous catheter and inject hydrogen peroxide: if duct is injured, visualize gas bubbles in wound.
    - Repair duct to prevent sialocele, or leave drain.
    - *If sialocele develops, aspirate and apply pressure dressing.
  - **Nerve injury**—can use nerve stimulator up to 48-72 hours later
    - Considerable crossover between zygomatic and buccal CN VII branches
    - Does not require repair if medial to lateral canthus
- **Nose**
  - Redundant arterial supply: lateral nasal, external nasal, septal, and columellar arteries
  - Septum composed of septal cartilage, vomer bone, perpendicular plate of ethmoid, maxillary crest, and premaxilla
  - **Septal hematoma**
    - Evacuate with needle aspiration or blade to prevent necrosis and septal perforation.
    - Place running quilted 4-0 gut suture or nasal packing.
  - **Laceration repair**
    - Mucosal lining: 4-0 chromic with knots in nasal cavity
    - Cartilage: 5-0 clear nylon or PDS sutures
    - Skin: 6-0 nylon in the skin
  - **Avulsion injuries:** consider composite graft (replantation if possible)
    - 50% failure
    - All grafted material must be within 5 mm of viable tissue
- **Ears**
  - Arterial supply: superficial temporal and postauricular arteries

- ○ Great auricular, auriculotemporal, Arnold, lesser occipital nerves provide sensation
- ○ **Otohematoma**
  - ▪ Evacuate with needle or blade to avoid "cauliflower ear"
  - ▪ Compression dressing
    - ▫ Xeroform bolster secured with 3-0 Prolene through and through mattress sutures
    - ▫ Remove in 1 week
- ○ **Lacerations**
  - ▪ May require figure-of-eight sutures in cartilage (clear nylon or absorbable monofilament)
  - ▪ Evert skin margins in key locations (eg, helix) with mattress sutures
- ○ **Amputation**
  - ▪ Partial amputation—suture repair
  - ▪ Complete amputation—attempt replantation
  - ▪ Consider leech therapy for venous congestion
  - ▪ Consider dermabrasion of ear part and banking cartilage in dermal pocket
- **Mouth**
  - ○ Anatomic landmarks: philtral columns, philtral dimple, Cupid bow, vermillion border, and white roll
  - ○ Lacerations: repair mucosa, orbicularis, and skin in layers. Mark white roll with methylene blue or marking pen prior to administration of local anesthetic to prevent distortion which can be prevented with regional nerve blocks
- **Tongue**
  - ○ Lingual block: insert needle **6-8 mm** inferior to the lingual gingival margin of the 2nd molar. Depth of injection is 5-8 mm.
  - ○ Small lacerations can be healed by secondary intention.
  - ○ Large (>2 cm) and through-and-through lacerations require suture repair with absorbable sutures (4-0 Vicryl or chromics).

FACIAL FRACTURE EVALUATION AND MANAGEMENT

MANDIBLE FRACTURES
- **Anatomy (Fig. 20-2)**
  - ○ **Mental nerve** (CN V_3)
    - ▪ Exits skull base from foramen ovale
    - ▪ Courses 2 mm below foramen
    - ▪ *Exits mental foramen at second premolar
    - ▪ Nerve is closest to buccal cortex at third molar, farthest from buccal cortex at first molar
  - ○ **Muscles of mastication** (CN V_3) exert deforming forces of mandible
    - ▪ *Lateral pterygoid: protracts (lowers) mandible
    - ▪ Medial pterygoid: closes mouth
    - ▪ Temporalis: elevates and retracts mandible
    - ▪ Masseter: elevates mandible
    - ▪ Geniohyoid, genioglossus, mylohyoid, digastric muscles: depress mandible
- **Clinical Presentation**
  - ○ Patient may endorse malocclusion
  - ○ Exam may show floor of mouth ecchymosis, step offs, tenderness over fracture site, open bite, premature contact
- **Management Considerations**
  - ○ The mandible is like a pretzel: difficult to break in only one location; look for second fracture.
  - ○ Classification of fracture—location on mandible, simple vs comminuted, open vs closed, and intracapsular/extracapsular.

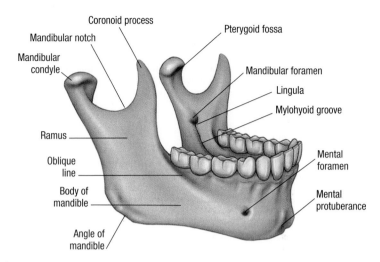

Figure 20-2 Mandible anatomy. (From Anatomical Chart Co., 2013.)

- Teeth in line of fracture should be retained if roots are not fractured.
- Maxillomandibular fixation (MMF; also called intermaxillary fixation, or IMF) may be used as a single modality (controversial) for 4-6 weeks.
• Principles of open reduction and internal fixation (ORIF)
  - Indications: displaced fracture with abnormal occlusion
  - MMF to restore occlusion
  - Subperiosteal dissection to expose fracture line
  - Reduction of fracture fragments
  - Rigid fixation using plates/screws, 2.0-mm plating systems
  - Early, active mobility
  - Tension band plate placed along alveolar border
  - Large reconstruction plate along inferior border
• General Management of Fracture Subtypes
  - **Symphyseal/parasymphyseal fractures.** Miniplate fixation with at least two points of fixation
  - **Body fractures.** Miniplate fixation
  - **Angle fractures.** Highest complication rate
    ▪ Isolated: treat with MMF and/or Champy plate (load sharing at oblique ridge), strut plate
    ▪ Complex: treat with MMF, two load-sharing plates, or one load-bearing plates
    ▪ If severe, may need external fixation
  - **Coronoid fractures**—MMF for 2 weeks is usually enough
  - **Condylar and subcondylar fractures**
    ▪ Intracapsular
      □ Condylar fractures (head and upper neck)
      □ Closed reduction and limited (2 weeks) MMF with early controlled mobilization; rarely ORIF
      □ **Open treatment warranted if:** (1) cannot reduce fracture and it precludes ranging the mandible, (2) a foreign body is present within the TMJ, (3) the condyle has displaced into the middle cranial fossa, and (4) bilateral condyle fractures with midface fractures to restore vertical height

- Extracapsular
  - Subcondylar fractures
  - IMF × 4-6 weeks, weekly observation of occlusion after release
- Pediatric mandible fractures
  - *Avoid immobilization, early active therapy, growth potential allows improvement of occlusion with time
  - May require MMF
  - In the absence of permanent dentition
    - Piriform drop wires
    - Circum-mandibular wires
- Edentulous mandible
  - Closed fractures with minimal displacement: no dentures, soft diet
  - Open fractures or those with displacement: ORIF with load-bearing plate, may require gunning splint
- Dislocations
  - Anterior displacement of condyle from glenoid fossa
  - Closed reduction necessary
    - Conscious sedation
    - Intraoral downward and posterior pressure at ramus
- **Indications for Tooth Removal**
  - Grossly mobile
  - Severe periodontal disease
  - Root fracture
  - Exposed apices
- **Common Complications**
  - Malocclusion/malunion/nonunion
  - Increased facial width, rotation of mandible
  - TMJ ankylosis: stiffness, pain, limited range of motion
  - Infection: often treated with I&D, hardware removal generally not required

ZYGOMA FRACTURES

- Anatomy
  - Zygoma has a quadrilateral shape: articulates with maxilla, sphenoid, temporal, and frontal bones; fractures are, therefore, "tetrapod fractures"
  - Muscle attachments: masseter, temporalis, zygomaticus major and minor
- Clinical Presentation
  - **Flattening of malar eminence with downslanting palpebral fissure:** lateral canthus attaches to zygoma via Whitnall tubercle.
  - Zygomatic arch fractures may limit the motion of coronoid, resulting in trismus.
  - Enophthalmos.
  - Infraorbital paresthesia.
- **ORIF:** required to restore facial width, malar projection, and orbital dystopia
  - **Approaches**
    - Upper blepharoplasty incision: access to zygomaticofrontal junction
    - Coronal incision: to expose entire arch and lateral orbital rim
    - Gillies approach
      - Temporal incision behind hair line
      - *Dissect deep to temporalis muscle fascia
      - Reduce posteriorly displaced arch fracture with outward force
    - Transconjunctival incision: access to zygomaticomaxillary junction (and orbital floor)
    - Intraoral incision: Dingman elevator placed under arch with outward force
  - Fixation: 1.5- or 2.0-mm plating systems.

- o Postoperative arch splint: may wrap tongue depressor in silk tape and bend into bridge shape, secure to face with tape as buttress to prevent infracturing during sleep (not needed when plated).
- o Zygomaticosphenoid articulation is the most important to assess reduction.

ORBITAL FRACTURES

- **Anatomy (Fig. 20-3)**
  - o Orbit is constructed of seven bones—maxilla, zygoma, sphenoid, frontal, palatine, lacrimal, and ethmoid.
  - o *Conical/pyramid shape: optic nerve is ~4 cm posterior to orbital rim.
  - o Thinnest region is medial wall (lamina papyracea).
- Ophthalmology consult if concern for ocular trauma
- Fractures most common in orbital floor and medial wall (lamina papyracea of ethmoid)
- Dystopia occurs if loss of bony support
- **Enophthalmos**
  - o Fractures of orbit result in increased intraorbital volume and disrupt ligamentous support of globe.
  - o During healing, periorbital takes on shape with smaller volume.
- **Clinical Presentation**
  - o Periorbital edema
  - o Periorbital ecchymosis
  - o Diplopia
  - o Infraorbtial nerve paresthesia
  - o Enophthalmos
  - o Orbital rim step-off
  - o Limited globe excursion from edema or entrapment
- **Indication for ORIF**
  - o Persistent diplopia (>2 weeks).
  - o Fractures that involve >50% orbital floor or >2 cm².
  - o Clinically significant enophthalmos.
  - o *Entrapment of extraocular muscles (requires emergent intervention, that is, <24 hours, to release ischemic muscle). Entrapment is determined by assessing extraocular movements or by forced duction testing (see above, under ED Evaluation and Physical Examination) if unconscious.

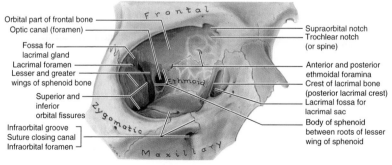

Anterior view

Figure 20-3 Skeletal orbital anatomy and the relationship of the superior and inferior orbital fissures and optic foramen. (From Dalley AF II, Agur AMR. *Moore's Clinical Oriented Anatomy*. 9th ed. Wolters Kluwer; 2023. Figure 8.44B.)

- **ORIF**
  - Subciliary, transconjunctival, inferior orbital rim incisions.
  - *Transconjunctival approach is associated with lowest rate of postoperative ectropion.
  - Medpor (porous polyethylene) implant or cranial bone grafts can be used to reconstruct the orbital floor: secured in place with screws at infraorbital rim.
  - Young children may present with a "trapdoor" floor fracture in which there is no defect but the fracture has entrapped the extraocular muscle (usually the inferior rectus muscle). The muscle can be released and the orbital floor usually needs no implant or reconstruction if it feels stable.
- **Associated Potential Ophthalmic Consequences**
  - Corneal abrasion
  - Hyphema: blood in anterior chamber
  - Sympathetic ophthalmia
  - Traumatic optic neuropathy: traumatic loss of vision
    - Requires surgical decompression, and high-dose steroids
  - *Superior orbital fissure syndrome
    - Effects oculomotor, trochlear, abducens, and trigeminal (lacrimal, frontal, and nasociliary branches) nerves and ophthalmic vein
    - Signs
      - Ptosis
      - Proptosis
      - Ophthalmoplegia
      - Numbness in VN V1
      - Dilation and fixation of ipsilateral pupil
  - *Orbital apex syndrome: same as superior orbital fissure syndrome but with loss of vision due to injury to optic nerve
  - Traumatic carotid cavernous sinus fistula
    - Proptosis
    - Ocular bruit
    - Ophthalmoplegia of CN III, IV, or VI
    - Treatment: surgical ligation of carotid artery or coils to block off fistula

NASAL BONE FRACTURES

- **Nasal Anatomy**
  - Upper one-third of the nose: paired nasal bones
    - Fractures common in thinner lower halves of paired nasal bones.
    - Younger patients experience fracture-dislocations of larger segments.
    - Older patients develop comminuted patterns.
  - Lower two-thirds of the nose: paired upper lateral cartilage, lower lateral cartilage
  - Septum consists of quadrangular cartilage, vomer, perpendicular
- **Treatment Goals**
  - Restoration of function and appearance.
  - Wait 6 months before considering revision rhinoplasty or secondary closed reduction plate of ethmoid bone.
  - Acutely before edema begins (uncommon) or after swelling resolves (3-5 days).
  - Closed reduction should be accomplished within 2 weeks of injury to avoid osteotomies.
- **Principles and Technique**
  - Look for septal hematoma.
  - Do not misdiagnose NOE for simple fx as NOE is hard to fix.
  - Usually treat closed except with complex facial fractures, inability to obtain good closed reduction, severe comminution.

- External nose anesthetized by regional block 0.5% lidocaine with 1:200 000 epinephrine.
- Internal nose anesthetized by Afrin-soaked pledgets.
- Reduce bridge with elevator and septum and Asch forceps or butter knife.
- Nasal bone must be mobilized before reduction.
- External thermoplast splint and internal nasal splints placed after reduction.

- **Complications**
  - Subperichondral fibrosis with partial obstruction
  - Synechiae
  - Obstruction of the nasal vestibule from malunited fractures or scar contractures from loss of vestibular lining
  - Osteitis
  - Malunion of nasal fractures with residual deviation

NOE FRACTURES

- **Fractures of** nasal bones, frontal processes of maxilla, lacrimal bone, and ethmoid bone
- **Markowitz Classification:** based on central fragment with medial canthal tendon
  - Type I: single, noncomminuted, central fragment without medial canthal tendon disruption
  - Type II: comminuted central fragment without medial canthal disruption
  - Type III: severely comminuted central fragment with disruption of medial canthal tendon
- **Clinical Presentation**
  - *Telecanthus (not always seen acutely): normal intercanthal distance is 30-34 mm
  - Foreshortened and depressed nose
  - Lack of nasal support on palpation
  - Subconjunctival hemorrhage
  - CSF rhinorrhea
  - Mobility of the medial canthus on bimanual exam
- **Commonly includes medial canthal ligament–bearing bone**
  - Fracture line through anterior and posterior lacrimal crest
  - Leads to traumatic telecanthus
  - Possible damage to nasolacrimal system, leading to epiphora
- **Septal Cartilage Fractures:** progressive deviation from warping forces due to perichondrium
- **Treatment**
  - Principles
    - Rule out brain injury (frontal lobes, dural tears, and bone fragments in the brain) and coordinate with neurosurgery
    - Early intervention (very difficult to fix if done as a late reconstruction)
    - Wide exposure; reduce and stabilize anterior orbital rim; restore internal orbital architecture with bone graft; reconstruct glabella, upper nasal region, medial canthi; and release soft tissue
  - Exposure
    - Usually required two to three separate incisions
    - Nasofrontal area: through laceration, midline nasal, or coronal incision (best exposure)
    - Subciliary or transconjunctival: with lateral canthotomy
    - Upper buccal sulcus: may be required to obtain adequate reduction
  - Technique
    - Subperiosteal dissection to inferior orbital rim and floor.
    - Asch forceps used intranasally to elevate and reduce nasal fragments.
    - Do not detach canthal ligament from bone fragment if avulsed.
    - Preserve medial canthal ligament attachments to the bone.

Section II: Craniofacial

- Preserve lacrimal sac and nasolacrimal duct attachment to the bone.
- Isolate segments containing canthal ligament, place in perfect anatomic reduction, and stabilize with rigid fixation.
- Preserve and attach all bone fragments.
- Reduction, rigid fixation.
  - Plates/screws if canthal-bearing segment is large enough
  - If canthus is avulsed from bone, reposition using transnasal wires
  - *Vector of wire fixation: posterior and superior
- Bone graft often needed for medial orbital wall and floor and for restoration of nasal dorsum height and contour (cantilever cranial bone graft or rib graft).
- External splinting 2 weeks.

FRONTAL BONE/SINUS FRACTURES

- **Anatomy**
  - Thick anterior table, thin floor (orbital roof), and thinner posterior table.
  - Nasofrontal duct is posterior medial in location and runs through anterior ethmoid bone.
  - Drains into middle meatus.
  - *Not present at birth, begins to develop at 2 years old, and does not reach adult size until 12 years old.
- **Fracture Classification**
  - Anterior table
  - Posterior table
  - Nasofrontal duct involvement
- Forces of 800-2200 lb are required for frontal sinus fractures, 2-3× greater than any other facial bone
- Frequently associated with NOE and midface fractures
- **Clinical Presentation**
  - Palpable deformity to frontal bone
  - CSF rhinorrhea
  - Paresthesia in pattern of supraorbital and supratrochlear nerves
  - Inferior globe displacement of orbital roof
- **Complications**
  - Mucocele; pyomucocele
  - Osteomyelitis
  - Infection of orbital contents
  - CSF rhinorrhea
    - Halo test/ring sign: fluid is placed on gauze and concentric rings of blood and CSF form, indicating CSF leak.
    - Fluid can be sent for beta transferrin level to confirm leak.
- **Indications for Operative Management**
  - Displaced anterior table (leads to contour deformity)
  - Nasofrontal duct involvement or obstruction (leads to mucocele)
  - Depressed posterior table
- **Treatment Goals**
  - Restoration of contour
  - Isolation of cranial cavity from upper airway
  - Construction of safe sinus
- **Operative Management**
  - **Displaced anterior table**
    - ORIF with low-profile miniplates
    - If comminuted, IO wiring may be needed
    - **Nasofrontal duct obstruction** or posterior table displacement with minimal or no CSF leak. Obliteration of sinus with bone, fat grafts, or pericranial flaps after exenteration of sinus mucosa

TABLE 20-2 Frontal Sinus Fracture Treatment Algorithm

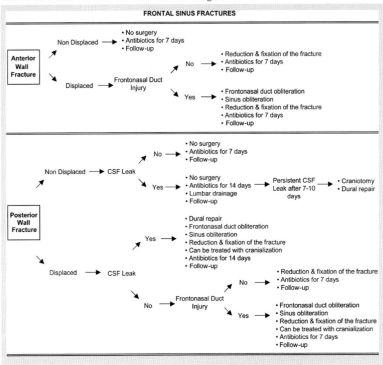

- ○ Posterior table fracture with CSF leak: cranialization
  - ▪ Exenterate sinus mucosa
  - ▪ Remove posterior table allowing the brain to fill potential space
- ○ **Nasofrontal duct obstruction** can result in mucopyocele. To test for patency: instill methylene blue into sinus and place cotton tip applicator (ie, Q-Tip) endonasally for confirmation of flow (**Table 20-2**)

MAXILLARY FRACTURES

- **Anatomy**
  - ○ Four processes: frontal, zygomatic, palatine, and alveolar
  - ○ Contains maxillary sinus
  - ○ Muscle attachments include facial expression muscles anteriorly and pterygoid muscles posteriorly
  - ○ Three major buttresses that provide strength (**Fig. 20-4**)
    - ▪ Nasomaxillary
    - ▪ Zygomatic
    - ▪ Pterygomaxillary
- *Le Fort Classification (Fig. 20-5)
  - ○ Alternating thick buttresses and thinner segments create distinct fracture patterns
  - ○ Usually involve pterygoid plates
  - ○ **Le Fort I: transverse**

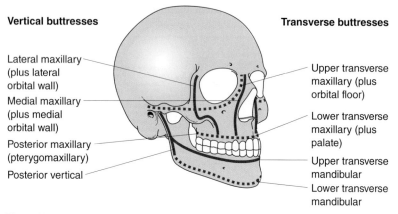

Vertical buttresses

Lateral maxillary
(plus lateral
orbital wall)

Medial maxillary
(plus medial
orbital wall)

Posterior maxillary
(pterygomaxillary)

Posterior vertical

Transverse buttresses

Upper transverse
maxillary (plus
orbital floor)

Lower transverse
maxillary (plus
palate)

Upper transverse
mandibular

Lower transverse
mandibular

Figure 20-4 Vertical and transverse buttresses of the facial skeleton. (From Mulholland MW, ed. *Greenfield's Surgery.* 5th ed. Lippincott Williams & Wilkins; 2011.)

- Fracture at the level of tooth apices above the palate and alveolus
- Separates tooth-bearing maxilla from midface
- Extends from pyriform aperture posteriorly through nasal septum, anterior maxillary wall, lateral nasal wall, and pterygoid plates
  ○ Le Fort II: pyramidal
    - Fracture crosses nasal bones along zygomaticomaxillary suture
    - May involve frontal sinus
    - Upper jaw and nasal bones mobile as single unit
  ○ Le Fort III: craniofacial disjunction
    - May be minimally displaced with subtle occlusion problems
    - Entire midface is mobile and detached from cranial base
    - Fracture though pterygoid plates at a high level

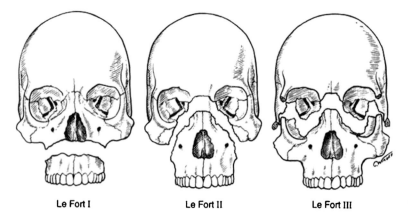

Le Fort I   **Le Fort II**   **Le Fort III**

Figure 20-5 Le Fort fracture patterns. (From Tasman W, Jaeger EA. Duane's *Ophthalmology.* 2006 ed. Lippincott Williams & Wilkins; 2005.)

- Simultaneous mobility of maxilla and nasofrontal and zygomaticofrontal regions
- **Vertical or Sagittal Fractures**
  - Fracture sections maxilla in AP plane
  - Split palate, less common than Le Fort
- **Initial Management**
  - ABCs: midfacial fractures are associated with high impact injury and **concomitant C-spine fracture (10%).**
  - IMF reduces fracture and decreases bleeding.
- **Treatment**
  - Alveolar fractures: apply arch bars, place segment in occlusion, place IMF wires, 2-0 plates to stabilize fracture
  - Le Fort fractures: primary bone grafts and rigid fixation
    - IMF 4-6 weeks
    - Ensure proper reduction of nasomaxillary and zygomaxillary buttresses
  - Surgical steps
    - MMF to reestablish proper occlusal relations. This will usually establish the known starting point, mandible to crania base (may be difficult in the presence of split palate, alveolar, or mandible fx).
    - Expose widely. May require multiple incisions—coronal, upper buccal sulcus, transconjunctival, depending on the location of fractures.
    - Reduce each segment anatomically starting from mandible → maxilla → zygoma → NOE, etc.
    - Stabilize with mini-plates. Le Fort II must stabilize nasofrontal jx and infraorbital rims; Le Fort III must stabilize zygomaticofrontal suture.
    - Primary bone grafting utilized in the acute setting. Bridge gaps >0.5 cm of maxillary buttresses, >1.5 cm of antral wall.
    - Soft tissue suspension of check to infraorbital rim.
    - Immobilization in MMF is not necessary for the healing of Le Fort fx if rigid fixation is utilized in the fx repair.
    - For the Le Fort fx without mobility (<10%), place in MMF with elastics. If occlusion is not restored in 3 days, do ORIF, otherwise keep in MMF for 6 weeks with soft diet.
    - If the patient is allowed to return to early fx, soft foods only as true rigid fixation in the midface is not completely attained due to the thin bones and corresponding thin plates and screws.
    - If the mandible is fractured at the condyle—cannot rely on mandible to establish proper facial height. ORIF midface first and star with the zygoma then place the patient in MMF and treat the mandible as indicated.
    - If the palate is fractured, it may be helpful to first wire the posterior aspect of the palate for stability before MMF or any midfacial plating is undertaken.
    - Most common complication of Le Fort is reduced facial height and projection.
  - **Common inadequate fixation sequelae:** enophthalmos, malocclusion, increased facial width, soft tissue descent, facial diastasis, and fat atrophy
  - **Complications:** hemorrhage, airway compromise, pneumocephalus, open bite, nonunion, and malunion

TEMPORAL BONE TRAUMA

- **Clinical Signs**
  - Facial palsy
    - 10%-50% of temporal bone fractures
    - Management:
      - □ Observation for incomplete paresis
      - □ Surgical exploration for complete paresis that is not recovering
  - Bruising over mastoid (Battle sign)

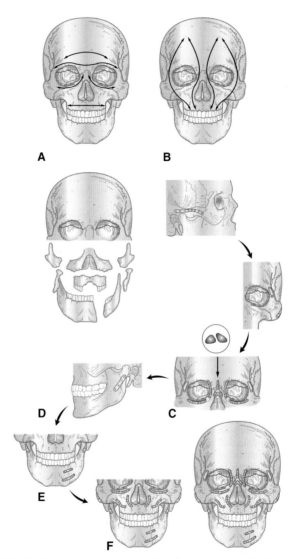

Figure 20-6 Panfacial fracture treatment protocol, based on reconstructing load-bearing structures of the facial skeleton. A. Projection of the midface is created by reconstructing the zygomatic arches, starting from the stable part of the temporal bone. **B.** The zygomas are fixed to the arches and to the frontal bone to create the final projection of the midface. **C.** The width of the midface is reconstructed by repositioning the central midface (orbits and nose) to its correct position, in relation to the zygomas and frontal bone. Concomitantly, canthopexy is fixed, and the frontal bone and sinus fractures are treated. (This procedure is independent of the occlusion.) **D.** The posterior vertical height of the face is reconstructed by positioning and fixing the condylar fractures. **E.** Intermaxillary fixation is applied, and the mandible is reconstructed. **F.** Finally, the Le Fort I-level fractures are positioned to natural occlusion. (Modified from Guyuron B, Eriksson E, Persing JA. *Plastic Surgery: Indications and Practice*. Vol. 1. 2009:633; Booth PW, Schendel SA, Hausamen JE. *Maxillofacial Surgery*. 2nd ed. 2007;Vol. 1:38.)

- Hemotympanum
- CSF leak
- Vestibular dysfunction

PALATE FRACTURES

- **Indications for Surgery**
  - Anterior-posterior–oriented fractures with large individual segments and no comminution.
  - Palatal splints are used for complex fractures to provide the best vault stabilization.
- **Surgical Approach**
  - Avoid devascularizing the buccal, gingival, or palatal mucosa during fracture exposure.
  - Full open reduction must include reduction and stabilization of the palatal vault, dental arch (alveolus and pyriform aperture), and the four anterior vertical buttresses of the maxilla.
  - Place the patient in MMF for 2-6 weeks.
  - Splints only to supplement fixation.

PANFACIAL FRACTURES

- **Definition:** facial fractures that involve the upper, middle, and lower (mandible) face
- **Goals**
  - Reestablish proper vertical columns and anterior facial projection via anatomic reduction and rigid fixation of the facial skeletons
  - Reestablish functional occlusion and orbital/oral/nasal volume
- **General Principles (Fig. 20-6)**
  - Systematic approaches either from "top down" or "bottom up"
    - Traditionally, a "bottom-up" approach by achieving anatomic reconstruction of the mandible is performed to provide a stable base. This provides the base to reconstruct the midface and up.
    - A "top-down" approach can also be used and sometimes can be helpful in presence of condylar fracture. This would avoid opening and fixating the condylar fractures (high ankylosis rate).
  - Working from known (ie, stable) area to unknown area and from inside to outside makes proper reduction more manageable and achievable.
  - Some degrees of malreduction above the dentition may be tolerated if functional occlusion, vertical facial height, and projection can be achieved.

QUESTIONS YOU WILL BE ASKED

1. The bones comprising the orbit.
   Maxilla, zygoma, sphenoid, palatine, ethmoid, lacrimal, and frontal (**see Fig. 20-3**).
2. Facial nerve branches.
   ("Two zebras bit my cat") temporal, zygomatic, buccal, marginal mandibular, and cervical.
3. Patterns of Le Fort fractures.
   See Figure 20-5. Le Fort I is horizontal maxillary fracture. Le Fort II is pyramidal maxillary fracture. Le Fort III is craniofacial disjunction. All involve pterygoid plates.
4. The ZMC "tetrapod."
   The zygoma has a quadrilateral shape. It articulates with maxilla, frontal, sphenoid, and temporal bones.
5. The facial buttresses and their importance.
   See Figure 20-4. Four transverse and four vertical paired structural units of thicker bone lend strength and stability and project the soft tissue envelope of face.
6. How to diagnose a CSF leak?
   Send fluid for β-transferrin.

Section II: Craniofacial

Recommended Readings

1. Fraioli RE, Branstetter BF IV, Deleyiannis FW. Facial fractures: beyond Le Fort. *Otolaryngol Clin North Am.* 2008;41(1):51-76. vi.
2. Haug RH, Buchbinder D. Incisions for access to craniomaxillofacial fractures. *Atlas Oral Maxillofac Surg Clin North Am.* 1993;1(2):1-29.
3. Sargent LA. Nasoethmoid orbital fractures: diagnosis and treatment. *Plast Reconstr Surg.* 2007;120(7 Suppl 2):16S-31S.
4. Sharabi SE, Koshy JC, Thornton JF, Hollier LH Jr. Facial fractures. *Plast Reconstr Surg.* 2011;127(2):25e-34e.
5. Yavuzer R, Sari A, Kelly CP, et al. Management of frontal sinus fractures. *Plast Reconstr Surg.* 2005;115(6):79e-93e. discussion 94e-95e.
6. Zide BM, Swift R. How to block and tackle the face. *Plast Reconstr Surg.* 1998;101(3):840-851. doi:10.1097/00006534-199803000-00041

21

Scalp and Calvarial Reconstruction

Alexandra O. Luby

SCALP RECONSTRUCTION

ANATOMY

- Anatomic Layers of the Scalp—Acronym Scalp (**Fig. 21-1**)
  - Skin.
  - Connective tissue
    - Hair follicles, sweat glands, and fat cells
    - Connective tissue fibers between the galea and skin
  - Aponeurotic layer or galea aponeurotica: a fibrous tissue layer that is continuous with the frontalis and occipitalis and temporoparietal (TP) fascia.
  - *Loose areolar tissue: this layer allows the scalp to move on the cranium and is the most common plane of scalp avulsion injuries.
  - Pericranium/periosteum: a thick collagenous layer with firm attachments to the skull.
- Scalp Vascular Supply (**Fig. 21-2**)
  - **Internal Carotid Artery Branches**
    - Supraorbital artery
    - Supratrochlear artery
  - **External Carotid Artery Branches**
    - Superficial temporal artery.
    - Postauricular artery.
    - Occipital artery.
    - Extensive interconnections are present between branches and across the midline. These anastomoses allow potential replantation of a scalp based on a single artery and vein.
- Scalp Innervation (**Fig. 21-3**)
  - **Motor**
    - Frontalis: frontal branch of CN VII
    - Occipitalis: posterior auricular branch of CN VII
    - Temporalis: deep temporal nerve of CN V
  - **Sensation**
    - Forehead and anterior scalp supplied by supratrochlear and supraorbital nerves (V_1)
    - Supraorbital nerve
      □ Superficial division: supplies skin of the forehead and anterior hairline
      □ Deep division: innervates frontoparietal scalp
    - Temporal region supplied by zygomaticotemporal nerve (V_2) and auriculotemporal nerve (V_3)
    - Posterior scalp supplied by greater and lesser occipital nerves (both are spinal nerves from C_2/C_3)
    - Ear and postauricular area supplied by great auricular nerve (cervical plexus from C_2/C_3)

---

*Denotes common in-service examination topics.

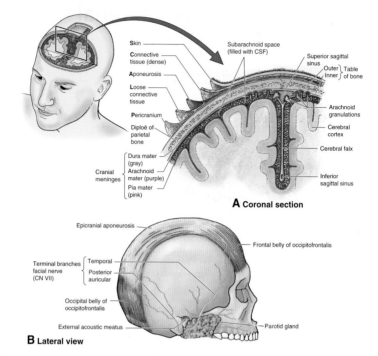

Figure 21-1 Anatomic layers of the forehead and scalp. (From Head. In: Dalley AF II, Agur AMR. *Moore's Clinically Oriented Anatomy.* 9th ed. Wolters Kluwer; 2023:839-999. Figure 8.15.)

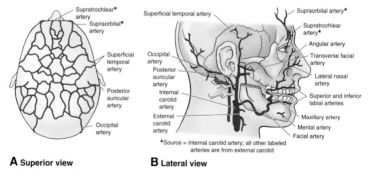

Figure 21-2 Arterial supply to the scalp and face. (From Head. In: Dalley AF II, Agur AMR. *Moore's Clinically Oriented Anatomy.* 9th ed. Wolters Kluwer; 2023:839-999. Figure 8.24.)

SCALP RECONSTRUCTIVE LADDER (FIG. 21-4)

- **Primary closure is an excellent option for defects <3 cm in diameter.**
  - ∘ Facilitated by wide undermining in the avascular subgaleal plane.
  - ∘ Scoring the galea allows additional advancement but may decrease the skin's blood supply.

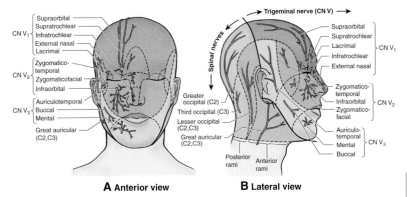

A Anterior view   **B** Lateral view

Figure 21-3 Sensory innervation to the scalp and face. (From Head. In: Dalley AF II, Agur AMR. *Moore's Clinically Oriented Anatomy.* 9th ed. Wolters Kluwer; 2023:839-999. Figure 8.20.)

- **Split-Thickness Skin Grafting** (STSG)
  - Indication: patients who are not candidates for extensive procedures and cosmesis are of low importance.
    - Design: can be placed directly on subcutaneous tissue, galea, or pericranium. If calvarial bone is exposed, STSG is contraindicated. If bare calvarium is present, the outer table can be burred and the STSG placed on the diploe.
    - Alternatively, Integra (a bilaminate bovine collagen construct) can be placed at the index procedure. At a second operation 2-3 weeks later to allow for neovascularization of the Integra, a thin STSG (approximately 8/1000 of an inch) can be placed
  - Disadvantages: no hair follicles, contour deformities, susceptible to trauma.
- **Local Flaps**
  - Indication: coverage of defects between 3 cm and up to 30% defects of the scalp
  - Design: rotation flaps: designed 4-6× as long as the defect is wide
    - Double-opposing rotation flaps (yin-yang) are also useful.
    - Orticochea three-flap and four-flap techniques are based on axial blood supply and can cover 30%.

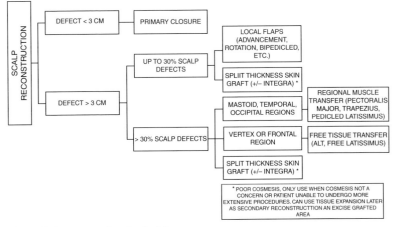

Figure 21-4 Reconstruction of scalp defects.

- Local flaps provide superior cosmesis as hair-bearing skin is brought into the defect.
- Flaps should be raised in the subgaleal plane, which keeps the pericranium as a "lifeboat" for STSG should the donor site break down.
- Galeal scoring can increase flap movement.
  ○ Disadvantage: STSG of the secondary defect may be necessary in order to cover the primary defect.
  ○ Local rotation and advancement flaps often create a dog ear at the base. Do not excise the dog ear as flap compromise may result. The majority of these will flatten out over time.
- **Local axial flaps can be used for specific indications.**
  ○ Galeal flaps can be based on one or multiple axial vessels.
    - The flap is thin and pliable with minimal donor site morbidity.
    - They are particularly useful for three-dimensional (3D) intracranial defects.
  ○ TP fascia flaps are based on the superficial temporal vessels and can carry vascularized calvarium. TP fascial flaps are useful for 3D defects or, if bone is included, for periorbital or facial defects.
  ○ Temporalis muscle flaps are based on the deep temporal arteries. Temporalis flaps have limited use as rotation flaps for anterior scalp and periorbital defects.
  ○ "Crane" flaps are interpolated flaps used to transfer soft tissue to the recipient site. Once vascularization occurs from the recipient site, the flap is raised in a more superficial plane, leaving adequate soft tissue at the recipient site. The flap is then replaced into the original donor site.
- **Tissue expansion** is often used in secondary scalp reconstruction and can replace hair-bearing skin with hair-bearing skin.
  ○ Tissue expansion requires a staged approach with 2-3 months between operations.
  ○ Tissue expansion goal is to generate flaps that are 50% wider and longer than the defect.
  ○ Multiple rounds of tissue expansion may be required for large defects.
  ○ *Up to 50% defects can be reconstructed with tissue expansion before getting alopecia.
  ○ Tissue expanders (TEs) are placed via incisions at the flap margin, often at the junction of normal scalp and skin graft.
    - Dissection in the subgaleal plane should be just large enough to allow TEs insertion.
    - Important not to have any sharp folds when placing TE.
    - A separate incision allows placement of a remote filling port over stable bone.
  ○ Hematoma, infection, and implant exposure are the most common complications of expansion. In children, pressure-related deformation of the cranial vault may occur.
- **Regional muscle transfers** are useful for defects in the mastoid, temporal, and occipital regions but cannot reach the frontal area or vertex.
  ○ Pectoralis major muscle.
  ○ Pedicled latissimus muscle can also be used for space-filling in orbital exenteration or other defects.
  ○ Trapezius muscle.
- **Free tissue transfer** is indicated for extensive wounds or wounds of the vertex and frontal region where regional muscle is not available.
  ○ Free latissimus flap and anterolateral thigh perforator flap are the workhorse flaps for scalp coverage due to its broad, flat size, and long vascular pedicle that allows anastomosis in the neck.
  ○ Free omentum, rectus abdominis flap, and parascapular flaps can also be used.
  ○ Inclusion of a skin island may result in a bulky reconstruction. Both muscle and omentum can be skin grafted.

SCALP TRAUMA

- All wounds should be irrigated and débrided.
- The scalp has robust blood supply and can bleed extensively.
- Closure of scalp wounds with full-thickness sutures or staples will provide hemostasis.
- Layered closure is usually unnecessary. For extensive wounds, closure of the galea may be necessary.
- Healing by secondary intention is acceptable for small wounds.
- *Scalp avulsion injuries most commonly occur in the loose areolar plane (eg, between galea and periosteum). Microvascular anastomosis is the standard of treatment for total and near-total scalp avulsions.
    - The scalp should be treated similarly to a replantable digit in the field: wrap in moist gauze, place in a plastic bag, and store on an ice slurry.
    - The entire scalp can often be replanted on one artery and vein. The superficial temporal system is preferred.
    - The ideal recipient vessels are contralateral to the zone of injury. Vein grafts are almost always necessary.
    - Contraindications to replantation include ischemia time >30 hours, failure to identify a suitable vascular pedicle, and medical condition precluding prolonged operation and potential blood loss.

OTHER CONSIDERATIONS IN SCALP RECONSTRUCTION

- In oncologic reconstruction of scalp, negative margins must be confirmed prior to reconstruction.
- If patient with previously reconstructed scalp with underlying hardware develops a wound or infection, infection of underlying hardware, native calvarium, bone flap, or alloplastic material must be considered. Suspicion should be especially high in the setting of recurrent wounds or infection.
    - Remove underlying material (hardware, implant, etc.).
    - Take intraoperative cultures (including from adjacent native bone).
    - Copiously irrigate wound.
    - Close wound over a drain.
    - Treat with antibiotics.
    - Delay reconstruction for at least 3-6 months.

CALVARIAL RECONSTRUCTION

ANATOMIC LAYERS OF THE CRANIUM

- The adult calvarium is composed of two layers of cortical bone, an external and internal table. Inner table is thin and weak, while the outer table is thick and strong.
- Between the inner and outer table is the spongy, cancellous diploe layer. Split calvarial bone grafts are raised at this level to harvest outer table.
- Periosteum covers the superficial surface of the external table and the deep surface of the internal table.
- Average bony vault thickness is 7 mm.
- Temporal bone is thinnest. Occipital bone is thickest.

PRINCIPLES OF CALVARIAL RECONSTRUCTION

- The goals are similar to all reconstructive efforts, namely, restoration of form and function. Specifically, this includes restoration of aesthetic contour and protection of the brain.
- The frontal region is important aesthetically because it is not covered with hair-bearing skin. Additionally, frontal bone contributes to the superior portion of the orbit.

- Thick temporalis muscle can camouflage contour defects in the temporal region. Defects of up to 10 cm^2 may not require reconstruction.
- The parietal and occipital regions require repair for protection of underlying structures; aesthetics in these areas are less of an issue.

OPERATIVE PLANNING AND TIMING

- Physical examination is critical in preoperative planning to examine defect size, location, and quality of local skin and soft tissue to ensure appropriate soft tissue coverage of cranioplasty material (ie, locations of previous incisions, previous irradiation, areas of skin laxity for advancement/rotation flaps if needed).
- Preinjury photographs are helpful when available.
- Noncontrast CT images are used in presurgical planning. 3D CT and 3D-printed anatomic models can also be used to assist in the planning process.
- Virtual surgical planning (ie, CAD/CAM) is another helpful tool to formulate reconstructive plans, especially when using a custom reconstructive implant.
- Appropriate timing for calvarial reconstruction after craniectomy remains debated.
- If no infection, recent studies suggest that early cranioplasty (<12 weeks) may be appropriate. Other studies advocate for cranioplasty once cerebral edema resolution on imaging.
- In the setting of infection, it is recommended that definitive reconstruction is delayed for a minimum of 3-6 months after infected implant or bone removal.
- For defects that involve the frontal or ethmoid sinus, delaying reconstruction for 1 year is preferable to minimize infection risk.

ALLOPLASTIC CRANIOPLASTY MATERIALS

- Alloplastic materials—for large calvarial defects for which adequate bone stock is not available; reduced operative time in the case of prefabricated implants and no associated donor site morbidity. However, majority of alloplastic materials do not incorporate and carry lifetime risk of infection.
- **Prefabricated polyether ether ketone and polymethyl methacrylate (PMMA) implants:** acrylic resins with smooth texture and good contour. Custom prefabricated using CAD/CAM prior to surgery; can decrease operative time. Not incorporated into surrounding bone. Can be very expensive.
- **Custom titanium:** titanium mesh is very pliable and can be easily contoured intraoperatively to fit defect size if unknown preoperatively. Will not be incorporated. Radiopaque and will cause scatter on imaging.
- Liquid PMMA, high-density porous polyethylene (MEDPOR), and hydroxyapatite are less commonly used to reconstruct calvarial defects.
  - Liquid PMMA: requires fabrication and curing in the operating room. Minimal integration. Cures in an exothermic reaction, which can burn the dura. Material is radiolucent. Relatively inexpensive material.
  - High-density porous polyethylene: allows for tissue in growth for incorporation.
  - Hydroxyapatite: capable of partial osseointegration, but use around frontal sinus is contraindicated due to increased risk of infection in this area.

AUTOLOGOUS CRANIOPLASTY MATERIALS

- **Bone** is considered to be the ideal cranioplasty material by many surgeons. Every attempt should be made to preserve the bone flap at the time of craniectomy (banking or freeze), except if grossly infected.
  - **Advantages** include the potential for revascularization, bony remodeling, and osseous healing to native calvarial bone. Once revascularized, infection risk is minimal. No additional expense.
  - **Disadvantages** include possible need for a second donor site if cranial bone grafts are not used. Harvest has a low but real risk of dural injury, CSF leak, and meningitis. Bone graft may reabsorb.

- **Split Rib Grafts**
  - Provide long, stable pieces of bone to bridge gaps.
  - Can be contoured with a Tessier bone bender to fit specific defects.
  - Donor site morbidity is minimal, and some bones may regenerate if the periosteum is left intact.
- **Calvarial Bone Graft**
  - Best harvested from the thick parietal region.
  - The outer and inner tables can be separated at the diploe layer using a side biting burr and osteotome.
  - Alternatively, a craniotomy can be performed and the bone flap split with a saw.
  - The sagittal sinus runs in the midline. This site should be avoided for bone graft harvest.
  - Bone dust, obtained by diffuse burring of calvarium, can be applied directly to dura or used as a final onlay for contouring.

SOFT TISSUE IN CRANIOPLASTY

- Some clinical circumstances require obliteration and infection control without cranial vault reconstruction.
- Microvascular-free tissue transfer may be required to provide soft tissue bulk. This technique is useful when there is a history of infection, extensive dead space, or communication between the intracranial cavity and sinuses.

PEARLS

1. The avascular loose areolar plane (subgaleal and supraperiosteal) is commonly dissected in scalp reconstruction. This plane is also where scalp avulsion injuries occur.
2. In a noninfected and nonurgent setting, tissue expansion is the ultimate method to replace up to 50% of the scalp with hair-bearing tissue.
3. Calvarial reconstruction requires thoughtful preoperative planning, often with a 3D CT and virtual surgical planning. Custom implant creation requires several weeks of advance notice.
4. Bone grafts (split rib or calvarial) are the preferred method for calvarium reconstruction when clinically appropriate.

QUESTIONS YOU WILL BE ASKED

1. How much of the scalp can be reconstructed with tissue expansion before noticing alopecia?
   50%.
2. What are the advantages of using autogenous bone over alloplastic material for calvarial reconstruction?
   Less risk of infection and extrusion.
3. At what level is the scalp commonly avulsed?
   Between the galea and periosteum.
4. What technique can be performed intraoperatively to improve rotation/advancement of scalp flaps?
   Scoring of the galea.

Recommended Readings
1. Chao AH, Yu P, Skoracki RJ, Demonte F, Hanasono MM. Microsurgical reconstruction of composite scalp and calvarial defects in patients with cancer: a 10-year experience. *Head Neck.* 2012;34(12):1759-1764.
2. Lin SJ, Hanasono MM, Skoracki RJ. Scalp and calvarial reconstruction. *Semin Plast Surg.* 2008;22(4):281-293.
3. Mehrara BJ, Disa JJ, Pusic A. Scalp reconstruction. *J Surg Oncol.* 2006;94(6):504-508.
4. Pasick C, Margetis K, Santiago G, Gordon C, Taub P. Adult cranioplasty. *J Craniofac Surg.* 2019;30(7):2138-2143.

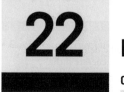

22 Ear Reconstruction

Chien-Wei Wang

Please refer to **Chapter 17: Reconstruction of Congenital Ear Deformities** for external ear anatomy

ETIOLOGIES AND CONSIDERATIONS

TUMOR

- Benign
  - Keloids
    - A fibroproliferative skin disorder characterized by abnormal collagen deposit with extension beyond the original wound border
    - Common site: ear lobe (ear piercing)
    - Etiology: dark skin tone, genetic deposition, age (second decade of life), traumatic wounds
    - Management
      - Conservative: pressure device, silicone gel/sheeting, corticosteroid injection (in combination with 5-FU and/or hyaluronidase)
      - Surgical: excision and tension-free closure +/− postoperative radiation (within 24 hours)
  - Chondrodermatitis nodularis chronica helicis
    - Common in elderly men related to trauma from sleeping
    - Presentation: a painful, inflammatory papule on the helix due to cartilage inflammation eroding through the overlying skin
      - Commonly mistaken for malignant skin tumor (usually not painful)
    - Treatment: excisional biopsy
      - The recurrence rate is high (11%-31%), so patients should avoid sleeping on the affected ear.
- Malignant
  - The external ear is prone to sun exposure and development of cutaneous malignancies (10% of all head and neck skin cancers).
  - **Squamous cell carcinoma** is the most common and has a higher rate of nodal metastasis compared to other head and neck sites.

TRAUMA

- **Hematomas** are caused by skin shearing from the cartilage
  - *Treatment involves immediate clot evacuation followed by a tie-over-bolster dressing to prevent fluid reaccumulation between the perichondrium and cartilage.
  - If the clot is not evacuated, it will undergo fibrosis and calcification resulting in a **cauliflower ear deformity.**
- **Simple lacerations** should be minimally debrided to remove avascular tissue prior to wound closure
  - Small lacerations can be easily closed using a single-layer technique (ie, skin-only closure).
  - Large lacerations should be closed using a double-layer technique by first reapproximating the cartilage to reduce tension on the wound edges.

---

*Denotes common in-service examination topics.

- **Avulsions and amputations** can be considered for replantation depending on the quality of the avulsed/amputated tissue, mechanism of injury, and the overall clinical status of the patient (ie, a sharp laceration near the base of the ear has the best chance of survival).

THERMAL INJURES

- Burn
  - Initial management includes fluid resuscitation, local wound care, pressure relief, avoidance of pillow friction, and topical application of **mafenide acetate** due to its superior cartilage penetration (**side effects include pain and hyperchloremic metabolic acidosis due to carbonic anhydrase inhibition**).
  - Allow injured tissues to demarcate (may take days to weeks) prior to definitive reconstruction.
  - Small burns may heal secondarily with dressing changes.
  - Large burns with exposed cartilage require well-vascularized soft tissue coverage, and the choice of donor site will depend on the zone of injury (eg, if the temporoparietal fascia is injured, then it is not available for use).
  - *Complete auricular loss will require total ear reconstruction in a delayed fashion using either a costal cartilage ear framework with a temporoparietal fascia flap or pre-expanded local flap for coverage (if the local tissue is not severely scarred), or an ear prosthesis with osseointegrated titanium implants.
- Frostbite
  - Initial management includes rapid rewarming, **use of nonsteroidal anti-inflammatory agents (reduces thromboxane production)**, and topical application of mafenide acetate.
  - Allow injured tissues to demarcate (may take weeks to months) prior to definitive reconstruction.

RECONSTRUCTION OF ACQUIRED AURICULAR DEFORMITIES

PARTIAL-THICKNESS DEFECTS

- **Presence of Perichondrium**
  - Small defects can heal secondarily with local wound care.
  - Full-thickness skin grafts are recommended for larger defects.
- **Absence of Perichondrium**
  - Small defects <1.5 cm near the helical rim can be converted to a full-thickness defect by wedge or shield excision and closed primarily.
  - Large defects require coverage with a local flap.
    - **Helical rim:** same flaps used for full-thickness defects of the upper and middle thirds
    - **Conchal bowl:** trapdoor flap, postauricular island "revolving door" flap, and bipedicle advancement flap
- **Involvement of the External Auditory Canal**
  - Stenosis is a common long-term complication
  - Treatment is application of a full-thickness skin graft over an acrylic mold used as a temporary stent

FULL-THICKNESS DEFECTS

- Can Be divided Into Thirds Based on Location
- **Upper Third Defects**
  - **Primary closure**
    - Indication: limited to defects <1.5 cm to avoid a significant size discrepancy with the contralateral side. Commonly performed after wedge or shield excision of skin cancers involving the helical rim.
    - To prevent buckling, a star-shaped resection pattern can be used.

- ○ Contralateral chondrocutaneous graft
  - Indication: defects up to 1.5 cm and is usually harvested from the contralateral helical rim or conchal bowl.
  - Design: the graft should be slightly larger than the defect to account for postoperative contraction.
  - **Predictable pattern of color changes during graft takes starting with white initially (ischemia), then blue for 24-72 hours (venous congestion), and finally pink after 3-7 days (neovascularization).**
- ○ Banner flap
  - Indication: for defects up to 2-3 cm.
  - A local transposition flap that can be based on either the pre- or postauricular skin
    - □ Can provide soft tissue coverage to the helical rim, antihelix, and triangular fossa
  - Design: performed with or without a cartilage graft; however, if the defect involves more than 25% of the helical rim, then costal cartilage is required for support.
- ○ Antia-Buch helical advancement (Fig. 22-1)
  - Indication: for defects up to 3 cm
  - Design: a transcartilaginous incision is made in the helical sulcus along its entire length from the scapha to the lobule preserving the integrity of the posterior skin
    - □ The posterior skin is then elevated off the remaining ear cartilage in a supraperichondrial plane until the entire helical rim is mobilized as a chondrocutaneous composite flap (based on the posterior skin).
    - □ Additional length can be gained by performing a V-Y closure at the root of the helix.
- ○ Chondrocutaneous composite flap (Fig. 22-2)
  - Indication: for defects involving the superior helical rim, especially when burn patients desire a stump to support their eyeglasses and other local options are not available.
  - Design: anterior skin and cartilage are rotated from the conchal bowl as a composite flap based on either the root of the helix (Davis) or the lateral helical rim (Orticochea).
  - The donor site is skin grafted or left to heal by secondary intention.
- **Middle Third Defects**

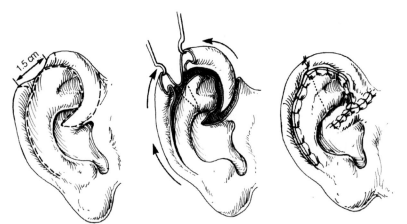

Figure 22-1 A-C. Antia-Buch helical advancement.

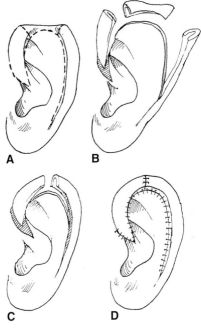

Figure 22-2 Chondrocutaneous composite flap of the ear. Helical rim defect (**A**). *Dotted lines* indicate incision to be made through both skin and cartilage. Helical root is advanced on soft tissue pedicle (**B**). Remaining helical rim is pedicled on lobule. Flaps advanced (**C**). Final wound closure (**D**). (From Urken ML. *Multidisciplinary Head and Neck Reconstruction.* Wolters Kluwer; 2010. Figure 11.6.)

○ Similar to full-thickness defects involving the upper third of the ear, reconstructive options include primary closure, contralateral chondrocutaneous graft, Banner flap, and Antia-Buch helical advancement.
○ **Tubed bipedicle flap**
  ▪ Based on the retroauricular skin and is performed with or without a cartilage graft in three stages.
  ▪ The flap is elevated and tubed with primary closure of the donor site. Three weeks later, one end of the tube is divided and transferred into the defect. Finally, after an additional 3 weeks, the other end of the tube is divided and transferred into the defect.
○ **Dieffenbach flap (Fig. 22-3)**
  ▪ Similar to the tubed bipedicle flap, this flap is based on the retroauricular skin and is also performed in multiple stages.
  ▪ A cartilage graft is harvested and placed into the helical rim defect. The anterior surface of the graft is then covered with a postauricular transposition flap. Three weeks later, the flap is divided at its base and inset using the additional length of the flap to cover the posterior surface of the graft.
  ▪ The donor site is skin grafted or closed by local tissue rearrangement.
○ **Converse "tunnel" technique**
  ▪ A prelaminated flap based on the retroauricular skin.
  ▪ A cartilage strut is tunneled beneath the retroauricular skin and secured to both ends of the helical rim defect. Three weeks later, the cartilage strut is elevated along with the retroauricular skin still attached.

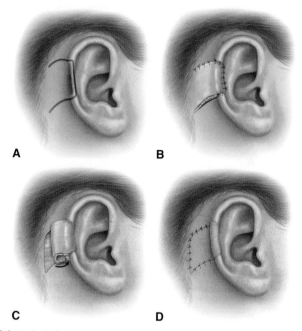

Figure 22-3 Method of reconstructing marginal ear defects with the postauricular flap, as originally described by Dieffenbach. The postauricular flap is initially elevated (**A**), and the flap is transposed from the posterior auricle to the anterior auricle during inset (**B**). A helical cartilage graft is strongly recommended to preserve the shape of the ear and give definition to the helix, although not included in the original description by Dieffenbach. At a second stage, the base of the flap is divided (**C**), and the flap donor site is skin grafted (**D**). (From Hanasono MM. Postauricular flap for ear reconstruction. In: Chung KC, Disa JJ, Gosain A, et al., eds. *Operative Techniques in Plastic Surgery*. Wolters Kluwer; 2020:1133-1137. Figure 3.30.2.)

- ▪ The donor site is skin grafted or closed by local tissue rearrangement.
- • **Lower Third Defects (Fig. 22-4)**
  - ○ Many techniques have been described to reconstruct the lobule, but the basic premise involves the use of local flaps folded over on themselves.
  - ○ The lobule normally does not contain any cartilage; however, contralateral auricular cartilage or nasal septal cartilage can be placed subcutaneously as a graft to provide additional support and contour.
  - ○ If the lobule on the contralateral side is enlarged, sometimes it can be surgically reduced to match the reconstructed side.
  - ○ For cleft lobules, our preferred technique is wedge excision and primary closure with eversion of the wound edges to prevent postoperative notching.

THE AMPUTATED EAR

NONMICROSURGICAL OPTIONS

- • Usually involves burying or banking cartilage in the temporal scalp, abdomen, or volar forearm for delayed reconstruction.
- • Many techniques have been described, but often the results are inconsistent and the cartilage loses its definition over time becoming flattened and warped.

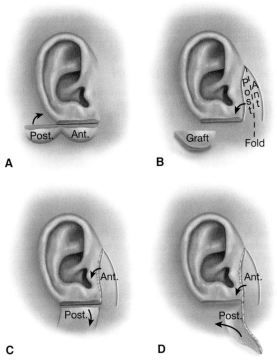

Figure 22-4 Some methods of ear lobe reconstruction with local flaps. A. Transversely oriented, bilobe flap originally described by Gavello. **B.** Inferiorly based preauricular flap that is folded longitudinally. A cartilage graft is needed to maintain ear lobe height. **C.** Double-opposing flap technique in which a postauricular flap becomes the posterior surface of the ear lobe and a preauricular flap becomes the anterior surface of the ear lobe. No cartilage graft is usually needed. The postauricular flap is divided at its base to release the ear lobe from the postauricular (mastoid) region, and the donor site is skin grafted at a second stage. **D.** Double-opposing flap technique in which a superiorly based postauricular (infra-auricular) flap becomes the posterior surface of the ear lobe and a preauricular flap becomes the anterior surface. The donor sites are closed primarily, and a second stage may not be necessary, although, in practice, a second stage is often needed to revise the anterior attachment of the reconstructed ear lobe. (From Hanasono MM. Reconstruction of the ear lobe. In: Chung KC, Disa JJ, Gosain A, et al., eds. *Operative Techniques in Plastic Surgery*. Wolters Kluwer; 2020:1138-1141. Figure 3.31.1.)

- **Baudet** recommended removing only the posterior skin from the amputated segment and fenestrating the cartilage to allow for greater imbibition and neovascularization. The cartilage was covered by a postauricular flap and later divided at 3 months.
- **Mladick** recommended dermablading the amputated segment, reattaching it, and then burying it beneath the retroauricular skin. Three weeks later, the reconstructed ear was removed from its "pocket," and the denuded areas eventually re-epithelialized.
- **Destro and Speranzini** recommended removing all the skin from the amputated segment except for the concha and then made small round perforations in the cartilage. The cartilage was covered by a postauricular flap and later divided at 3 months.

○ **Park** recommended removing all the skin from the amputated segment except for the helical rim. The cartilage was then sandwiched between two flaps: a skin flap anteriorly and a fascial flap posteriorly, both based on the mastoid region. The skin on the helical rim later necrosed but was salvaged with additional operations.

MICROVASCULAR REPLANTATION

- **Microvascular replantation provides a more natural-appearing reconstructed ear and is preferred to other forms of delayed reconstruction.**
- It is a technically demanding operation due to the small caliber of the vessels, and often venous outflow is a problem.
- Microvascular anastomosis is performed to either the posterior auricular artery or the superficial temporal artery. Both can restore the blood supply to the entire amputated segment given the numerous interconnections that are present between these two arterial networks.
  ○ If no vein can be found, or the veins are small, have a low threshold for starting leeches postoperatively.

PEARLS

1. Ears are usually operated on between the ages of 6 and 7 when ear growth is nearly complete.
2. For the burned ear, mafenide acetate is preferred due to its superior cartilage penetration. Complications of mafenide use include pain and beware of hyperchloremic metabolic acidosis from carbonic anhydrase inhibition.
3. Microvascular replantation may sacrifice the superficial temporal artery, which would impair the use of the temporoparietal fascial flap in the future.
4. Costal cartilage is often stiffer and more calcified in adults compared to children; thus, the cartilaginous ear framework used for total ear reconstruction in adults is usually carved en bloc.

QUESTIONS YOU WILL BE ASKED

1. What is the most common reason ear replantations fail?
   Poor venous outflow.
2. Why is it more difficult to use autogenous cartilage in the elderly for total ear reconstruction?
   Calcification of the rib cartilage.

Recommended Readings
1. Antia NH, Buch VI. Chondrocutaneous advancement flap for the marginal defect of the ear. *Plast Reconstr Surg.* 1967;39(5):472-477.
2. Baker SR. *Local Flaps in Facial Reconstruction.* Elsevier; 2022.
3. Brent B. The acquired auricular deformity. A systematic approach to its analysis and reconstruction. *Plast Reconstr Surg.* 1977;59(4):475-485.
4. Pribaz JJ, Crespo LD, Orgill DP, Pousti TJ, Bartlett RA. Ear replantation without microsurgery. *Plast Reconstr Surg.* 1997;99(7):1868-1872.

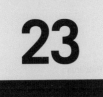

23 Eyelid Reconstruction

Jane S. Kim and Peter M. Kally

OVERVIEW

EYELID ANATOMY AND PHYSIOLOGY (FIG. 23-1)

- The primary function of the eyelids is to protect the globe and to maintain adequate lubrication of the ocular surface.
- The movement of the upper eyelid is dynamic, whereas the lower eyelid acts as a static sling.
- The eyelid is composed of three lamellae (see Fig. 23-2, Table 23-1)
  - ○ Anterior lamella: well-vascularized external coverage
  - ○ Middle lamella: central structural support
  - ○ Posterior lamella: deep structural support with a mucosal lining
- Ligamentous Structures of the Eyelid (Fig. 23-3)
  - ○ Medial canthal tendon (MCT)
    - Originates at the medial margin of the superior and inferior tarsal plates
    - Crura fuse as a tripartite common tendon prior to insertion on the medial orbital wall
      - □ Anterior limb: passes anterior to the lacrimal sac

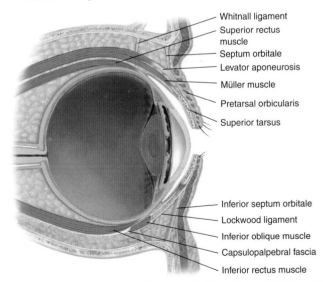

Figure 23-1 Cross section of the upper and lower eyelids. (From Shahzad F, Mehrara BJ, Fay A. Lower eyelid reconstruction with palatal grafts. In: Chung KC, Disa JJ, Gosain A, et al., eds. *Operative Techniques in Plastic Surgery*. Wolters Kluwer; 2020:1094-1098. Figure 3.23.1A.)

---

*Denotes common in-service examination topics.

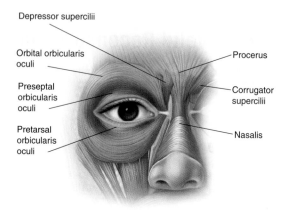

Figure 23-2 Periorbital musculature. (From Thorne CH, ed. *Grabb and Smith's Plastic Surgery*. 7th ed. Lippincott Williams & Wilkins; 2014. Figure 46.3A.)

- Inserts onto the frontal process of the maxillary bone (anterior lacrimal crest)
- Provides majority of MCT strength and contributes to punctal position
□ Posterior limb: passes posterior to the lacrimal sac
- Inserts onto the posterior lacrimal crest
- Thinner and weaker than the anterior limb but contributes to lid-globe apposition
□ Superior limb: forms the roof of the lacrimal sac
- Inserts onto the orbital process of the frontal bone
- Functions in the lacrimal pump mechanism and provides greater contribution to lid-globe apposition
- Function: provides support for the eyelids, particularly with punctal position and lid-globe apposition
○ Lateral canthal tendon (LCT)
- Originates at the lateral margin of the superior and inferior tarsal plates
- Upper and lower crura fuse as a Y-shaped common tendon that inserts onto Whitnall tubercle
- Function: provides support for the eyelids
- Transected in lateral canthotomy/cantholysis procedure to relieve orbital compartment syndrome (ie, retrobulbar hemorrhage)
○ Whitnall (superior transverse) ligament
- Formed by condensation of fibrous tissues surrounding the levator palpebrae superioris
- Medially anchored to connective tissues surrounding the trochlea and laterally to the lacrimal gland and lateral orbital rim (10 mm above Whitnall tubercle)
- Function: provides support for the upper eyelid, lacrimal gland, and surrounding tissues. Acts as a fulcrum for the levator palpebrae superioris
○ Lockwood (suspensory) ligament
- Formed by fusion of the sheath of the inferior rectus muscle, the inferior tarsal muscle, and the check ligaments of the medial and lateral rectus muscles
- Medially anchored to the MCT and laterally to Whitnall tubercle
- Function: provides support for the globe and the anteroinferior orbit (like a hammock)

TABLE 23-1 Structures of the Eyelid

	Anterior lamella		Middle lamella	Posterior lamella	
Upper and lower eyelid (tarsal)	Skin • Very thin skin (~1-mm thick)	Pretarsal orbicularis oculi • Action: spontaneous (involuntary) blink • Innervation: CN VII		Tarsus • Dense connective tissue containing meibomian glands • Provides structural support and rigidity to eyelids • Attached to medial and lateral canthal tendons • Height: upper lid, 10-11 mm; lower lid, 4-5 mm • Length: 29 mm • Thickness: 1 mm	Conjunctiva • Nonkeratinized squamous epithelium • Lines the inner surface of the lid from lid margin (palpebral) to fornix (forniceal) and extends onto the globe (bulbar)
Upper eyelid (supratarsal)		Preseptal orbicularis oculi • Action: voluntary and partial involuntary eyelid closure • Innervation: CN VII *Orbital portion encircles the preseptal orbicularis and allows for forced voluntary eyelid closure (Fig. 23-2)	Septum • Anatomic boundary between eyelid and orbit • Origin: orbital rim • Insertion: levator aponeurosis (fuses at ~2-3 mm above superior tarsal border) Fusion point is lower in an Asian eyelid	Orbital (postseptal) fat • Medial and central (preaponeurotic) fat pads (2) • The trochlea, superior oblique tendon, and medial horn of the levator separate the medial and central fat pads • The medial fat pad is lighter in color than the central fat pad	Levator palpebrae superioris • Origin: lesser wing of sphenoid, then transitions into aponeurosis at Whitnall ligament • Insertion: anterior surface of superior tarsus and dermis (forms lid crease) • Action: upper lid excursion (15 mm) • Innervation: superior division of CN III	Müller (superior tarsal) muscle • Origin: undersurface of levator at Whitnall ligament • Insertion: superior tarsal border • Action: 1-2 mm of upper lid elevation • Innervation: sympathetic

(continued)

TABLE 23-1 Structures of the Eyelid (*Continued*)

	Anterior lamella	Middle lamella		Posterior lamella	
Lower eyelid (infratarsal)		**Septum** • Anatomic boundary between eyelid and orbit • Origin: orbital rim • Insertion: CPF (fuses at ~4-5 mm below inferior tarsal border)	**Orbital (postseptal) fat** • Medial, central, and lateral fat pads (3) • The inferior oblique muscle divides the medial and central fat pads (Fig. 23-3)	**Capsulopalpebral fascia (CPF)** • Origin: inferior rectus sheath, splits at inferior oblique muscle, then reunites as Lockwood (suspensory) ligament • Insertion: inferior tarsal border with septum • Action: 1-2 mm lower lid excursion on downgaze	**Inferior tarsal muscle** • Origin: posterior to CPF • Insertion: inferior tarsal border • Action: coupled with CPF • Innervation: sympathetic

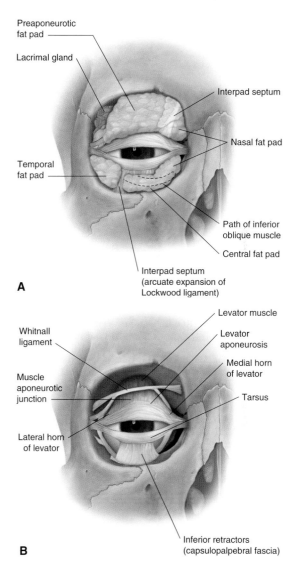

Preaponeurotic fat pad

Lacrimal gland

Interpad septum

Nasal fat pad

Temporal fat pad

Path of inferior oblique muscle

Central fat pad

Interpad septum (arcuate expansion of Lockwood ligament)

A

Whitnall ligament

Levator muscle

Levator aponeurosis

Medial horn of levator

Muscle aponeurotic junction

Tarsus

Lateral horn of levator

Inferior retractors (capsulopalpebral fascia)

B

Figure 23-3 A. Fat compartments of the eyelids. **B.** Ligamentous support of the eyelids. (From Thorne CH, ed. *Grabb and Smith's Plastic Surgery*. 7th ed. Lippincott Williams & Wilkins; 2014. Figures 46.6 and 46.5.)

- ○ **Orbicularis-retaining (orbitomalar) ligament**
  - ▪ Arises from the arcus marginalis of the inferior orbital rim and inserts onto the dermis of lower eyelid skin, forming the nasojugal fold
  - ▪ Laterally becomes lateral orbital thickening, which should be released when elevating the lateral brow
  - ▪ Transected in fat transposition technique for lower eyelid blepharoplasty

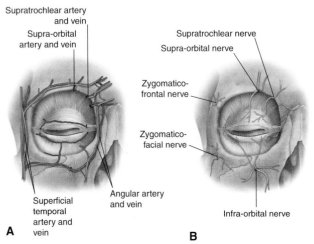

Figure 23-4 Vascular supply (**A**) and sensory innervation (**B**) of the eyelids. (From Nguyen J, Fay A. Tenzel semicircular rotational flap. In: Chung KC, Disa JJ, Gosain A, et al., eds. *Operative Techniques in Plastic Surgery.* Wolters Kluwer; 2020:1084-1088. Figure 3.21.1CD.)

- **Periocular Fat**
  - **Retro-orbicularis oculi fat (ROOF):** sub-brow fat and superior preseptal fat that lie deep to the orbicularis oculi muscle and superior to the orbital (postseptal) fat
  - **Suborbicularis oculi fat (SOOF):** inferior supraperiosteal fat that lies deep to the orbicularis oculi muscle and the superficial malar fat pad
- **Vascular Supply of the Eyelid (Fig. 23-4)**
  - **Dual blood supply** from both external (ECA) and internal carotid arteries (ICA)
  - **Upper eyelid:** primarily supplied by branches of the ophthalmic artery (ICA)
    - The peripheral arterial arcade is located between the levator palpebrae superioris and Müller muscle just above the superior tarsal border.
    - The marginal arterial arcade is located 2-3 mm from the lid margin.
  - **Lower eyelid:** primarily supplied by branches of the facial artery (ECA)
    - The marginal arterial arcade is located 2-3 mm from the lid margin.
- **Sensory Innervation of the Eyelid (Fig. 23-4)**
  - Upper eyelid: ophthalmic division (V1) of CN V
  - Lower eyelid: maxillary division (V2) of CN V
- **Motor Innervation of the Eyelid**
  - Orbicularis oculi: CN VII
  - Levator palpebrae superioris: superior division of CN III
  - Müller (superior tarsal) muscle and inferior tarsal muscle: sympathetic

PREOPERATIVE ASSESSMENT

- **Goal:** to restore form and function of the eyelids and periocular structures including the medial and LCTs as well as the tear ducts
- **Examination**
  - **Assess visual acuity** for both eyes.
  - Perform a basic **slit lamp exam.**
    - **Dry eyes**
      - Add 2% fluorescein dye to the eye and observe if there is any staining.
    - **Tear film break-up time**
      - Add 2% fluorescein dye to the eye and observe how quickly the tear film breaks up or evaporates.

□ The longer the time it takes to evaporate, the more stable the tear film.
- Normal: >10 seconds
- Abnormal: <5 seconds
○ *Assess tear production.
  ▪ **Schirmer test**
    □ Place paper strip in inferior fornix for 5 minutes.
      - Topical anesthetic can prevent reflexive tearing (false positive).
    □ The more wet the paper strip, the less dry the eye.
      - Normal: >10 mm
      - Abnormal: <10 mm
○ **Assess lid laxity.**
  ▪ **Snap-back test**
    □ Pull the lower eyelid away from the globe. Upon release, it should immediately return to its normal position without blinking.
    □ If this takes longer than 1 second, then significant laxity is present.
○ **Assess laxity, ptosis, and overall structural support of surrounding tissues.**
  ▪ Mobility of tissues adjacent to defect
  ▪ Presence of midface ptosis
  ▪ **Vector**
    □ Refers to the position of the anterior surface of the globe in relation to the most anterior point of the inferior orbital rim on lateral view.
      - Neutral vector: vertical line (no inclination) from the cornea to the rim
      - **Negative vector**: posteriorly inclined line from the cornea to the rim (increased risk of postoperative lower lid retraction and ectropion)

RECONSTRUCTION OF EYELID AND CANTHAL DEFECTS

PARTIAL-THICKNESS EYELID DEFECTS (FIG. 23-5)

- **Anterior Lamellar Defects**
  ○ Adjacent tissue transfer (preferred) or full-thickness skin graft (preferred site for FTSG: contralateral upper eyelid)
  ○ Consider frost sutures and/or lateral canthopexy or canthoplasty to reduce risk of postoperative lid retraction
- **Posterior Lamellar Defects**
  ○ If involves conjunctiva only
    ▪ Primary repair by 1-3 widely spaced, buried, interrupted 7-0 or 8-0 Vicryl sutures for smaller defects
    ▪ Amniotic membrane grafts or buccal/gingival mucosal grafts for larger defects
  ○ If involves tarsus and conjunctiva
    ▪ Primary repair for smaller defects. Ensure parallel apposition of both edges of tarsus to prevent kinking or notching.
    ▪ Tarsal alternatives for larger defects: ear cartilage, nasal chondromucosal graft (septal cartilage), or hard palate mucosal graft.

FULL-THICKNESS EYELID DEFECTS (FIG. 23-5)

- **Less than 33%**
  ○ **Primary closure** (after converting to pentagonal wedge) with meticulous lid margin repair; lateral canthotomy ± cantholysis may be required. In elderly patients, preexisting laxity may allow for closure of larger defects.
    ▪ **Lid margin repair (Fig. 23-6)**
      □ **Align lid margin** using a vertical-mattress 6-0 Vicryl suture at the gray line.
        - Evert wound edges to prevent postoperative notching.
        - Secure long suture ends under skin sutures away from the cornea or bury the suture ends.
      □ **Repair the tarsal wound** using buried interrupted 6-0 Vicryl sutures.

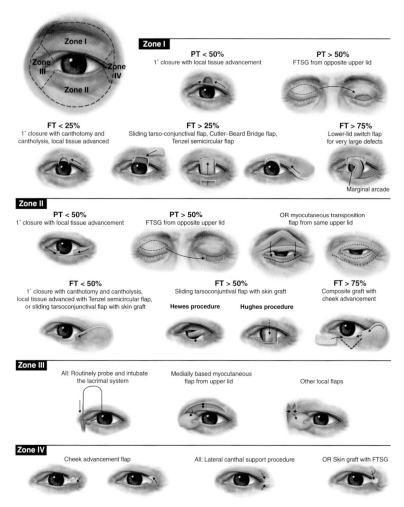

Figure 23-5 Eyelid reconstruction. FT, full thickness; PT, partial thickness. (Adapted from Spinelli HM, Jelks GW. Periocular reconstruction: a systematic approach. *Plast Reconstr Surg.* 1993;91(6):1017-1024; Thorne CH, ed. *Grabb and Smith's Plastic Surgery.* 7th ed. Lippincott Williams & Wilkins; 2014. Figure 32.2.)

- Partial-thickness bites protect the cornea from suture irritation.
- Bury all suture knots closer to the skin/orbicularis oculi than to the conjunctiva.
□ **Close skin** using 6-0 nonabsorbable or absorbable suture (conjunctival closure is not required).
- Remove skin sutures in 5-7 days. Lid margin sutures can either be left alone or removed in 7-10 days.
□ **Complications:** notching (most common), trichiasis, and madarosis.

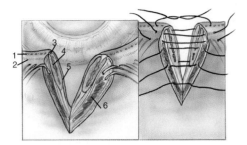

Figure 23-6 Full-thickness eyelid margin repair. (From Johnson J. *Bailey's Head and Neck Surgery*. 5th ed. Wolters Kluwer; 2014. Figure 75.7.)

- **Between 33% and 50%**
  - ○ **Tenzel semicircular flap**: advancement of any remaining lateral eyelid along with a myocutaneous flap (incision oriented inferiorly for an upper eyelid defect and superiorly for a lower eyelid defect). Medially, a full-thickness lid repair is performed. Laterally, the lateral commissure is reformed with a buried interrupted 6-0 Vicryl suture, and the flap is secured to periosteum along the lateral orbital rim at the level of the newly formed lateral canthal angle.
  - ○ **SOOF or midface lift** for lower eyelid defects: elevation of the SOOF or midface can be helpful in supporting the lower eyelid in addition to adjacent tissue transfer.
- **Greater Than 50%**
  - ○ ***Cutler-Beard flap for upper eyelid defects**
    - ▪ **First stage**: full-thickness flap is developed in the ipsilateral lower eyelid ~1-2 mm below the inferior tarsal border and passed beneath the lower lid margin into the upper lid defect (may include cartilage for additional support).
    - ▪ **Second stage**: flap is divided and inset 3-4 weeks later. Consider longer interval in smokers (ie, 6-8 weeks).
  - ○ **Hughes tarsoconjunctival flap with full-thickness skin graft** for lower eyelid defects
    - ▪ **First stage**: tarsoconjunctival flap is developed from the ipsilateral upper eyelid, leaving 4 mm for upper eyelid support, and is transferred into the lower eyelid defect. Müller muscle is also included in smokers. A full-thickness skin graft covers the tarsoconjunctival flap (preferred site for FTSG: contralateral upper eyelid skin, pre- or postauricular skin).
    - ▪ **Second stage**: flap is divided and inset 3-4 weeks later. Consider longer interval in smokers (ie, 6-8 weeks).
  - ○ **Free tarsoconjunctival graft** from contralateral upper eyelid **with overlying myocutaneous flap** (preferred in monocular patients)
    - ▪ Can also consider ear cartilage, nasal chondromucosal graft (septal cartilage), or hard palate mucosal graft for posterior lamellar defect, with myocutaneous flap for anterior lamellar defect
  - ○ **Paramedian forehead flap** for large lower eyelid and medial canthal defects
  - ○ **Mustardé cheek rotation flap** for large vertical lower eyelid defects
    - ▪ Elevate in a subcutaneous plane for a thinner flap. Consider deep plane elevation in smokers to reduce risk of distal flap necrosis.
    - ▪ Anchor flap to the deep temporal fascia and the periosteum of the infraorbital rim to reduce risk of postoperative ectropion.
    - ▪ Can combine with a free posterior lamellar graft or amniotic membrane graft for total lower eyelid defects.
  - ○ **Unipedicled myocutaneous Fricke transposition flap** for large lower eyelid and lateral canthal defects: temporally based supraciliary forehead flap transposed into a lower eyelid defect.
  - ○ **Bipedicled myocutaneous Tripier transposition flap**: medially and temporally based upper eyelid flaps transposed into a lower eyelid defect. Requires redundant or lax upper eyelid skin. Typically for narrow lower eyelid defects.

LATERAL CANTHAL DEFECTS

- **Canthopexy** for LCT laxity (**Fig. 23-7**)
- **Canthoplasty** for any disruption or loss of LCT
  - Depending on tissue laxity and presence of medial LCT stump, can either suture to periosteum at inner aspect of lateral orbital rim or use a lateral tarsal strip (**Fig. 23-8**) or periosteal flap
- A **local flap**, regional flap, or full-thickness skin graft can be used for soft tissue coverage.

MEDIAL CANTHAL DEFECTS

- **Rule out any injury to the canalicular system and perform a canalicular repair as needed** (see below).
- **Canthoplasty** for any disruption or loss of MCT
  - Depending on tissue laxity and presence of any MCT stump, can either suture to remaining MCT or periosteum of the medial orbital wall.
  - If there is complete avulsion, can still suture to periosteum if it is intact. For deeper defects with loss of periosteum, consider bone fixation using a microplate or transnasal wiring.
- A **local flap**, regional flap, or full-thickness skin graft can be used for soft tissue coverage.

RECONSTRUCTION OF THE CANALICULAR SYSTEM

LACRIMAL APPARATUS (FIG. 23-9)

- Lacrimal Gland
  - Located within the lacrimal fossa in the superolateral orbit.
  - Lateral horn of the levator aponeurosis separates the orbital and palpebral lobes with ~10-12 ducts passing from the orbital lobe through the palpebral lobe into the superior fornix.
  - Supplied by the lacrimal artery, a branch of the ophthalmic artery.
  - The lacrimal vein empties into the superior ophthalmic vein.
  - Lacrimal nerve via ophthalmic division of CN V provides sensation.
  - Pterygopalatine ganglion provides parasympathetic innervation.
  - Superior cervical ganglion provides sympathetic innervation.
- Tears
  - *The tear film is trilaminar
    - **Outer lipid layer:** produced by meibomian glands, accessory sebaceous glands of Zeis and Moll; provides tear film stability, limits contamination of ocular surface, and reduces tear evaporation.
    - **Middle aqueous layer:** produced by lacrimal gland, accessory lacrimal glands of Krause and Wolfring; lubricates ocular surface, nourishes cornea, contains proteins and glycoproteins with antimicrobial activity, washes away foreign bodies and debris, and provides 90% tear film volume.
    - **Inner mucoprotein layer:** produced by goblet cells; lubricates ocular surface (hydrophilic), reduces friction during blinking, contributes to tear film stability, and prevents pathogen adhesion.
  - **Tear drainage**
    - Tears are produced in the lacrimal gland and travel medially, with each blink.
    - Tears enter the puncta, which open into the superior and inferior canaliculi at the medial end of the upper and lower eyelids, respectively.
    - Both canaliculi travel 2 mm vertically and then 8 mm horizontally before uniting to form the common canaliculus. (The common canaliculus is absent in 2% of patients.)

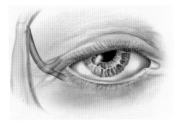

A Eyelid droop due to lateral canthal tendon attenuation

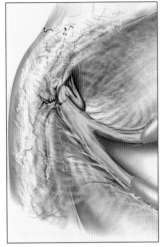

Line of division
of lateral retinaculum
for common canthoplasty

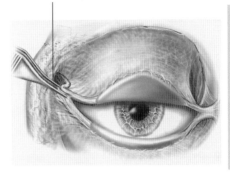

B Common canthal tendon is retracted laterally and superiorly anchored to periosteum

Close-up of common canthopexy

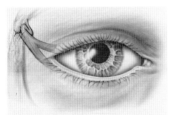

C Effect of completed repair

Figure 23-7 Lateral canthopexy. (From Spinelli HM. Eyelid malpositions. In: Spinelli HM, ed. *Atlas of Aesthetic Eyelid and Periocular Surgery*. Elsevier; 2004:47.)

- The common canaliculus empties into the lacrimal sac through the valve of Rosenmüller.
- The lacrimal sac empties into the nasolacrimal duct, which travels 12-18 mm inferiorly before entering the inferior meatus.
- The opening of the nasolacrimal duct is covered by a mucosal fold (valve of Hasner) to prevent reflux of air and intranasal contents.

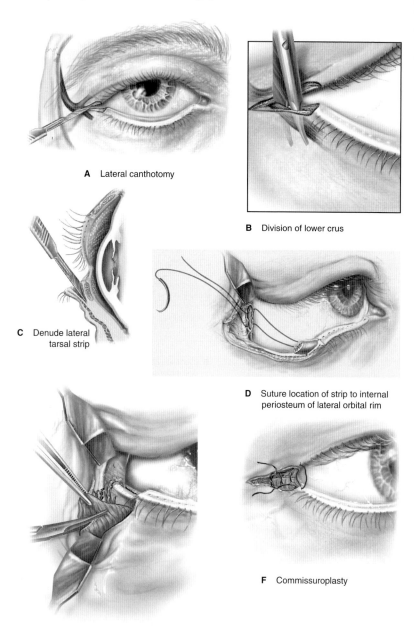

A Lateral canthotomy

B Division of lower crus

C Denude lateral tarsal strip

D Suture location of strip to internal periosteum of lateral orbital rim

F Commissuroplasty

E Trim excess skin and/or orbicularis muscle

Figure 23-8 Lateral tarsal strip. (From Spinelli HM. Eyelid malpositions. In: Spinelli HM, ed. *Atlas of Aesthetic Eyelid and Periocular Surgery*. Elsevier; 2004:47.)

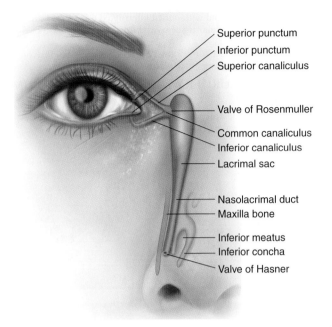

Superior punctum
Inferior punctum
Superior canaliculus

Valve of Rosenmuller

Common canaliculus
Inferior canaliculus

Lacrimal sac

Nasolacrimal duct
Maxilla bone

Inferior meatus
Inferior concha
Valve of Hasner

Figure 23-9 Nasolacrimal system. (From Zepeda EM, Jacobs SM, Chambers CB. Nasolacrimal duct obstruction. In: Chung KC, Disa JJ, Gosain A, et al., eds. *Operative Techniques in Plastic Surgery*. Wolters Kluwer; 2020:2870-2876. Figure 8.42.1.)

- **Lacrimal pump mechanism**
  - When the eyelids close, the orbicularis oculi muscle contracts. Contracture of the pretarsal orbicularis closes the puncta and canaliculi. Contracture of the preseptal orbicularis opens the lacrimal sac, creating negative pressure to draw tears into the sac.
  - When the eyelids open, the orbicularis oculi muscle relaxes, opening the puncta, relaxing the canaliculi, and collapsing the lacrimal sac. The tears are pushed down the nasolacrimal duct, and the canaliculi are refilled with more tears.

CANALICULAR REPAIR (FIG. 23-10)

- Should always be performed when there is canalicular compromise to prevent postoperative epiphora.
- Identify both proximal and distal ends of the lacerated canaliculus.
  - Irrigate the area and gently use cotton-tip applicators to find the white lumen of the distal end, which can be more difficult to identify (usually more posterior).
  - Irrigation of the uninjured canaliculus aids in the identification of the distal end by observing for backflow of saline. Can use fluorescein-tinted saline when performing lacrimal irrigation.
- Pass a 00 Bowman probe first to confirm proper identification of the distal end, and then pass the lacrimal stent to bridge the laceration (**Fig. 23-10A and B**). Bicanalicular silicone stents are preferred, and alternatively, annular pigtail probe can also be used for bicanalicular intubation with silicone stenting (**Fig. 23-10C-F**). Monocanalicular silicone stent can be used if the laceration is small.

- Reapproximate the tarsal wound with buried interrupted 6-0 Vicryl sutures. Reapproximate the pericanalicular tissues with buried interrupted 7-0 or 6-0 Vicryl sutures.
- The stent should be left in place for at least 12 weeks. Patients should avoid sneezing or blowing the nose while the stent is in place.

LACRIMAL BYPASS SURGERY FOR A BLOCKED LACRIMAL DRAINAGE SYSTEM

- Silicone Tube Intubation: obstructions at the lacrimal puncta
- Conjunctivodacryocystostomy: obstructions at the canalicular level

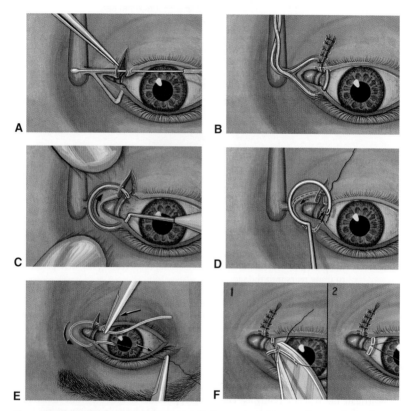

Figure 23-10 Canalicular laceration repair. A, B. Pass stent on wire introducer through punctum and into proximal opening of transected canaliculus. Thread stent down nasolacrimal duct and into nose. Pass other end of silicone stent through opposite canalicular system and into nose. Repair eyelid wound. **C-F.** Alternatively, pass a pigtail probe through the intact punctum and canaliculus and out the proximal cut end of lacerated canaliculus. Thread a suture through hole of the probe and pull the probe so suture passes from cut canaliculus to intact punctum. Pass pigtail probe through punctum and distal cut end of canaliculus. Thread tubing over suture. Pull suture and tubing through canalicular system so free ends emerge from two puncta. Cut tubing and tie suture. Repair eyelid wound. Rotate silicone loop so knot lies in common canaliculus. (From Repair of canalicular lacerations. In: Dutton J, ed. *Atlas of Oculoplastic and Orbital Surgery.* 2nd ed. Wolters Kluwer; 2019. Figures 84.3-6, 84.9, 84.12.)

- Conjunctivodacryocystorhinostomy: also for obstructions at the canalicular level, or in patients with congenital absence of the lacrimal sac—requires use of a permanent Pyrex glass tube (Jones tube)
- *Dacryocystorhinostomy (DCR): obstructions at the nasolacrimal duct
- Canaliculodacryocystorhinostomy: obstructions at the junction of the common canaliculus and lacrimal sac—combination of DCR and microsurgical repair of the stenotic common canaliculus

PEARLS

1. A lateral canthotomy ± cantholysis may facilitate primary closure of eyelid defects.
2. A lateral canthopexy/canthoplasty and/or SOOF or midface lift may help to reduce risk of postoperative lower lid retraction and ectropion. Frost suture tarsorrhaphy may also be helpful.
3. For 33%-50% eyelid defects, a Tenzel semicircular flap is effective.
4. For >50% eyelid defects, consider a Cutler-Beard flap for upper eyelid defects and a Hughes tarsoconjunctival flap for lower eyelid defects. If the defects are larger than the horizontal length of the eyelid, then transposition flaps may be required.
5. The presence of a negative vector places a patient at increased risk for what postoperative complications?

QUESTIONS YOU WILL BE ASKED

1. What is the most common complication following lower lid procedures?
   Lower lid ectropion.
2. What structure attaches to the superior margin of the tarsus and is often visualized in cases of levator dehiscence?
   Müller muscle.
3. What lower lid structure is analogous to the levator palpebrae superioris in the upper lid?
   Capsulopalpebral fascia.
4. What lower lid structure is analogous to Müller muscle in the upper lid?
   Inferior tarsal muscle.
5. Patients with a negative vector are at increased risk for what postoperatively?
   Lower lid retraction, ectropion, and dry eye syndrome.

Recommended Readings
1. Becker BB. Tricompartment model of the lacrimal pump mechanism. *Ophthalmology.* 1992;99(7):1139-1145.
2. Codner MA, McCord CD, Mejia JD, Lalonde D. Upper and lower eyelid reconstruction. *Plast Reconstr Surg.* 2010;126(5):231e-245e.
3. DiFrancesco LM, Codner MA, McCord CD. Upper eyelid reconstruction. *Plast Reconstr Surg.* 2004;114(7):98e-107e.
4. Holds JB. Lower eyelid reconstruction. *Facial Plast Surg Clin North Am.* 2016;24(2):183-191.
5. Sand JP, Zhu BZ, Desai SC. Surgical anatomy of the eyelids. *Facial Plast Surg Clin North Am.* 2016;24(2):89-95.
6. Section 2—Fundamentals and Principles of Ophthalmology, Part 1—Anatomy, Chapter 1—Orbit and Ocular Adnexa. *BCSC 2020-2021 Series.* https://www.aao.org/bcscsnippetdetail. aspx?id=4e50a7ba-97a9-4136-8099-89aa8487488b
7. Spinelli HM, Jelks GW. Periocular reconstruction: a systematic approach. *Plast Reconstr Surg.* 1993;91(6):1017-1024. discussion 1025-1026.

24 Eyelid Malposition

Jane S. Kim and Peter M. Kally

ECTROPION

- Definition: eversion of the lid margin and loss of normal lid-globe apposition leading to scleral show, keratinization of the cornea and conjunctiva, and ultimately loss of vision.

MANAGEMENT

- **Nonsurgical Management of Ectropion**
  - Protect the cornea and lubricate the ocular surface by using artificial tears, punctal occlusion, moisture chambers, taping or patching the eyelid closed, etc.
  - If there is a corneal ulcer, treat the infection with topical antibiotic drops. A culture is often obtained prior to starting topical antibiotics.
- **Surgical Management of Ectropion**
  - **Involutional (senile)**
    - Most common type of ectropion, due to horizontal lid laxity related to aging
    - Surgical repair
      - □ **Lateral tarsal strip procedure (lateral canthoplasty) (see Fig. 24-1)**
        - ▪ Preferred method, as lateral canthopexy often cannot adequately address the underlying horizontal lid laxity if lower lid ectropion is present. Suborbicularis oculi fat (SOOF) or midface lift is often performed in conjunction if there is midface descent.
        - ▪ Lateral canthotomy followed by cantholysis of the inferior crus.
        - ▪ A strip of lateral tarsus is then denuded and sutured to the periosteum of the inner aspect of the lateral orbital rim with slight overcorrection.
        - ▪ Excess skin and orbicularis oculi muscle are excised, and the lateral commissure is reformed.
        - ▪ The skin is closed with running 6-0 plain gut suture.
      - □ **Pentagonal wedge resection**
        - ▪ A full-thickness pentagonal wedge is excised, and full-thickness lid margin repair is performed (see **Chapter 23: Eyelid Reconstruction, section on Full-Thickness Eyelid Defects**).
      - □ **Medial spindle procedure** for punctal or medial lower lid ectropion
        - ▪ Medial conjunctiva and lower lid retractors are excised in a diamond-shaped pattern parallel to the inferior tarsal border.
        - ▪ The lower lid retractors are reapproximated to the inferior tarsal border.
  - **Cicatricial**
    - Due to scarring of the anterior lamella.
    - Surgical repair. If conservative measures fail (eg, digital massage, intralesional corticosteroid, or 5-FU injections), then treatment involves surgical release of the scar and lengthening of the anterior lamella.
      - □ Additional tissue is often needed in the form of a local flap, regional flap, or full-thickness skin graft (preferred).
      - □ Temporary traction suture (Frost suture) is used postoperatively to counteract downward pull of tissue edema.
      - □ Consider addition of SOOF/midface lift.

*Denotes common in-service examination topics.

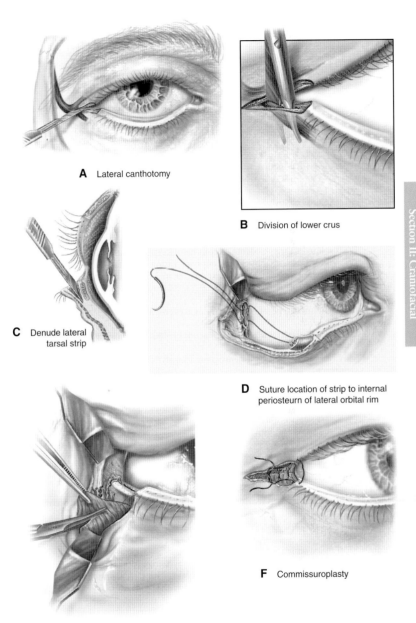

A Lateral canthotomy

B Division of lower crus

C Denude lateral tarsal strip

D Suture location of strip to internal periosteurn of lateral orbital rim

E Trim excess skin and/or orbicularis muscle

F Commissuroplasty

Figure 24-1 The lateral tarsal strip procedure. (From Spinelli HM. Eyelid malpositions. In: Spinelli HM, ed. *Atlas of Aesthetic Eyelid and Periocular Surgery.* Elsevier; 2004:39.)

Section II: Craniofacial

- Neurogenic (paralytic)
  - Due to a deficit in CN VII function
  - Results in exposure keratopathy, often with neurotrophic keratopathy secondary to absent corneal sensation
  - Surgical repair
    - Mild to moderate cases: lateral tarsal strip ± SOOF/midface lift.
    - Severe cases: a static sling is recommended.
    - If poor Bell phenomenon, a permanent lateral tarsorrhaphy can be helpful.
    - If lagophthalmos with upper lid retraction, also consider gold/platinum weight, blepharotomy, or botulinum toxin of the levator palpebrae superioris.
- Mechanical
  - Due to mass, excess skin, severe facial ptosis, etc., weighing down lower lid, typically with concurrent horizontal lid laxity
  - Can also be caused by tissue edema in the early postoperative period
  - Surgical repair
    - If related to lower lid mass, excise the offending lesion and perform eyelid reconstruction as outlined in **Chapter 23: Eyelid Reconstruction.**
    - If related to excess lower lid skin and midface descent, perform lower lid blepharoplasty with SOOF/midface lift or face-lift.
    - If related to tissue edema, recommend keeping head of bed elevated, avoiding any straining, bending over, lifting weights >5 lb, etc. Can also perform lymphatic massage. Improves in 2-3 months when new lymphatic channels form.
- Congenital
  - Least common type of ectropion, due to vertical deficiency of the anterior lamella
  - Usually associated with euryblepharon, blepharophimosis syndrome, Down syndrome
  - May be complicated by a neurogenic (paralytic) component (eg, Möbius syndrome)
  - Surgical repair
    - Manage initially with ocular lubrication.
    - Consider small lateral tarsorrhaphies if progressive.
    - Severe cases require full-thickness skin grafts or local flaps in conjunction with horizontal lid tightening.

ENTROPION

- Definition: inversion of the lid margin.
- Posteriorly directed lashes (trichiasis) cause ocular surface irritation and corneal compromise, with increased tearing, mucoid discharge, eye redness, and discomfort. If not addressed, can lead to irreversible corneal scarring and vision loss.

MANAGEMENT

- **Nonsurgical management of entropion**
  - It is important to lubricate the ocular surface by using artificial tears (ie, drops, gel, ointment). Consider use of bandage contact lens, with topical antibiotic prophylaxis.
  - If there is a corneal ulcer, treat the infection with topical antibiotic drops. A culture is often obtained prior to starting topical antibiotics.
  - Eyelid can be taped to assist with everting the lid margin.
  - Botulinum toxin injection can be used in cases of spastic entropion.
- Trichiatic lashes can be electroepilated. Typically requires multiple sessions.**surgical management of entropion**
  - **Involutional (senile)**
    - Most common type of entropion, due to horizontal lid laxity, lower lid retractor disinsertion, and overriding preseptal orbicularis related to aging.

- Surgical repair.
  - Lateral tarsal strip is often required due to horizontal lid laxity.
  - Reinsertion of lower lid retractors is also recommended.
- A small strip of overriding orbicularis and/or skin can also be excised.
  - Quickert procedure: multiple double-armed absorbable sutures are placed in a horizontal mattress fashion to tighten the lower lid retractors and evert the lid margin. Results are temporary, and recurrence is expected.
  - Weis procedure: full-thickness rotational procedure of the lid margin involving a transverse blepharotomy and a lateral tarsal strip.

  ○ Spastic
  - Due to ocular irritation or inflammation, leading to sustained contraction or overactivity of the orbicularis oculi muscle
    - Nonsurgical approaches. Temporizing measures include eyelid taping, local anesthetic infiltration, or botulinum toxin injection into the orbicularis oculi muscle, which can break the spasm.
  - Surgical approaches
    - Quickert procedure.
    - If horizontal or vertical lid laxity also exist, then a lateral tarsal strip procedure and/or reinsertion of the lower lid retractors should be performed.

  ○ Cicatricial
  - Due to scarring of the posterior lamella (eg, trachoma, Steven-Johnson syndrome/toxic epidermal necrolysis, chemical burns)
  - Surgical repair
    - Do not operate if the conjunctiva is actively inflamed.
    - Treatment involves surgical release of the scar and rotation of the lid margin.
      - Consider Weis procedure.
      - Conjunctiva may need to be grafted using either amniotic membrane graft or buccal mucosa.
      - If the tarsus is also missing or deformed, it can be fractured and repositioned or replaced with an interpositional graft (**See Chapter 23: Eyelid Reconstruction, section on Partial Thickness Eyelid Defects**).

  ○ Congenital
  - Least common type of entropion; due to vertical deficiency of the posterior lamella. Can be caused by dysgenesis of the lower lid retractors or structural abnormalities of the tarsus
  - Can be secondary to facial nerve palsy in children
  - Surgical repair
    - Transverse blepharotomy with marginal rotation
    - Transverse blepharotomy and tarsotomy at the level of deformed tarsus
    - Tarsal kink wedge resection with primary closure
  - **Frequently confused with epiblepharon**
    - A fold of skin with underlying orbicularis muscle overriding the lower eyelid margin and pushing lashes vertically along the medial lower lid. More common in Asian and Hispanic children.
    - Often asymptomatic, even if there is cornea-lash touch.
    - No rotational abnormality exists. Typically resolves spontaneously as the patient grows older, which differs from congenital entropion.
    - If there is corneal compromise, excision of an ellipse of redundant infraciliary skin and underlying orbicularis, typically with lash rotation and tarsal fixation.

LID RETRACTION

- Definition: superior displacement of the upper lid or inferior displacement of the lower lid.
- Lagophthalmos from retraction can cause exposure keratopathy, which may lead to corneal ulceration, thinning, perforation, and visual loss.

- Possible causes (eg, hyperthyroidism) depending on accompanying sign/symptoms.

MANAGEMENT

- **Nonsurgical management of lid retraction**
  - ○ Protect the cornea and lubricate the ocular surface by using artificial tears, punctal occlusion, moisture chambers, taping or patching eyelid closed, contact lens.
  - ○ If there is a corneal ulcer, treat the infection with topical antibiotic drops. A culture is often obtained prior to starting topical antibiotics.
  - ○ For lid retraction secondary to anterior lamellar deficiency, treat the underlying medical cause.
  - ○ For retraction secondary to thyroid disease, treatment may improve lid retraction. Avoid smoke exposure. Consider teprotumumab.
  - ○ For lid retraction secondary to ipsilateral CN VII palsy, consider botulinum toxin injection into the levator palpebrae superioris to induce ptosis for a temporary "tarsorrhaphy."
  - ○ For mild lid retraction, hyaluronic acid filler injections may improve lid position.
- **Surgical Management of Lid Retraction**
  - ○ **Mechanical**
    - ■ Due to globe prominence or exophthalmos
      - ▫ In a young child, consider buphthalmos due to elevated intraocular pressure. Recommend ophthalmology evaluation to reduce risk of irreversible visual loss!
      - ▫ If unilateral, consider orbital mass and obtain neuroimaging.
    - ■ Surgical repair
      - ▫ Posterior spacer graft ± SOOF/midface lift for prominent globes if causing ocular irritation and/or corneal pathology
      - ▫ Orbital fat and/or bony decompression
      - ▫ Excision or debulking of orbital mass (as appropriate)
  - ○ **Anterior lamellar deficiency**
    - ■ Shortage of eyelid skin (atopic dermatitis, rosacea, ichthyosis, periocular burns, radiation, surgery, trauma). Retraction increases with mouth opening or upgaze.
    - ■ Surgical repair
      - ▫ Full-thickness skin graft (preferred donor is contralateral upper lid, pre- or postauricular skin, supraclavicular skin) in combination with lateral canthoplasty, suture tarsorrhaphy, ± SOOF/midface lift
      - ▫ May require release of scar if also involving middle lamella
  - ○ **Middle lamellar deficiency**
    - ■ Due to scarring of orbital septum, related to prior surgery, burns, or trauma
    - ■ Surgical repair
      - ▫ Complete release of cicatrix in middle lamella.
      - ▫ Depending on the extent of scarring, typically requires full-thickness skin graft or adjacent tissue transfer for anterior lamellar involvement and posterior spacer graft for posterior lamellar involvement.
      - ▫ Suture tarsorrhaphy and SOOF/midface lift may also be necessary to optimize postoperative outcomes.
  - ○ **Posterior lamellar deficiency**
    - ■ Due to **scarring of tarsus and/or conjunctiva** (eg, trachoma, Steven-Johnson syndrome/toxic epidermal necrolysis, chemical burns), often with cicatricial entropion
    - ■ Surgical repair—similar to cicatricial entropion repair (see section Entropion, Cicatricial)
  - ○ **Neuromuscular**
    - ■ Most commonly due to thyroid eye disease, less commonly due to other inflammatory conditions (sarcoidosis), dorsal midbrain lesions (Collier sign), and orbicularis weakness due to facial nerve palsy
    - ■ Surgical repair

- □ For upper eyelid retraction secondary to thyroid eye disease, perform disinsertion of the levator palpebrae superioris and Müller muscle.
- □ For upper eyelid retraction secondary to ipsilateral CN VII palsy, implant gold or platinum weight or perform blepharotomy.
- ○ **Congenital**
  - ▪ Rare but requires work-up as appropriate for symptoms/signs. Should be seen by a pediatric ophthalmologist.
  - ▪ Surgical repair—if causing corneal compromise and/or amblyopia, consider blepharotomy or levator recession.
- ○ **Pseudoretraction**
  - ▪ Due to contralateral ptosis (Hering law). Requires systematic evaluation of ptosis
  - ▪ Surgical repair—if involutional, perform ptosis repair on the contralateral upper eyelid. May also require correction of ipsilateral upper eyelid (**see Chapter 59: Periocular Rejuvenation: Blepharoplasty, Eyelid Ptosis, and Brow Lift**)

PEARLS

1. Lubricate the ocular surface well to reduce the risk of corneal compromise, infection, and vision loss.
2. The surgical approach should always address the underlying etiology of lid malposition.
3. Ectropion, or eversion of the lid margin, can be involutional (senile), cicatricial, neurogenic (paralytic), mechanical, or congenital.
4. The most common type of ectropion is involutional, which is typically repaired by the lateral tarsal strip procedure.
5. Entropion, inversion of the lid margin, can be involutional (senile), spastic, cicatricial, or congenital.
6. Epiblepharon is different from congenital entropion and may resolve spontaneously as the patient grows older.

QUESTIONS YOU WILL BE ASKED

1. What is the most common etiology of lower lid ectropion?
   Involutional.
2. What is the preferred method to surgically repair involutional lower lid ectropion?
   Lateral tarsal strip procedure.
3. What is the best approach to surgically repair cicatricial lower lid ectropion?
   Full-thickness skin graft with Frost suture tarsorrhaphy.
4. What are the hallmark features of involutional entropion?
   Horizontal lid laxity, lower lid retractor disinsertion, and overriding preseptal orbicularis.

Recommended Readings
1. Guthrie AJ, Kadakia P, Rosenberg J. Eyelid malposition repair: a review of the literature and current techniques. *Semin Plast Surg*. 2019;33(2):92-102.
2. Hahn S, Desai SC. Lower lid malposition: causes and correction. *Facial Plast Surg Clin North Am*. 2016;24(2):163-171.
3. Kooistra LJ, Scott JF, Bordeaux JS. Cicatricial ectropion repair for dermatologic surgeons. *Dermatol Surg*. 2020;46(3):341-347.
4. Nelson ER, AAO/ASOPRS Oculofacial Plastic Surgery Education Center. *Eyelid Retraction*. https://www.aao.org/oculoplastics-center/eyelid-retraction
5. Pereira MG, Rodrigues MA, Rodrigues SA. Eyelid entropion. *Semin Ophthalmol*. 2010;25(3):52-58.
6. Sand JP, Zhu BZ, Desai SC. Surgical anatomy of the eyelids. *Facial Plast Surg Clin North Am*. 2016;24(2):89-95.
7. Woo KI, Kim YD. Management of epiblepharon: state of the art. *Curr Opin Ophthalmol*. 2016;27(5):433-438.

Section II: Craniofacial

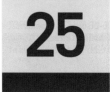

25 Nasal Reconstruction

Alisa Yamasaki

PREOPERATIVE CONSIDERATIONS

ASSESSING THE DEFECT

- **Location, size, and depth of defect** are considered when determining reconstructive options.
  - ○ Match the color, thickness, and texture of skin/tissue when determining donor site.
  - ○ Soft tissue defects up 1.5 cm can typically be reconstructed with a local flap.
  - ○ Flap design should align with nasal aesthetic units as best as possible.
  - ○ *If more than 50% of a subunit is involved, generally the remainder of the subunit is removed to camouflage scars along depressions and shadows at the junction of subunits, as well as create a whole unit (subunit principle). This concept is less popular currently.
  - ○ Contralateral/normal side should be used as a template for reconstruction.
  - ○ Composite wounds of the nose (ie, involving other facial units such as cheek and lip) should be reconstructed separately from the nose to maintain facial anatomic landmarks.
- **Determine missing tissue types** that will require reconstruction (eg, skin, cartilage/bone, mucosa)
  - ○ Structural support: perichondrium/cartilage and periosteum/bone
  - ○ Internal nasal lining (mucosa)
  - ○ External nasal cover: skin, subcutaneous fat, and submuscular aponeurotic system (SMAS)
- **Trauma, ischemic necrosis, and infection:** wound must be stabilized prior to reconstruction
  - ○ Débride necrotic tissue until clear demarcation of healthy tissue.
  - ○ Achieve source control for wound infections.

HISTORY AND PHYSICAL

- Prior to reconstruction, patient and wound should be assessed for readiness.
- Patient comorbidities such as diabetes, immunosuppression, smoking, hypothyroidism, nutritional deficiency, history of keloids, and history of prior radiation can significantly compromise wound healing and preoperative work-up should be performed to optimize comorbidities.
- **Skin Cancer:** must have clear oncologic margins before reconstruction.
  - ○ **Immediate reconstruction** is possible and preferred after Mohs excision (delay allows for scar contraction and increased infection risk).
  - ○ **Delayed reconstruction** performed for non-Mohs or melanoma resection.
  - ○ **History of prior radiation** may limit reconstructive options due to compromised soft tissue quality and vascularity.

---

*Denotes common in-service examination topics.

NASAL ANATOMY

NASAL SUBUNITS

- Distinctive convexities and concavities separate the **nine different subunits of the nose** (**Fig. 25-1**).
  - o Dorsum
  - o Sidewall (2)
  - o Tip
  - o Soft tissue triangle (2)
  - o Ala (2)
  - o Columella

LAYERS (SUPERFICIAL TO DEEP)

- Skin (sebaceous skin near tip, thinner skin at rhinion)
- Subcutaneous fat
- SMAS ± musculature
- Deep fatty layer
- Perichondrium/periosteum
- Cartilage/bone (septal cartilage, upper and lower lateral cartilage; nasal bone)
- Mucosa/mucoperichondrium

RELEVANT VASCULAR SUPPLY

Major nerves and blood vessels of the external nasal covering run deep to the SMAS, with few exceptions (**Fig. 25-2**).

- **External Carotid Artery Branches**
  - o **Angular artery**
    - ▪ Branch of facial artery that is superficial to/within SMAS
    - ▪ Supplies lateral surface of caudal nose

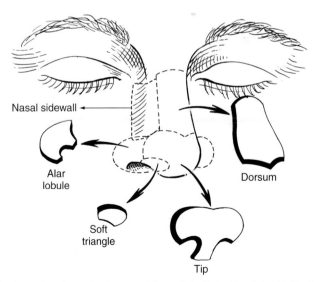

Nasal sidewall

Alar lobule

Dorsum

Soft triangle

Tip

Figure 25-1 Nasal aesthetic subunits. (From Thorne CH, ed. *Grabb and Smith's Plastic Surgery.* 7th ed. Lippincott Williams & Wilkins; 2014. Figure 33.1.)

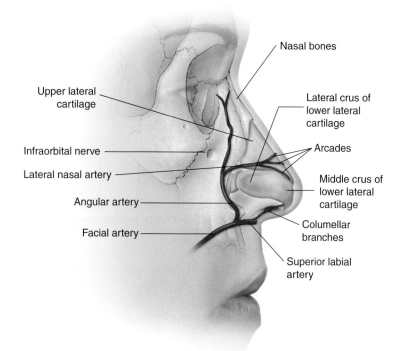

Figure 25-2 Arterial supply of external nasal cover. (From Thorne CH, ed. *Grabb and Smith's Plastic Surgery.* 7th ed. Lippincott Williams & Wilkins; 2014.)

- ○ **Superior labial artery**
  - ■ Within the orbicularis oris muscle, or between the mucosa and muscle
  - ■ Supplies nasal sill, septum, and base of columella
- ○ **Infraorbital artery**
  - ■ Branch of internal maxillary artery
  - ■ Supplies dorsum and lateral nasal side walls
- **Internal Carotid Artery Branches**
  - ○ **Dorsal nasal artery**
    - ■ Terminal branch of ophthalmic artery
    - ■ Supplies dorsum and lateral nasal skin
  - ○ **Supratrochlear arteries**
    - ■ Branch of ophthalmic artery
    - ■ 1.7-2.2 cm from midline
    - ■ Runs between corrugators and frontalis layers at orbital rim, becoming superficial to frontalis at mid-forehead level
  - ○ **Supraorbital arteries**
    - ■ Branch of ophthalmic artery

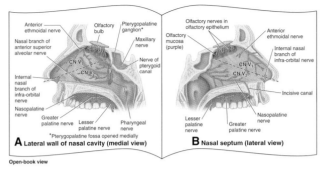

Open-book view

Figure 25-3 Innervation of nasal cavity. A. Sensory innervation of the lateral wall of the nasal cavity. **B.** Sensory innervation of the medial wall and the nasal septum. (From Dalley AF II, Agur AMR. *Moore's Clinically Oriented Anatomy.* 9th ed. Wolters Kluwer; 2023. Figure 8.108.)

- 2.9 cm from midline
- Runs through a notch or foramen with a superficial branch coursing superficial to SMAS and a deep branch coursing deep to or within the SMAS
- **Septal Vasculature:** branches of the anterior ethmoidal artery, posterior ethmoidal artery, sphenopalatine artery, and superior labial artery.
- **Lateral Nasal Wall Vasculature:** branches from anterior ethmoidal artery, posterior ethmoidal artery, and sphenopalatine artery.
- **Venous Drainage:** parallels arterial supply. Note—the angular vein becomes the anterior facial vein and communicates with the ophthalmic veins and cavernous sinus.

INNERVATION (FIG. 25-3)

- **Sensory**
  - External cover: branches from the ophthalmic (V_1) and maxillary (V_2) divisions of the trigeminal nerve
    - Supratrochlear, infratrochlear, and external nasal branches of the anterior ethmoidal nerve (derive from V1)
    - Infraorbital nerve (derives from V_2)
  - Septum: branches of the anterior ethmoidal (V_1) and nasopalatine nerves (V_2)
  - Lateral nasal wall: branches of the anterior ethmoidal (V_1) and branches of the pterygopalatine nerve (V_2)
- **Motor innervation** to superficial mimetic muscles of the face is supplied by branches of the facial nerve (VII).

APPROACHES TO NASAL RECONSTRUCTION

GENERAL PRINCIPLES

Depending on the defect, one or more of these objectives will need to be achieved.
- Establish bony/cartilaginous foundation.
- Restore internal nasal lining.
- Resurface nasal surface with external covering.
- Maintain nasal airway patency.
- Optimize aesthetic result.

BONE/CARTILAGE RECONSTRUCTION

- **Septal Reconstruction**
  - **L-shaped septal strut**: fabricated from septal cartilage/bone, autologous rib, outer table calvarium.
  - **Cantilevered graft**: fabricated from septal cartilage/bone, autologous rib, outer table calvarium) and secured to the remaining nasal bones or frontal bone.
  - **Septal hinge and pivot flaps** (see below "Intranasal flaps for lining").
  - **Alloplastic materials** such as vitallium, titanium, or porous polyethylene are not recommended due to the high rate of exposure and infection.
- **Lateral Bony/Cartilaginous Framework Reconstruction** (e.g., Nasal Bones, Upper Lateral Cartilage, Lower Lateral Cartilage)
  - Use **septal, conchal, or autologous rib cartilage.**
  - Reconstruct native cartilage anatomy when possible.
  - Use cartilage grafting to stabilize areas that are prone to collapse/retract (eg, sidewalls, ala, columella).

RECONSTRUCTION OF NASAL LINING

- Nasal lining must be restored or wound contraction from secondary healing will result in significant scar that can distort the nose and/or cause nasal obstruction.
- **Nasal Vestibular Skin Advancement**
  - A few mm of residual nasal vestibular skin may be advanced toward the caudal nostril margin and combined with a cartilage graft for rigid support to prevent retraction.
  - Bipedicled vestibular skin advancement flap can be used for full-thickness ala or unilateral tip defects <1 cm (cranial-caudal) using an extender intercartilaginous incision from anterior septal angle to lateral vestibular floor until the caudal edge of the defect is reached with 1-2 mm of redundancy. The donor site may need coverage with a full-thickness skin graft.
- **Intranasal Flaps for Lining** (Use With Caution for Smokers and Patients on Anticoagulation) (**Fig. 25-4**)
  - **Ipsilateral septal composite mucoperichondrial hinge flap**
    - Indication: large full-thickness defects involving the internal lining of the tip and/or columella, or dorsum.
    - Includes septal mucoperichondrium. Hinged on the caudal cartilaginous septum based on axial septal blood supply (septal branch of the superior labial artery).
    - Can be designed up to 3 cm wide × 4.5 cm long.
    - Full-thickness alar defects also require cartilage framework at caudal nostril margin.
    - Septal cartilage can also be harvested for additional grafting material as needed, though auricular cartilage contour can be more favorable.
    - Flap is divided in 3 weeks during second stage procedure.
  - **Contralateral/bilateral septal composite mucoperichondrial hinge flap**
    - Indication: used to resurface the roof and lateral wall of the middle vault.
    - Contralateral mucoperichondrial flap is hinged on the dorsum and reflected across the midline via the septal perforation necessitated by use of two flaps.
  - **Septal composite chondromucosal pivotal flap**
    - Indication: large full-thickness defects of the central nose or for full-thickness loss of the nasal tip and columella.
    - Typically 3 cm wide × 5 cm long and includes the entire length of cartilaginous septum with bilateral mucosal and may include bony septum.
    - For tip/columellar defects, wedge of caudal septal cartilage is removed to allow flap to pivot 90° anterocaudally, and flap is secured to remaining cartilaginous dorsum.

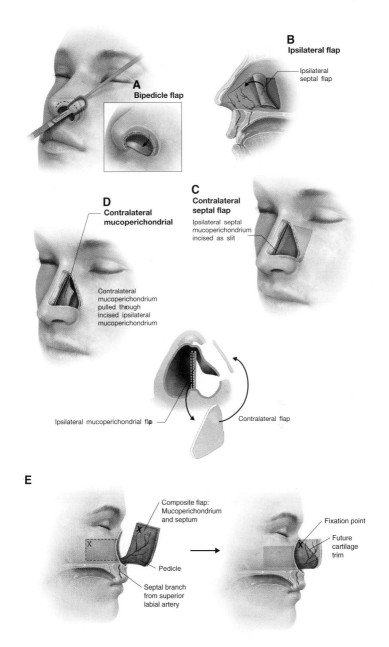

Figure 25-4 Intranasal lining flaps. A. Bipedicle flap. **B.** Ipsilateral mucoperichondrial flap. **C.** Contralateral mucoperichondrial flap. **D.** Contralateral septal flap. **E.** Composite flap. (From Thorne CH, ed. *Grabb and Smith's Plastic Surgery.* 7th ed. Lippincott Williams & Wilkins; 2014. Figure 33.2.)

- For dorsal defects, flap is pivoted 45° anterocaudally to reconstruct the region of the anterior septal angle and upper lateral cartilages. Excess caudal septal cartilage may need to be removed at posterior septal angle.
  - Turbinate mucoperiosteal flap
    - Indication: small mucosal defects can be reconstructed with inferior or middle turbinate.
    - Blood supply from lateral descending branch of the sphenopalatine artery.
    - Turbinate is medialized and bone is removed to fashion an anteriorly based mucosal flap.
- Flap techniques for internal lining that are combined with paramedian forehead flap (see reconstruction of nasal cutaneous defects for details on the paramedian forehead flap)
  - Full-thickness skin graft
    - Indication: used to line a full-thickness forehead flap.
    - Reconstruction typically performed in three stages, and cartilage grafts are inserted under skin-grafted areas during subsequent stages.
  - Folded forehead flap
    - Indication: full-thickness unilateral and bilateral nasal defects. Can replace internal lining defects ≤3.5 cm.
    - The most distal edge of the flap—often designed obliquely along the hairline to minimize hair-bearing scalp—is folded over on itself.
    - If cartilage grafts are required, a three-stage reconstruction is typically performed with cartilage grafts placed during the second stage.
  - Prelaminated forehead flap
    - Indication: small- to medium-sized rim defects when vascular supply and/or to patient morbidity are a concern (minimizes the time skin bridge is in place).
    - First stage involves application of a full-thickness skin graft to the distal deep surface of the flap under the frontalis muscle along the proposed nostril margin of the planned forehead flap. Cartilage graft may also be placed between the frontalis muscle and overlying external skin if needed.
    - Second stage involves flap elevation and inset.
  - Turnover flap
    - Indication: used when external nasal covering is being reconstructed with a forehead flap.
    - Distal flap is turned in to be used as lining.
    - Disadvantages are soft tissue bulk (native nasal lining is very thin) and potential flap necrosis given that the distal component of the flap is used for turnover.
  - Bilateral paramedian forehead flaps
    - Indication: large full-thickness defects in which one flap is used for external covering and one flap is used for internal lining.
    - May perform structural grafting and internal lining at the first stage if bony/cartilaginous framework of the nose require reconstruction, followed by staged second forehead flap for external lining.
    - Additional cartilage grafts (eg, at alar rim) and flap thinning may be performed during subsequent stages.

RECONSTRUCTION OF NASAL CUTANEOUS DEFECTS

- Technical Pearls
  - Square off defects to provide sharp edges for tissue alignment and avoid concentric contraction that can occur with circular defects.
  - Incisions should follow natural relaxed skin tension lines when possible.
    - Separate reconstruction for nose vs cheek.
    - Respect borders of nasal subunits.
    - Avoid incisions on concavities.

- **Full-Thickness Skin Graft**
  - Indication: ideal for superficial, smaller defects in thin-skinned areas of the nose (eg, cephalic sidewall, dorsum).
  - May be used at the nasal tip in select patients with thin and fair skin (eg, older patients with atrophic skin; skin grafts may be used almost anywhere on the nose for superficial defects in these patients).
  - May be combined with cartilage grafting when close to the caudal nostril margin.
  - Graft typically remains lighter in color than native nasal skin.
- **Composite Auricular Cartilage Graft**
  - Indication: for full-thickness defects ≤1 cm involving the alar margin or soft tissue triangle.
  - Reported survival rates ranging from 50% to 90% (avoid in patients with compromised vasculature/healing; e.g., smokers, diabetic patients).
  - *Graft is initially white; turns blue at 24-72 hours; gradually becomes pink over subsequent days.
  - Intermittent icing the graft in the first 48 hours (decreases metabolic demand) and the use of Medrol dose pack may increase graft survival.
- **Nasal Cutaneous Flaps**
  - **Transposition flap**
    - Indication: nasal tip, dorsum, or sidewall defects ≤1.0 cm
    - Must ensure skin is mobile and skin thickness matches native skin of defect
    - Less applicable for thicker, less mobile skin of caudal nose
  - **Dorsal nasal flap (Rieger flap)**
    - Indication: redundant glabellar skin is used to repair defects of nasal tip, dorsum, and sidewall ≤2.5 cm.
    - Use pinch test to assess adequate skin laxity to accommodate mobilization.
    - Can elevate/distort nasal tip and unfavorably distort/medialize brow.
  - **Bilobe flap**
    - Indication: nasal tip or caudal sidewall defects ≤1.5 cm (max size varies proportionally with size of nose).
    - Typically based laterally with standing cutaneous deformity designed along alar groove.
    - Two lobes designed along 90°-110° arc with first lobe transposed into defect, second lobe transposed into first lobe defect, and second lobe closed primarily.
  - **V-to-Y island advancement flap**
    - Indication: ala and tip defects ≤1.0 cm
    - Triangular flap designed with apex positioned laterally
  - **Melolabial interpolation flap (Fig. 25-5)**

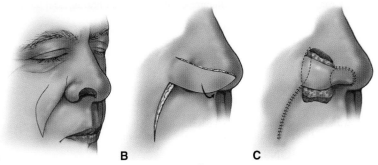

Figure 25-5 A-C. Two-stage nasolabial flap. (From Nose reconstruction. In: Kaufman A. *Practical Facial Reconstruction.* Wolters Kluwer; 2017:95-163. Figure 5.11BCE.)

A   B   C

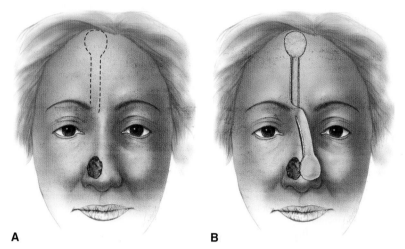

A   **B**

Figure 25-6 Forehead flap. A. Arteries of the forehead. This richly anastomotic network provides the basis for the paramedian forehead flap (**B**). (From Nose reconstruction. In: Kaufman A. *Practical Facial Reconstruction.* Wolters Kluwer; 2017:95-163. Figure 5.12BC.)

- Indication: lateral nasal tip or alar defects ≤3.0 cm.
- Designed along nasolabial fold with blood supply based on subcutaneous fat pedicle.
- Flap is brought over the alar facial sulcus into the defect.
- May require concomitant cartilage grafting if defect is close to caudal nostril margin.
- Flap detachment performed 3 weeks later in second stage.
  - Paramedian forehead flap (Fig. 25-6)
    - Indication: larger nasal defects ≥ 2.5 cm.
    - Axial flap based on supratrochlear artery located 1.7-2.2 cm lateral to midline with 1.5 cm pedicle width.
    - Template is created from the defect and placed at anterior hairline with flap centered over the supratrochlear artery.
    - Elevated in a subfascial plane with blunt dissection used near the brow to avoid injury to the pedicle.
    - May extend obliquely (minimize extension into hair-bearing skin) for flaps wider than 3 cm.
    - Flap detachment performed 3 weeks later in second stage.
    - Can be combined with other reconstructive techniques depending on tissues involved in defect (see above "Combined flap techniques for internal lining").
- Free Flap
  - Used for large, full-thickness defects with multiple donor options, including radial forearm free flap and temporoparietal fascia flap
  - Requires staged reconstruction using multiple techniques (eg, initial stage with reconstruction of internal nasal lining and bony/cartilaginous framework followed by reconstruction of external nasal covering)

COMPLICATIONS

- **Infection** should be treated aggressively and possible bacterial seeding of underlying structural grafts should be assessed.

- Systemic antibiotics.
- Any abscess must be washed out.
- Persistent drainage suggests infection of structural grafts; investigate for internal lining defects.
- **Flap necrosis** can be mitigated by protecting the vascular supply during flap elevation and ensuring the medical risk factors are optimized in at-risk patients.
  - Ensure pedicle width is adequate and there is no kinking of pedicle in interpolated flaps (eg, pedicles that are too wide may kink with rotation, flaps that are too short may have excess tension).
  - Avoid excessive thinning that can compromise subdermal blood supply to the skin.
  - Patient factors
    - **Smoking**: three-stage approach is safer in smokers; avoid "intranasal flap" options for internal lining; may consider delaying >3 weeks for subsequent stages.
    - **Anticoagulation**: intranasal flap options may lead to uncontrolled bleeding.
    - **Diabetes.**
    - **Radiation**: can lead to severe atrophy, induration, or ulceration.
  - If necrosis occurs, débride involved areas.
  - If flap cannot be salvaged with acceptable structural support and/or aesthetic result, stabilize the wound prior to planning next steps in reconstruction.

RHINOPHYMA

FEATURES AND ETIOLOGY

- Stages of Rosacea
  - Prerosacea: frequent facial flushing
  - Vascular rosacea: thickened skin/telangiectasias/erythrosis
  - Inflammatory rosacea
  - Late rosacea (**rhinophyma—the most advanced stage of rosacea**)
- Rosacea is diagnosed by presence of at least one primary and secondary feature.
  - Primary features: transient erythema (blushing), non-transient erythema (persistent redness), papules, pustules, telangiectasia
  - Secondary features: facial skin hypersensitivity, plaques, edema, ocular manifestations, non-facial involvement, phymatous changes (skin thickening, pore enlargement, surface nodularities)
- Predominantly male disease; prevalent among English/Irish ancestry, peak presentation at later than age 50, no proven association with alcohol.
- Disease begins with vascular instability of the skin; fluid is lost into interstitium; inflammation and fibrosis follow. Dermal and sebaceous gland hypertrophy develop. Sebaceous ducts become plugged, resulting in dilation, edema, and eventual gland fibrosis. Erythema, telengiectasia, and thickening of nasal skin results that progressively disfigures nose. Nasal obstruction can occur with bulky disease.
- **Differential diagnosis includes cutaneous malignancies** (e.g., basal cell carcinoma, squamous cell carcinoma), sarcoidosis, lymphoma, and other granulomatous disease.

MANAGEMENT

- **Nonsurgical treatments:** topical and oral antibiotics and isotretinoin, which will slow progression but do not provide cure.
- **Surgical treatments:** goal is to remove involved skin and resculpt the nose to its native contour. **Oral retinoids (isotretinoin/Accutane) should be discontinued 6-12 months prior to surgery as they compromise re-epithelialization.**
  - Dermaplaning
  - Dermabrasion

- Excision (full-thickness removal with flap/graft reconstruction vs partial-thickness removal)
- Electrocautery
- Coblation
- CO_2 laser (also: diode laser, Nd:YAG, KTP)
- Plasma and radiofrequency ablation

PEARLS

1. If the blood supply to the columella is disrupted, the nasal tip relies on the lateral nasal arteries for its blood supply.
2. The forehead flap should become thicker when dissecting distal to proximal (subcutaneous to submuscular to subperiosteal), as the vessels are deeper proximally/inferiorly.
3. The forehead donor site of the forehead flap heals well by secondary intention in cases of large flap donor sites that cannot be closed primarily (be sure to leave periosteum down).
4. The maximum rotation of a bilobed flap is 100°.
5. Reconstruction of the nasal ala should often include a cartilage framework (alar batten graft) to prevent retraction and notching of the rim (despite the absence of cartilage in this location natively).

QUESTIONS YOU WILL BE ASKED

1. What three structural elements are considered in cases of nasal reconstruction? Lining, support, and coverage.
2. What is the subunit principle of nasal reconstruction?
   If 50% or more of a subunit is missing, then the remaining portion of the subunit is removed to follow subunit boundaries and optimize the aesthetic outcome. This is not a "hard and fast" rule.
3. How far on either side of the midline are the supratrochlear and supraorbital arteries located (on average)?
   1.7 and 2.7 cm, respectively.
4. When should isotretinoin be discontinued in relation to nasal resurfacing procedures?
   At least 6 months prior to surgery.

THINGS TO DRAW

Draw the nasal aesthetic subunits (Fig. 25-1).

Recommended Readings
1. Burget GC, Menick FJ. Nasal support and lining: the marriage of beauty and blood supply. *Plast Reconstr Surg.* 1989;84(2):189-202.
2. Guo L, Pribaz JR, Pribaz JJ. Nasal reconstruction with local flaps: a simple algorithm for management of small defects. *Plast Reconstr Surg.* 2008;122(5):130e-139e.
3. Joseph AW, Truesdale C, Baker SR. Reconstruction of the nose. *Facial Plast Surg Clin North Am.* 2019;27(1):43-54. doi:10.1016/j.fsc.2018.08.006
4. Menick FJ. The evolution of lining in nasal reconstruction. *Clin Plast Surg.* 2009;36(3):421-441.
5. Menick FJ. Nasal reconstruction. *Plast Reconstr Surg.* 2010;125(4):138e-150e. doi:10.1097/PRS.0b013e3181d0ae2b
6. Rohrich RJ, Griffin JR, Adams WP Jr. Rhinophyma: review and update. *Plast Reconstr Surg.* 2002;110(3):860-869. quiz 870.
7. Zitelli JA. The bilobed flap for nasal reconstruction. *Arch Dermatol.* 1989;125(7):957-959.

Lip and Cheek Reconstruction

Chien-Wei Wang

LIP RECONSTRUCTION

OVERVIEW

- **Etiology of Lip Defects**
  - Most common cause (>90%): cancer resection
    - Most common neoplasm overall: squamous cell carcinoma
      - Most commonly on lower lip
    - Most common neoplasm of upper lip: basal cell carcinoma.
    - *Vermillion cancers (anterior to wet-dry border) behave like cutaneous tumors, but those posterior to this landmark behave like intraoral tumors (higher risk of metastasis).
    - Resection typically done by Mohs micrographic surgery.
    - If Mohs surgery is not available
      - Recommended surgical margin for squamous cell carcinoma: 7-10 mm
      - Recommended surgical margin for basal cell carcinoma: 2-4 mm
  - Other causes: trauma and burns
- **Lip Anatomy**
  - **Layers:** skin, subcutaneous tissue, orbicularis oris muscle, and mucosa
  - **Vermilion**
    - Unique tissue consisting of modified mucosa with relatively few underlying minor salivary glands
    - **White roll:** junction of the vermilion and the lip skin
      - *Continuity is critical during reconstruction because even a 1 mm step off is noticeable at conversational distance.
    - Wet-dry border: the posterior vermilion line
      - Upper and lower lips meet when the mouth is closed.
      - Transition from oral mucosa to vermilion mucosa.
  - **External anatomy (Fig. 26-1)**
    - The lips are divided into four subunits
      - **Philtrum:** between the philtral columns. The tubercle is the central portion of vermilion inferior to the philtrum.
      - **Lateral wings:** between each philtral column and nasolabial fold.
      - **Lower lip:** the entire lower lip is a single subunit.
    - The labiomental fold separates the lower lip from the chin.
    - The nasolabial folds confine the lateral extents of the upper lip.
    - The normal intercommissural distance in an adult at rest is 5-6 cm.
      - Approximately the distance between the medial limbi of the corneas
      - Ideally should equal the distance from the stomion to the menton
  - **Muscular anatomy (Fig. 26-2)**
    - **Orbicularis oris muscles**
      - Function: the primary muscles for closure of the lips as a sphincter for the oral cavity. It everts the lips.
      - Origin: medial aspects of maxilla and mandible, modiolus.
      - Insertion: upper and lower lips.

---

*Denotes common in-service examination topics.

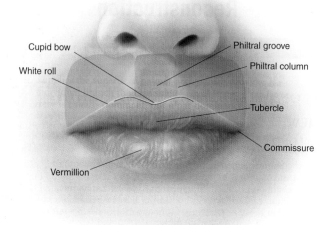

Figure 26-1 External lip anatomy includes four subunits. Medial aesthetic subunit of the upper lip is depicted by the shaded *red area*, and the lateral aesthetic subunits are depicted by shaded *blue areas*. (From Sando IC, Brown DL. Reconstruction of acquired lip and cheek deformities. In: Chung KC, ed. *Grabb and Smith's Plastic Surgery*. 8th ed. Wolters Kluwer; 2020:408-419. Figure 41.1.)

- In the upper lip, the muscles cross the midline and insert into the opposite philtral column.
  □ Innervation: buccal branches of the facial nerve
- **Paired mentalis muscles**
  □ Function: principal elevators of the lower lip
  □ Origin: lower border of the mandible
  □ Insertion: soft tissues of the chin below the level of the labiomental crease
  □ Innervation: marginal mandibular branch of the facial nerve

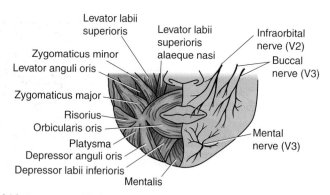

Figure 26-2 Arrangement of the facial muscles around the lips and the sensory nerve supply of the lips. (From Wineski LE. *Snell's Clinical Anatomy by Regions*. 10th ed. Wolters Kluwer; 2019. Figure 12.75.)

- **Lip elevators**
  - Muscles: paired levator anguli oris, levator labii superioris, zygomaticus major, and zygomaticus minor muscles
  - Innervation: zygomatic and buccal branches of the facial nerve
- **Lip depressors**
  - Muscles: paired depressor anguli oris and depressor labii inferioris muscles.
  - Innervation: marginal mandibular branch of the facial nerve.
  - *The paired platysma muscles also provide some lateral lower lip depression (eg, during full denture smile) and are innervated by the cervical branch of the facial nerve.
  - **Sensation (Fig. 26-2)**
    - **Upper lip:** innervated by infraorbital nerves
      - Terminal branch of the maxillary division of the trigeminal nerve (V_2) and exits the maxilla at the infraorbital foramen in line with the pupil and 1 cm inferior to the infraorbital rim
    - **Lower lip:** innervated by mental nerves
      - Terminal branch of the mandibular division of the trigeminal nerve (V_3) and exits the mandible at the mental foramen at the level of the **second premolar**
  - **Blood supply**
    - **Arterial**
      - Branches of facial artery: the superior and inferior labial arteries.
      - *The labial artery usually lies between the orbicularis oris muscle and mucosa within the vermilion portion of the lip.
      - Superior labial artery is 10 mm from superior lip margin.
      - Inferior labial artery is 4-13 mm from lower lip margin.
    - **Venous:** superior and inferior labial veins drain to the ipsilateral facial vein.
  - **Lymphatic drainage**
    - **The upper lip and lower lateral lip segments drain into the submandibular nodes.**
    - The central lower lip drains into the submental nodes.
- **Lip Reconstruction Goals**
  - **Functional goals:** restore oral competence
    - Primary goal in lip reconstruction
      - Suboptimal cosmesis is more well tolerated than loss of function.
    - Maximizing oral aperture, mobility, sensation, and preservation of lower lip sulcus
      - Around <50% preoperative stoma size significantly impairs lip functions.
      - Loss of functions lead to dribbling of saliva or food.
  - **Aesthetic and social goals:** restores static and dynamic symmetry
    - The lips are essential for facial expression and communication.

EVALUATION AND CONSIDERATIONS

- **What Tissue Is Missing:** vermilion, skin, orbicularis muscle, and/or mucosa.
- **How Much of the Lip Is Missing:** the proportion of total lip tissue missing is often described in thirds, partial vs full-thickness defect, involvement of commissure, and involvement of the philtrum.
- **Patient Factors:** age of patient, tissue elasticity, lip redundancy, need for dentures, radiation, previous scars, tolerance for complex reconstruction, and general health status.
- **Lip defects that involve >30%** of the lip may result in microstomia if closed primarily. Microstomia is a difficult condition that impedes eating, use of dentures, and adequate oral hygiene.
  - **Optimal repair:** re-approximation of the orbicularis oris muscle, mucosa, white roll, dermis, and epidermis is crucial

APPROACHES TO PARTIAL-THICKNESS LIP DEFECTS

- **Superficial Defects of the Skin:** usually do not cause functional deficits
  - ○ **Skin grafts** can provide efficient coverage of superficial lip defects but can result in inferior aesthetic results.
    - ▪ Split-thickness skin grafts contract more than full-thickness grafts.
    - ▪ Severe cases of retraction can lead to lip eversion and decreased oral competence.
  - ○ **Local tissue rearrangement** techniques generally offer the best match in tissue thickness, color, and texture.
    - ▪ Small defects (<1.5 cm) can be closed with O-to-T plasty.
      - □ Larger defects make the excision of standing cone cutaneous deformity excision in O-to-T plasty not favorable due to extension into normal structure.
    - ▪ Cheek advancement flaps combined with perialar excisions and lateral V-Y advancement flaps are commonly used for upper lip skin defects.
    - ▪ Lower lip defects are often resurfaced with rotational flaps (eg, bilobed) and transposition flaps (eg, rhomboid).
    - ▪ If the defect is confined to the philtrum, consider healing by secondary intention or full-thickness skin grafting.
- **Vermilion Defects (Fig. 26-3)**
  - ○ General principles
    - ▪ Before infiltrating area with local anesthetic, use a fine-tipped pen and mark the superior and inferior edges of the white roll.
    - ▪ Lesions of the vermillion are preferentially excised perpendicular to the white roll to facilitate alignment of this landmark.
    - ▪ Local tissue rearrangements that involve skin only will require the use of one of the following techniques to repair the vermillion.
  - ○ Techniques for reconstruction
    - ▪ **Small/superficial vermilion defects**
      - □ Generally can be closed with V-Y advancement flaps of labial or buccal mucosa (generally horizontally oriented)
      - □ If unable to close with V-Y advancement flaps, consider:
        - ▪ For superficial vermillion defects <30% of the lip, the vermillion-skin border can be incised, and the vermilion can be directly advanced along the lip.
        - ▪ For more complex vermillion defects <30% of the lip, full-thickness excision of the defect can be performed and closed with vermilion advancement flap (based on labial pedicles).
    - ▪ **Large defects**
      - □ Defects usually occur after vermillionectomy for precancerous lesions and involve the entire vermillion.
      - □ Resurface with a retrolabial mucosal advancement flap.
        - ▪ Tip: dissect to the sulcus at a level between the orbicularis oris muscle and the accessory salivary glands, which are included in the mucosal flap.
      - □ Staged procedures that borrow mucosa from the upper lip (eg, bipedicled mucosa flap, cross lip mucosa flap).
      - □ Staged tongue flap: dorsal tongue for upper lip and volar tongue for lower lip.

APPROACHES TO FULL-THICKNESS LIP DEFECTS (FIG. 26-4)

- Requires approximation/replacement of skin, muscle, and mucosa
- **Defects up to One-Third of the Lip:** primary closure is most appropriate
  - ○ **Shield or wedge excision:** preferred design around lip lesion for excision. Can be modified into a "W" on the lower lip to limit the length of closure and prevent disruption of the labiomental or nasolabial creases.

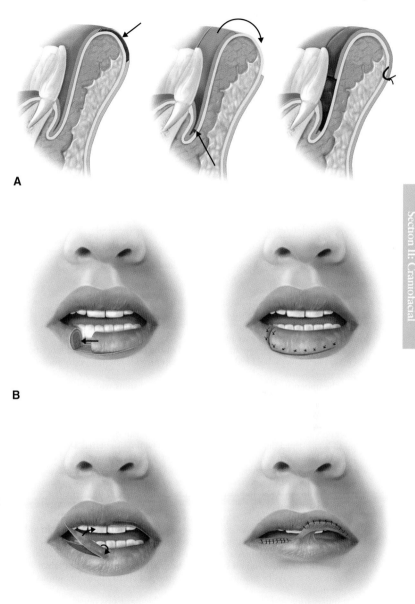

Figure 26-3 Vermilion reconstruction. Bipedicle flap released from gingivobuccal sulcus (**A**). Musculomucosal advancement flap (**B**). Unipedicle vermilion lip switch flap (**C**). (From Thorne CH, Gurtner GC, Chung KC, et al., eds. *Grabb and Smith's Plastic Surgery*. 7th ed. Wolters Kluwer; 2014. Figure 34.3.)

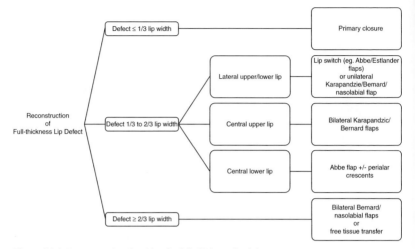

Figure 26-4 Reconstructive algorithm for full-thickness lip defects.

- Central upper lip defects involving the philtrum can be reconstructed with an Abbe flap to maintain aesthetic subunits.
- **Defects of One-Third to Two-Third of the Lip**
    - Primary closure with skin excisions
        - For defects slightly larger than one-third of the lower lip, bilateral labiomental crease excisions (Schuchardt procedure) can provide enough laxity for primary closure.
        - For the upper lip, bilateral perialar crescentic excisions with cheek advancement (Webster flaps) may allow for primary closure.
    - Lip-sharing techniques
        - **Abbe flap** (Fig. 26-5): a two-staged lip-switch procedure where a full-thickness flap of up to one-third of the donor lip can be used to reconstruct up to a two-third defect of the recipient lip. The flap is rotated 180° on its pedicle (labial artery) and remains for about 3 weeks, when the pedicle is divided.
            - □ Indication: can be utilized with upper and lower lip defects. In the upper lip, an Abbe flap can be used for either philtral or lateral lip reconstruction.
            - □ Flap design: flap borders parallel to relaxed skin tension lines. The height of the flap should match that of the defect. The width of the flap should be about half of the defect (to allow for proportional reduction of both lips).
            - □ Pedicle: based on either a medial or lateral pedicle. Artery is located at level of the white roll on sagittal section. Several millimeters of labial mucosa should be maintained around the pedicle to allow for venous drainage.
            - □ Innervation: despite denervation of the orbicularis oris muscle during harvest, motor and sensory function improves over the first year.
            - □ Can be performed in conjunction with labiomental crease incisions or perialar crescent excisions for larger defects.
        - **Estlander flap** (Fig. 26-6): a medially based lip-switch technique that is indicated in lip defects that demonstrate commissure involvement
            - □ Indication: commissure involvement

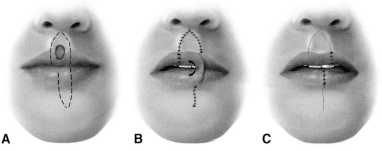

Figure 26-5 Abbe flap. A. An upper lip defect is being prepared. Complete excision of the lesion will produce a full-thickness lip defect that can be reconstructed with an Abbe flap. Markings are shown. **B.** The Abbe flap has been rotated into the defect. The flap is perfused by the labial vessels. **C.** After 2 or 3 weeks, the flap is divided and *inset*. (From Sando IC, Brown DL. Reconstruction of acquired lip and cheek deformities. In: Chung KC, ed. *Grabb and Smith's Plastic Surgery*. 8th ed. Wolters Kluwer; 2020:408-419. Figure 41.6.)

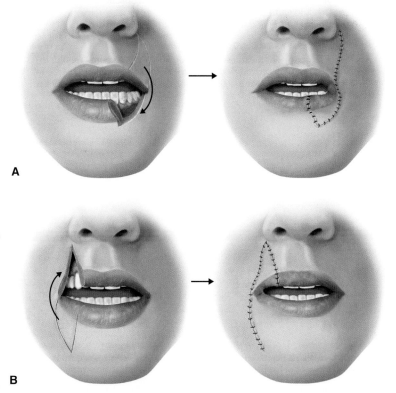

Figure 26-6 A. Estlander flap. **B.** Reverse Estlander flap. (From Thorne CH, Gurtner GC, Chung KC, et al., eds. *Grabb and Smith's Plastic Surgery*. 7th ed. Wolters Kluwer; 2014. Figure 34.7.)

□ Flap design: principles of design similar to the Abbe flap. Again, the flap width should be about half the defect width for deficit balance. Incisions lie within the nasolabial fold and are used with upper and lower lip defects.

□ Pedicle: blood supply more tenuous than the Abbe flap because it comes from contralateral labial artery. Cuff of muscle should be maintained at rotation point to improve vascularity to flap.

□ Innervation: flap is not innervated and oral animation can be distorted.

□ Despite being a one-stage reconstruction, there is often **blunting of the reconstructed commissure** and patients often require commissuroplasty.

○ Karapandzic flap (**Fig. 26-7**): a modification of the Gillies fan flap, **this one-stage technique preserves motor and sensory function through meticulous dissection of the neurovascular pedicles**

■ Indication: large central defects of up to 80% of the lower lip. May be used in cases with commissure involvement as the rotating donor lip tissue creates a new commissure.

■ Flap design
□ For lower lip defects, circumoral incisions are made extending from the defect and curve up around the commissures to include the nasolabial folds.
□ For upper lip defects, incisions are made along the nasolabial creases and extend down to the labiomental crease.
□ Bilateral opposing flaps are created and the incisions are limited to skin and subcutaneous tissue superficially and separate incisions to release the mucosa.

■ Pedicle/innervation: the intervening neurovascular structures are bluntly dissected out with scissors and preserved as the soft tissues are released to provide laxity to close the defect. Motor and sensory function preserved.

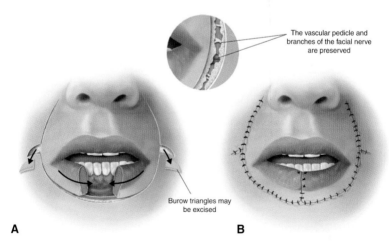

The vascular pedicle and branches of the facial nerve are preserved

Burow triangles may be excised

A   **B**

Figure 26-7 Karapandzic flap. The flap elements are incised and elevated (*left*, **A**). Small Burow triangles may be excised to facilitate rotation. The blood vessels and facial nerve branches are preserved (*inset*). The flaps are rotated into position and closed (*right*, **B**). (From Sando IC, Brown DL. Reconstruction of acquired lip and cheek deformities. In: Chung KC, ed. *Grabb and Smith's Plastic Surgery*. 8th ed. Wolters Kluwer; 2020:408-419. Figure 41.9.)

- Because it is often used for large lip defects, the Karapandzic flap may lead to blunting of the commissures and microstomia, which may require the use of lip-stretching appliances.

APPROACHES TO SUBTOTAL AND TOTAL LIP DEFECTS

- **Combination of Flaps**
  - Lower lip: two lateral Abbe flaps are used to reconstruct the lower lip while perialar crescent excisions with cheek advancement are used to close the upper lip Abbe donor sites.
  - Upper lip: an Abbe flap from the lower lip is used to reconstruct the philtrum in addition to bilateral perialar crescent excisions with cheek advancement.
- **Karapandzic Flap:** appropriate for very large defects if patients demonstrate sufficient tissue laxity.
- **Bilateral Opposing Cheek Advancement:** many eponyms exist, but all are based on horizontal advancement of cheek skin with removal of Burow triangles. Excisions involve skin and subcutaneous excisions only to protect neurovascular structures and preserve as much oral competence as possible. Buccal mucosa is used to reconstruct the vermillion.
  - **Bernard-Burow for lower lip (Fig. 26-8):** two large Burow triangles are excised lateral to the upper lip
  - **Webster modification** of Bernard-Burow for lower lip: places triangular skin excisions adjacent and parallel to the bilateral nasolabial folds, resulting in scars that are within natural skin creases and avoids violating the aesthetic region of the chin.
  - **Bernard-Burow's for upper lip:** four triangular skin excisions are needed, two perialar and two lateral to the lower lip.
- **Nasolabial Flap:** a long segment of skin and subcutaneous tissue is transposed to reconstruct full-thickness defects of the upper or lower lip.
  - Requires a skin graft to line the inner surface at the first stage.
  - Flaps have a random blood supply and can be delayed if necessary.
  - Must account for significant contraction and, therefore, flaps should be made larger than the lip defect.
  - Reconstruction of the vermillion is necessary at a second stage.

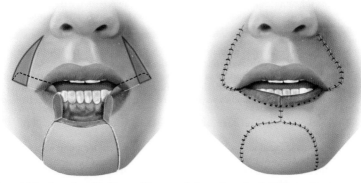

Figure 26-8 Bilateral modified Bernard-Burow technique. (From Sando IC, Brown DL. Reconstruction of acquired lip and cheek deformities. In: Chung KC, ed. *Grabb and Smith's Plastic Surgery.* 8th ed. Wolters Kluwer; 2020:408-419. Figure 41.10.)

Section II: Craniofacial

- Due to these limitations, this is not a preferred choice for subtotal or total lip reconstruction.
- Blood supply thought to be from perforators off angular artery off of facial artery.
- **Temporoparietal Scalp Flap**
  - A regional option best suited for male patients providing full-thickness reconstruction.
  - Bilateral flaps based on the superficial temporal artery can be used for full lip reconstruction.
  - Like nasolabial flaps, a skin graft is needed to line the deep surface and the flaps can be delayed.
- **Free Tissue Transfer** (eg, radial forearm with palmaris longus tendon for static support for oral competence).

POSTOPERATIVE CARE

- Nutrition: proper-sized pieces, or pureed diet
- Oral hygiene: Peridex rinse, soft brush

CHEEK RECONSTRUCTION

CHEEK ANATOMY

- **Anatomic Boundaries of the Cheek**
  - Lateral: preauricular skin
  - Medial: nasal sidewall and nasolabial fold
  - Superior: lower eyelid and temple
  - Inferior: mandibular border
- **Subunits of the Cheek**
  - Suborbital: between the nasolabial fold and anterior sideburn, lower eyelid, and gingival sulcus
  - Preauricular: between ear and malar eminence, includes masseteric and parotid fascia
  - Buccomandibular: between the gingival sulcus and the border of the mandible, includes oral lining
- *Muscle: the muscles of facial expression are connected by a contiguous fibrous sheet known as the superficial musculoaponeurotic system (SMAS), which lies just deep to the subcutaneous layer. Superiorly, it is continuous with the temporoparietal fascia (also known as superficial temporal fascia), and inferiorly, it is continuous with the platysma.
- **Innervation**
  - **Sensation** to the cheek is mediated by branches of the maxillary (V_2) and mandibular (V_3) divisions of the trigeminal nerve.
  - **Motor function** to the muscles of facial expression is imparted by the facial nerve (VII), which travels underneath the superficial lobe of the parotid gland. More anteriorly, the distal branches are found just deep to the parotid masseteric fascia.
- **Blood Supply**
  - The cheek is supplied predominantly by the facial artery, which gives off the angular artery.
  - The transverse facial artery branches from the superficial temporal artery and supplies the cheek superiorly.
  - Distally, these anastomose with the infraorbital artery and infratrochlear artery.
- **Retaining Ligaments**
  - There are two areas along the cheek where the skin and soft tissues are relatively fixed to the underlying bone.

○ The zygomatic ligament is found on the zygoma, just posterior and inferior to the malar eminence.
○ The mandibular ligament is found along the jaw line just posterior to the chin.
○ These ligaments resist advancement of cheek skin and may require release to allow for closure of cheek defects.

PREOPERATIVE CONSIDERATIONS

• Patient factors such as smoking, diabetes mellitus, immunosuppression, history of radiation, and prior scars may compromise wound healing or cause necrosis of local flap.
• Defect size, complexity, surrounding skin quality, skin laxity, hair-bearing status, and orientation of relaxed skin tension lines all affect the selection of the most appropriate reconstruction.
• After excision of aggressive tumors (eg, melanoma), a simpler reconstruction such as healing by secondary intention, primary closure, or skin grafting may be preferred initially to allow for tumor surveillance.
• Increased tension across the cheek will affect the appearance of neighboring facial units. For example, scar contractures of the cheek commonly result in traction on the lower eyelid or upper lip, causing ectropion.

RECONSTRUCTIVE OPTIONS

• **Secondary Healing**
  ○ Indication: reserved for selected cases where the defect is small and there is a reason to not perform primary closure.
  ○ Larger defects left to heal secondarily risk significant scar contraction that will lead to distortion and asymmetry.
  ○ Secondary healing leads to superior results in flat or concave areas (eg, temple, preauricular) as opposed to convex areas (eg, malar eminence).
• **Primary Closure**
  ○ Indication: small defects <1 cm in size can be reliably closed primarily, especially with skin undermining.
  ○ Elderly patients demonstrate increased skin laxity and, therefore, primary closure is often appropriate even for larger cheek defects.
  ○ In general, undermining up to 4 cm beyond the defect borders increases recruitment of surrounding tissue; further undermining does not contribute significantly to decreased wound closure tension.
  ○ Lesion excision and primary closure should be designed ideally along the relaxed skin tension lines.
  ○ Some lesions are positioned perpendicular to the relaxed skin tension lines: in these cases, it is better to accept an unfavorably oriented scar than to create a much longer scar within the relaxed skin tension lines.
• **Skin Grafts:** often the most efficient technique for covering larger cheek defects, skin grafts usually result in a poorer cosmetic outcome compared to local flap reconstruction
  ○ Skin grafts are considered in unhealthy patients who cannot tolerate more complex reconstructive surgical options and patients who require surveillance for recurrence of aggressive tumors.
  ○ Healed skin grafts on the cheek will demonstrate a patchlike appearance, color mismatch, and contour deformity. However, skin grafting is a preferred technique for temporal defects.
  ○ Full-thickness skin grafts will result in less secondary contraction and should be used whenever possible. When split-thickness grafts must be used, a thick nonmeshed graft should be harvested to optimize cosmesis.
• **Local Tissue Rearrangement (see Chapter 3: Flaps):** local flaps are useful for moderate (2-3 cm) and large (>3 cm) cheek defects. When designing a local flap, it is

critical that the vector of maximum tension after closure of the donor site is not in an unfavorable direction (eg, pulling down the lower eyelid predisposing to ectropion). Often, many surgical options will serve to close a cheek defect; the most appropriate reconstruction depends of the aforementioned preoperative considerations.

- o **Transposition flaps:** these versatile reconstructions capitalize on the substantial mobility of the cheek skin. Skin and subcutaneous tissue are borrowed from adjacent areas of relative laxity and the donor site is closed primarily. With careful planning of incisions and donor site tension, drawbacks such as complex scarring, trapdoor deformity, and irregularity in hair pattern can be minimized.
  - ▪ **Banner flap**
    - □ Simple transposition flap.
    - □ Design: final scar is placed along the relaxed skin tension lines of the cheek and the apex of the banner is usually excised.
    - □ Disadvantage: not the ideal choice because it typically results in a standing cutaneous deformity.
  - ▪ **Rhomboid flap (see Chapter 3: Flaps; Table 3-1)**
    - □ Indication: commonly used for coverage of defects on the lateral cheek and jawline.
    - □ Design: the classic rhomboid flap requires conversion of the defect to a rhombus with 60 and 120° angles. The donor flap is drawn from one of the 120° angles. The flap must be designed so that the vector of maximum tension after donor site closure is placed favorably.
    - □ Disadvantage: multiple incisions create one or more scars that lie perpendicular to lines of relaxed skin tension.
  - ▪ **Bilobed flap (see Chapter 3: Flaps; Table 3-1)**
    - □ Indication: may be used along the lateral and inferior cheek.
    - □ Design: modification of the banner flap, the bilobed flap uses a second secondary flap to help close the donor site of the primary flap. A pivotal arc of 90°-110° is commonly used.
    - □ Disadvantage: given the complex scarring, these flaps are generally not a first choice in cheek reconstruction.
- o **Cheek advancement flap**
  - ▪ Indication: useful for preauricular defects, a flap of cheek tissue can be directly advanced into the defect with excision of Burow triangles at the base.
  - ▪ Design: variations of this advancement technique may be utilized depending on defect characteristics. One example is the O-T flap, where a circular defect is converted into two opposing advancement flaps and the intervening standing cutaneous deformity is excised.
- o **V-Y advancement flap**
  - ▪ Indication: appropriate for defects of the medial cheek, alar base, and along the nasolabial fold, this flap survives on perforators within the subcutaneous pedicle.
  - ▪ Design: the flap may be designed with curved limbs that lie along the natural rhytids. With care, this flap is well suited for infraorbital defects, with low rates of ectropion and significant advantages over Mustardé-type flaps.
  - ▪ Sufficient subcutaneous dissection around the V-Y flap is required to achieve adequate mobilization for closure.
- • **Regional Flaps**
  - o **Cervicofacial flap**
    - ▪ Indication: large (>4 cm) medial cheek defects that are inappropriate for other local tissue rearrangement options can be repaired with a cervicofacial flap.
    - ▪ Design: various designs of cervicofacial flaps may be used depending on the size and location of the defect and flaps may be based superiorly or inferiorly.
    - ▪ Often a standing cutaneous deformity will need excision.

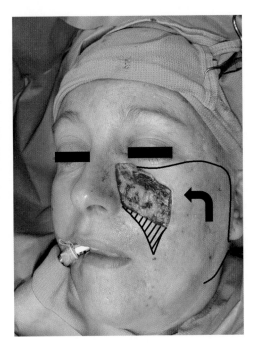

Figure 26-9 Mustardé cervicofacial flap.

○ **Mustardé flap (Fig. 26-9)**
  ▪ Indication: for defects close to or including the lower eyelid.
  ▪ Design: the incision may be carried into either the subciliary line or the inferior orbital rim. The incision is then taken beyond the lateral canthus and curves superiorly before extending inferiorly into the preauricular crease.
  ▪ The flap should be anchored to the deep temporal fascia above the lateral canthus to reduce tension on the repair and to prevent ectropion.
○ **Cervicopectoral flap**
  ▪ Indication: useful for very large cheek defects requiring significant advancement and rotation of donor tissue.
  ▪ Design: incisions are similar to a Mustardé flap but are extended onto the lower neck posteriorly and then over the clavicle anteriorly.
  ▪ Anchoring sutures to inferior orbital rim periosteum and temporary frost sutures can help prevent ectropion.
• **Tissue Expansion**
  ○ Provides skin that has good color and texture match and is well vascularized and sensate to resurface large cheek defects.
  ○ Tissue expansion in the head and neck region is associated with high complication rates.
  ○ Usually, lateral cheek and upper neck skin can be expanded to resurface defects resulting from excision of scars, large benign lesions, or previous skin grafts.
• **Free Flaps**
  ○ Reserved for complex cheek defects involving multiple tissue layers or patients who are not suitable candidates for local tissue rearrangements, such as patients with facial burns, patients who have had neck dissection, or patients demonstrating significant radiation dermatitis.
  ○ A classic choice is the radial forearm free flap, which is usually harvested with palmaris longus tendon for lip support.

PEARLS

1. When planning lip reconstruction, think about: What tissue is missing (layers)? How much of the lip (% width) is missing? What are the relevant patient factors?
2. Before injection of local anesthetic into a lip or around a skin lesion, always mark the white roll (above and below) and the edges of the lesion.
3. When a cheek defect is close to the lower eyelid, always consider the vector of pull and the risk of ectropion.
4. Be able to sketch various options for local flap designs (and their resultant scars) to reconstruct defects of the lip and cheek.
5. For any given cheek defect, be able to list several possible reconstructive choices; know the pros and cons of each option.

QUESTIONS YOU WILL BE ASKED

1. In the elderly, why is it important to consider oral stoma size when planning the reconstruction?
   To ensure postoperative denture placement.
2. In order to reduce the risk of postoperative ectropion, what structure can the cervicofacial flap be anchored to?
   Deep temporal fascia.
3. What is the most common complication of the Karapandzic flap?
   Microstomia.
4. What secondary procedure do Estlander flaps sometimes require?
   Commissuroplasty to correct rounded commissure.

THINGS TO DRAW

Draw the surface anatomy of the lips, including location of the labial artery in relation to skin, muscle, and mucosa.
See **Figure 26-1**.

Recommended Readings

1. Anvar BA, Evans BCD, Evans GRD. Lip reconstruction. *Plast Reconstr Surg.* 2007;120(4):57-64. doi:10.1097/01.prs.0000278056.41753.ce
2. Langstein HN, Robb GL. Lip and perioral reconstruction. *Clin Plast Surg.* 2005;32(3 SPEC. ISS.):431-445. doi:10.1016/j.cps.2005.02.007
3. Rapstine ED, Knaus WJ, Thornton JF. Simplifying cheek reconstruction: a review of over 400 cases. *Plast Reconstr Surg.* 2012;129(6):1291-1299. doi:10.1097/PRS.0b013e31824ecac7
4. Sanniec K, Harirah M, Thornton JF. Lip reconstruction after mohs cancer excision: lessons learned from 615 consecutive cases. *Plast Reconstr Surg.* 2020;145(2):533-542. doi:10.1097/PRS.0000000000006509
5. Sugg KB, Cederna PS, Brown DL. The V-Y advancement flap is equivalent to the Mustardé flap for ectropion prevention in the reconstruction of moderate-size lid-cheek junction defects. *Plast Reconstr Surg.* 2013;131(1):28-36. doi:10.1097/PRS.0b013e3182729e22

27 Head and Neck Masses and Neoplasms

Rebecca W. Gao

Section II: Craniofacial

OVERVIEW

- **Signs and Symptoms**
  - Localized pain, dysphagia (difficulty swallowing), odynophagia (painful swallowing), otalgia (referred ear pain), hoarseness, dyspnea, stridor, hemoptysis.
  - Fluctuating size → more likely nonneoplastic.
  - Constitutional: fever, chills, night sweats, or weight loss.
  - Hyper/hypothyroidism: changes in energy, mood, temperature sensitivity, bowel movements.
  - Trismus (inability to fully open the mouth) indicates possible involvement of pterygoid muscle, masseter muscle, and/or infratemporal fossa.
  - Middle ear effusion → nasopharyngeal mass.
- **Associations**
  - Exposures: TB, cats, radiation, or nickel
  - Recent infections: URI, sinusitis, dental problems/procedures
- **Family History**
  - *Multiple endocrine neoplasia
    - Type I: pancreatic tumors, parathyroid hyperplasia, and pituitary adenoma
    - Type IIA: medullary thyroid cancer, parathyroid hyperplasia, pheochromocytoma
    - Type IIB: medullary thyroid cancer, marfanoid habitus, mucosal neuromas, pheochromocytoma
  - Li-Fraumeni syndrome: p53 mutation, malignancies at young age
  - Basal cell nevus (Gorlin) syndrome: many basal cell carcinomas, odontogenic keratocysts, frontal bossing
  - Neurofibromatosis
- **Social History**
  - Tobacco: head and neck squamous cell carcinoma (SCC) is six times more likely in smokers.
  - EtOH: increases risk of carcinoma in patients who are also smokers.

DIFFERENTIAL DIAGNOSIS OF NECK MASSES

- **"80% Rule"**
  - 80% of nonthyroid neck masses in adults are neoplastic, 80% of these are malignant, 80% of these are metastases, and 80% of these are from primaries above the clavicles.
  - 80% of neck masses in children are inflammatory or benign.
- *The type of neck mass is predicted by location.
  - Midline: teratoma, dermoid, thyroglossal duct cyst, thyroid
  - Lateral neck/anterior triangle: branchial cleft anomaly, lymph nodes
  - Posterior triangle: lymph nodes

---

*Denotes common in-service examination topics.

- **Lymphadenitis**
  - ○ **Nodes >1-1.5 cm** in diameter are abnormal.
  - ○ Bacterial—*Streptococcus*, *Staphylococcus*, *Mycobacterium* (purple), catscratch fever (*Bartonella*), tularemia, and *Actinomyces* (sulfur granules and fistula tracts).
  - ○ Viral—Epstein-Barr virus, cytomegalovirus, herpes simplex virus, HIV, rhinovirus, adenovirus, toxoplasmosis.
  - ○ Fungal infections → coccidioidomycosis.
  - ○ **Treatment → empiric antibiotics** for 10-14 days. Persistence of adenitis >2 weeks → additional work-up.
- **Congenital Neck Masses**
  - ○ **Branchial cleft anomalies**
    - ▪ May include cysts, fistulas, or sinuses
    - ▪ **Cleft I: external auditory canal**
    - ▪ **Cleft II**
      - ▫ Most common
      - ▫ **Runs under sternocleidomastoid and over CN IX**
      - ▫ Runs under ECA and over internal carotid, exist/opens into the tonsillar fossa
    - ▪ Cleft III: similar to cleft II but runs under ICA
    - ▪ Treated by complete tract excision
  - ○ **Thyroglossal duct cyst**
    - ▪ *Remnant from descent of thyroid gland →occurs anywhere from the foramen cecum of the tongue to the suprasternal notch
    - ▪ May be patient's only thyroid tissue → pre-op ultrasound to check that patient has a normal thyroid in the usual location as well
    - ▪ Midline, moves when patient swallows, patients <30 years old
    - ▪ Treat by completely excising the cyst tract; decreased recurrence rate if hyoid bone is also excised (Sistrunk procedure)
  - ○ **Dermoid cyst**
    - ▪ Teratoma-like contain two rather than three (teratoma) germ layers.
    - ▪ *Midline doughy mass in a young adult, often in nasal cavity.
    - ▪ Need CT to rule out:
      - ▫ Extension of dermoid through posterior table into the brain (requires neurosurgery)
      - ▫ **Glioma or encephalocele**
- **Thyroid Masses**
  - ○ Solitary nodule: functional (benign) vs nonfunctional (benign vs malignant).
  - ○ Multinodular goiter.
  - ○ Inflammatory/autoimmune: Riedel thyroiditis, Hashimoto thyroiditis, and de Quervain thyroiditis.
  - ○ Malignancy: papillary, follicular, Hürthle cell, medullary, and anaplastic. The majority of thyroid cancers are low grade (papillary and follicular) and treated surgically.
    - ▪ Anaplastic → very poor prognosis, rapidly aggressive, not surgically resectable.
    - ▪ Medullary → from parafollicular C cells; check calcitonin levels.

DIAGNOSTIC STUDIES

- **Ultrasound:** primary imaging choice for thyroid pathologies.
- **MRI:** best for palate, parotid, and retro- and parapharyngeal spaces and cranial nerves/concern for perineural invasion.
- **CT with contrast:** evaluation of nodes >1.5 cm, especially with necrotic center. Helpful for stone identification in duct obstruction.
- **FNA**—diagnostic method of choice for neck masses concerning for malignancy. Accuracy is dependent on operator and cytopathologist experience.

- **Nuclear medicine studies:** thyroid uptake scans determine whether a mass is actively sequestering iodine (and therefore likely benign). Warthin tumor and oncocytoma usually have positive uptake of technetium-99.
- **Positron emission testing (PET):** tissues with high metabolic rates (such as tumors) demonstrate increased uptake of radioactive 18-fluorodeoxyglucose (FDG avidity).
  - Differentiate post-radiation changes from tumor, workup of occult nodal disease, pulmonary metastasis, and secondary primaries
  - Used for post-chemoradiation response evaluation (12 weeks after completion)
- **Indications for open biopsy** of a neck mass
  - Persistent for >3 weeks
  - Negative endoscopy with multiple random biopsies
  - Negative FNA with high clinical suspicion for malignancy
  - Concern for lymphoma

SALIVARY GLAND NEOPLASMS

SALIVARY GLAND ANATOMY

- Glands develop during the 6th-8th week of gestation.
- **Parotid Gland**
  - **Parotid = preauricular cheek extending to the upper neck** (tail) with deep and superficial lobes. The facial nerve and retromandibular vein separate the lobes.
  - Serous acini make up the gland.
  - *Stenson duct arises from the anterior border of the parotid and enters the oral cavity at the level of the maxillary second molar.
- **Submandibular (Submaxillary) Gland**
  - *Mucous and serous acini (along with parotid) are responsible for the majority of saliva production.
  - Wharton duct → enters the oral cavity in the anterior floor of mouth (FOM).
  - Closely associated with the lingual nerve, which sends autonomic fibers to the gland.
- **Sublingual Gland**
  - Anterior FOM just below the mucosa
  - Made up of mucous acini
- **Minor Salivary Glands**
  - 600-1000 glands are located just below the submucosal layer of the oral cavity.

BENIGN SALIVARY NEOPLASMS

- *Pleomorphic Adenoma
  - The most common salivary gland tumor (the most common malignant salivary tumor is mucoepidermoid carcinoma).
  - 65% of parotid/submandibular and 40% of minor gland tumors. Age 30-50 years, painless and slowly growing mass.
  - Rare malignant transformation (see below).
  - *Treated with excision with wide margins. Do NOT just enucleate → spillage and pseudopod extensions cause 30% recurrence.
- **Canalicular and Basal Cell Adenoma** (previously monomorphic adenoma)
  - **Rule of 75%:** Canalicular adenomas → upper lip in 75% of cases. Basal cell adenomas present in the parotid gland in 75% of cases.
  - May resemble a mucocele, which is rare in the upper lip.
  - Surgical excision is usually curative. Recurrence is rare and may be multifocal disease.
- *Warthin Tumor (papillary cystadenoma lymphomatosum)
  - Second most common salivary tumor. Most common site is the parotid gland.
  - Rule of 10s

- 10% are bilateral.
- 10× risk in smokers.
- Male to female ratio is 10:1.
  ○ Treat with superficial parotidectomy.

MALIGNANT SALIVARY NEOPLASMS

- *Mucoepidermoid Carcinoma
  ○ Most common salivary malignancy in children and adults (however, the most common salivary neoplasm is pleomorphic adenoma).
  ○ Most (70%) are found in the parotid gland.
  ○ Treatment is based on grade.
    - Low/intermediate: surgical excision; 90% cure rate
    - High (more solid components): excision, neck dissection, postoperative radiation
- Adenoid Cystic Carcinoma
  ○ Rare in the parotid; most common malignancy in the submandibular and minor glands.
  ○ Cribriform (best prognosis), tubular, and solid (worst) histopathologic types.
  ○ *Perineural spread/facial paralysis is common, seen on MRI.
  ○ Treat with surgery and radiation; 5-year survival is 70%, but 15-year survival is ~10% due to distant metastasis presenting many years later.
- Polymorphous Low-Grade Adenocarcinoma
  ○ Minor glands of the hard/soft palate
  ○ 70% female; commonly presents in 6th-8th decade of life
  ○ Perineural invasion common → wide surgical excision
- Acinic Cell Carcinoma
  ○ Rare (1%), low grade, 95% in parotid, excision curative
- Malignant Mixed Tumors
  ○ Most common: carcinoma ex pleomorphic adenoma.
    - Results from malignant degeneration of pleomorphic adenoma (10% degenerate)
    - Rapid growth in previous slow-growing lesion
  ○ Pain and facial nerve involvement, aggressive, high grade.
  ○ Treated with excision, neck dissection, and radiation therapy. Five-year survival is 50%.

MALIGNANT SALIVARY NEOPLASM MANAGEMENT

- Surgical Treatment
  ○ Gland removal
  ○ Neck dissection for:
    - High-grade primary tumor
    - Known positive lymph nodes
    - Large primary lesion size
- Postoperative Radiation Therapy
  ○ Indications: high-grade, residual, or recurrent disease; T3 or T4; invasion of adjacent structures; close or positive surgical margins
- Postoperative Complications of Salivary Tumor Excision
  ○ Sialocele
    - Presents as postoperative swelling with fluid collection
    - *Aspiration with placement of pressure dressing
    - Botulinum toxin injection for recurrent sialoceles
  ○ Facial nerve damage (see Chapter 19: Facial Palsy)
    - Transected nerves should be immediately repaired, if noted intraoperatively, or grafted, if a branch is intentionally resected for malignant disease.

- Loss of the marginal mandibular or temporal branches → most significant long-standing deformity due to lack of arborization; the zygomatic and buccal branches have extensive arborization, and distal branches will often recover function.
- The frontal/temporal branch is most important for eye closure and may need reconstruction if inadequate arborization from the buccal/zygomatic branch.
  - *Frey syndrome (auriculotemporal syndrome)
  - Caused by reinnervation of sympathetic sudomotor (sweat) fibers by severed parasympathetic (salivomotor) fibers normally directed to parotid gland
  - Preauricular gustatory sweating (sweating in response to salivary stimulation)
  - Minor starch-iodine test (topical starch/iodine powder mix turns blue with sweating)
  - Initial treatment = topical antiperspirant prior to meals
  - Long-term treatment = botulinum toxin injections

SQUAMOUS CELL CARCINOMA OF THE HEAD AND NECK

EPIDEMIOLOGY

- Squamous cell carcinoma (SCC) is the most common cancer involving head and neck mucosal sites (90% of malignancies).
- 60s-70s, incidence increases with age.
- Male to female ratio 2:1.
- Risk Factors
  - Tobacco (including smokeless/chewing tobacco)
  - Alcohol: synergizes with tobacco; increases risk by 10- to 15-fold
  - Human papilloma virus (HPV): oropharyngeal SCC
  - Epstein-Barr virus: associated with nasopharyngeal SCC
  - Poor dental hygiene
  - Chronic irritation (ie, ill-fitting dentures)
  - Plummer-Vinson syndrome (achlorhydria, iron deficiency anemia, dysphagia, mucosal atrophy)
  - Syphilis
  - Lichen planus
  - Chronic immunosuppression
  - Betel nuts: common in Indian population

PATHOLOGY

- Premalignant Lesions
  - Biopsies of the following lesions are required to rule out invasive component.
  - Leukoplakia—white patchy mucosa
    - Epithelial hyperplasia, usually secondary to trauma
    - Can represent dysplasia, carcinoma *in situ*, or invasive SCC
  - Erythroplakia—red "velvetlike" mucosal patches
    - Higher incidence of associated SCC compared to leukoplakia
  - Lichen planus
    - White, flat inflammatory papule involving oral mucosa.
    - 5% undergoes malignant transformation.
- SCC Histology
  - Well differentiated → increased amounts of keratin, better prognosis.
  - Nasopharyngeal carcinoma has a separate classification. Type III includes lymphoepithelioma, anaplastic, and clear cell variants.

- **Verrucous carcinoma** (Ackerman tumor)
  - Rare, less aggressive variant of SCC
  - Buccal/gingival mucosa
  - Treatment → surgery; evaluate final specimen for focal invasive SCC
- **Metastatic Disease**
  - **Regional spread** to cervical lymph nodes
    - Midline tumors can drain to bilateral nodal basins.
    - Poor prognostic factors → multiple lymph node involvement, extracapsular spread, perineural invasion, and matted nodes.
  - *Distant metastasis → most often to the lung

ANATOMY

- **Oral Cavity**
  - Extends from the skin-vermilion lip junction posteriorly to the junction of the hard and soft palate and circumvallate papillae.
  - The oral cavity subsites
    - Lips
    - Buccal mucosa
    - Upper and lower alveolar ridge
    - Retromolar trigone (RMT)
    - FOM
    - Hard palate
    - Anterior two-third of the tongue
- **The Pharynx** (nasopharynx, oropharynx, hypopharynx)
  - **Nasopharynx:** skull base superiorly to the soft/hard palate inferiorly; from the nasal choanae to posterior pharyngeal wall. Subsites include the following:
    - Fossa of Rosenmüller
    - Torus and orifice of the eustachian tube
    - Lateral and posterior walls
  - **Oropharynx**
    - Anterior border: circumvallate papillae
    - Lateral borders: tonsil, tonsillar fossa, and tonsillar pillars
    - Posterior border: posterior pharyngeal wall
    - Inferior border: floor of vallecula (space between base of tongue [BOT] and epiglottis)
    - Superior border: soft palate
    - Waldeyer ring, within oropharynx; lymphoid tissue of palatine and lingual tonsils
  - **Hypopharynx:** extends from floor of vallecula and aryepiglottic folds to inferior border of cricoid cartilage; contains three subsites:
    - Pyriform sinuses
    - Posterior pharyngeal wall
    - Postcricoid region/pharyngoesophageal junction (least common)
- **Larynx** (supraglottis, glottis, subglottis)
  - **Supraglottis** (30% of laryngeal SCC)
    - Separated from glottis by horizontal plane through ventricle (space between true and false vocal cords)
    - Includes epiglottis, aryepiglottic folds, arytenoids, false vocal cords, and ventricles
  - **Glottis** (50%-70% of laryngeal SCC)
    - From ventricle to 1 cm below the free edge of the true vocal cord
    - Includes true vocal cords and anterior and posterior commissure
  - **Subglottis:** glottis to inferior border of cricoid ring
- **Lymphatic Drainage Levels of the Neck**
  - **Level IA (submental triangle):** triangle created by anterior digastric muscle bellies and hyoid. Floor is the mylohyoid.
  - **Level IB (submandibular triangle):** triangle bound between the anterior and posterior digastric muscles and mandible.

- Level II (**upper jugular**): bound by skull base superiorly, mandible/hyoid medially, and laterally by lateral border of sternocleidomastoid muscle (SCM). IIA is anterior to CN XI, and IIB is posterior to CN XI.
- Level III (**midjugular**): from hyoid superiorly to inferior border of cricoid cartilage inferiorly. Carotid medially and lateral SCM laterally.
- Level IV (**lower jugular**): from inferior border of cricoid cartilage superiorly to the clavicle. Carotid medially and lateral SCM laterally.
- Level V (**posterior triangle**): between SCM and anterior border of trapezius muscle from skull base to below the cricoid (VA) and inferiorly to the clavicle (VB).
- Level VI (**upper mediastinum**): between hyoid superiorly and suprasternal notch inferiorly, and between the lateral borders of both common carotid arteries.

EVALUATION

- Comprehensive history and physical examination.
- **Duration of lesion or mass,** and rapidity of enlargement, should be determined.
- **Associated symptoms may include the following:**
  - Localized pain
  - Odynophagia (painful swallowing)
  - Otalgia (referred ear pain)
  - Hoarseness (indicating glottic involvement)
  - Dysphagia (difficulty swallowing)
  - Weight loss
  - Shortness of breath/stridor
  - Hemoptysis
- **Social History**
  - **Tobacco use** (type; number of years)
  - **Alcohol** (type; daily amount consumed)—patient may require prophylaxis with benzodiazepines to prevent delirium tremors if hospitalization planned
- **Past Medical History**
  - Past history of head and neck SCC
  - Previous exposure to radiation

PHYSICAL EXAMINATION

- **Tympanic Membranes:** middle ear effusion may indicate nasopharyngeal mass.
- **Oral Cavity**
  - State of dentition is important for radiation and reconstructive considerations. Teeth may need to be extracted if they have excessive caries prior to radiation therapy (post-XRT extraction can be inciting event in osteoradionecrosis).
  - Note size and location of suspicious lesions.
  - Comment on fixation of lesion to surrounding bone.
  - Describe extension of tumor by noting all structures involved.
  - Deviation of the tongue on protrusion indicates involvement of hypoglossal nerve (CN XII) ipsilateral to the deviation.
  - Trismus (inability to fully open the mouth) indicates possible involvement of pterygoid muscle, masseter muscle, and/or infratemporal fossa.
- **Oropharynx**
  - Note size and location of suspicious lesions.
  - Comment on fixation to surrounding bone.
  - Describe extension of tumor.
  - Palpate BOT and RMT because lesions can infiltrate and/or be difficult to visualize.
- **Larynx**
  - Perform indirect examination with mirror visualization.
  - Direct visualization with flexible laryngoscopy should be performed.
  - Assess airway, nasal portion of the soft palate, vocal cord mobility, pyriform sinuses, epiglottis, and vallecula.
  - Anticipate potential need for surgical airway prior to treatment.

- **Neck**
  - Careful palpation for cervical lymphadenopathy is performed.
    - Comment on node size, location, and fixation.
    - "Lymph nodes" >3 cm are likely matted nodes.
  - A neck mass can also represent direct tumor extension.
  - Fixation of the larynx (loss of laryngeal crepitus and ability to move the larynx side-to-side) is indicative of extralaryngeal tumor extension.
- **Imaging** (CT head/neck, PET scan)
- **FNA** → biopsy of neck mass to evaluate if it is a metastatic lymph node.
- **Direct laryngoscopy** → evaluation of tumor extension under general anesthesia with biopsies. Can do esophagoscopy/bronchoscopy at the same time to evaluate for second primary lesions.
- **HPV/p16 status** for oropharynx cancers. Positive HPV more favorable prognosis.
- **Nutrition:** if dysphagia/odynophagia will be problematic, consider feeding tube placement.
- **Dental examination:** Patients undergoing radiation will need poor dentition extracted prior to treatment to avoid infections and osteoradionecrosis.
- **Pulmonary function tests (PFTs)** if a patient is being considered for laryngeal conservation surgery (hemilaryngectomy, supracricoid, etc.).

TREATMENT

- **Oral Cavity and Pharynx (Excluding Nasopharynx)**
  - **Single modality treatment** (surgery or radiation therapy) for T1/T2 lesions
  - **Surgery for oral cavity tumors**
    - Better locoregional control and overall survival vs radiation
  - **Surgery vs radiation for oropharynx lesions**
    - Chemoradiation for HPV+ advanced oropharynx SCC with excellent survival rates.
    - Areas with high rate of occult nodal metastasis (eg, oropharynx) should include radiation to neck fields.
    - Disadvantages of XRT: the patient will miss 2 months of work, tumor recurrence may be difficult to detect in the setting of postradiation changes.
  - **Multimodality treatment for T3/T4 lesions**
    - Surgery with postoperative radiation +/− chemotherapy
    - Concurrent chemotherapy (usually cisplatin and 5-FU) and radiation with salvage surgery for any residual disease
- **Nasopharynx**
  - *Radiation to primary lesion and bilateral necks.
  - Concomitant chemotherapy decreases the development of distant metastasis and improves both disease-free and overall survival for advanced disease.
  - Salvage neck dissection for persistent nodal disease following chemoradiation.
- **Larynx**
  - **Glottic SCC *in situ***
    - Initial → vocal cord stripping and close follow-up.
    - Recurrence → repeat stripping, excision, radiation, or partial laryngectomy.
  - **Glottic T1/T2 SCC**
    - Primary radiation with 70 Gy preserves voice quality compared to surgery.
    - Surgery alone, overall cure rate of 80%-85%.
    - Neck metastases are rare (8%) due to limited lymphatics in glottic region.
  - **T3/T4 laryngeal tumors**
    - Partial vs total laryngectomy (depending on tumor location and pulmonary status) with postoperative radiation.
    - Concurrent chemotherapy (usually cisplatin and 5-FU) and radiation have equal survival rates vs primary surgery with postoperative radiation.

- Subglottic SCC
  - Nodal/cartilage involvement common because presentation is late.
  - Total laryngectomy with bilateral neck dissections and post-op radiation.
  - Stomal recurrence is common.
- Speech rehabilitation
  - **Esophageal speech:** air released from esophagus. "Burping" voice.
  - **Tracheoesophageal puncture** = a one-way valve is placed through posterior tracheal wall into the esophagus.
    - Pulmonary air is diverted through the valve to vibrate against esophageal-pharyngeal wall and produce speech.
    - Complications: leakage, granulation tissue, and *Candida* infections.
  - **Artificial larynx** (electrolarynx)

MANAGEMENT OF THE NECK

- **Selective Neck Dissection**
  - Preservation of one or more lymph node groups (eg, levels I-III, I-IV)
- **Modified Radical Neck Dissection**
  - Removes all ipsilateral cervical lymph node groups (levels I-V)
  - Preserves at least one of the following vital structures: the internal jugular vein (IJV), SCM, or spinal accessory nerve (CN XI)
- **Radical Neck Dissection**
  - Removal of all ipsilateral cervical lymph node groups (levels I-V)
  - Removal of all three: IJV, SCM, and CN XI
- **Extended Neck Dissection:** involves additional lymph node groups beyond levels I-V or other nonlymphatic structures such as the hypoglossal nerve

COMPLICATIONS

- **Surgical**
  - Infection, potential for carotid artery exposure and carotid blowout
  - Nerve paresis/paralysis (especially marginal mandibular branch of CN VII and spinal accessory nerve)
  - Pharyngocutaneous fistula
  - Chronic aspiration
  - Trismus (limited mouth opening) and scarring
- **Radiation**
  - Xerostomia (dry mouth secondary to salivary gland dysfunction).
  - Mucositis: patient may require feeding tube.
  - Laryngeal and esophageal scarring/stenosis.
  - Osteoradionecrosis: treatment requires débridement, local wound care; ± antibiotics; may eventually require free tissue transfer.
  - Dental caries.
  - Chronic aspiration.

FOLLOW-UP

- **Routine appointments** imperative because HNSCCA has a high rate of locoregional recurrence and of second primary tumor development
  - First 1-2 years: every 2 months
  - Third year: every 3-4 months
  - Fourth and fifth year: every 6 months
  - Yearly thereafter
- **Yearly Chest X-ray** (CT chest for smokers who smoked within the last 15 years) to evaluate pulmonary metastasis
- **Radiated Patients:**
  - **Yearly TSH** because of risk for hypothyroidism
  - **Carotid ultrasound** to evaluate for stenosis

PEARLS

1. 80% of neck masses in adults are neoplastic, 80% of these are malignant. 80% of neck masses in children are inflammatory or benign.
2. Most common salivary neoplasm = pleomorphic adenoma (benign). Most common salivary malignancy in children and adults = mucoepidermoid.
3. Midline neck mass = teratoma, dermoid, thyroglossal duct cyst, thyroid cancer. Lateral neck mass = branchial cleft anomaly, infectious/metastatic lymph nodes.
4. Postoperative complications of salivary tumor excision = sialocele, facial nerve damage, Frey syndrome (gustatory sweating).
5. Generally, treatment of early SCC = surgery +/− radiation. Treatment of advanced SCC = chemoradiation +/− salvage surgery for residual disease.

QUESTIONS YOU WILL BE ASKED

1. What is the course of frontal branch of facial nerve?
   A line from the lobule to 1.5 cm above the lateral eyebrow. Crosses the zygoma 1.5 cm anterior to the tragus, within the temporoparietal fascia (superficial temporal fascia).
2. What is the relation of marginal mandibular nerve to facial vessels?
   The marginal mandibular nerve crosses superficial to the facial vein and artery.
3. Name five ways to find the main trunk of the facial nerve.
   a. The tympanomastoid suture 6-8 mm lateral to the stylomastoid foramen.
   b. 10 mm inferior and 10 mm deep to the tragal pointer.
   c. Identify distal branches and follow proximally.
   d. At the level of the digastric muscle (in the superficial to deep dimension).
   e. Drill out the mastoid to identify the descending (intratemporal) segment.
4. What are branches of the external carotid artery?
   Superior thyroid, ascending pharyngeal, lingual, occipital, facial, posterior auricular, maxillary, and superficial temporal.
5. What is the relationship of CN XI to sternocleidomastoid?
   The accessory nerve travels ~1 cm superior to Erb point.
6. What is the difference between a modified and radical neck dissection?
   Radical neck dissection sacrifices CN XI, IJV, and SCM. A modified radical neck dissection spares one or more of these three structures.

Recommended Readings
1. Haugen BR, Alexander EK, Bible KC, et al. 2015 American Thyroid Association Management Guidelines for Adult Patients with Thyroid Nodules and Differentiated Thyroid Cancer: The American Thyroid Association Guidelines Task Force on Thyroid Nodules and Differentiated Thyroid Cancer. *Thyroid*. 2016;26(1):1-133.
2. Jackson DL. Evaluation and management of pediatric neck masses: an otolaryngology perspective. *Physician Assist Clin*. 2018;3(2):245-269. doi:10.1016/j.cpha.2017.12.003
3. Marur S, Forastiere AA. Head and neck squamous cell carcinoma: update on epidemiology, diagnosis, and treatment. *Mayo Clin Proc*. 2016;91(3):386-396. doi:10.1016/j.mayocp.2015.12.017

28 Principles of Head and Neck Reconstruction

Rebecca W. Gao

GENERAL PRINCIPLES

- Patients are often debilitated and long-term survival may be poor.
- Many cancer patients must also undergo postoperative radiation or chemotherapy. Therefore, the goal is rapid reconstruction with optimization of function and low morbidity, accomplished as a one-stage procedure whenever possible.
- Specific principles guide head and neck reconstructive planning.
  - Attempt to restore symmetry.
  - Maintain structural integrity of the nose and ears, for both aesthetic and functional reasons (eg, support for glasses, nasal airflow).
  - Maintain competence of the oral and ocular openings, with particular attention paid to the risk of late scar contractures.
  - Replace entire anatomic subunits when possible for the best aesthetic outcome.
  - Maintain or restore independent speech, breathing, and swallowing functions.

RECONSTRUCTION BY ANATOMIC REGION

THE MIDFACE

- Goals
  - Restore the contour and projection.
  - Recreation of the maxilla and the occlusive surfaces.
  - Separation of the oral and nasal cavities.
  - Provide support for the eye or a prosthetic replacement.
  - Maintain flow through the lacrimal system.
- Prosthetics: used extensively in the midface, either alone or in combination with tissue transfers. Maxillectomy defects that do not involve the buttresses or the orbits can be managed effectively with a palatal obturator.
- Regional Flaps: the deltopectoral flap, the temporalis muscle flap, and the forehead flap can be used to address medium-sized defects.
- Nonvascularized Bone Grafts: used to fill bony gaps. The graft must be covered with adequate well-vascularized tissue and be rigidly fixed in position for success.
- Free Tissue Transfer
  - Radial forearm osteocutaneous flap: a vascularized piece of radius up to 10 cm in length can be harvested with the flap.
  - Scapular osteocutaneous flaps, with or without a skin paddle, may include a portion of the latissimus muscle. They are based either on the descending or on the transverse branches of the circumflex scapular artery and the angular branch thereof.
  - Fibula, rectus abdominis muscle, or omental flaps less commonly used in the midface.

---

*Denotes common in-service examination topics.

THE MANDIBLE

- Goals
  - ○ Restore facial contour.
  - ○ Maintain tongue mobility.
  - ○ Restore mastication and speech.
- **Reconstruction of large defects** should be immediate unless there is question as to surgical margin or if the patient's health demands it.
- **Choice of reconstructive technique** depends on the defect size and location.
  - ○ Small bony defects, especially lateral ones, may be addressed with either no repair or with autologous bone graft. Nonvascularized bone grafts tolerate radiation poorly.
  - ○ Metallic implants (such as mandibular reconstruction bars) can serve as spacers to maintain position, but they often fail or lead to exposure and infection.
- **Vascularized bone flap** is the method of choice for most bony defect reconstruction, particularly anterior ones. Such flaps promote healing, resist resorption, and permit dental restoration with osseointegrated implants.
  - ○ **Free fibula flap (Fig. 28-1)**
    - Segment of bone up to 40 cm long available, along with the overlying skin.
    - Based on perforators from the peroneal artery (2 mm diameter, 6-10 mm length).
    - Minimal functional debility (eg, foot drop).
    - Leave at least 6-10 cm of distal fibula to avoid destabilization of ankle.
    - Leave cuff of soleus and flexor hallucis longus to avoid disruption of periosteum.
    - Important to identify and preserve common peroneal nerve at head of fibula and superficial peroneal between fibula and extensor digitorum longus.
    - Often secured in place with large mandibular plate and screws. These can be prefabricated preoperatively based on CT imaging. Screws should be unicortical and on opposite side of pedicle to avoid injury.
    - CT angiography or magnetic resonance angiogram (MRA) is used preoperatively to assess the arterial anatomy. The leg opposite the defect is usually chosen to allow for optimal skin paddle and pedicle placement in the recipient neck.
    - Allows for osseointegrated implants in the future.
  - ○ **Iliac crest bone flaps**
    - Based on the deep circumflex iliac artery (1-3 mm diameter, 5-7 cm length).
    - Both iliac crests can be used to perform a total mandibular reconstruction.
    - Can provide 16 cm length, and for mandible should use 2 cm height.
    - Inner cortex usually sufficient and allows for decreased donor site morbidity.
    - Skin paddle marked over anterior iliac crease from ASIS to posterior axillary line.
  - ○ **Scapula**
    - Pedicle: subscapular artery (3-4 mm diameter, 4-6 cm length)
    - Bone size up to 15 cm
    - Very large skin paddle and quality bone
    - Requires intraoperative repositioning to harvest
  - ○ **Radius, rib, and metatarsal** are other vascularized bone options for the mandible.

THE NECK

- Goals
  - ○ Protect vital neck structures (eg, carotid, internal jugular, trachea).
  - ○ Prevent regional complications (eg, chylous fistula, oropharyngocutaneous fistula, carotid artery blowout, and wound infection due to intraoral contamination).

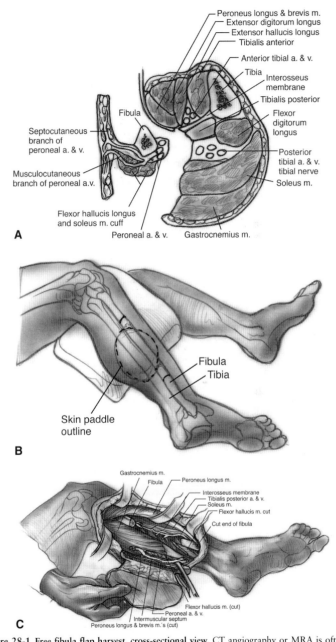

Figure 28-1 Free fibula flap harvest, cross-sectional view. CT angiography or MRA is often used preoperatively to assess the arterial anatomy. The leg opposite the defect is usually chosen to allow for optimal skin paddle and pedicle placement in the recipient neck.

- **Pedicled Pectoralis Major Flap:** useful for neck coverage
  - Origin: medial clavicle, sternum, anterior ribs (2-6), external oblique, and rectus abdominis.
  - Insertion: upper humerus, 10 cm from humeral head on lateral side of intertubercular sulcus.
  - Function: adduction and medial rotation of arm.
  - Dominant pedicle: thoracoacromial artery off axillary artery.
  - Secondary: internal mammary perforators, intercostal perforators, and lateral thoracic artery.
  - Overlying skin may be transferred with the flap.
  - Flap is dependable, but bulky.
  - **Innervation: medial and lateral pectoral nerves (named for origin in brachial plexus rather than region of pectoralis muscle innervated).**
- **Pedicled Latissimus Dorsi Flap**
  - Thinner flap than the pectoralis, and the skin paddle is more likely hairless.
  - Paddle up to 10 cm wide can be harvested with primary closure of the skin.
  - Disadvantage: must reposition patient intraoperatively.
  - Origin: broad aponeurosis from thoracolumbar fascia and spine of lower sixth thoracic vertebrae, sacral vertebrae, supraspinal ligament, and posterior iliac crest.
  - Insertion: intertubercular groove of humerus.
  - Dominant pedicle: thoracodorsal branch of the subscapular artery, the flap may be tunneled either below pectoralis major or subcutaneously along the anterior chest.
  - Secondary pedicles: posterior intercostal perforators, lumbar artery perforators.
  - Innervation: thoracodorsal nerve (C6-C8).
  - Complication: seroma formation at the donor site; drains are mandatory.
- **Trapezius Flap:** three different flaps can be raised:
  - Superior trapezius flap: based on the occipital artery and paravertebral perforators. The most reliable. Its skin paddle extends laterally across the top of the scapula.
  - Inferior trapezius flap: descending branch of the transverse cervical artery (also called dorsal scapular). Either as a muscle or as a myocutaneous flap. Its point of rotation is posterior, at the base of the neck.
  - Lateral trapezius flap: based on the superficial transverse cervical artery over the acromion. Useful for small lateral defects.
- **The Deltopectoral Flap**
  - Supplied by first four perforators from the internal mammary artery.
  - A delay procedure will permit more lateral skin to be used safely.
  - Flap is thin and can reach the oral cavity.
  - Can raise up to a 10- × 20-cm fasciocutaneous flap.
  - Donor site often requires skin graft and less aesthetic closure.

THE ORAL CAVITY

- **Goals**
  - Maintenance of oral competence
  - Provision of support for the floor of the mouth
  - Prevention of aspiration by maintaining or restoring sensation and mobility
- **Tongue Flaps:** can be used for small intraoral defects; care is taken not to tether the tongue.
- **Palatal or Palatopharyngeal Flaps:** can be used to fix small defects in the palate.
- **The Free Radial Forearm Flap**
  - First choice for larger intraoral defects.
  - Based on the radial artery and venae comitantes and/or cephalic/basilic veins.
  - Ideal for intraoral lining due to flap thinness. It can be made sensate by attaching the lingual nerve to the lateral antebrachial cutaneous nerve.

- **The Pedicled Latissimus Dorsi Flap:** can be used for extensive oral cavity defects
  - Advantage of large size, but the arc of rotation can limit its use in the oral cavity.
  - Alternatively, it can be used as a free flap.
  - Based on thoracodorsal artery.
- **The Gastro-Omental Free Flap:** provides a secreting mucosal surface useful in preventing postradiation xerostomia.

THE TONGUE

- **Goals:** maintenance/restoration of mobility, preserve speech, and swallowing function
- **Partial Glossectomy**
  - Reconstruction may not be necessary if the defect volume is low. The tongue heals exceptionally well; infection, scarring, and tissue loss are rare.
  - Can heal by secondary intention or full-thickness skin grafting to limit tongue tethering.
- **Hemiglossectomy or Anterior 2/3 Glossectomy**
  - Radial forearm free flap: pliable tissue can be designed in a "rectangle tongue template" to achieve oral cavity obliteration and premaxillary contact for oral intake.
- **Total glossectomy reconstruction requires larger volume.** Primary goal to restore speech and swallowing function. Adequate bulk in the oral cavity will help food propulsion and can seal against the palate. Choices for reconstruction are as follows:
  - **Rectus Abdominis Free Flap:** the large volume flap permits creation of two or three separate cutaneous islands for complex reconstructions. A perforator-based rectus can help tailor the volume of free tissue transferred.
  - **Latissimus Dorsi:** either a free or a pedicled flap.

THE HYPOPHARYNX

- Hypopharyngeal and esophagopharyngeal defects are either partial or circumferential (total).
- **For partial defects, options are as follows**
  - **Primary closure**
    - Do not narrow the lumen excessively.
    - Width of mucosa must be at least 3 cm for primary closure (pharynx must permit passage of at least a 34 French catheter for swallowing).
  - **Skin or dermal grafts:** may be used for partial defects of the lining of esophagus or pharynx. They are initially secured with a stent to allow adherence and prevent strictures.
  - **Pectoralis, latissimus, or trapezius muscles** can be used to fill larger defects.
- **Circumferential Reconstruction**
  - **Free jejunum:** the historical flap of choice. A proximal segment is isolated on its mesentery and transferred to the neck, where it is placed in an isoperistaltic orientation. Complications include a "wet" voice, halitosis, and dysphagia.
  - **Tubed radial forearm flap:** particularly useful when jejunal harvest is not advisable. High incidence of stricture formation if adequate dimensions are not harvested.
  - **Gastric transposition or gastro-omental flaps:** for patients with tumors with significant inferior extension. Outside the scope of plastic surgery; typically performed by thoracic surgeons.

COMPLICATIONS

CHYLE LEAK

- Dissection low in level IV places thoracic duct at risk
- Presents with milky JP drain output within 24-48 hours of when PO intake starts

- *Low output → treat with no fat diet or medium chain fatty acids, pressure dressing
- **High output (>200 mL/8 hours)**
  - ○ Replace fluid loss and frequently check electrolytes.
  - ○ Neck exploration vs intrathoracic ligation.
  - ○ Octreotide.

PHARYNGOCUTANEOUS FISTULA

- Much higher incidence if previously radiated field.
- Usually presents with doughy erythematous skin around POD 4,7 before frank salivary communication to skin.
- Can be managed conservatively with NPO, irrigations/local wound care, and antibiotics.
- If carotid/jugular at risk, salivary diversion (bypass tube) and/or tissue coverage required.
- Assess thyroid and nutritional status to optimize healing.
- Delayed fistula (months/years postoperatively) must raise suspicion for recurrence.
- Carotid blowout must be in the differential of bleeding in any head and neck patient, especially with a history of radiation.

CAROTID BLOWOUT

- Sentinel bleed—smaller volumes may herald a large volume bleed.
- Acute rupture—high morbidity and up to 50% mortality.
- Acute management: large bore IV, secure airway, neck pressure.
- Interventional radiology for carotid embolization.
- In exposed carotid or sentinel bleed, can assess stroke risk with balloon occlusion for possible elective embolization or ligation.
- Surgical ligation for life-threatening rupture (but high risk of stroke).

PEARLS

1. Head and neck cancer patients will often require postoperative radiation. Reconstruction should take this into account, favoring one-step reconstructions, feeding tube placement at time of reconstruction, vascularized free flaps, and neck tissue coverage to protect the carotid/jugular vessels.
2. Scapula, iliac crest, radial forearm, and fibula free flaps are common options for maxillary and mandibular reconstructions.
3. Radial forearm free flaps can be used for smaller mandibular reconstructions, oral cavity, hemiglossectomies, and hypopharynx (tubed).
4. Trapezius flaps can be raised superiorly (based on occipital and paravertebral), inferiorly (based on descending branch of transverse cervical), or laterally (based on superficial transverse cervical artery over the acromion).
5. Acute management of carotid blowouts include large bore IVs, neck pressure, and securing the airway with carotid embolization vs ligation.

QUESTIONS YOU WILL BE ASKED

1. How do you diagnose and treat a chyle leak?
   Send drain fluid for triglycerides. Nonfat or medium-chain triglyceride diet. Apply pressure dressing to supraclavicular fossa. Octreotide. If high output, consider fluid replacement of losses. If >200 mL/shift, then consider returning to OR to identify/ ligate the leak.
2. How do you treat a fistula after a jejunal free flap?
   NPO and tube feeds. Irrigate and pack the wound. Optimize thyroid and nutrition. Divert saliva to protect the great vessels (a salivary bypass tube is sometimes used).

Recommended Readings
1. Cordeiro PG, Santamaria EA. Classification system and algorithm for reconstruction of maxillectomy and midfacial defects. *Plast Reconstr Surg.* 2000;105:2331-2346.
2. Disa JJ, Pusic AL, Hidalgo DA, et al. Microvascular reconstruction of the hypopharynx: defect classification, treatment algorithm, and functional outcome based on 165 consecutive cases. *Plast Reconstr Surg.* 2003;111:652-663.
3. Haughey BH. Tongue reconstruction: concepts and practice. *Laryngoscope.* 1993;103:1132-1141.
4. Hidalgo DA, Pusic AL. Free flap mandibular reconstruction: a 10-year follow up study. *Plast Reconstr Surg.* 2002;110:438-449.
5. Makitie AA, Beasley NJ, Neligan PC, et al. Head and neck reconstruction with anterolateral thigh flap. *Otolaryngol Head Neck Surg.* 2003;129:547-555.

Section II: Craniofacial

29 Hand and Wrist Anatomy and Examination

Jennifer C. Lee and Widya Adidharma

EVALUATION OF THE PATIENT

HISTORY

- **General History:** ABCs (airway, breathing, circulation), AMPLE (allergies, medications, past medical history, last meal, and events leading to injury), time, and mechanism of injury
- **Focused History:** handedness, prior hand injuries/surgeries, vocation/avocations, smoking history, diabetes, or vascular diseases
- Tetanus and rabies prophylaxis and antibiotics if needed

THE QUICK HAND EXAM

- The hand is composed of vessels, nerves, bones/joints, muscle/tendon, and overlying soft tissue. Test for the integrity of each of these components.
- **Skin/Overlying Soft Tissue:** inspect and palpate for wounds, deformities, signs of infection (erythema, induration, fluid collections), and discoloration.
- **Vascular Exam**
    - Assess color, temp, capillary refill, pulse/Doppler.
    - Capillary refill should be 2 to 3 seconds; check nail bed or eponychial fold.
    - **Allen test:** compress radial and ulnar arteries at the wrist, have the patient make a tight fist (to exsanguinate hand), and then relax; release one vessel to check patency of the palmar arch and blood supply to the hand via that artery.
    - A digital Allen test can be done to isolate the radial or ulnar vessel of a finger.
- **Neurology Exam**
    - Median nerve: sensation at the volar tip of IF (light touch and two-point discrimination); ability to make "OK" sign: demonstrates FPL, FDP, and OP
    - Ulnar nerve: sensation at the volar tip of SF; ability to abduct/adduct/cross fingers. Test AdP
    - Radial nerve: sensation at the dorsal first web space; give "thumbs up" (EPL)
- **Muscle/Tendon:** assess muscle tone/bulk, wrist tenodesis effect, ability to close hand into a fist and open (quickly assesses overall range of motion)—fingers not ranging like the others can be a sign of tendon injury. For specific tendon exam, see **Tendons and Muscles Section.**
- **Bone/Joint:** assess for deformities, asymmetry, angulation, rotation. Examine the joint(s) proximal and distal to any injury.
    - **Finger cascade:** fingers should converge toward the scaphoid tubercle when flexed at PIPJ and MCPJ. Fingers that do not converge likely have abnormal alignment.
    - **Imaging:** treat X-rays like a portion of the physical exam. Three-view X-rays can evaluate for bony fractures, dislocations, and other abnormalities.
- Special Tests (**Fig. 29-1; Table 29-1**)

---

*Denotes common in-service examination topics.

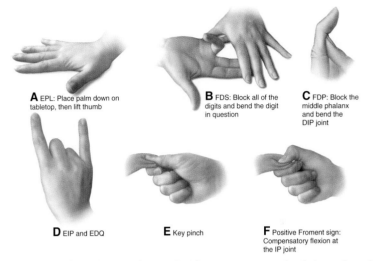

A EPL: Place palm down on tabletop, then lift thumb

B FDS: Block all of the digits and bend the digit in question

C FDP: Block the middle phalanx and bend the DIP joint

D EIP and EDQ

E Key pinch

F Positive Froment sign: Compensatory flexion at the IP joint

Figure 29-1 Specific hand exam techniques. Specific movements are used to isolate and test the functions of the hand.

TABLE 29-1 Special Hand Tests

Flexor tests	
FDS	Lay the hand flat on table and palm up. Hold other fingers in extension (blocks FDP), test active flexion at each proximal interphalangeal joint (PIPJ). Also test against resistance
FDP	PIPJ held in extension (pressure on middle phalanx), test active dorsal interphalangeal joint (DIPJ) flexion
FPL	Check active flexion of interphalangeal joint (IPJ) with metacarpophalangeal blocked (pressure on proximal phalanx). Also check against resistance
Extensor tests	
EIP, EDM	Independent extension of the IF or SF with other fingers flexed
EPL	Check the ability to raise the thumb up with the hand prone and flat on table
Intrinsic tests	
AdP	Key pinch (thumb to side of IF) by having the patient hold a piece of paper deep in the web space and resist the paper from being pulled away. If FPL takes over (DIPJ flexes), this is a positive "Froment sign" and implies AdP function is absent or diminished (compare to the opposite side)
Interosseous	Abduction/adduction of fingers with and without resistance
Intrinsic Tightness	With the wrist neutral, hyperextend the MPJ to relax the extrinsics. Measure passive flexion of PIPJ ("intrinsic tightness"). Classify as mild (60°-80°), moderate (20°-59°), or severe (<20°)
Extrinsic tightness	With wrist neutral, flex the MPJ to relax the intrinsics. Check passive PIP motion, which will indicate "extrinsic tightness"

VASCULATURE

ARTERIAL SUPPLY (FIG. 29-2)

- Radial artery supplies the deep palmar arch, which gives off princeps pollicis. This branches to proper digital artery to the thumb and radialis indices to index finger.
- Ulnar artery supplies the superficial palmar arch, which provides the common digital arteries and individual branch to ulnar side of small finger.
- **The radial artery is usually dominant,** but ulnar dominance and codominance are common (and some studies indicate ulnar dominance is more common).
- *"Kaplan cardinal line" is a line drawn across the palm from the first web space to the hook of the hamate, indicating approximate location of the superficial palmar arch. Deep arch is 1 cm proximal.
- Dorsal carpal arch is fed from radial, ulnar, and interosseous arteries and gives rise to dorsal metacarpal arteries.
- Relationship between paired arteries and nerves
  - In the palm: arteries are volar to nerves
  - In the digits: arteries are dorsal to nerves (**Fig. 29-3**)

VENOUS DRAINAGE

- Dorsal (subcutaneous) venous network and palmar venous arch
- Drains to cephalic vein (originates radially) and basilic vein (originates on the dorsoulnar aspect of the hand)

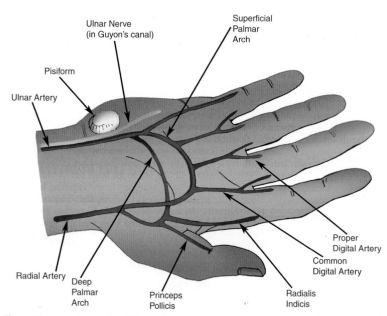

Figure 29-2 Arterial supply of the hand. The ulnar artery becomes the superficial palmar arch, while the radial artery becomes the deep palmar arch. (From Dalman R. *Operative Techniques in Vascular Surgery.* Wolters Kluwer; 2016. Figure 11.1.)

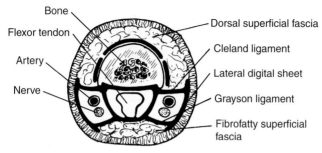

Figure 29-3 Cross section of the digit.

NERVE

- Radial, median, and ulnar nerve anatomy (**Table 29-2**)
- Cutaneous sensory innervation distribution (**Fig. 29-4**)
- Median nerve cross-innervation can mask an ulnar nerve injury
  - **Martin-Gruber anastomosis:** an anatomic variant in which the median nerve crosses over to contribute to the ulnar nerve. The two most common variations are as follows:
    - Median nerve in the proximal forearm contributes to the ulnar nerve in the distal forearm.
    - AIN contributes to the ulnar nerve.
  - **Riche-Cannieu anastomosis:** more distal, ulnar fibers contribute to median nerve branches in the palm
- **Nerve blocks** (**Table 29-3**)

TABLE 29-2 Hand Nerve Anatomy Table

| | Path in the forearm | Branches | | |
		Nerve	Forearm innervation	Distal innervation
Radial	Enters between the BR and the ECRL/ECRB (innervates these three muscles)	Divides 1-3 cm distal to the lateral epicondyle, deep to BR		
		Posterior interosseous	Passes between the heads of the supinator; innervates supinator, EDC, ECU, EDM, APL, EPB, EPL, and EIP (in order)	Sensory branch to the wrist capsule (deep within the fourth dorsal compartment of the wrist)
		Superficial radial	Exits between BR and ECRL tendons approximately two-third down the forearm	Sensory to dorsum of the thumb, first web space, dorsal IF, MF, and radial RF up to the PIPJs (Fig. 29-1)

(continued)

TABLE 29-2 **Hand Nerve Anatomy Table** *(Continued)*

	Path in the forearm	Nerve	Forearm innervation	Distal innervation
Median	Enters lateral to the brachial artery, emerging between the heads of the PT; innervates the PT, FCR, FDS, and PL	Divides at junction of the two heads of PT, ~6 cm distal to elbow		
		Anterior interosseous (AIN)	Runs with anterior interosseous artery on interosseous membrane; innervates FPL, PQ, radial two FDPs (IF and MF)	Sensory to wrist capsule
		Rest of median nerve runs between FDS and FDP		
		Palmar cutaneous	Branches ~5 cm proximal to wrist	Sensory to palm
		Enters carpal tunnel and branches		
		Recurrent motor		Abductor pollicis brevis, flexor pollicis brevis, opponens pollicis, and 2 lumbricals (in order)
		Digital nerves		Sensory to thumb, IF, MF, and radial RF
Ulnar	Enters behind the medial epicondyle through the cubital tunnel under Osborne band/ ligament; innervates FCU and ulnar two FDPs (RF and SF)	Travels under FCU to wrist		
		Dorsal sensory	Branches ~6-8 cm proximal to ulnar head	Sensory to dorsum of SF and ulnar RF
		Enter Guyon canal and branches		
		Deep branch		ADM, FDM, ODM, deep head of FPB, all interosseous muscles, ulnar lumbricals (2), and AdP (terminal branch)
		Superficial branch		PB, sensory palmar digital nerves to SF and ulnar RF

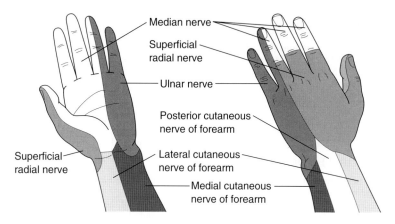

Figure 29-4 Cutaneous sensory innervation of the hand, volar, and dorsal surfaces.

TABLE 29-3 Nerve Blocks

	Needle placement	Technique
Median	Distal wrist crease between PL and FCR	Enter at 45° angle to the forearm. Often a "pop" is felt when deep fascia is penetrated. If unsure of depth, insert until paresthesias occur or bone is encountered, then withdraw slightly and inject 3-5 mL local anesthetic
Ulnar	Just proximal to the ulnar styloid	Enter behind the FCU tendon with the needle directed from ulnar to radial in the coronal plane. Once needle is just beyond FCU, inject anesthetic (3-5 mL). Must inject dorsally on the wrist to get dorsal sensory branch
Radian	Proximal to the radial styloid	Enter and inject the subcutaneous tissue. Extend the field block volar and dorsal around the distal forearm. Must block a wide area
Digital (dorsal)	Just proximal to each webspace	Subcutaneous wheal over extensor tendon to block dorsal nerve. Advance needle until the tip approaches the palmar skin. Inject slowly while withdrawing
Digital (volar)	Midpoint of the base of the finger where it joins the palm	Subcutaneous wheal directly over the flexor tendon. Slightly deeper on each side, near the digital neurovascular bundles
Digital (sheath)	Just distal to distal palmer crease, volar down into the flexor tendons	With slight pressure on the plunger, withdraw needle slowly until there is a loss of resistance = injection into potential space of flexor sheath. Sometimes, fluid wave can be felt distally in the finger over the sheath. Reliably results in digital anesthesia but is not as effective in cases of sheath violation (eg, distal amputation)

TENDONS AND MUSCLES

- **Common abbreviations (Fig. 29-5)**
- **Active and Passive ROM**—approximate normal ranges below
  - Finger MPJ: 0°-45° hyperextension, 90° flexion
  - Finger PIPJ: 0° extension, 100° flexion
  - Finger DIPJ: 0° extension, 70°-80° flexion
  - Thumb MPJ: 10° hyperextension, 55° flexion, 90° in full range of radial adduction/abduction
  - Thumb IPJ: 15° hyperextension, 80° flexion
  - Wrist: 70° extension, 75° flexion, 20° radial deviation and 35° ulnar deviation

FLEXOR TENDONS

- **Five flexor tendon zones (Fig. 29-6; also see Chapter 38: Tendon Injury and Tendonitis).**
- Flexor muscles originate largely at the medial epicondyle of the humerus, with some deeper compartment muscles originating on radius and ulna.
- **Superficial:** PT, FCR, FCU, PL; **intermediate:** FDS; **deep:** FDP, FPL
- Carpal tunnel contains median nerve and nine tendons: FDP(4), FDS(4), and FPL **(Fig. 29-5)**
  - FDS is superficial to the FDP in carpal tunnel.
  - FDS MF and RF are volar to FDS IF and SF.
- **FDS**
  - Innervated by median nerve
  - Muscle bellies divide in forearm, which leads to less power, but better independent function than FDP (note: 15% of people do not have independent FDS to SF because FDS to RF and SF may be joined).
  - Tendon splits into radial and ulnar slips prior to inserting into the volar base of the middle phalanx.
- **FDP**
  - Dually innervated (IF/MF median n., RF/SF ulnar n.).
  - Common muscle belly affords more power but less independent function—IF branches off first but can only get ~30° of IF flexion before other digit FDPs begin to engage.

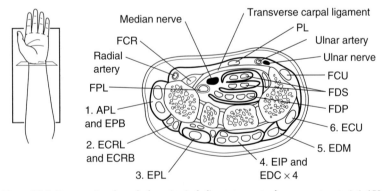

Figure 29-5 Cross section through the wrist, including extensor tendon compartments 1-6. APL, abductor pollicis longus; ECRB, extensor carpi radialis brevis; ECRL, extensor carpi radialis longus; ECU, extensor carpi ulnaris; EDC, extensor digitorum communis; EDM, extensor digiti minimi; EIP, extensor indicis proprius; EPB, extensor pollicis brevis; EPL, extensor pollicis longus; FCR, flexor carpi radialis; FCU, flexor carpi ulnaris; FDP, flexor digitorum profundus; FDS, flexor digitorum superficialis; FPL, flexor pollicis longus; PL, palmaris longus.

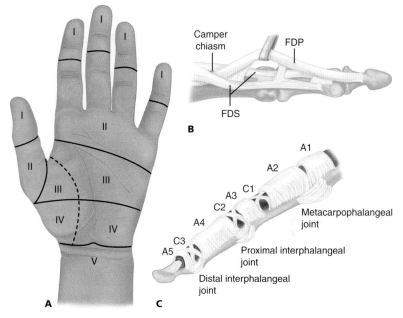

Figure 29-6 A. Flexor tendon zones I-V. **B.** Flexor tendon anatomy in zone II. **C.** Flexor sheath pulley anatomy and distribution in zones I and II. (From Wiesel SW, Albert T. *Operative Techniques in Orthopaedic Surgery.* 3rd ed. Wolters Kluwer; 2022. Figure 6.48.1.)

- o FDP passes between the two FDS slips, also known as "Camper chiasm," and inserts into proximal volar aspect of the distal phalanx.
- **FPL** inserts into distal phalanx of the thumb
- **Pulleys:** prevent tendon bowstringing, increase mechanical effectiveness of pull across joints (**Fig. 29-6**)
  - o Fingers have five annular pulleys (A1-A5), three cruciate pulleys (C1-C3). A2 and A4 are usually considered most critical to finger function.
  - o Thumb has three pulleys: A1 (MPJ), A2 (IPJ), and oblique (over proximal phalanx). Oblique pulley is most mechanically important.

EXTENSOR TENDONS

- **Nine Extensor Tendon Zones.** The odd-numbered zones (1-7) lie over joints, with the even-numbered zones in between.
- Extensor muscle mass (aka "mobile wad") originates largely at the lateral epicondyle.
- **Superficial:** EDC, EDM, ECU; **deep:** APL, EPB, EPL, EIP; **lateral/radial:** ECRL, ECRB, BR.
- **Juncturae Tendinae:** interconnect tendons on back of the hand. May mask an extensor tendon rupture, as pull from another finger can be transmitted via juncturae to the distal extensor tendon of the injured finger.
- **Dorsal (or extensor) Wrist Compartments 1-6** (see **Fig. 29-6**).
- **EIP and EDM** are ulnar to their accompanying EDC tendons.
- **Extensor Mechanism** (**Fig. 29-7**)

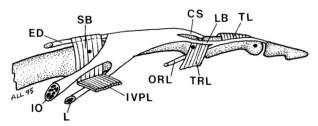

Figure 29-7 **Extensor tendon anatomy in the digit.** CS, central slip; ED, extensor digitorum; IO, interosseous; L, lumbrical; LB, lateral band; ORL, oblique retinacular ligament; SB, sagittal band; TL, triangular ligament; TRL, transverse retinacular ligament; VPL, volar plate ligament.

- EDC (plus EIP and EDM) expands over MPJ to form extensor hood for each digit. Most extrinsic tendon function translated to the MPJ.
- Sagittal bands help stabilize the extensor tendon across the MPJ and form a "bucket handle" with insertions on volar plate.
- Lumbrical and interosseous tendons join the hood laterally to add MPJ flexion and provide IPJ extension.
- Extensor hood divides into three components over the proximal phalanx
  - Central slip inserts on the base of the middle phalanx for PIPJ extension
  - Two lateral bands continue distally and fuse, inserting on the base of the distal phalanx (terminal tendon) for DIPJ extension
- Oblique and transverse retinacular ligament (**Table 29-4**).

INTRINSIC MUSCLES

- **Thenar:** opponens pollicis (OP), APB, flexor pollicis brevis (FPB) (dual innervation)
- **Hypothenar:** ODM, FDM, ADM, PB
- **Interosseous Muscles**
  - Three palmar and four dorsal
  - Palmar interossei adduct IF/RF/SF and dorsal interossei abduct IF/MF/RF/SF. [Think PAd and DAb.]
  - Innervated by the ulnar nerve

TABLE 29-4 Ligaments of the Extensor Mechanism

	Description	Movement	Pathology
Oblique retinacular ligament (of Landsmeer)	Cord that runs from flexor tendon sheath at the proximal phalanx to the terminal extensor tendon	When PIP joint is flexed, ligament relaxes allowing DIP flexion whereas extension tightens ligament facilitating DIP extension, thus linking motion of PIP and DIP joints	Contractures cause Boutonnière deformity
Transverse retinacular ligament	Cord that runs from flexor tendon sheath at the proximal phalanx to the fused lateral bands	With PIP flexion, pull lateral bands volarly over PIP. With PIP extension, prevents excessive dorsal translation of lateral bands	Attenuation leads to dorsal translation of lateral bands and a resulting swan neck deformity

- **Lumbricals**
  - Origin of each lumbrical is on the radial side of FDP tendon in the palm.
  - In the palm, the radial digital nerve runs on volar aspect of the lumbrical muscle belly to that digit.
  - Lumbricals are innervated by the same nerve as the FDP they originate from—IF/MF by median and RF/SF ulnar.

BONE AND JOINTS ANATOMY

WRIST

- Radius and ulna articulate with each other and with the carpus.
- Conceptually, the radius rotates around the fixed ulna at the wrist, sliding distally with pronation.

CARPUS

- **Eight Bones:** radial to ulnar—proximal row: scaphoid, lunate, triquetrum, pisiform; distal row: trapezium, trapezoid, capitate, hamate. Mnemonic: "So Long To Pinky Here Comes The Thumb."
- **Pisiform** is a sesamoid bone imbedded in the FCU tendon.
- **Radiocarpal and midcarpal joints stabilized by ligaments**
  - All ligaments are intracapsular.
  - The interosseous ligaments are intra-articular as well.
  - Ligament integrity is critical for the normal wrist motion and stability, as no tendons insert directly on the carpal bones but rather attach through these ligaments and joint capsules.
- **Normal Alignment:** the capitate is collinear with the lunate and the third metacarpal.
- **Gilula Lines**
  - Arcs formed by the outlines of the carpal bones, seen on AP radiographs of the wrist
  - The proximal row forms the proximal arc, and the proximal edge of the distal row forms the distal arc
  - The arcs should be smooth and continuous
- **Scapholunate Interval:** on AP view of the wrist, if space between the scaphoid and the lunate is >2-3 mm, this indicates possible scapholunate dissociation (may need to compare with contralateral side radiograph)—"Terry Thomas sign"
- *Scapholunate Angle: measured on lateral radiograph. Normal is 30°-60°.
  - >60° indicates possible dorsal intercalated segment instability (DISI) deformity
  - <30° indicates possible volar intercalated segment instability (VISI) deformity

FINGERS

- **Five metacarpals, 14 phalanges** (3 per finger, 2 in thumb)
- **"Protected splinting position" also known as intrinsic-plus places the wrist gently extended at 30°**, PIPJ and DIPJ fully extended
  - A cam effect is created over the ovoid contour of the metacarpal head. As a result, the collateral ligaments are tight in flexion but lax in extension and must be protected from shortening by flexing the MPJ.
  - At the IPJ, the issue is different
    - When flexed, the volar plate can become adherent to the tendon or periosteum and result in flexion contracture.
    - When flexed, the extensor mechanism is stressed. Prolonged stress (especially with surrounding inflammation) can result in disruption of transverse retinacular ligaments, allowing lateral bands to slip, and causing boutonniere deformity.

TOURNIQUET USE

- Never place a digital tourniquet without an obvious reminder to remove it (eg, hemostat and sterile glove) to avoid digital loss.
- Blood pressure cuffs make good arm tourniquets in the ER. Arm tourniquet should be wide to distribute pressure.
- Try to wait on inflating the arm tourniquet until you have done an exam. Minimize cycles of placing/removing a tourniquet during the acute evaluation of a traumatized limb. If possible, use direct pressure to stop bleeding until exam is complete.
- **Tourniquet pressure should be 125-150 mm Hg above systolic pressure** (usually set around 230-250 mm Hg). Always inflate fully!
- **Limit continuous tourniquet time to 2 hours** to prevent permanent damage and minimize patient discomfort from tourniquet.
  - ○ Nerves are the most vulnerable to pressure/hypoxia.
  - ○ **Blood flow should be returned to the ischemic part for 5 minutes for every 30 minutes of ischemia (ie, deflate tourniquet for 20 minutes every 2 hours).**
  - ○ Do not progressively loosen a tourniquet: either have it fully inflated, or let it down completely and use pressure to control bleeding as needed.

INCISIONS ON THE HAND

- **When planning incisions, avoid crossing flexion creases at a right angle.**
  - ○ Mid-axial incisions: with the finger fully flexed, mark the radial and ulnar extent of the flexion crease at each finger joint. Connect these dots.
  - ○ Bruner incisions: incisions on the flexor surface that diagonally connect mid-axial point to mid-axial point.
- **Extensor surface with less risk of scar contracture limiting function.** Longitudinal, curvilinear, and transverse incisions usually all acceptable.

PEARLS

1. Develop a system for the hand exam that goes through the key anatomical components and use it every time—avoid shortcuts and stay organized so nothing gets missed.
2. Always document the neurovascular exam BEFORE injecting local anesthetic, and if possible before inflating a tourniquet.
3. Test function against RESISTANCE—may detect a partial injury that is otherwise compensated.
4. Whenever in doubt, compare the injured hand to the uninjured one to help identify abnormalities.
5. Always incorporate a "removal reminder" when applying a tourniquet.

QUESTIONS YOU WILL BE ASKED

1. What structures on the extensor surface of the finger might mask an extensor tendon injury?
   a. Junctura tendinae.
2. What is maximum tourniquet time? How long must you release the tourniquet if the case is longer than the maximum and you wish to use another tourniquet run?
   a. 2 hours.
   b. 5 minutes for every 30 minutes of tourniquet time.
3. What is the standard protected position for splinting the hand and wrist? Why?
   a. Intrinsic plus with thumb in palmar abduction.
   b. See Section V, subsection C.

4. What is the last muscle innervated by the ulnar nerve? How is it tested?
   a. Adductor pollicus.
   b. Key pinch/Froment sign. See Section II, subsection D.
5. In the finger, how are nerve and artery related in position?
   Nerve is volar to artery (opposite orientation in the palm).
6. Relative position of extensor indicis and the corresponding extensor digitorum to the index finger?
   EIP is ulnar to EDC tendon.
7. Of the different pulleys in the flexor system, which are the most important to preserve? Why?
   a. A2 and A4.
   b. Prevent bowstringing of the tendon overlying the proximal (A2) and middle (A4) phalanx.

THINGS TO DRAW

1. Cross section of the carpal tunnel
2. Bruner incision pattern on a digit
3. Identify and mark Kaplan cardinal line

Recommended Readings
1. Mazurek MT, Shin AY. Upper extremity peripheral nerve anatomy: current concepts and applications. *Clin Orthop Relat Res*. 2001;383:7-20.
2. Moore KL, Dalley AF, Agur AMR. *Clinically Oriented Anatomy*. Lippincott; 2009.

30 Basics of Fixation

Atticus Coscia

GENERAL CONCEPTS

- Fracture healing
  - Factors affecting healing
    - Too much or too little strain across a fracture can prevent bony union.
      - Motion as measured by strain across fracture: = $\Delta L/L$.
      - Increasing stress (ie, force per cross-sectional area) increases ΔL.
      - Increasing rigidity of fixation decreases ΔL under the same stress.
      - Increasing distance increases L and decreases strain.
    - Blood supply: inadequate blood supply can prevent healing.
      - Sources
        - Endosteal: supplies inner 2/3 of cortical bone
        - Periosteal: supplies outer 1/3 of cortical bone
      - May be disrupted or limited by
        - Initial trauma
        - Surgical exposure, implants
        - Inherent properties of particular bones or fracture fragments (eg, articular fragments have limited blood supply as they lack periosteum)
  - Types of healing (for details, please **see Chapter 1: Complex Wound Care, section "Bone Healing"**)
    - Primary (Haversian remodeling)
      - **Intramembranous ossification:** normal bony remodeling as if no fracture were present (ie, no cartilage intermediate)
      - Cutting cones of osteoclasts migrate across the fracture site, followed by osteoblasts that form new bone
      - Requirements:
        - Anatomic reduction (denominator in strain definition $\Delta L/L$ must be small)
        - Absolute stability (<2% strain: because L must be small, ΔL must be extremely small)
    - Secondary
      - **Endochondral ossification:** a cartilaginous model is created first and replaced by bony remodeling
      - Sequence:
        - Inflammation: hematoma and granulation tissue form across the fracture.
        - Repair: soft callus (cartilage) is remodeled to hard callus (woven bone).
        - Remodeling: woven bone is replaced by mature lamellar bone.
      - Requires more strain than primary: 2%-10%
- Factors influencing fixation method
  - **Fracture pattern**
    - Predictable patterns result from combinations of compression, tension, and shearing forces.
      - Three-point bending produces tension on one side (resulting in a transverse fracture line) and compression on the other (two 45° oblique lines around a "butterfly" fragment).
      - Torsion around the long axis (eg, a phalanx) produces a spiral fracture.

---

*Denotes common in-service examination topics.

- Fixation failure and displacement (leading to nonunion or malunion) typically reproduce the displacement seen in the original injury.
- Implants are chosen to specifically neutralize the forces manifested by the fracture pattern.
- Comminuted fractures distribute stress over a longer distance (L is large) so less rigid fixation may be required to achieve acceptable strain (ΔL must be proportionally larger).

- **Energy transferred during injury**
  - High-energy injuries damage surrounding soft tissues and bony blood supply increasing the risk of nonunion, delayed union, and wound problems.
  - The fracture pattern belies the energy imparted during injury.
    - Bone is strongest in compression and weakest in shear.
    - Increasing energy results in increasing comminution.
  - Surgical approach and fixation should respect angiosomes and limit damage blood supply.
- **Deforming forces**
  - Soft tissue attachments to fractures produce predictable deforming forces. Examples
    - Base of the thumb metacarpal fractures (eg, Bennett's) are shortened and radially and dorsally deviated by abductor and extensor pollicis longus m. and adducted and supinated by the adductor pollicis m.
    - Proximal phalanx fractures angulate volar due to interossei flexing the proximal fragment and the extensor central slip extending the distal fragment.
  - Implants should be selected to specifically resist deforming forces.
- **Affected region of bone and desired healing type**
  - Articular surfaces are typically fixed with anatomic reduction and absolute stability.
    - Articular fluid may prevent secondary bone healing.
    - Malreduction of articular surfaces can produce arthritis from instability or point loading.
  - Diaphyseal fractures typically only require restoration of the length, alignment, and rotation.
    - Restore the relative positions of adjacent joints.
    - Restore appropriate tension on surrounding soft tissues.
- **Expected stress across the fracture**
  - Increasing stress requires increasingly rigid fixation constructs to control motion.
  - Stress may be affected by:
    - The bone: some bones see more stress under physiologic load than others
    - Surrounding tissues: ligaments and muscles can apply stress across a fracture or resist displacing forces.
    - Activity: early motion to prevent joint contractures or rehabilitate tendon repairs may demand more rigid fixation of surrounding fractures.
- **Reduction methods**
  - **Direct**: visualizing and manually manipulating the fracture fragments
    - Typically required to achieve anatomic reduction.
    - Associated surgical trauma to surrounding soft tissues can compromise blood supply.
    - Often paired with absolute stability to achieve primary bone healing.
  - **Indirect**: positioning fracture fragments in space without directly manipulating them
    - May be achieved by manipulating two ends of a bone without exposing the fracture itself
    - Relies on surrounding muscles, ligaments, and periosteum to get fragments close to each other
    - Often paired with relative stability to achieve secondary bone healing

FIXATION METHODS

- **Pins and Wires**
  - Cylindrical metal rod, often with a sharp tip to facilitate insertion through cortical bone.
  - Typically varies in diameter from <1mm to several mm in diameter.
  - May be smooth or partially or fully threaded.
  - Can be placed percutaneously.
  - Typically provide relative stability.
  - Tension may be applied along the axis of a wire to increase its bending resistance.
  - Example uses
    - Provisionally maintain alignment while applying definitive fixation
    - Definitive percutaneous fixation of small fracture fragments or joints
    - Transmit external traction applied perpendicular to the axis of the pin to a transfixed bone
    - As a guide over which a cannulated screw may be inserted
    - As part of a tension band
    - As part of an external fixator
    - Malleable wire may be wrapped around a bone as a cerclage (does not resist torsional or longitudinal forces)
    - As an intramedullary nail (see below)
- **Screws**
  - A threaded metal cylinder that converts rotational to linear force
  - Components and terms
    - Head: larger diameter end, acts as a stop to further linear motion.
    - Tip: may be self-drilling and self-tapping.
    - Threads: inclined plane wrapping around the central core.
    - Cannulation: an open tube along the central long axis of the screw.
    - Inner diameter (ID): the diameter of the central core, affects resistance to bending and shear forces.
    - Outer diameter (OD): the diameter of the threads (a 3.5-mm screw has a 3.5 mm OD and a 2.5 mm ID).
    - Pitch: the longitudinal distance between thread.
    - Pullout strength: the primary property is the difference between the inner and outer diameters.
  - Lag screw vs locking screw
    - **Lag screw**: compresses two fragments of bone against each other
      - The hole in the near fragment equals the OD (the head pushes it as the screw advances), and the hole in the far fragment equals the ID (so the threads pull the far fragment toward the near fragment).
      - By design: the screw is partially threaded so a smooth shank slides through the near fragment and threads are only engaging the far fragment.
      - Particularly useful to obtain fixation and compression across amenable fractures (eg, oblique or spiral metacarpal shaft fractures).
    - **Locking screw**: threads in the head engage the screw holes of a plate such that the two act as a single fixed angle device. Particularly useful in osteoporotic bone, short segments where it is impossible to fit an adequate number of screws, and where screws cannot be placed bicortically.
- **Plates**
  - Rigidity of the fixation construct is affected by intrinsic properties of the plate such as width and thickness but also how it is applied, and the load shared (or not) by the fracture.
  - They may be held in place by friction produced from compressing the plate to the bone or by inserting "locking" screws that thread into both the bone and threads in the plate's screw hole.

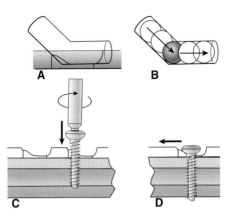

Figure 30-1 Illustration of dynamic compression plating mechanism. The screw head is eccentrically inserted into a scalloped plate hole (**A**) and slides like a ball down a ramp (**B**) on the scalloped edge as it is tightened. As the screw is tightened (**C**), the plate slides (**D**), resulting in compression across the fracture as the plate is already fixed to the other fracture fragment. (From Bishop JA, Behn AW, Gardner MJ. Principles and biomechanics of internal fixation. In: Tornetta P, Ricci W, Court-Brown CM, McQueen MM, McKee M, eds. *Rockwood and Green's Fractures in Adults.* 9th ed. Wolters Kluwer; 2020. Figure 11.12.)

- ○ The holes may be scalloped at the edge to permit an eccentrically inserted screw to cause the plate to slide along the bone as the screw is inserted. This can be used to compress fracture lines perpendicular to the axis of the plate (see "compression plating" below) (**Fig. 30-1**).
- ○ Modern plates provide a high degree of modularity, allowing multiple screw types to be placed through different holes in the same plate (eg, standard cortical screw, cortical screw placed in compression mode, fixed or variable angle locking screws).
- ○ May be **"load sharing"**, as when applied to anatomically reduced fractures with interfragmentary compression (eg, simple oblique metacarpal shaft fracture fixed with a dorsal plate), or **"load bearing"**, as when bony apposition is not achieved (eg, segmental distal radius fracture fixed with a bridge plate). Fatigue risk and motion are likely to increase when applied loads are not shared with the bone.
- ○ Application to the tension side of the bone is generally preferred so the bone shares applied loads such that strain and risk of hardware fatigue are reduced.
- ○ Common use cases
  - ■ **Neutralization** (aka "protection plating")
    - □ Used to protect lag screws from torsional or bending forces.
    - □ Independent lag screw(s) may be placed outside of the plate, or, depending on plate placement and fracture angle, a lag screw may be placed through the plate.
    - □ Supports absolute stability by preventing motion while compression is achieved with interfragmentary lag screws.
  - ■ **Compression**
    - □ Use of eccentrically placed screws in scalloped plate holes to generate compression along the long axis of the plate.
    - □ For transverse fractures, a convex bend should be placed in the plate (ie, pre-contoured away from the bone) so that excess compression applied on the near cortex does not generate gapping of the far cortex (**Fig. 30-2**).
    - □ For oblique fractures, the plate is first secured to the fragment that generates an acute angle with the plate (ie, an axilla is created between the fracture and the plate) into which the cortical spike of the other fragment can be compressed.
    - □ Used to produce absolute stability through interfragmentary compression.
    - □ Stiffness is increased (and motion thereby reduced) by permitting the bone to absorb some of the applied loads.

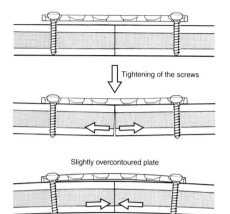

**Figure 30-2 Illustration of rational for overcontouring (ie, pre-contouring a convexity bend)
compression plates prior to application in order to avoid excess compression at near cortex and
resultant gapping at far cortex.** (From Bishop JA, Behn AW, Gardner MJ. Principles and biomechanics of internal fixation. In: Tornetta P, Ricci W, Court-Brown CM, McQueen MM, McKee M, eds.
Rockwood and Green's Fractures in Adults. 9th ed. Wolters Kluwer; 2020. Figure 11.13.)

- **Buttress or antiglide**
  - Resists shear forces that are produced along the oblique fracture line by axial loads.
  - May be used to achieve reduction and provide interfragmentary compression.
  - As the plate is secured to one fracture fragment with a cortical screw, the unsecured portion of the plate drives reduction of a cortical spike in the other fragment into an acute axilla formed between the plate and the first fragment.
  - The most important, and first applied, screw is at the apex of the fracture.
  - Use of the term "buttress" may be reserved for cases in which a depressed articular fragment is being supported and compressed to the intact metadiaphysis.
  - May be used in combination with other techniques including compression through the plate (see compression plating above) and interfragmentary lag screws.
  - Used to achieve absolute stability.
- **Tension band**
  - Application to the tension side of eccentrically loaded bones (eg, olecranon, patella, femur) to move the hinge point of the fracture such that loads induce compression rather than fracture gapping.
  - Applied loads that are not coaxial with the anatomic axis of the bone create torque at the fracture site and produce a bending moment, which hinges on the compression side and gaps the tension side. The plate moves the hinge point to the cortex underneath it thereby preventing the tension side from gapping and inducing compression on the far cortex under the eccentric load.
  - This technique is not exclusive to plating. For example, a tensioned wire applied to the one side of the bone could function in the same way.
  - Used to generate absolute stability with dynamic interfragmentary compression.
- **Bridging**
  - Plate spans a (typically comminuted) fracture without concern for achieving anatomic reduction or fragment apposition *per se.*
  - Maintains relative distance, alignment, and rotation of the joints on either side.
  - Often combined with indirect reduction, percutaneous application, or both.

- May be accomplished with cortical screws, locking screws, or a combination.
- The fractured bone does not typically share a significant portion of the applied loads, and therefore motion at the fracture site is often relatively high.
- If the working length is too short, strain will be too high to permit bone healing.
- Usually reserved for diaphyseal or metaphyseal fractures with comminution or for situations in which the morbidity of dissection precludes anatomic reduction.
- Produces relative stability.
- Example: A plate may be secured to the diaphysis of the radius and second or third metacarpal to partially reduce and immobilize through ligamentotaxis a comminuted intra-articular distal radius fracture that is not amenable to direct reduction and fixation.

- **Intramedullary nail**
  - Markedly improved axial, torsional, and bending stability is achieved with the use of interlocking screws inserted through both cortices of the bone and holes in the nail.
  - Typically used for relative stabilization of metaphyseal or diaphyseal fractures.
  - Reaming of the intramedullary canal may be performed prior to insertion.
    - Permits passage of a larger diameter nail
    - Increases the length of the bone over which the nail achieves a tight intramedullary fit (ie, increases working distance)
    - Stimulates periosteal blood supply and deposits local bone graft at the fracture site
  - Other devices may be used in a similar fashion. For example:
    - A screw may be inserted longitudinally in the metacarpal medullary canal.
    - A Kirschner wire inserted percutaneously through the longitudinal axis of the distal phalanx.
    - "Elastic" nails placed in pediatric both-bone forearm fractures; intramedullary fit is achieved by three-point interference between the canal and the elastic recoil of the flexible nail.

- **External fixator**
  - A rigid device external to the body
  - Typically modular and assembled intraoperatively with components consisting of
    - Pins and wires
    - Bars or struts: external connections between the pins and wires
    - Clamps and rings: connections between pins and bars
  - The most commonly used systems include
    - Simple mono-lateral frames: constructs built with bars, pin-bar clamps, bar-bar clamps, and pins
    - Small wire circular frame fixation: small-diameter wires, circular rings, connecting rods
    - Hybrid fixator: construct uses pins, wires, bars, and circular rings (ie, a combination of the above)
  - Most commonly used for temporary fixation in complicated and/or high-energy injuries (significant soft tissue compromise, open wounds, compartment syndrome, gross contamination, bony devascularization)
  - May also be used for definitive fixation, but complications including pin tract infections and loss of reduction are common

- **Interfragmentary compression**
  - Compression, by creating friction between opposing surfaces, helps to prevent motion and thereby promote absolute stability and primary bone healing.
  - Should be applied perpendicular to facture line. Otherwise, compressive force is lost as shear.
  - The mode of application is typically determined by the fracture type and pattern.
    - Oblique fractures: lag screws, compression plating, buttress plating, bone clamps prior to fixation
    - Transverse fractures: compression plating, tension band, bone clamps applied prior to fixation

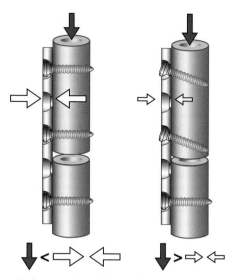

Figure 30-3 Compression between plate and bone (*white arrows*) is the key element of stability in conventional plating. As long as the friction generated by compression of the plate to bone is greater than load applied (*blue arrows*) to the fracture site the implant will remain stable (eg, fixation construct pictured on the *left*). In the fixation construct on the *right*, the load applied is greater than compression generated between the plate and bone, resulting in hardware failure and fracture displacement. (From Bishop JA, Behn AW, Gardner MJ. Principles and biomechanics of internal fixation. In: Tornetta P, Ricci W, Court-Brown CM, McQueen MM, McKee M, eds. *Rockwood and Green's Fractures in Adults.* 9th ed. Wolters Kluwer; 2020. Figure 11.9.)

- Plating with articulating tensioning device and contouring fixed angle devices may be used
  ○ Compression between plate and bone is the key element of stability in conventional plating (**Fig. 30-3**).

PEARLS

1. The particular fracture pattern predicts the intrinsic stability of the bone after reduction.
2. Stability of fixation represents a continuum from complete rigidity with no motion to no stability at all.
3. Rigid fixation is chosen when anatomic reduction is achieved and has the goal of primary bone healing.
4. Less rigid fixation, affording relative stability, is chosen when anatomic reduction is not achieved and the distance between fracture fragments is larger. The goal in this case is secondary bone healing.
5. Nonunion is most likely to result when elements of each strategy are combined. Direct anatomic reduction with relative stability and nonanatomic reduction with absolute stability are both recipes for failure.

Recommended Readings
1. Bishop JA, Behn AW, Gardner MJ. Principles and biomechanics of internal fixation. *Rockwood and Green's Fractures in Adults.* Wolters Kluwer; 2020:362-390.
2. Rüedi TP, Buckley RE, Moran CG. *AO Principles of Fracture Management.* Thieme; 2007:5.
3. Tencer AF, Johnson KD. *Biomechanics in Orthopedic Trauma: Bone Fracture and Fixation.* Taylor & Francis; 1994:18.
4. Thakur AJ. *The Elements of Fracture Fixation.* 2nd ed. Elsevier India; 2012:43.

31 Congenital Upper Extremity Anomalies

Alfred P. Yoon and Jennifer Waljee

OVERVIEW

- Incidence
  - Approximately 0.2% of all live births, 95% sporadic
  - Most common: syndactyly, polydactyly, and camptodactyly
  - Frequently associated with cardiac, hematopoietic, and tumorous conditions due to simultaneous development
- Embryologic Development
  - *The arm bud (consisting of mesenchyme and covered by ectoderm): appears at 30 days of gestation and is complete by 8 weeks (ossification continues throughout gestation)
  - Development: Hox genes (A, B, C, and D) and directed by signaling proteins including sonic hedgehog (SHH), fibroblast growth factor, and Wnt-7a
  - Development occurs in three planes: proximal to distal axis, dorsal to palmar axis, and anteroposterior (preaxial/postaxial) axis
    - *Apical ectodermal ridge: thickening of ectoderm at the leading edge of the limb bud; controls proximal to distal differentiation
      - Controlled by fibroblast growth factors (FGF-2, FGF-4, FGF-8)
    - Dorsal ectoderm: differentiation along dorsal to palmar plane (flexor and extensor regions)
      - Controlled through Wnt7a and induction of Lmx1b
    - *Zone of polarizing activity: anterior-posterior (radial/ulnar) differentiation and is a group of mesenchymal cells on the preaxial (radial) aspect of the upper limb
      - Controlled by SHH
  - 4th week: limb buds appear
  - 5th week: apical ectodermal ridge appears, hand plates develop
  - 6th week: digital separation by apoptosis
  - 7th week: mesenchymal differentiation and chondrogenesis
  - 8th week and beyond: ossification of the skeleton
- Developmental Milestones: ideally, reconstruction should be performed after 1 year and usually by age 4 prior to school entry for socialization and to match developmental milestones (Table 31-1)
  - 9 months: small object pinch (functional grasp)
  - 2 years: three-digit pinch
  - 3-4 years: hand preference established, hand-eye coordination
- Ossification centers: see tips of distal phalanx by 7 weeks of gestation, metacarpals and proximal phalanx by 9-10 weeks, and middle phalanx by 10-12 weeks. Wrist: first form capitate (0-6 months postnatal) and then hamate (0-6 months). Then the following order: triquetrum→lunate→scaphoid→trapezium→trapezoid→pisiform

TABLE 31-1 Development Milestones of Upper Extremity Hand Function

Timeline	Motor skills
Birth	Grasp reflex
3 mo	Power grip with ulnar digits
5 mo	Finger grip with adducted thumb; raking grasp
7 mo	Thumb opposition
9 mo	Small object pinch, bimanual palmar grasp
10 mo	Fine pinch
1-2 y	Tripod pinch
3-4 y	Hand-eye coordination and hand dominance established

- Classification of congenital hand anomalies (Table 31-2)
  - International Federation of Societies for Surgery of the Hand classifies congenital hand anomalies into seven distinct groups (failure of formation, failure of differentiation, duplication, overgrowth, undergrowth, constriction ring syndrome, generalized skeletal deformities)

TABLE 31-2 Classification of Congenital Hand Anomalies by the American Society for Surgery of the Hand and the International Federation of Societies for Surgery of the Hand

Type	Subtype	Examples
I. Failure of formation	Transverse arrest	Vascular disruption resulting in deficiency and proximal hypoplasia anywhere from the shoulder to the phalanges
	Longitudinal arrest	Radial deficiency
		Ulnar deficiency
		Central ray deficiency "cleft hand"
II. Failure of differentiation	Soft tissue	Simple syndactyly
	Skeletal	Complex syndactyly
		Radioulnar synostosis
	Congenital tumors	
III. Duplication		Pre/postaxial polydactyly Central polydactyly Mirror hand
IV. Overgrowth		Macrodactyly
V. Undergrowth		Thumb hypoplasia
VI. Constriction ring syndrome		
VII. Other skeletal anomalies	Flexion deformities	Camptodactyly

FAILURE OF FORMATION

TRANSVERSE FAILURE OF FORMATION (CONGENITAL AMPUTATION)

- **General concepts**
  - Etiology unknown but likely due to intrauterine vascular compromise at the apical ectodermal ridge or developing limb bud
  - Timing of apical ectodermal ridge removal may determine level of truncation
- **Epidemiology**
  - Usually unilateral, and most commonly at the proximal forearm
  - Sporadic
- **Associated syndromes:** usually not associated with other abnormalities
- **Presentation**
  - Most commonly presents with arrest at the proximal forearm
  - Elbow flexion and extension intact, but difficulty with pronation and supination
- **Treatment**
  - Surgical intervention rarely indicated. Children function well with active and passive prosthetic options.

RADIAL DEFICIENCY

- **General concepts**
  - Most common type of longitudinal failure of formation.
  - Involve radial side of the forearm, including the radius, radial carpus, and thumb.
  - Hypoplasia of some or all elements, including thumb hypoplasia, absence of the scaphoid and trapezium, camptodactyly of the radial digits, and absence of radial artery and nerve.
  - Radiographs of the hand and wrist are needed to determine the extent of malformation.
  - Associated with reductions in apical ectodermal ridge associated FGF.
- **Epidemiology**
  - 1:30 000-1:100 000 live births
  - More common among male infants and Caucasians
  - 50% are bilateral; unilateral: right more affected than left
- **Associated syndromes**
  - Genetic syndromes: children should be evaluated by a geneticist and undergo a thorough workup, including spinal radiographs, echocardiogram, and a renal ultrasound.
  - *Fanconi anemia: radial deficiency with polydactyly, syndactyly, clinodactyly, atrial septal defect (ASD), and pancytopenia (autosomal recessive)
  - TAR syndrome: thrombocytopenia, absent radius
  - Holt-Oram syndrome: ASD with radial deficiency (autosomal dominant)
  - VATERL association (vertebral anomalies, anal atresia, cardiac anomalies, tracheoesophageal fistula, renal defects, limb anomalies)
  - Chromosomal anomalies (trisomies 13 and 18)
  - Nager syndrome: radial deficiency/acrofacial dysostosis (autosomal dominant)
  - Mobius syndrome: congenital facial paralysis, limb abnormalities in 25% of cases
- **Presentation**
  - Fibrotic muscle bellies result in bowing of the ulna
  - Shortened ulna and hypoplastic distal humerus result in elbow stiffness
  - Hand assumes flexed and radially deviated position
  - Extensor indicis proprius (EIP) may be deficient, flexors abnormal, thumb muscles affected
  - Nerve: radial nerve ends after triceps; median nerve innervates radial forearm skin
  - Vessels: ulnar artery may be only vessel; interosseous artery may replace radial artery

- **Treatment (Table 31-3)**
  - Stretching
  - Serial casting
  - External soft tissue distraction
  - Centralization of the wrist on the ulna
    - Radially placed Z-plasty incision to release skin tightness.
    - Median nerve is usually present and can be easily injured during surgical exposure due to aberrant anatomy.
    - Carpus released from the radial-sided wrist flexors and extensors (brachioradialis [BR], flexor carpi radialis [FCR], extensor carpi radialis longus [ECRL]).
    - Carpus is centralized on the ulna, and a Steinmann pin is used to fix the middle metacarpal, carpus, and ulna.
    - Tendon transfers are used to maintain a centralized wrist position: fused mass of FCR, ECRL, extensor carpi radialis longus brevis, and BR is transferred to extensor carpi ulnaris to become ulnar deviator, thus balancing the wrist.
    - Corrective osteotomy of the ulna may also be performed.
    - Soft tissue coverage achieved via local tissue rearrangement (eg, bilobed flap).
    - Sometimes can use distraction lengthening to stretch soft tissues to permit tension-free centralization.
  - **Contraindications to reconstruction**
    - Older patients who have adapted to the deformity or in patients with poor elbow flexion.
    - In these cases, radial deviation and flexion of the hand assist with activities of daily living among patients with severe elbow stiffness.
  - **Long-term outcomes**
    - Recurrent radial deviation, wrist stiffness.
    - Centralization improves appearance, but the extent to which it improves long-term function is not known.

ULNAR DEFICIENCY

- **General concepts/presentation**
  - The ulna is absent, and a fibrocartilaginous "anlage" is present that inserts on the ulnar aspect of the carpus and distal radius rather than the ulna and fails to grow commensurately with the child.
  - Flexor carpi ulnaris typically absent.
  - Median and ulnar nerves present, but ulnar artery usually absent.
  - Unlike radial deficiency, the carpus is stable; however, the elbow may be unstable due to radial head dislocation.
  - Associated with disruption of zone of polarizing activity (ZPA) in the posterior region of limb bud.
- **Epidemiology**
  - Less common than radial deficiency.
  - Approximately 1/100 000 births.
  - Usually sporadic and unilateral, and rarely associated with other syndromes.
  - About 50% of patients have another musculoskeletal anomaly (eg, proximal femoral focal deficiency, fibular deficiency, phocomelia, and scoliosis); 90% have associated hand anomalies (eg, syndactyly, absent digits, and thumb abnormalities).
  - Malformations range from hypoplasia to total absence with radiohumeral synostosis.
- **Associated syndromes**: usually not associated with systemic syndromes
- **Treatment**
  - Depending on the associated hand anomalies, may require syndactyly release, first web space deepening, opponensplasty, pollicization, and thumb metacarpal rotational osteotomy.

TABLE 31-3 Classification and Treatment of Radial Deficiency

Type	Thumb	Carpus	Radius	Treatment options
N	Hypoplastic/absent	Normal	Normal	Thumb reconstruction as indicated, stretching and splinting
0	Hypoplastic/absent	Elements fused, hypoplastic, or absent	Normal distal radius Proximal radius normal, with radioulnar synostosis, or congenital dislocation of the radial head	Thumb reconstruction as indicated, stretching and splinting
1	Hypoplastic/absent	Elements fused, hypoplastic, or absent	Shortened radius compared with the ulnar Attenuation of the distal epiphysis Proximal radius normal, with radioulnar synostosis, or congenital dislocation of the radial head	Thumb reconstruction as indicated, stretching and splinting
2	Hypoplastic/absent	Elements fused, hypoplastic, or absent	Attenuation of the proximal and distal epiphyses, diminutive radius, ulnar bowing, poor support of the carpus	Thumb reconstruction as indicated, stretching and splinting in mild cases Radial lengthening and centralization in more severe cases
3	Hypoplastic/absent	Elements fused, hypoplastic, or absent	Absence of the physis, and hypoplastic proximal or middle radius with ulnar bowing and poorly supported carpus	Thumb reconstruction as indicated, serial casting or soft tissue distraction followed by centralization and transfer of aberrant radial wrist extensors; for cases of unilateral deficiency, consider distraction osteogenesis to lengthen the ulna following centralization
4	Hypoplastic/absent	Elements fused, hypoplastic, or absent	Complete absence of radius; unsupported hand with severe radial displacement	Thumb reconstruction as indicated, serial casting or soft tissue distraction followed by centralization and transfer of aberrant radial wrist extensors; for cases of unilateral deficiency, consider distraction osteogenesis to lengthen the ulna following centralization

○ Serial casting and splinting to improve elbow posture.
○ Excision of fibrous anlage when there is 30° or more of angulation or progressive ulnar angulation. May be combined with radial osteotomy to further straighten the forearm axis.
○ Loss of elbow function may be improved with resection of the radial head and osteosynthesis of the distal radius to the proximal ulna (ie, one bone forearm).
○ Derotational osteotomy of the humerus for children with severe internal rotation and radiohumeral synostosis.
○ **Outcomes:** following treatment, long-term function is improved but less pronounced in patients with radiohumeral synostosis and absent or stiff digits.

CENTRAL RAY DEFICIENCY "CLEFT HAND"

• **General concepts:** longitudinal deficiency of central hand elements
• **Epidemiology:** autosomal dominant with variable penetrance and expression
• **Associated syndromes**
  ○ Ectrodactyly-ectodermal dysplasia-cleft syndrome
    ▪ Autosomal dominant
    ▪ Triad of ectrodactyly, ectodermal dysplasia, and facial clefts
• **Presentation**
  ○ A V-shaped deformity is present with or without absence of digits
  ○ Typical
    ▪ Failure of development of the middle digit and metacarpal leading to a deep V-shaped cleft
    ▪ Border digits may have syndactyly
    ▪ Autosomal dominant
    ▪ May involve multiple extremities including feet
  ○ Atypical
    ▪ Broad and flat, U-shaped cleft with missing or shortened central digits
    ▪ Vestigial remnants may be present
    ▪ Sporadic
    ▪ One extremity involved
    ▪ Thumb and ulnar digits are present
    ▪ Variation of symbrachydactyly
  ○ Involvement of the first web space is predictive of hand function
• **Treatment**
  ○ Cleft hands frequently function well, despite aesthetic appearance
  ○ Progressive deformity may result from syndactyly or the presence of transverse bones within the cleft
    ▪ Removal of transverse bones
    ▪ Syndactyly release
    ▪ First web space release
    ▪ Cleft closure
  ○ Snow-Littler procedure: first web space is released, and the index metacarpal is transposed to the base of the middle finger metacarpal position.
  ○ Absence of the thumb
    ▪ Second toe transfer
    ▪ Pollicization of available digit

FAILURE OF DIFFERENTIATION

SYNDACTYLY

• **General concepts**
  ○ Fusion of soft tissue and sometimes bony elements of the digits
  ○ Interdigital apoptosis is under the control of bone morphogenic proteins and associated regression of FGF signaling in the overlying apical ectodermal ridge

- **Epidemiology**
  - *Occurs in ~1 in 2000-3000 births
  - 50% bilateral
  - 10%-40% present with a family history of syndactyly suggesting autosomal dominance with variable penetrance
- **Associated syndromes**
- Poland syndrome—absent/underdeveloped pectoralis muscle, syndactyly
- Apert syndrome—craniosynostosis, exophthalmos, mental retardation, complex syndactyly
  - Upton classification type 1: spade hand
    - Incomplete syndactyly of first web
    - Digit and palm can be flattened
    - Good digital MCP joints
  - Upton classification type 2: mitten (spoon) hand
    - Complete simple syndactyly of first web
    - Palmar concavity of the digit and palm
    - Fusion of fingertips
    - Synechia of central nails
    - Proximal metacarpal splayed
  - Rosebud (hoof) hand
    - Complete complex syndactyly of first web
    - Thumb incorporated into mass
    - Hand tightly cupped
    - Index ray with skeletal abnormalities
    - Synechia of central nails
- **Presentation**
  - *Most common between the middle and ring finger, followed by the ring and small finger
  - Simple: skin fusion only
  - Complex: bony fusion and skin fusion. Most commonly involves the distal phalanx. Can be identified with preoperative radiographs
  - Complete: fusion along the entire length of the digit
  - Incomplete: fusion along the portion of the digit not including the nail folds
  - Complicated: fusion of multiple digits (eg, Apert syndrome)
- **Treatment**
  - Release is indicated to enhance aesthetic appearance, limit functional limitations, and prevent growth restriction and deformity.
  - Release is usually performed between age 12 and 18 months unless growth restriction and angular deformity is evident earlier.
    - Border digits usually treated earlier at ~6 months
  - Contiguous web spaces are released in a staged fashion to avoid vascular compromise.
  - Surgical options
    - *A proximally based, dorsal rectangular skin flap is designed between the two metacarpal heads to incorporate the perforating metacarpal artery vessel is advanced into the web space. Interdigitating triangular flaps are designed to resurface the digits, and a full-thickness skin graft is often harvested from the groin to complete coverage (one variation shown in Fig. 31-1).
  - Postoperative complications
    - Skin flap loss and delayed wound healing, scar contracture, web space creeping (most common), joint instability, skeletal deformity, keloid formation

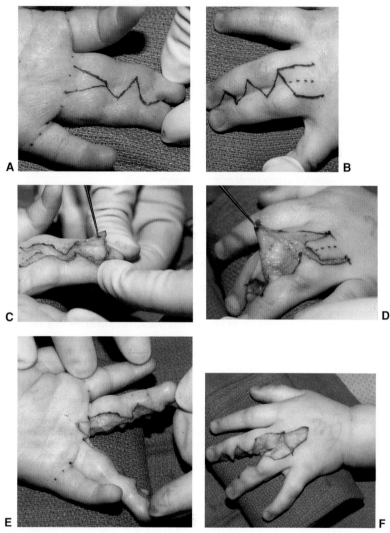

Figure 31-1 One method of syndactyly reconstruction. There are countless methods of syndactyly reconstruction. Most rely on a dorsal quadrilateral flap, as illustrated in this example. **A.** A volar zig-zag incision is designed to prevent scar contractures over the joints. If a straight line incision were used, then a contracted scar would develop. Some use a triangular flap at the volar base of the release as shown here. Many do not. **B.** A dorsal quadrilateral flap is designed to provide full-thickness coverage in the web. **C** and **D.** The zig-zag flaps are raised in a subcutaneous plane. **E** and **F.** The digits are fully separated, including the neurovascular bundles. **G.** The dorsal flap may be split, as shown in this example, by the volar flap. Many authors do not use a volar flap and thus inset the dorsal flap without splitting it. The zig-zag flaps are inset. **H.** Following release of the tourniquet, the fingertips have a pink color, indicating adequate circulation. **I** and **J.** Areas not covered by the flaps are resurfaced with full-thickness skin grafts. (From James MA. Release and Reconstruction of Digital Syndactyly. In: *Master Techniques in Orthopaedic Surgery: The Hand.* 2nd ed. Wolters Kluwer; 2005:171-196. Figure 12.1.)

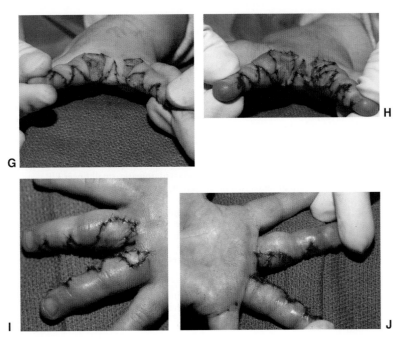

Figure 31-1 *(Continued)*

RADIOULNAR SYNOSTOSIS

- **General concepts:** failure of separation of the proximal radius and ulna
- **Epidemiology**
  - 60% bilateral
  - Majority sporadic, but autosomal dominant inheritance has been described
- **Associated syndromes:** may be associated with other upper extremities in 30% of affected children (eg, thumb hypoplasia) and associated with Apert syndrome and arthrogryposis
- **Presentation**
  - Children present with lack of forearm rotation and presence of elbow flexion contractures, resulting in difficulty with hand positioning and dexterity.
  - Radial head subluxation or dislocation may also be present.
  - Children may compensate through rotation at the shoulder, radiocarpal, intercarpal, and carpometacarpophalangeal (CMC) joints.
- **Treatment**
  - Indications
    - Functional impairment due to lack of supination and pronation.
    - Forearm is fixed in more than 60° of pronation.
    - Bilateral deformity.
  - Options
    - Derotational osteotomy at synostosis or at the diaphysis with placement of forearm in neutral or slight pronation.

- Resection of synostosis and interposition of autologous tissue (vascularized or nonvascularized grafts) or allograft between the radius and ulna.
  ○ Outcomes
    - Complications: chronic wrist and elbow pain, compartment syndrome, and neurovascular injury.
    - Recurrent deformity is common.

CAMPTODACTYLY

- **General concepts:** congenital flexion contracture at the PIP joint, which can be reducible or irreducible
- **Epidemiology:** can be sporadic or inherited in an autosomal-dominant fashion with variable penetrance
- **Presentation**
  ○ Majority of patients present with mild or asymptomatic, small finger PIP contractures with minimal functional deficit, usually bilateral
  ○ Classification
    - Type 1: flexion contracture presents in infancy
    - Type 2: presents gradually in school age; may progress to severe contractures
    - Type 3: bilateral involvement of multiple digits, usually associated with other congenital syndromes
  ○ Flexor digitorum superficialis (FDS) is contracted with atrophic or absent muscle belly.
- **Treatment**
  ○ Nonoperative management (serial casting and splinting) is indicated for those patients with mild deformity and minimal functional impairment.
  ○ Operative release of the PIP joint considered for severe PIP joint contractures (>60°).

CONGENITAL CLASPED THUMB

- **General concepts:** lack of passive metacarpophalangeal (MP) joint extension due to soft tissue deficiency, extrinsic tendon hypoplasia or absence, intrinsic muscle contracture, and MP joint contracture
- **Presentation**
  ○ Type 1: thumb flexible, absence or hypoplasia of extensor mechanism
  ○ Type 2: joint contracture, collateral ligament abnormality, first web space contracture, thenar muscle abnormality
  ○ Type 3: fixed flexion and adduction deformity at the IP, MP, and CMC joints; arthrogryposis
- **Associated syndromes**
  ○ May be associated with ulnar-deviated fingers (ie, windblown hand), arthrogryposis, Freeman-Sheldon syndrome
- **Treatment**
  ○ For type 1, conservative management preferred
  ○ For types 2 and 3:
    - Intrinsic muscle contracture: release adductor pollicis, thenar muscles, and palmar fascia
    - Deficiency of the soft tissue: Z-plasty techniques
    - Extrinsic tendon abnormalities
      □ Extensor pollicis longus (EPL)/extensor pollicis brevis (EPB) hypoplasia or absence: transfer of EIP or FDS to EPL
      □ Flexor pollicis longus (FPL) contracture: stepwise lengthening of FPL

CLINODACTYLY

- **General concepts**
  ○ Bony deformity resulting in radioulnar angulation of the digit distal to the MP joint >10°
  ○ Middle phalanx most affected because last bone to ossify

- **Epidemiology**
  - ○ Autosomal dominant with variable penetrance
  - ○ Bilateral
  - ○ Incidence is variable from 1% to 20%
  - ○ More common in males
- **Associated syndromes**
  - ○ Down syndrome
  - ○ Apert syndrome
- **Presentation**
  - ○ Growth deformity due to insult at the epiphyseal growth plate that restricts growth along one side of the bone: results in a triangular or "delta" phalanx.
  - ○ Most commonly seen as radial inclination of the small finger due to triangular or trapezoidal shape of the middle phalanx.
  - ○ Deviation may interfere with pinch and grip.
- **Treatment**
  - ○ Surgical intervention is indicated for severe shortening and angulation, resulting in severe functional limitations (eg, severe clinodactyly of the thumb or index finger that impairs pinch).
  - ○ Corrective osteotomy with/without bone grafting at skeletal maturity; may combine with Z-plasty or local flaps if there is a deficit of soft tissue.
  - ○ Partial/bracket epiphyseal resection and fat grafting to prevent fusion across the growth plate.

DUPLICATION

- Second most common congenital hand anomaly

THUMB DUPLICATION

- **General concepts: preaxial polydactyly involving duplication of varying elements of the thumb**
- **Epidemiology**
  - ○ 1/3000 live births
  - ○ Most common in Asian descent (2.2/1000), Native Americans (0.25/1000), and African Americans and Caucasians (0.08/1000)
  - ○ Inheritance: usually sporadic and does not require genetic counseling with the exception of triphalangeal thumb, which is inherited in an autosomal dominant fashion
  - ○ **Associated syndrome:** type VII could be associated with Holt-Oram syndrome, Fanconi anemia, Blackfan-Diamond syndrome
- **Presentation**
  - ○ Usually unilateral
  - ○ Wassel-Flatt classification is based on the level of duplication and number of elements (**Table 31-4**)
  - ○ Type IV is most common
- **Treatment**
  - ○ Reconstruction usually performed around the ages of 12-24 months to correspond with the development of pinch grasp.
  - ○ Reconstruction depends on the degree of hypoplasia, joint stability, and thumb alignment.
  - ○ Unusual connection between FPL and EPL tendon on radial side of thumb, called pollex abductus, need to be released to prevent postoperative angulation.
  - ○ Types I and II
    - ▪ Resection of radial duplication
    - ▪ Central resection of bone, soft tissue, and nail and fusion of elements (Bilhaut-Cloquet procedure)

TABLE 31-4 Wassel-Flatt Classification of Thumb Duplications

Type		Frequency (%)	
I	Incomplete, bifid duplication of the distal phalanx	4	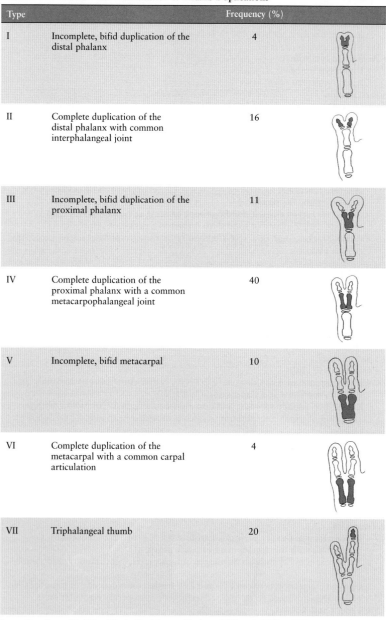
II	Complete duplication of the distal phalanx with common interphalangeal joint	16	
III	Incomplete, bifid duplication of the proximal phalanx	11	
IV	Complete duplication of the proximal phalanx with a common metacarpophalangeal joint	40	
V	Incomplete, bifid metacarpal	10	
VI	Complete duplication of the metacarpal with a common carpal articulation	4	
VII	Triphalangeal thumb	20	

Images From Berger RA, Weiss AC, eds. *Hand Surgery*. Lippincott Williams & Wilkins; 2004.

- o Types III and IV
  - ▪ Ablation of the radial duplicate
  - ▪ *Radial collateral ligament reconstruction
- o Types V and VI
  - ▪ Ablation of the radial duplicate
  - ▪ *Radial collateral ligament reconstruction
  - ▪ *Intrinsic muscle reattachment
  - ▪ *Corrective osteotomy
- o Type VII complex, multistage reconstruction

ULNAR POLYDACTYLY

- **General concepts:** accessory digit is present on the postaxial aspect of the hand
- **Epidemiology**
  - o *Most common presentation of polydactyly
  - o Autosomal dominant with variable penetrance
  - o More common in African Americans (1 in 143 births) compared with Caucasians (1 in 1400 births)
- **Associated syndromes:** chondroectodermal dysplasia (Ellis-van Creveld syndrome)
- **Presentation:** may be well developed (type A), or rudimentary and pedunculated (type B)
- **Treatment**
  - o Operative ablation or excision is preferred rather than bedside ligation in order to minimize long-term deformity.
  - o Well-developed accessory digits may require transfer of the ulnar collateral ligament and abductor digiti minimi, and identification and ablation of the accessory neurovascular bundle.

CENTRAL POLYDACTYLY

- **General concepts:** duplication of digits within the central aspect of the hand
- **Epidemiology:** much less common than preaxial and postaxial polydactyly (5%-15% of all polydactyly)
- **Associated syndrome:** not enough reported in the literature to ascertain
- **Presentation**
  - o Ring finger is most commonly duplicated
  - o May present in conjunction with syndactyly and can be discerned on radiographs
- **Treatment**
  - o Functional accessory digit without syndactyly may not require surgical intervention.
  - o Accessory digit with stiffness or functional limitation should undergo ray resection. If present with syndactyly, may require only partial resection with reconstruction to maintain function.

MIRROR HAND

- **General concepts:** symmetric duplication of the hand at the midline
- **Presentation**
  - o Central digit with three digits along the radial and ulnar aspect (duplicated middle, ring, and small fingers) and an absent thumb.
  - o Ulna is duplicated and radius is absent; ulnar carpal elements are duplicated.
  - o Hand is radially deviated; wrist extensor tendons may be absent and extension is weak. Limited pronation and supination.
- ***Pathophysiology:** duplication of the ZPA
- **Treatment:** reduce accessory digits to four digits and pollicization to create a thumb

OVERGROWTH

MACRODACTYLY

- **General concepts:** overgrowth of all digital structures
- **Epidemiology**
  - ○ Most seen in radial digits, especially index finger
  - ○ Very rare. Most cases are unilateral
- **Associated syndromes:** majority are sporadic cases but can be associated with neurofibromatosis, Ollier disease, Maffucci syndrome, Proteus syndrome, and Klippel-Trenaunay-Weber syndrome
- **Presentation**
  - ○ Usually progressive, disproportionate growth and stiffness
  - ○ Growth ceases with physeal closure at skeletal maturity
  - ○ Static type: digit large at birth, affected digit grows at the same rate as other fingers
  - ○ Progressive type: digit large at birth, and grows disproportionately
- **Treatment**
  - ○ Challenging to recreate normal appearing digit and frequently requires multiple procedures
  - ○ Growth-limiting procedures: epiphysiodesis
  - ○ Digit reduction: soft tissue debulking
  - ○ Amputation

UNDERGROWTH

THUMB HYPOPLASIA/ABSENCE (FIG. 31-2)

- **General concepts**
  - ○ Spectrum of thumb abnormalities ranging from mild hypoplasia to complete absence of soft tissue and skeletal elements
- **Epidemiology:** often seen in conjunction with radial longitudinal deficiency
- **Associated syndromes**
  - ○ Holt-Oram syndrome
  - ○ Fanconi anemia
  - ○ TAR
  - ○ VACTERL
- **Presentation**
  - ○ Blauth classification: five degrees of thumb hypoplasia (Table 31-5)
    - ▪ Type 1: smaller thumb but normal functioning
    - ▪ Types 2 and 3a present with a stable CMC joint
    - ▪ *Type IIIb, Type IV, and Type V: CMC joint absent
- **Treatment**
  - ○ Consider treatment within 2 years of age as pinch grip and opposition is developing
  - ○ Type I: no surgical treatment indicated
  - ○ Type II and Type IIIa
    - ▪ Deepening first web space with Z-plasty techniques
    - ▪ Opponensplasty using abductor digiti minimi (Huber transfer) or FDS from the ring finger
    - ▪ EIP to EPL transfer
  - ○ *Type IIIb, Type IV, and Type V: ablation of the remnant thumb if present, and index finger pollicization
    - ▪ General pollicization steps
      - ▫ Index finger elevated as an island flap on radial and ulnar neurovascular pedicles, dorsal veins, and tendons
        - ▪ Metacarpal osteotomized at the level of the distal epiphyseal plate

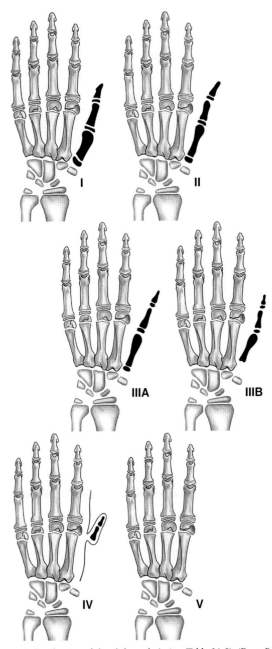

Figure 31-2 Blauth classification of thumb hypoplasia (see Table 31-5). (From Berger RA, Weiss AC, eds. *Hand Surgery*. Lippincott Williams & Wilkins; 2004.)

TABLE 31-5 Blauth Classification of Thumb Hypoplasia

Classification		Features	Treatment options
I		Mild hypoplasia with all elements present	No treatment
II		Absence of intrinsic thenar muscles, narrowing of first web space, UCL insufficiency	No treatment First web space release Opponensplasty (abductor digiti quinti, ring FDS)
III	A: Stable CMC joint	Type II features as well as extrinsic tendon deficiencies, hypoplastic metacarpal	No treatment First web space release Ulnar collateral ligament stabilization Opponensplasty (abductor digiti quinti, ring FDS)
	B: Unstable CMC joint		Pollicization
IV		Absent metacarpal and rudimentary phalanges; skin bridge with neurovascular bundle "Pouce flottant"	Pollicization
V		Total absence	Pollicization

CMC, carpometacarpophalangeal; FDS, flexor digitorum superficialis; UCL, ulnar collateral ligament.

- ▢ Finger pronated between 140° and 160°
- ▢ Metacarpal fixated in 45° abduction palmar to base of the index finger metacarpal
- ▢ Functional elements following pollicization
  - ▪ Index metacarpal head → new thumb CMC joint
  - ▪ First dorsal interosseous muscle → new abductor pollicis brevis
  - ▪ First palmar interosseous muscle → new adductor pollicis
  - ▪ Index finger EDC → new Abductor pollicis longus
  - ▪ EIP → new EPL

BRACHYDACTYLY

- **General concepts**
  - ○ Shortened digits with all elements present
  - ○ Index and small finger most commonly affected digits
  - ○ Middle phalanx most commonly affected bone
- **Epidemiology**: rare, except for type A3 (brachydactyly-clinodactyly) and D (stub thumb), which have a prevalence of 2%
- **Associated syndromes**
  - ○ Frequently inherited in autosomal dominant fashion
  - ○ Could be associated with Treacher Collins, Apert syndrome, Poland syndrome, Cornelia de Lange and Bloom syndromes
- **Presentation**
  - ○ Often seen in conjunction with other congenital hand anomalies (syndactyly, clinodactyly, and camptodactyly) and syndromes (eg, Poland syndrome, Apert syndrome, orofaciodigital syndrome)
  - ○ Can be associated with syndactyly (eg, Poland syndrome due to disturbance in development of the subclavian artery)

- Treatment
  - ○ Considered if significant functional limitation is present
    - ■ Lengthening:
      - □ Osteotomy and nonvascularized bone grafting (eg, toe proximal phalanx graft)—inconsistent results
      - □ Distraction osteogenesis—can produce 1-4 cm increased length
      - □ Microsurgical toe to hand transfer
      - □ Syndactyly release if present
  - ○ Common postoperative complications include digital stiffness and joint contracture

CONGENITAL CONSTRICTION BAND SYNDROME

CONSTRICTION RING SYNDROME/AMNIOTIC BAND SYNDROME (FIG. 31-3)

- **General concepts:**
  - ○ Circumferential constriction of the extremity or digits due to amniotic disruption and band formation
  - ○ Intrinsic mechanism: vascular disruption in the embryo
  - ○ Extrinsic mechanism: amniotic bands encircle and strangulate parts of limb in utero
- **Epidemiology**
  - ○ 1:1200-1:15000 births
  - ○ Usually affect distal extremities
  - ○ Prenatal risk factors: prematurity <37 weeks, low birth weight <2500 g, maternal drug exposure, maternal illness or trauma during pregnancy
- **Associated syndromes**
  - ○ No evidence of hereditary disposition
  - ○ Can occur with other deformities such as club foot, leg length discrepancy, cleft lip and palate, body wall defect

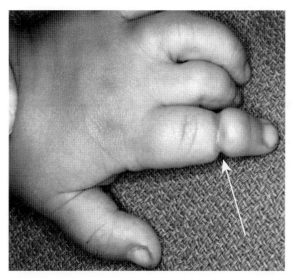

Figure 31-3 Constriction (amnionic) band syndrome. *Arrow* points to constriction band of the index finger. (From Berger RA, Weiss AC, eds. *Hand Surgery*. Lippincott Williams & Wilkins; 2004.)

- **Presentation**
  - Index, middle, and ring fingers most commonly affected
  - Extremity or digit is hypoplastic or absent distal to the band, and amputation, lymphedema, and acrosyndactyly
- **Treatment**
  - Elective release at 1 year of age is indicated to improve function (grip and pinch) and hand appearance; emergent release is indicated for arterial or venous compromise.
  - Constriction ring
    - Z-plasty release of constriction band along the lateral aspect of the digit to minimize scarring.
    - Advancement of adipofascial flap to recontour irregularities along the aspect of the digit.
  - Acrosyndactyly
    - Digits may be released using syndactyly release techniques to reconstruct the commissure.

GENERALIZED SKELETAL DEFORMITIES

CONGENITAL TRIGGER FINGER

- **General concepts**: flexion deformity due to either thickening of the flexor tendon and/or narrowing of the tendon sheath that is most commonly seen in the thumb and more rarely seen in the other digits.
- **Epidemiology**
  - Appears to occur shortly after birth, may not truly be congenital
  - Prevalence of 3 in 1000 children
- **Associated syndrome**: usually occurs sporadically without associated syndromes
- **Presentation**
  - Most commonly presents as a flexion deformity at the IP joint and **rarely with classic triggering**
  - Notta node: thickening of FPL tendon, which may present as a palpable nodule where tendon cannot pass distally through the tight pulley system
- **Treatment**
  - Several studies suggest nonsurgical treatment such as stretching lead to resolution in 6 months in 50% of children.
  - A1 pulley release is typically performed if deformity has failed to resolve by 1-3 years of age.
  - Notta node or FPL thickening does not require resection or debulking.

ARTHROGRYPOSIS

- **General concepts**
  - **Multiple** nonprogressive joint contractures due to a lack of fetal development
  - Thought to be secondary to mutations in at least five genes that code contractile apparatus of myofibers (TNNI2, TNNT3, TPM3, MYH3, and MYH8)
- **Epidemiology**: in 3000 births
- **Associated syndromes**: etiology is variable and can be related to genetic syndromes (eg, Beals syndrome and Freeman-Sheldon syndrome) or sporadic.
- **Presentation**
  - *Most commonly present with bilateral, symmetric contractures of the upper extremity, including shoulder adduction and internal rotation, elbow extension, forearm pronation, wrist flexion and ulnar deviation, and finger flexion.
  - Muscle atrophy is often present.
- **Treatment**
  - Nonoperative
    - Passive range of motion; stretching beginning in infancy
    - Static progressive splinting or serial casting if needed

- ○ Operative
  - ▪ Shoulder: corrective osteotomy of the humerus
  - ▪ Elbow: posterior capsulotomy and triceps lengthening to achieve passive elbow flexion
  - ▪ Wrist: proximal row carpectomy, soft tissue distraction, and corrective osteotomy

OTHER DEFORMITIES

MADELUNG DEFORMITY

- **General concepts**
  - ○ Excessive radial and palmar angulation of the distal radius due to a growth disturbance at the ulnar aspect of the physis.
  - ○ Growth disturbance at the physis may be due to a bony lesion or due to abnormal ligamentous tethering of the lunate to the distal radius.
  - ○ Associated with an abnormally short volar radioulnar ligament (Vickers ligament) that restricts growth across the volar-ulnar physis. As the remaining physis grows, radius deforms with increasing radial inclination and volar tilt. Unaffected ulna continues to grow creating ulnar positive variance. Eventually, DRUJ fails to form and distal ulna is unstable.
- **Epidemiology:** more common in females, usually bilateral
- **Associated syndromes:** Leri Weill dyschondrosteosis: genetic disease characterized by short stature, bilateral wrist deformity
- **Presentation**
  - ○ Patients typically present at school age, from 6 to 13 years
  - ○ Deformity includes dorsal prominence of the ulna and ulnar positive variance
  - ○ Concave, foreshortened appearance of the forearm
  - ○ The degree of functional impairment varies. Patients asymptomatic or complain of pain with ulnar deviation and wrist extension
- **Treatment**
  - ○ No treatment indicated for painless deformity
  - ○ Symptomatic deformity:
    - ▪ Release of Vickers ligament and physiolysis of the radius
    - ▪ Radial dome osteotomy
    - ▪ Ulnar shortening osteotomy

CONGENITAL DISLOCATION OF THE RADIAL HEAD

- **General concepts**
  - ○ Most common congenital elbow deformity
  - ○ Usually bilateral
  - ○ Posterior dislocation of radial head most common
  - ○ Associated with congenital radioulnar synostosis
- **Epidemiology:** very rare (<1 in 100 000 births)
- **Associated syndrome**
  - ○ *Nail-patella syndrome: genetic disorder with small, poorly developed nails and patella
  - ○ Antecubital pterygium
  - ○ Ulnar dysplasia
- **Presentation**
  - ○ Radial head may be dislocated anteriorly, posteriorly, or laterally, and patients present with a lack of forearm rotation.
  - ○ Diagnosis may be confused with traumatic dislocation.
  - ○ Majority of patients are asymptomatic with minimal functional limitations.
- **Treatment**

○ Observation
  ▪ Open reduction and reconstruction of the annular ligament can be considered in symptomatic patients but often unreliable and unpredictable results.
  ▪ Radial head excision can be considered for symptomatic patients with degenerative changes.

PEARLS

1. Significant congenital anomalies—more than a simple syndactyly or ulnar polydactyly—warrant evaluation by a geneticist.
2. Reconstructions in children–keep in mind that the extremity is growing and may need multiple procedures for a final outcome.
3. Never release syndactyly on both sides of the same digit at the same operation due to the risk of devascularization.

QUESTIONS YOU WILL BE ASKED

1. Incision designs:
   a. Syndactyly release incisions, particularly if full-thickness skin grafting is not planned.
   b. Pollicization incisions, Buck-Gramcko versus Ezaki.
2. Wassel-type thumb duplications.
   See Table 31-4.
3. What is the most common location of syndactyly?
   Between the middle and ring fingers followed by the ring and small fingers.
4. What is the most important variable when determining treatment of a hypoplastic thumb?
   Carpometacarpal ligament stability.

Recommended Readings
1. Bates SJ, Hansen SL, Jones NF. Reconstruction of congenital differences of the hand. *Plast Reconstr Surg.* 2009;124(1):128e-143e.
2. Comer GC, Potter M, Ladd AL. Polydactyly of the hand. *J Am Acad Orthop Surg.* 2018;26(3):75-82.
3. Goldfarb CA. Congenital hand anomalies: a review of the literature, 2009–2012. *J Hand Surg Am.* 2013;38(9):1854-1859.
4. Kozin SH. Upper-extremity congenital anomalies. *J Bone Joint Surg Am.* 2003;85-A(8):1564-1576.

32 Brachial Plexus Injuries

Ayobami L. Ward and Shay Nguyen

Section III: Upper Extremity

OVERVIEW

ANATOMY (TABLE 32-1, FIG. 32-1)

- Mnemonic: Read That Dang Cadaver Book → Root, Trunk, Division, Cord, Branch
- **Roots** (Preganglionic, Supraclavicular)
  - Ventral rami of C5-T1
  - Dorsal scapular n. (C5) → rhomboid minor and rhomboid major m.
  - Long thoracic n. (C5-C7) → serratus anterior m.
  - Scalene branches (C5-C8) → scalene m.
- **Trunks** (Postganglionic, Supraclavicular)
  - Upper (C5-C6; convergence at Erb point)
    - Direct branches
      - Suprascapular n. → supraspinatus and infraspinatus m.
      - Subclavian n. → subclavius m. (Useful landmark during brachial plexus exposure)
  - Middle (C7)
  - Lower (C8-T1)
- **Divisions** (Postganglionic, Retroclavicular)
  - Anterior
    - From upper and middle trunk → lateral cord
    - From lower trunk → medial cord
    - Go to the flexor region of the arm
  - Posterior: all three posterior divisions form the posterior cord and go to the extensor side of the arm.
- **Cords** (Postganglionic, Infraclavicular)
  - Lateral
    - Becomes musculocutaneous n. and part of median n.
    - Direct branch: lateral pectoral n. → pectoralis major m.
  - Posterior
    - Becomes radial n. and axillary n.
    - Direct branches (proximal to distal):
      - Upper subscapular n. → subscapularis m.
      - Thoracodorsal n. → latissimus dorsi m.
      - Lower subscapular n. → subscapularis and teres major m.
  - Medial
    - Becomes ulnar n. and part of median n.
    - Direct branches (proximal to distal)
      - Medial pectoral n. → pectoralis major and minor m.
      - Medial brachial cutaneous n. → sensory to the medial distal one-third of arm
      - Medial antebrachial cutaneous n. → sensory to the medial forearm and skin overlying the olecranon

---

*Denotes common in-service examination topics.

TABLE 32-1 Brachial Plexus Anatomy

Roots	Trunks	Divisions	Cords	Terminal branches
C5	Upper	Anterior	Lateral	Musculocutaneous n.
C6		Posterior		
C7	Middle	Anterior	Posterior	Axillary n.
		Posterior		Radial n.
C8	Lower	Anterior	Medial	Median n.
T1		Posterior		Ulnar n.

- Branches (Postganglionic, Infraclavicular)
  - See Chapter 29: Hand and Wrist Anatomy and Examination for innervation and function
  - Musculocutaneous n. (C5-C7)
  - Radial n. (C5-C8)
  - Median n. (C6-T1)
  - Axillary n. (C5-C7)
  - Ulnar n. (C8-T1)
- Vascular associations
  - Supraclavicular Region: subclavian artery is in close proximity to lower roots/lower trunk.
  - Infraclavicular Region: cords surround the axillary artery (cords are named with respect to the axillary artery).

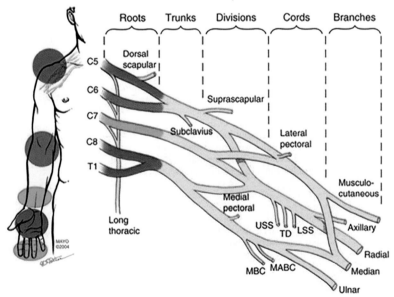

The brachial plexus

Figure 32-1 Brachial plexus. (Used with permission of Mayo Foundation for Medical Education and Research, all rights reserved.)

EPIDEMIOLOGY

- Brachial Plexus Birth Palsy
    - ○ Incidence is 0.4-5.1 per 1000 births, with incidence thought to be decreasing over time.
    - ○ Risk factors: macrosomia, shoulder dystocia, and instrumented birth.
    - ○ Most commonly involve upper trunk.
- Traumatic Brachial Plexus Injury
    - ○ Incidence between 0.17/100 000 and 1.6/100 000 per year.
    - ○ More common in young males. Most are closed lesions caused by motor vehicle accidents involving the supraclavicular plexus. Open lacerations and gunshot wounds are less common.

PATHOLOGY

- Classification of Nerve Injuries: see **Chapter 45: Nerve Injuries, Neuromas, and Compression Syndromes.**
- **Trauma**
    - ○ Traction injury: mild stretch to rupture or avulsion
        - ▪ 2/3 supraclavicular, 1/3 retroclavicular/infraclavicular.
        - ▪ C8-T1 are more likely to avulse, while C5-C6 are more likely to stretch/rupture (stronger supporting tissue).
        - ▪ Low-energy injuries: typically stretch injuries with potential for spontaneous regeneration; may interfere with microcirculation and cause ischemic injury.
        - ▪ High-energy injuries: may include rupture of plexus or avulsion of nerve roots. Early surgical interventions can improve function.
        - ▪ Associated injuries such as dislocations, fractures, and vascular injuries can contribute to brachial plexus injury.
    - ○ Gunshot injury: most gunshot wounds associated brachial plexus injury are in continuity and should be observed.
    - ○ Penetrating injury: plexus elements likely transected → typically requires nerve exploration.
    - ○ May be associated with vascular injuries
        - ▪ Axillary artery and vein injuries are often associated with plexus injury.
        - ▪ Pseudoaneurysm can form over time and compress the plexus, leading to progressive loss of function.
    - ○ **Common patterns**
        - ▪ **Erb-Duchenne palsy** 15%, C5-C6 injury. Due to head/shoulder distraction. Most common in motorcycle accidents and shoulder dystocia. Deficits in shoulder stability, abduction, and external and internal rotation; deficits in elbow flexion and forearm supernation. Sensory deficit in C5-C6 distributions.
        - ▪ **Erb-plus:** 20%-35%, C6-C7 injury. Erb-Duchenne plus variable C7 involvement such as weakness of elbow, wrist, and finger extensors, as well as sensory deficit in proximal arm, thumb, index and middle fingers.
        - ▪ **Klumpke palsy:** 10%, C8-T1 injury. Due to traction on an abducted arm. Weakness of the hand intrinsics, extrinsics, and finger extensors. Sensory loss in the ulnar digits, medial forearm, and distal arm. May result in Horner syndrome (ptosis, miosis, anhidrosis).
        - ▪ **Pan-plexus (C5-T1):** 50%-75%; completely flail arm and insensate hand.
        - ▪ First rib fractures may cause lower trunk injuries.
        - ▪ Clavicular fracture may cause injuries to the posterior cord, axillary n. or suprascapular n.
        - ▪ Mid-humeral fractures are often associated with radial n. injury.
- **Thoracic Outlet Syndrome (TOS)**
    - ○ **Neurogenic: 95% of TOS.** Compression of C8/T1 nerve roots associated with cervical rib or compressive band arising from the first rib. May present with Gilliatt-Sumner hand (wasting of the thenar and hypothenar muscle groups).

- Vascular: pain or sensory symptoms predominate. Can elicit cessation of radial pulse with Wright test or Adson test. Usually no cervical rib present.
- **Tumor**
  - Schwannomas: well-defined margins that allows for total resection
  - Neurofibromas: associated with NF1. Margins often indistinct
- **Neuropathy**
  - Compression: for example, Pancoast syndrome. C8-T1 more common. Workup should include apical lordotic chest x-ray.
  - Diabetes: typically distal symmetric sensory polyneuropathy, although can mimic brachial plexopathy with asymmetric and/or truncal presentation.
  - Vasculitis: rare cause of brachial neuritis.
  - Idiopathic brachial neuritis (Parsonage-Turner syndrome): acute onset of intense shoulder pain followed by shoulder weakness that improves spontaneously by 3-4 weeks after onset. Upper trunk predominant. Presumably immune mediated.
  - Post irradiation: for example, postmastectomy radiation. Can cause fibrosis and edema of the brachial plexus. Sensory loss and pain predominant.
  - Inherited: for example, hereditary neuropathy with pressure palsies. Rare. Painless brachial plexus palsies.
  - Posttraumatic.

PREOPERATIVE EVALUATION

HISTORY

- Trauma: follow standard trauma evaluation guidelines and patient should be stabilized. Ask about the injury mechanism, associated injuries, loss of consciousness, paresthesia, and weakness of affected and nonaffected limbs. Severe pain in an anesthetic extremity may be seen in root avulsion injuries.
- Chronic: ask about time course of symptoms and pain, autonomic changes, and occupational and recreational risk factors.

PHYSICAL EXAM

- The goal is to determine the location and severity of injury.
- Exam should include detailed motor and sensory exam, examining the unaffected limb, range of motion (ROM), evaluation for atrophy, reflexes, and pulses.
- Specific Exam Findings
  - *Winged scapula: serratus anterior weakness (long thoracic n.) or rhomboid weakness (dorsal scapular n.) indicates preganglionic injury to upper nerve roots (C5-C7). Trapezius weakness and rotator cuff instability can mimic scapula winging.
  - Horner syndrome: ipsilateral ptosis, miosis, and anhidrosis. Associated with C8 and/or T1 nerve root avulsion.
  - "Waiter's tip" deformity: shoulder internal rotation, elbow extension, wrist flexion. Suggestive of an upper plexus lesion (C5-C6) such as Erb-Duchenne palsy.
  - "Claw hand" deformity: MP joints extension, IP joint flexions. Suggestive of lower plexus lesion such as Klumpke palsy or TOS.
- Differentiating Between C8 vs Ulnar Nerve Injury
  - C8 root injury: loss of all intrinsic hand muscles (both ulnar and median)
  - Ulnar nerve injury: sensory loss over ulnar aspect of the fourth and all of the fifth fingers
- Evaluate Distal CN XI (Spinal Accessory N.): innervates trapezius m. Frequently used for nerve transfer.

DIAGNOSTIC STUDIES

- Radiographs: obtain in patients with high-energy trauma to rule out fractures and dislocations

- Paralyzed (elevated) diaphragm: phrenic n. (C3-C5) injury. Indicates proximal brachial plexus injury.
- Cervical transverse process fractures: associated with plexus avulsions.
- Rib fractures: first or second ribs associated with brachial plexus injuries. Rib fractures may be important if considering intercostal nn. for nerve transfer.
- Ultrasound: noninvasive. Can image portions of the plexus and be used in guidance for plexus/nerve blocks.
- Computed Tomography (CT) Myelogram: most reliable for identifying root avulsion and traumatic pseudomeningoceles. Typically performed at least 3-4 weeks after the injury to allow for potential blood clots to dissolve and pseudomeningocele to form.
- Magnetic Resonance Imaging (MRI): can identify masses, large neuromas, root abnormalities, inflammation, edema, and traumatic pseudomeningoceles.
- Electromyography/Nerve Conduction Studies (EMG/NCSs): can localize and characterize the nerve lesion. Can be used to assess recovery.
  - Usually obtained at least 3-4 weeks after injury when Wallerian degeneration has occurred; nerve may still respond to electrical stimulus prior to this time.
  - Normal sensory nerve action potentials with dermatomal anesthesia and absence of motor nerve conduction suggest preganglionic root avulsion.
  - Nascent motor unit potentials: low amplitude, polyphasic, variable. Suggests reinnervation.
- Compound Nerve Action Potentials (CNAPs): more sensitive than EMG. Often used intraoperatively for operative decision making. Absence of CNAPs 2-6 months after injury: likely complete transection.

MANAGEMENT

GENERAL TREATMENT CONCEPTS

- Obstetric Palsy: 66%-92% of cases resolve over time. Repair generally not considered until older than 6 months.
- Laceration injuries in proximity to the brachial plexus require immediate surgical exploration and repair.
- Gunshot injuries should be observed because in most cases, the plexus is in continuity and has the potential to spontaneously recover. If there is no evidence of clinical or EMG recovery, then surgery is indicated.
- **Traction Injuries**
  - If there is clear evidence of complete nerve root avulsion or nerve rupture, surgery is indicated without the observation period.
  - Otherwise, observe for spontaneous recovery. If there is no evidence of clinical or EMG recovery, then surgery is indicated.
  - Timing for delayed surgery
    - Timing is based on multiple factors, including history/mechanism of injury, physical exam, electrophysiologic studies, imaging studies, and surgeon's preference.
    - Should rarely wait for more than 6 months.
- **Neurolysis**
  - Indicated if there is intraoperative finding of a postganglionic neuroma-in-continuity and a positive CNAP.
  - Removal of scar tissue from around the nerve or between the fascicles.
  - Start with uninjured portion of nerve and move toward injured segment.
- **End to End Repair**
  - Possible if short nerve gap is present (eg, after resection of surrounding neuroma or with sharp transection).
  - Preferred over grafting, as it produces better functional results.

○ Avoid tension across the repair. May need to mobilize the nerve proximally or distally.
- **Nerve Grafting**
  ○ Indicated for postganglionic nerve ruptures or postganglionic neuromas that do not conduct a CNAP, when the gap is to too large to perform direct end to end repair
  ○ Length of graft = length of gap + 10% of distance
  ○ Possible donor grafts: sural (most commonly used), superficial radial, or medial antebrachial cutaneous, lateral antebrachial cutaneous, and dorsal ulnar cutaneous nn.
- **Nerve Transfer** (Also Known as Neurotization or Nerve Crossing)
  ○ Indicated in preganglionic injuries (nerve grafting cannot adequately repair avulsions) and some postganglionic injuries
  ○ Advantages over nerve grafting
    ▪ Closer to end organ → more rapid and reliable recovery
    ▪ Delivers large number of "pure" axons
    ▪ Repair is outside of injured and scarred zone
    ▪ One repair site instead of two repair sites
  ○ Common nerve transfers
    ▪ Descending cervical plexus or spinal accessory nerve to suprascapular nerve to restore shoulder abduction in upper trunk avulsion injuries
    ▪ Medial pectoral or thoracodorsal nerve to musculocutaneous or axillary nerve to restore elbow flexion and/or shoulder abduction
    ▪ Medial pectoral or intercostal nerve to musculocutaneous nerve to restore elbow flexion

POSTOPERATIVE CARE

- Recovery may take years.
- Must preserve ROM with physical therapy. Nerve transfers require motor retraining.

ADJUNCT PROCEDURES

- Tendon transfer, functional muscle transfer, wrist fusion
- Can be done at any time.
- Considered in patients with late presentation (ie, >12 months after injury, with severe muscle atrophy), failed brachial plexus reconstructions, global avulsions, wrist palsy.
- Upper extremity amputation followed by prosthesis can be done for painful flail arm.

PEARLS

1. Preganglionic (avulsion) injury is more common at C8-T1.
2. Peripheral nerves regenerate approximately 1 mm/day or 1 in/month.
3. Laceration-induced nerve injuries should be explored and repaired within 3 days, due to significantly better outcomes.
4. Lesions in continuity should be observed (up to 6 months) to evaluate for spontaneous recovery.
5. C5-C6 neonatal brachial plexus injuries have better outcomes than other brachial plexus injuries in this group.
6. Motor nerve regeneration must take place prior to atrophy of the target muscle.
7. The sensory roots of the median nerve come from C5-C7, while the motor roots come from C8-T1.
8. Repairs of C5-C6 root injuries generally have better outcomes than C8-T1 or panbrachial plexus injuries.

QUESTIONS YOU WILL BE ASKED

1. What is the best timing for repair of traction injuries of the plexus?
   If no recovery is seen after 3-6 months, intervention and reconstruction are indicated.
2. Which nerve roots supply the brachial plexus?
   C5-C8, T1.
3. Which part of the cord is most affected by obstetrical brachial plexus injury?
   The upper plexus.
4. A patient presents with numbness/tingling in the ring and small fingers, weakness of interossei, adductor pollicis, and the abductor pollicis brevis. Where is the most likely cause of symptomatology, cubital tunnel syndrome (ulnar nerve) or C8 radiculopathy?
   C8 radiculopathy. The median nerve innervates the LOAF muscles—lumbricals 1 and 2, opponens pollicis, abductor pollicis brevis, and the flexor pollicis brevis muscles. The ulnar nerve innervates the rest of the hand intrinsic muscles. Ulnar n. innervates all the rest of hand intrinsics. By comparision, C8 innervates all the hand intrinsics (both median and ulnar).
5. What is the clinical presentation of an upper cord injury?
   Adducted shoulder, medially rotated arm, extended elbow, and palm up.
6. Anterior interosseous nerve (AIN) dysfunction presents as the inability for a patient to make what common sign with the fingers?
   "Ok sign." AIN innervates the flexor pollicis longus and flexor digitorum profundus muscles to the index and middle fingers. Thus, patients cannot appropriately flex the distal tip of the thumb and index finger.

Recommended Readings
1. Shin AY, Pulos N. *Operative Brachial Plexus Surgery: Clinical Evaluation and Management Strategies.* Springer; 2021.
2. Spinner RJ, Shin AY, Elhassan BT, Bishop AT. *Traumatic Brachial Plexus Injury. Green's Operative Hand Surgery.* 8th ed. Elsevier; 2022:34, 1304-1362. ISBN 0-323-69794-1

Distal Radius and Ulna Fractures

Cecilia M. Pesavento and Alexander N. Khouri

DISTAL RADIUS FRACTURES

OVERVIEW

- **Epidemiology**
  - Most commonly fractured bone in the human body
  - Accounts for 17% of all fractures treated in the emergency department and 75% of all forearm fractures
  - 4× more common in females
  - Bimodal distribution of patients
    - Young males (age 6-10) suffer high energy, athletic injuries.
    - Elderly females (age 60-70) suffer osteoporotic fractures after a fall on an outstretched hand (FOOSH).
- **Anatomy (Fig. 33-1)**
  - Normal anatomy—**rule of 11's (Table 33-1)**.
  - Ulnar variance is the relative length of the distal ulna compared to the distal radius
    - Positive ulnar variance (0 to +2 mm) leads to greater relative distribution of compressive load through the ulna compared to negative ulnar variance (−2 mm to 0).
  - Normal wrist motion: 120° flexion/extension, 50° radial/ulnar deviation.
  - Distal radius has three concave articular surfaces: scaphoid fossa, lunate fossa, and sigmoid notch.
  - Brachioradialis (BR) is the only tendon to insert onto the distal radius, attaches to the radial column, and is immediately volar to the first dorsal compartment. Pulls distal radius in dorsoradial direction, intraoperative release commonly performed to mobilize the fracture.
  - Lister tubercle: palpable bony protuberance on the dorsal distal radius, which separates the second and third extensor compartments and acts as a pulley for the extensor pollicis longus (EPL) tendon.
- Eponyms and Fracture Patterns
  - **Colles fracture**: extra-articular fracture with "dinner fork" deformity (dorsal displaced distal fragment), radial shortening, and associated ulnar styloid fracture
  - **Smith fracture** (reverse Colles): extra-articular fracture with "garden spade deformity" (volar displaced distal fragment)
  - **Barton fracture**: intra-articular shear fracture with fracture-dislocation of radiocarpal joint
  - **Chauffeur fracture**: intra-articular radial styloid fracture due to high energy mechanism
  - **Essex-Lopresti injury**: fracture of the radial head with disruption of the forearm interosseous membrane and distal radioulnar joint dislocation
  - **Monteggia fracture**: ulnar shaft fracture with associated radial head dislocation
  - **Die-punch fracture**: Intra-articular fracture of the lunate facet due to compression of the radius from the lunate
- Many different classification systems exist (AO, Fernandez, Mayo, Melone) but none is universally accepted, and they do not provide prognostic information.

---

*Denotes common in-service examination topics.

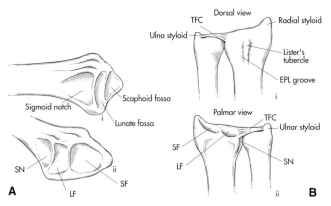

Figure 33-1 Anatomy of the articular surface of the distal radius. A. Three articular surfaces can be involved in distal radius fractures: scaphoid fossa (SF), lunate fossa (LF), and sigmoid notch (SN). (Axial [ii] and oblique [i] views.) **B.** Topographic landmarks of the distal radius. i, Dorsal view with palpable landmarks of the radial styloid, Lister's tubercle with ulnar-side groove for the extensor pollicis longus tendon (EPL groove), ulnar styloid, and triangular fibrocartilage (TFC). ii, Palmar view demonstrates palmar tilt (14°) of the articular surfaces of the distal radius, scaphoid fossa (SF), lunate fossa (LF), and sigmoid notch (SN). (From Cooney WP. *The Wrist: Diagnosis and Operative Treatment.* 2nd ed. Wolters Kluwer; 2011. Figure 12.1.)

EVALUATION

- **Presentation:** typically presents after FOOSH with compressive loading on a dorsiflexed wrist
- **History**
  - Age, gender, hand dominance, mechanism of injury, timing of injury, previous history of hand trauma or surgery
  - Past medical history: diabetes mellitus, steroids, peripheral arterial disease, systemic sclerosis or Raynaud disease, smoking status
  - Social determinants of health: baseline level of activity, avocation, occupation, and ability to participate in therapy
- **Physical Exam**
  - May present as classic "dinner fork deformity" with wrist pain and swelling or appear anatomically normal.
  - Perform a standard hand and wrist examination including motor/sensory function, circulation, and range of motion assessment.

TABLE 33-1 Normal and Radiographic Surgical Indications for Distal Radius Fractures—Rule of 11's

Measurement	Normal	Indication for surgery
Radial height	11 mm	>5 mm radial shortening
Radial inclination	22°	<15°
Volar tilt	11°	<5° angulation
Articular step-off	Congruous	>2 mm step-off

Surgical candidacy should also consider patient's overall health, baseline degree of activity, and presence of associated ipsilateral extremity injuries.

- o Palpate the anatomical snuffbox to assess for an associated scaphoid fracture.
- o Examine the entire upper extremity to rule out associated elbow or shoulder injuries.
- o Rule out associated carpal tunnel syndrome or compartment syndrome.
- **Diagnostics (Fig. 33-2)**
  - o PA view: evaluate radial inclination, radial height, ulnar variance, congruity of sigmoid notch and radiocarpal joint, scapholunate width, and baseline osteoarthritis.
  - o Lateral view: evaluate volar tilt, teardrop angle, extent of dorsal comminution. **Teardrop angle**: angle between line down long axis of radius and line drawn through center of lunate facet (normal 70°).
  - o Computed tomography (CT) and magnetic resonance imaging (MRI) are rarely ordered to assess carpal bone injury or better characterize a comminuted articular fracture.
- Characterize the Fracture: open vs closed, intra-articular vs extra-articular, displaced vs nondisplaced, comminuted, etc.
- Associated injuries outlined in **Table 33-2.**

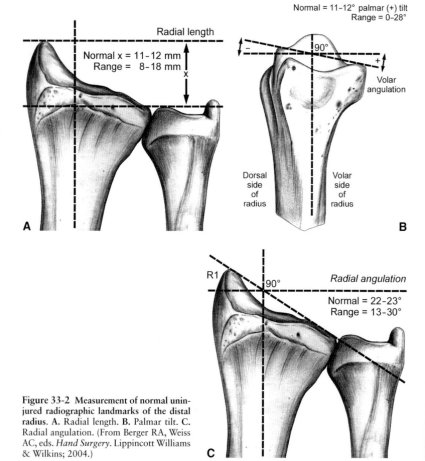

Figure 33-2 Measurement of normal uninjured radiographic landmarks of the distal radius. A. Radial length. B. Palmar tilt. C. Radial angulation. (From Berger RA, Weiss AC, eds. *Hand Surgery.* Lippincott Williams & Wilkins; 2004.)

TABLE 33-2 Distal Radius Fracture Commonly Associated Injuries

Associated injury	Comment
Median nerve injury	Indication for urgent reduction, often a self-limiting neuropraxia
Ulnar styloid fracture	Examine distal radioulnar joint (DRUJ) stability
Ligamentous injury	Examine for scapholunate ligament, lunotriquetral ligament, and/or radioulnar ligament injury
Vascular injury	Rare in closed fractures. Ulnar or radial artery injury can occur with high energy displaced fractures. Indication for emergent reduction and vascular evaluation if impairment persists after reduction
Compartment syndrome	<1% of DRFs result in compartment syndrome, associated with high energy trauma. Requires urgent reduction

TREATMENT

- General Principles
  - Goal is anatomic reduction to maintain wrist biomechanics
  - Restore "ARMS": angular congruity, radial alignment, motion, stability
- **Procedural Tips: closed bedside reduction**
  - Supplies: 10-mL syringe, 18 g and 27 g needles, povidone-iodine solution, 1% plain lidocaine without epinephrine, finger traps/kerlix and weight, splinting material, +/− c-arm (if available).
  - Perform a hematoma block by inserting a 10-mL syringe into the dorsal wrist angled distally toward the fracture site. Aspirate until blood is seen in the needle hub and inject 10 mL of 1% plain lidocaine into the fracture site.
  - Place the patient in finger traps. Position the arm with shoulder abducted 90° and elbow flexed 90°. Apply 5 to 10 lb of weight to the elbow. Patient may require additional IV morphine or valium to assist with forearm muscle relaxation.
  - First recreate the injury mechanism to disimpact the fragment and then apply axial traction and push distal segment in a dorsal, opposite direction to reduce the fracture. Avoid flexion and extreme ulnar deviation of the wrist to prevent carpal tunnel syndrome (Cotton-Loder positioning).
  - Use c-arm to assess postreduction radial height and volar tilt, if available.
  - Re-evaluate for carpal tunnel or compartment syndrome symptoms.
  - Apply a splint. Traditionally a sugar tong splint has been used if the distal radial ulnar joint (DRUJ) is involved to prevent supination/pronation. If the DRUJ is not involved or surgery is anticipated, volar resting splint is preferable for patient comfort.
  - Obtain postreduction films, elevate the extremity, and establish outpatient follow-up.
- **Management**
  - **Nonoperative management:** splint +/− closed reduction
    - Indications
      - Nondisplaced fracture
      - Extra-articular fracture that can be reduced to an acceptable deformity
      - <5 mm radial shortening
      - Dorsal angulation <5° or within 20° of contralateral distal radius
      - Poor surgical candidate due to baseline activity or medical comorbidities

- Nondisplaced extra-articular fractures may not require closed reduction and can be treated with splinting alone.
- Obtain rigid immobilization (or removable splint if minimally displaced) and establish serial clinic appointments for ongoing radiographic evaluation.
- Current research strongly supports nonoperative management in select adults >60 years.
  - Surgical management
    - Suggested criteria for surgery
      - Intra-articular displacement or step-off >2 mm
      - Radial shortening >3 mm or inclination <15°
      - Dorsal tilt >10°
      - Extensive comminution
      - Open fractures
      - Carpal, radiocarpal, or DRUJ instability
      - Associated neurovascular injury, including acute carpal tunnel syndrome
      - Ipsilateral extremity injury
    - Surgery commonly performed in young, active patients with high functional needs.
    - Open reduction internal fixation with volar-locking plate is the most performed technique.
    - In patients with high energy, severely comminuted, and unstable distal radius fracture patterns, dorsal bridge plating can be performed to provide additional stability across the carpus.
    - Rarely, closed reduction and percutaneous K-wire fixation for reducible extra-articular fractures with good bone quality or very distal fracture lines, or closed reduction and external fixation for patients unable to undergo a lengthy procedure, are performed.
  - Common surgical complications outlined in **Table 33-3.**

TABLE 33-3 Common Complications After Distal Radius Fracture

Complication	Significance	Management
Malunion	Common in comminuted fractures managed nonoperatively Often asymptomatic or may result in ulnocarpal impaction, weakness, decreased range of motion	Treat with corrective osteotomy and bone grafting
Nonunion	Uncommon unless overdistracted in external fixator	Treat with ORIF and bone grafting
Tendon rupture	*Most commonly an attritional rupture of extensor pollicis longus (EPL) weeks after a nondisplaced distal radius fracture	Treat with extensor indicis propius (EIP) transfer to EPL
Posttraumatic arthritis	Articular step off of >1 mm leads to radiographic arthritis	Often clinically asymptomatic
Complex regional pain syndrome	Incidence reported between 22% and 39%. May present as persistent pain, cold intolerance, autonomic dysfunction, and/or trophic changes	Prevent with prophylactic vitamin C (ascorbic acid) 500 mg × 50 days

ASSOCIATED DISTAL RADIAL ULNAR JOINT INJURIES

OVERVIEW

- **General Principles**
  - The DRUJ forms an anatomically complex unit that allows for rotation of the forearm.
  - The triangular fibrocartilage complex (TFCC) is the major stabilizer of the DRUJ.
  - Intermediate column and radioulnar ligaments also contribute to DRUJ stability.
  - DRUJ injuries can occur separately or in conjunction with distal radius fractures. Galeazzi fracture is fracture of the distal third of the radial shaft with associated DRUJ injury.
- **Anatomy**
  - Articulation between ulnar head and sigmoid notch allows radius and carpus to pivot smoothly around the ulna.
  - Stabilized primarily by the TFCC, specifically the volar and dorsal radioulnar ligaments.
  - Joint movement also includes axial and translational motion.

EVALUATION

- **Presentation**
  - Patients present with ulnar-sided wrist pain and joint instability.
  - Physical exam may demonstrate crepitus, decreased grip strength, pain with proximal rotation of the forearm, positive fovea sign, and laxity in supination vs pronation. Special exam maneuvers include piano key sign, press test, and TFCC compression test to assess DRUJ stability.
- **Diagnostics**
  - X-ray can identify most DRUJ instability: widening of DRUJ (AP) and dorsal displacement of ulnar head (lateral).
  - Dynamic CT can assist with diagnosing subtle chronic DRUJ instability.
  - MRI is useful in the identification of TFCC or other ligamentous injuries.

MANAGEMENT

- After completing distal radius ORIF, assess DRUJ stability
  - If the DRUJ is unstable in both supination and pronation, then consider ORIF of large ulnar styloid base fractures and/or TFCC repair.
  - If the DRUJ is positionally unstable (usually supination), immobilize the extremity in stable position for 6 weeks with a long-arm cast.
  - If the DRUJ is stable, no need for further surgical management.
- **Nonoperative management.** Closed reduction and immobilization is appropriate for purely ligamentous injury
  - Forearm is placed in supination for dorsal instability injuries.
  - Forearm is placed in pronation for volar instability injuries.
- **Surgical management**
  - Indicated for a highly unstable DRUJ injury or Galeazzi fracture.
  - Surgical options include DRUJ pinning and radioulnar ligament repair.

ULNAR STYLOID FRACTURES

- **General Principles**
  - Ulnar styloid fractures accompany more than 50% of distal radius fractures.
  - Often these fractures are asymptomatic; however, they have been associated with DRUJ instability, disruption of the TFCC complex, stylocarpal impaction, and ECU tendonitis.

- **Management**
  - Ulnar styloid fractures with initial displacement more than 2 mm should be treated with ORIF. Fixation can be performed with a single K-wire, tension band wiring, wire loop/suture, or screw fixation.
  - If the ulnar styloid fracture is nondisplaced or is reducible with ORIF distal radius, patients can be treated with an above elbow cast ×6 weeks.
  - Ulnar styloid fractures commonly progress to nonunion, which is typically asymptomatic but can present with ulnar sided wrist pain and tenderness over the ulnar styloid.

PEARLS

1. Restoring anatomic alignment does not improve outcomes in elderly patients with distal radius fractures.
2. Less than 1% of DRFs result in compartment syndrome, but it is a surgical emergency and requires urgent reduction.

QUESTIONS YOU WILL BE ASKED

1. What are the normal radiographic parameters for a distal radius and what are the indications for surgery?
   See **Table 33-1** and **Figure 33-2**.
2. What is the most common tendon rupture after distal radius fracture and how is it managed?
   EPL tendon rupture occurs, on average 7 weeks after a nondisplaced distal radius fracture and is treated with EIP tendon transfer.

Recommended Readings
1. Diaz-Garcia RJ, Oda T, Shauver MJ, Chung KC. A systematic review of outcomes and complications of treating unstable distal radius fractures in the elderly. *J Hand Surg.* 2011;36A:824-835.
2. Logan AJ, Lindau TR. The management of distal ulnar fractures in adults: a review of the literature and recommendations for treatment. *Strategies Trauma Limb Reconstr.* 2008;3(2):49-56. doi:10.1007/s11751-008-0040-1
3. Schneppendahl J, Windolf J, Kaufman RA. Distal radius fractures: current concepts. *J Hand Surg.* 2012;37A:1718-1725.
4. Wolfe SW, Hotchkiss RN, Pederson WC, et al. *Green's Operative Hand Surgery.* 6th ed. Elsevier; 2011

34 Carpal Fractures and Dislocations

Davin C. Gong and Stefano Muscatelli

OVERVIEW

- There are eight carpal bones (Fig. 34-1A)
  - The pisiform is a sesamoid bone within the flexor carpi ulnaris (FCU) tendon.
- Gilula Lines (Fig. 34-1B)
  - Curve marking the proximal aspect of proximal carpal row (scaphoid, lunate, triquetrum)
  - Curve marking the distal aspect of proximal carpal row
  - Curve marking the proximal aspect of the distal carpal row (capitate, hamate)
- Wrist Ligaments
  - Intrinsic ligaments
    - Connect carpal bones within a carpal row
    - Most important are scapholunate (SL) and lunotriquetral (LT) ligaments
  - Extrinsic ligaments
    - Connect bones between carpal rows (spans midcarpal joint)
    - Volar extrinsic ligaments stronger than dorsal extrinsic ligament
  - Carpal dislocations are rare, only 5% of carpal injuries.

CARPAL FRACTURES

SCAPHOID FRACTURES

- Epidemiology
  - 60% of all carpal bone fractures
  - Fall on pronated, extended, and ulnar deviated wrist, common in young men—age 15-25 years
  - 10% affect proximal pole, 70% waist, 20% distal pole
- Pertinent Anatomy
  - Shape: 80% surface covered in articular cartilage; Greek "skaphos" meaning "boat"
  - Articulations: spans both carpal rows, thus having less mobility; articulates with trapezium, trapezoid, radius, lunate, and capitate
  - Blood supply
    - Superficial palmar (supplies distal 20%) and dorsal carpal (supplies proximal 80%) branches of radial artery.
    - *Dorsal carpal branch flows retrograde to supply proximal pole (Fig. 34-2).
- Evaluation
  - Physical exam
    - Anatomic snuffbox tenderness is highly sensitive (~90%) but nonspecific.
    - Watson test (tenderness with volar pressure at distal tubercle while moving the wrist from ulnar to radial deviation) is more specific.
    - Scaphoid compression test (tenderness with axial load through thumb metacarpal).

---

*Denotes common in-service examination topics.

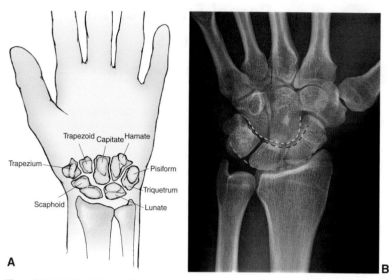

A

B

Figure 34-1 **A. The eight carpal bones. (From Oatis CA.** *Kinesiology: The Mechanics and Pathomechanics of Human Movement.* 3rd ed. Wolters Kluwer; 2017. Figure 14.8.) **B.** Gilula line. (From Wiesel SW, Albert T. *Operative Techniques in Orthopaedic Surgery.* 3rd ed. Wolters Kluwer; 2022. Figure 6.1.5.)

○ **Imaging**
- *Wrist x-rays: standard films with a "scaphoid view" (PA with wrist in ulnar deviation).
- Computed tomography (CT) scan: more sensitive than x-rays for scaphoid fractures. Useful in assessing bony union in postoperative period.
- MRI: best for occult fractures. T1 sequence can assess proximal pole vascularity to evaluate for AVN. Also evaluates ligamentous injuries.

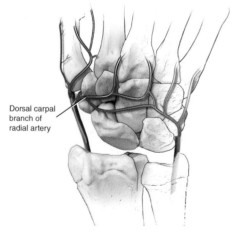

Dorsal carpal
branch of
radial artery

Figure 34-2 Branches of the radial artery supplying the radial wrist. The dorsal carpal branch supplies the proximal pole of the scaphoid. (From Diaz-Garcia RJ, Imbriglia FE. Partial scaphoid excision of scaphoid nonunions. In: Hunt TR III, ed. *Operative Techniques in Hand, Wrist, and Elbow Surgery.* 2nd ed. Wolters Kluwer; 2016:368-379.)

- **Management**
  - If normal radiographs but high clinical suspicion, then place in a thumb spica splint and repeat x-rays in 2 weeks.
  - Nonoperative cast immobilization (**most cases**)
    - Distal pole fractures
    - Nondisplaced waist fractures
    - 90% union rate if displacement is <1 mm
  - ORIF
    - Indications
      - >1 mm of displacement
      - **Proximal pole fractures**
      - Humpback deformity >35° intrascaphoid angle
      - Comminution
      - Perilunate fracture-dislocation
    - Screw fixation technique (includes percutaneous): countersink (spreads load of screw head across cortical surface of bone and prevents screw head irritation by burying it), long screw as centered as possible
      - Dorsal approach for proximal pole fractures, take care to **avoid EPL tendon**
      - Volar approach, waist and distal pole fractures, take care to **avoid STT joint cartilage**
      - Open volar approach visualize entire scaphoid, treat humpback deformity, less screw prominence compared to percutaneous
- **Complications**
  - **Nonunion**
    - Defined as a failure to heal after 6 months
    - Risk factors include proximal pole fractures, delay in diagnosis >4 weeks, displaced fractures
    - Can lead to **scaphoid nonunion advanced collapse (SNAC)** wrist
      - Stage 1: arthrosis of scaphoid and radial styloid
      - Stage 2: arthrosis of scaphocapitate and stage 1
      - Stage 3: arthrosis of periscaphoid, spares radiolunate articulation
    - Treatment—ORIF with bone grafting if no signs of arthritis, otherwise salvage procedures such as proximal row carpectomy, subtotal wrist fusion (ie, scaphoid excision and four corner fusion), and total wrist fusion
  - Malunion
    - Usually heals in apex dorsal angulation (humpback deformity)
    - Leads to dorsal intercalated segmental instability and arthritis
    - Treatment—ORIF with bone grafting (nonvascularized graft OK if no AVN, but must assess presence of punctate bleeding of the proximal pole intraoperatively)
  - **Avascular Necrosis (AVN)**
    - Increasing incidence as fracture is more proximal
      - Proximal fifth—100% rate of AVN
      - Proximal third—33% rate of AVN
    - Appears as sclerosis of proximal fragment on x-ray
    - Treatment—**vascularized bone grafting**, many options
      - Local 1, 2 intercompartmental supraretinacular artery
      - Free medial femoral condyle or free medial femoral trochlea
      - Free iliac crest

OTHER CARPAL FRACTURES

- Rare injuries, representing 1%-2% of all fractures
- Usually a result of a fall on outstretched hand
- **Triquetrum**

- ○ *Most common carpal bone fracture after scaphoid
- ○ Majority are dorsal cortical fractures either from impaction (wrist hyperextended and ulnarly deviated) or avulsion (palmar hyperflexion and radial deviation from radiotriquetral and triquetroscaphoid ligaments)
- ○ Treatment: immobilization
- **Trapezium**
  - ○ Third most common carpal bone fracture. Fall onto thumb with compression of trapezium by the metacarpal base
  - ○ Treatment: ORIF for displaced body fractures; excision for painful low demand patients
- **Lunate**
  - ○ Fourth most common carpal bone fracture. Incidence is 1%-6% of all carpal fractures (6% includes cases of Kienbock disease, collapse of lunate from AVN)
  - ○ Fall on hyperextended wrist, risk of carpal instability (LT or SL ligament disruption)
  - ○ Treatment: immobilization for nondisplaced fractures; ORIF for volar lip, displaced fractures, or any evidence of carpal instability
- **Capitate**
  - ○ High energy injuries, commonly associated with greater arc injury
  - ○ Scaphocapitate fracture syndrome: **trans-scaphoid transcapitate perilunate fracture dislocation,** often resulting in 180° rotation of proximal capitate and high incidence of AVN
  - ○ Treatment: ORIF
- **Hamate**
  - ○ Associated with sports requiring grip, that is, baseball, golf, and may be associated with ulnar nerve paresthesias
  - ○ Body fractures treated with immobilization if extra-articular; ORIF if intra-articular. Hook fractures treated with immobilization, can also be excised for faster return to play
- **Pisiform**
  - ○ Rare carpal bone fracture, can be symptomatic with radial or ulnar wrist deviation due to pisiform embedded in FCU tendon
  - ○ Treatment: ulnar gutter splint immobilization for nondisplaced; excision for symptomatic nonunion

CARPAL DISLOCATIONS

KINEMATICS

- Wrist motion is complex and occurs primarily at radiocarpal and midcarpal interface.
- Proximal carpal row flexes with radial deviation of wrist and extends with ulnar deviation. This function is impaired with SL and LT ligament disruptions.

PERILUNATE INJURY

- **Occurs progressively** as ligaments sequentially fail around the lunate—Mayfield classification
  - ○ **Stage I:** scaphoid fracture or SL ligament tear
  - ○ **Stage II:** lunocapitate ligament tear
  - ○ **Stage III:** lunotriquetral ligament tear (dorsal perilunate dislocation)
  - ○ **Stage IV:** dorsal radiolunate ligament tear (volar lunate dislocation)
- **Greater Arc Injury** (Involves Carpal Fracture)
  - ○ Combines carpal bone fracture with perilunate dislocation
  - ○ Fractures occur as injury pattern involves an arc of greater radius around lunate that passes through surrounding osseous structures

- ○ Trans-scaphoid perilunate fracture-dislocation
  - Most common type of greater arc injury
  - Immediate treatment: closed reduction and splinting to minimize damage to neurovascular structures
  - Definitive treatment: ORIF with dorsal approach for ligament repair, K-wires for maintenance of reduction of dislocation, compression screw across scaphoid
- ○ Transradial styloid perilunate fracture-dislocation
  - Immediate treatment: closed reduction and splinting
  - Definitive treatment—ORIF
- Lesser Arc Injury (Purely Ligamentous Injury)
  - ○ Immediate treatment
    - Attempted closed reduction and splinting to minimize damage to neurovascular structures
    - Open reduction often required in volar lunate dislocations
  - ○ Definitive treatment
    - ORIF via combined dorsal (between third and fourth compartments) and volar (via carpal tunnel) approaches
    - Repair volar ligament injury
    - Percutaneous pinning to restore carpal bones anatomic alignment
    - Pins remain in place for 8-12 weeks
  - ○ Outcomes from surgical intervention
    - 60% of contralateral wrist motion
    - 75% of contralateral grip strength

PEARLS

1. An occult scaphoid fractuer can be easily missed on initial Xrays, so one should have a low threshold based on the physical exam to either immobilize and obtain repeat x-rays, or to order advanced imaging (CT scan).
2. Immobilization is necessary for fracture healing but results in joint stiffness, so timing must be judicious.
3. Carpal dislocations are associated with poor functional outcomes despite definitive surgical management.

QUESTIONS YOU WILL BE ASKED

1. What is the main blood supply to the scaphoid?
   The Dorsal carpal branch of the radial artery.
2. What neurovascular injury is associated with Mayfield IV perilunate instability?
   Median nerve compression in the carpal tunnel.
3. What is a scaphoid humpback deformity?
   Apex dorsal angulation of the scaphoid after a scaphoid waist fracture.

Recommended Readings
1. Catalano LW III, Minhas SV, Kirby DJ. Evaluation and management of carpal fractures other than the scaphoid. *J Am Acad Orthop Surg.* 2020;28(15):e651-e661.
2. Clementson M, Björkman A, Thomsen N. Acute scaphoid fractures: guidelines for diagnosis and treatment. *EFORT Open Rev.* 2020;5(2):96-103.
3. Muppavarapu RC, Capo JT. Perilunate dislocations and fracture dislocations. *Hand Clin.* 2015;31(3):399-408. doi:10.1016/j.hcl.2015.04.002

Section III: Upper Extremity

35 Phalangeal and Metacarpal Fractures and Dislocations

Matthew T. Rasmussen and Evangeline F. Kobayashi

OVERVIEW

CLASSIFICATION OF FRACTURES
- Thorough Understanding of Anatomy (**Fig. 35-1**)
- Universal Descriptive System
  - Open vs closed
  - Fracture orientation (transverse, oblique, spiral)
  - Anatomic location (base, shaft, neck, head, condyle, articular)
  - Displacement (rotation, angulation, shortening)
  - Degree of comminution
- Salter-Harris Classification for Pediatric Physeal Fractures (**Fig. 35-2**)
  - Type I: fracture through the physis
  - Type II: fracture through the physis and metaphysis
  - Type III: fracture through the physis and epiphysis
  - Type IV: fracture extends from the metaphysis, through the physis, and into the epiphysis
  - Type V: physeal crush injury
  - The amount of injury to the growth plate and possible growth disturbance increases from type I to type V—continue to observe closely
  - Mnemonic for fracture location in relation to growth plate: "**SALTER**" – Straight across (type I), **A**bove (type II), **L**ower (type III), **T**hrough **E**verything (type IV), c**R**ush (type V)

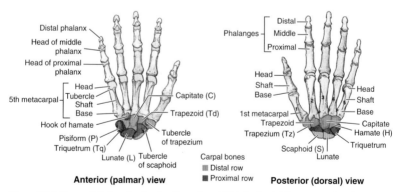

Figure 35-1 Bones of the hand and wrist. (From Agur AMR, Dalley AF II. *Grant's Atlas of Anatomy.* 15th ed. Wolters Kluwer; 2021. Figure 2.90A.)

---

*Denotes common in-service examination topics

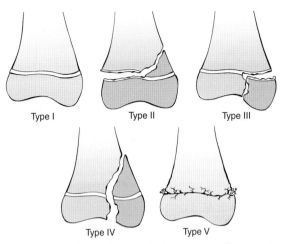

Figure 35-2 The Salter-Harris classification of pediatric physeal fractures. As the injury goes up in type, there is greater injury to the physis and greater chance of growth disturbance. (From Rathjen KE, Kim HKW, Alman BA. The injured immature skeleton. In: Waters PM, Skaggs DL, Flynn JM, eds. *Rockwood and Wilkins' Fractures in Children.* 9th ed. Wolters Kluwer; 2020:13-39.)

GENERAL TREATMENT

- Influenced by Fracture Displacement, Stability, and Location
- Goals of Treatment
  - Anatomic reduction
  - Appropriate immobilization
  - Maximizing range of motion (ROM) and function following healing
- Treatment Options
  - **Closed reduction and splint/cast immobilization**
    - Indication: stable fracture patterns that are easily reduced and remain anatomically aligned
    - Requires longer course of immobilization
  - **Closed reduction and percutaneous pinning (CRPP)**
    - Indication: unstable fracture patterns that are easily reduced
    - Requires longer course of immobilization
    - Increased risk of pin-tract infections
  - **Open reduction and internal fixation (ORIF)**
    - Indication: comminuted and/or complex fracture patterns, polytrauma patients
    - Requires anatomic reduction
    - Promotes early, active ROM
    - Risks of increased edema, infection, and predisposition to stiffness
  - **External fixation**
    - Indication: open fractures with significant contamination and periarticular fractures with comminution
    - Can result in sensory neuritis and pin-tract infections

POSTOPERATIVE CARE

- Duration of Immobilization
  - Dependent on multiple factors
    - Fracture pattern, location, and stability
    - Treatment (eg, ORIF < CRPP)

- ○ Most fractures are stable enough for activity by 8 weeks.
- ○ Wean patients from splint to slowly increase the stress on the fracture site and reduce stiffness.
- Assessment of Healing
  - ○ Serial radiographs (assessment of fracture callus or resolution of fracture lucency)
  - ○ Physical examination (loss of tenderness over fracture site reflects bony union and precedes radiographic changes)
- Therapy and Further Interventions
  - ○ Therapy (with a certified hand therapist, physical therapist, or occupational therapist) after immobilization or operative intervention is often valuable to regain ROM.
  - ○ Activity progression from gentle active ROM to passive ROM to strengthening programs.
  - ○ Patients should maximize their outcomes from therapy prior to contemplating further procedures (ie, tenolysis, capsulotomies, etc.).
  - ○ Preoperative counseling is paramount to set expectations for final outcomes.

PHALANGEAL FRACTURES

DISTAL PHALANX FRACTURES

- Most common hand fracture, with thumb and middle finger most common.
- **See Chapter 37: Fingertip and Nail Bed Injuries** for discussion of distal phalanx fractures and complications.

MIDDLE AND PROXIMAL PHALANX FRACTURES

- **Evaluation**
  - ○ Angulation or malrotation: when malrotation is present, the normal finger cascade is lost and affected digit can scissor over the adjacent digit.
    - ▪ Normal finger cascade: when all digits align with scaphoid tubercle upon flexion at metacarpophalangeal (MCP) joint and proximal interphalangeal (PIP) joint
  - ○ Shortening: shortening >2-4 mm can alter tendon balance and cause swan neck/boutonniere deformity.
- Assess for closed vs open injury, swelling, tenderness, ROM, extension/flexion lag, and malrotation ("scissoring").
- Obtain radiographs (three views, PA/oblique/lateral).
- **General Management**
  - ○ Stable and nondisplaced fractures can be treated with "buddy taping" or a short course of immobilization.
  - ○ Outcomes are influenced by many factors, including patient age, motivation/compliance, associated injuries, duration of immobilization, and articular involvement.
  - ○ Digits should be immobilized ≤4 weeks to minimize stiffness.
- **Extra-articular Fractures**
  - ○ Neck fractures
    - ▪ Usually seen in children
    - ▪ Often treated by reduction and splinting or K-wires
    - ▪ Open reduction (typically from dorsal approach) if closed reduction fails
  - ○ Shaft fractures
    - ▪ Varied orientation: transverse, oblique, spiral, or comminuted.
    - ▪ Proximal phalanx fractures often have apex volar angulation based on intrinsic pull.
    - ▪ Treatment
      - ▫ Stable fractures are treated with intrinsic plus splinting (metacarpophalangeals [MPs] flexed and interphalangeals [IPs] extended) and buddy taping.
      - ▫ Unstable fractures require fixation with K-wires, lag screws, or mini plate.

- **The PIP Joint**
  - Bicondylar hinge joint responsible for up to 85% of motion needed for functional grasp
  - Stabilized by collateral ligaments, tongue-in-groove joint surfaces, volar plate (**Fig. 35-3A-C**)
  - Radiographic assessment: is volar lip, dorsal lip, or both involved? Dislocation only vs fracture-dislocation?
  - **Dorsal dislocation:** more common than volar dislocation
    - Likely associated with volar plate avulsion
    - Classification of dorsal dislocations
      - Type I: partial or complete avulsion of volar plate locking middle phalanx in hyperextension
      - Type II: dorsal dislocation with avulsion of volar plate and significant tear of collateral ligaments
      - Type III: fracture-dislocation with avulsion fracture of volar middle phalanx base with volar plate
  - **Volar dislocation**
    - Likely avulsion of central slip.
    - Lack of active extension of the middle phalanx against gentle resistance indicates central slip rupture (Elson test).
  - **Treatment**
    - **Volar lip fracture-dorsal dislocation (Fig. 35-3D)**
      - If <30% of lip (stable): closed reduction, extension block splint, early ROM.
      - If >30% of lip (tenuous/unstable): ORIF, usually small screw if large fragment. If >3 fragments, consider hemi-hamate arthroplasty.
    - **Dorsal lip fracture-volar dislocation**
      - Fracture fragments approximate: closed reduction, splint in extension
      - Irreducible or recurrent dislocation: CRPP vs ORIF
    - **Pilon fracture:** involve both volar and dorsal cortices
      - Dynamic distraction external fixation or ORIF
- **Other Articular Fractures**
  - Condylar fractures
    - Inherently unstable: err on the side of operative intervention
    - Benefit from transverse K-wire fixation or lag screw placement
    - Bicondylar or comminuted fractures often require ORIF
    - Comminuted head fractures: associated with soft-tissue injury that is best treated nonoperatively
  - Base fractures
    - Often result from avulsion of central tendon or collateral ligaments.
    - Stable joints can be treated nonoperatively.
    - Significantly displaced corner fracture may be unstable, requiring ORIF.
    - Comminuted pilon fractures can be treated with skeletal traction or ORIF.
- Complications: malunion, nonunion, PIPJ extensor lag, infection

METACARPAL FRACTURES

EVALUATION

- Assess for closed vs open injury, swelling, tenderness, ROM, extension/flexion lag, and malrotation (scissoring).
- Obtain radiographs (three views, PA/oblique/lateral).
- No prospective studies comparing nonoperative with operative fixation.
- General indications for operative management: open fractures, segmental loss, clinically significant angulation, +/− multiple displaced fractures.
  - Shortening >5 mm weakens the flexion force of the finger and can lead to extensor lag (**Table 35-1**).

TABLE 35-1 Acceptable Metacarpal Fracture Angles

	Acceptable shaft angulation (°)	Acceptable neck angulation (°)
Index and long finger	<10	15-20
Ring finger	10-15	30-40
Little finger	10-15	40-50

METACARPAL HEAD FRACTURES

- Rare and usually intra-articular
- Most commonly involve the index finger due to the immobile carpometacarpal (CMC) joint
- **Treatment**
  - Nondisplaced fractures: immobilize MCP joint in 70° flexion and Interphalangeal (IP) joint in extension × 3 weeks
  - Operative indications: >25% of articular surface or >1 mm of step-off
    - Repair collateral ligaments if involved
  - "Fight bite": open fractures due to a clenched fist injury, require operative débridement, must evaluate for tendon injury

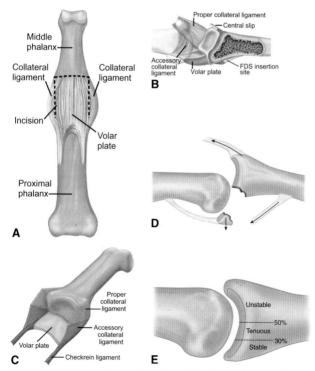

Figure 35-3 A-C. PIP joint stabilizers. (From Wiesel SW, Albert T. *Operative Techniques in Orthopaedic Surgery*. 3rd ed. Wolters Kluwer; 2022. Figure 6.7.1.) **D, E.** Unstable volar lip PIP fracture—dorsal dislocation. Tenuous fractures (30%-50% of joint surface)—if joint does not stay reduced with <30° flexion, it is considered "unstable." (From Wiesel SW, Albert T. *Operative Techniques in Orthopaedic Surgery*. 3rd ed. Wolters Kluwer; 2022. Figure 6.8.1.)

METACARPAL NECK FRACTURES

- Common fracture when clenched MCP joint strikes a solid object.
- Cause little functional deficit in the absence of "pseudoclawing" or malrotation.
- *Mobility of CMC joint allows some residual deformity to be tolerated (see Table 35-1). The increased mobility of ring and small finger CMC joint allows for greater degree of acceptable deformity.
- Treatment
  - Closed reduction
    - Ulnar digital block commonly used for the fifth metacarpal, may need hematoma block for the fourth metacarpal
    - *Jahss maneuver: passively flex the MCP joint and IP joints to 90° and push metacarpal (MC) head dorsally to counteract the apex dorsal displacement (Fig. 35-4)
    - Splint with ulnar gutter splint in intrinsic plus position. Some centers now using buddy taping for the fifth metacarpal fractures with <70° flexion and no malrotation
  - CRPP if reduction cannot be maintained or greater than acceptable degree of angulation
  - ORIF if closed reduction unsuccessful or fixation needed in setting of poor bone quality or comminution

METACARPAL SHAFT FRACTURES

- Types of Fractures
  - Transverse fractures: cause apex dorsal angulation due to forces from interosseous muscles
  - Oblique: due to torsional forces, can lead to malrotation
  - Comminuted: direct impact, can lead to shortening
- Treatment
  - Reduction and immobilization: works well for most shaft fractures, wrist in 30° of extension, MCP joints flexed >80°, and IP joints extended
  - CRPP
    - Can be antegrade or retrograde but may interfere with extensor tendons
    - Should be in place at least 4 weeks in adults

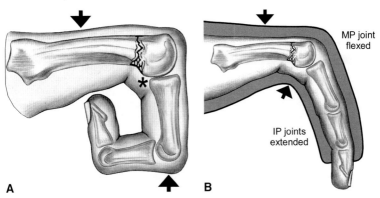

MP joint flexed

IP joints extended

A **B**

Figure 35-4 A. Schematic of the Jahss maneuver for closed reduction of metacarpal neck fractures. B. Schematic of cast immobilization of a metacarpal neck fracture. Asterisk indicates the site of reduction. Note the position of the interphalangeal (IP) joints. MP, metacarpophalangeal. (From Berger RA, Weiss AC, eds. *Hand Surgery.* Lippincott Williams & Wilkins; 2004.)

○ ORIF
  ▪ Can be done with plate/screws (≥2 mm) or with lag screws (long oblique fractures)
  ▪ Need to start active ROM at first post-op appointment to prevent adhesions/stiffness
○ Operative indications
  ▪ Open fractures: need thorough débridement and fixation
  ▪ Multiple fractures: difficult to obtain acceptable reduction with adjacent fractures
  ▪ Unstable fractures: particularly true in border digits
  ▪ Malalignment: malrotation is poorly tolerated as it is magnified distally, some sagittal angulation tolerated
  ▪ Significant shortening: opinions vary, >3 mm shortening believed to result in intrinsic dysfunction

METACARPAL BASE FRACTURES

• **Index, Middle, and Ring Finger**
  ○ Rare given lack of motion at these CMC joints, usually fracture avulsion injuries (extensor carpi radialis longus and extensor carpi radialis brevis from base of index and middle metacarpals).
  ○ Can usually be treated nonoperatively. However, displaced fractures involving the articular surface should be fixed to restore joint congruity.
• **Small Finger Fracture-Dislocation of the CMC Joint**
  ○ Relatively the most common given mobility of CMC and unprotected location of small finger
  ○ Relatively unstable with dorsal and proximal subluxation of the metacarpal due to the deforming forces of the extensor carpi ulnaris insertion
  ○ Eponym is "Baby Bennett" or "reverse Bennett fracture"
  ○ **Treatment**
    ▪ Displaced fractures and dislocations: reduction with pressure over dorsal MC base
    ▪ Usually requires closed reduction and K-wire fixation

THUMB METACARPAL FRACTURES

• **Extra-articular**
  ○ Typically midshaft or epibasal
  ○ Usually apex dorsal
    ▪ Distal fragment adducted and flexed due to pull of adductor, abductor pollicis brevis, and flexor pollicis brevis
  ○ Usually treated nonoperatively with thumb spica cast
  ○ Can tolerate up to 30° of deformity due to motion at CMC joint
• **Intra-articular Fracture**
  ○ *Bennett fracture: two-piece intra-articular fracture dislocation
    ▪ Single volar-ulnar fracture fragment remains due to anterior oblique ligament, abductor pollicis longus pulls on metacarpal base radially, proximally, and dorsally
    ▪ Usually treated with CRPP
    ▪ *Reduction performed by longitudinal traction, pressure at thumb metacarpal base (palmar abduction), and pronation
  ○ **Rolando fracture**: comminuted fracture of the base of the thumb metacarpal. Usually requires ORIF with plate and screws to restore articular surface.

COMPLICATIONS

• Malunion: may result in loss of "knuckle," which is unaesthetic, pseudoclaw with digital extension, or palmar prominence, which may be painful with grasping
• Infection

- Nonunion: uncommon in closed injuries
- Tendon adhesions: usually a result of ORIF
- Intrinsic muscle dysfunction: can result from significant shortening

DISLOCATIONS

GENERAL CONSIDERATIONS

- May be pure dislocation or associated with a fracture fragment (see above sections)
  - Small volar or dorsal fragment may indicate an avulsion fracture.
  - Fracture fragments involving >20%-30% of the articular surface are often unstable and may require operative intervention.
- Analgesia
  - Digital blocks are commonly sufficient for finger dislocations.
  - Thumb reductions may require median and radial nerve blocks.
- Reduction Maneuvers
  - Stabilize patient's hand and use other hand to grip the finger or thumb.
  - Exaggerate deformity and apply traction.
- Splinting
  - Dorsal dislocations require extension blocking splints with finger splinted in slight flexion.
  - Volar dislocations are splinted in extension.
  - Can use aluminum padded or plaster splint.
- Postreduction images

DISTAL INTERPHALANGEAL (DIP) JOINT DISLOCATIONS

- Usually a dorsal dislocation, secondary to a hyperextension injury
- Treatment
  - **Reducible:** closed reduction
    - Digital block.
    - Maneuver: exaggerate deformity and then apply traction.
    - Check radiographs to confirm joint congruity and rule out associated fracture.
    - Splint for 2 weeks.
  - **Irreducible:** open reduction is required
    - Possible causes include interposition of the profundus tendon (implies disruption of at least one collateral ligament), volar plate, or displaced articular fracture fragment.

PIP JOINT DISLOCATIONS

- See section Middle and Proximal Phalanx Fractures → PIP Joint above.

MCP JOINT DISLOCATIONS

- Anatomy
  - Volar plate
    - Laterally supported by deep transverse MC ligament that allows stabilization to adjacent MCP joint
    - Floor of joint
  - *Cam effect: collateral ligaments taut in flexion and lax in extension—the MCP joint allows for some abduction-adduction when the joint is in extension.
- Evaluation
  - Notable deformity with marked MCP Joint hyperextension
  - Dorsal vs volar dislocation

- **Treatment**
  - **Dorsal dislocation**
    - **Incomplete dislocation** (proximal phalanx locked at 60°-80° hyperextension): closed reduction
      - Tip: flexing the wrist will relax the flexor tendons. Hyperextend the MCP joint and then apply dorsal pressure to proximal phalanx base while flexing the MCP joint.
      - Splint with MCP joint in 50°-70° flexion for 1 week followed by buddy taping.
    - **Complete and irreducible dislocation:** open reduction and A1 pulley release
      - *Cannot be reduced due to interposition of volar plate and/or trapping of MC head between lumbrical (radially) and flexor tendon (ulnarly)
  - **Volar dislocation:** most are managed with closed reduction. Open reduction if not successful

PEARLS

1. Indications for operative management include intra-articular fractures, displaced fractures, and malrotation.
2. PIP dislocations often occur dorsally due to disruption of the volar plate.
3. PIP fracture-dislocations with <30% involvement of the volar P2 base fragment can be treated nonoperatively with a dorsal blocking splint.
4. Irreducible MCP, PIP, and DIP joint dislocations are often due to the interposition of the volar plate into the joint.

QUESTIONS YOU WILL BE ASKED

1. What structures provide stability to the PIP joint?
   The Lateral and proper collateral ligaments and the volar plate.
2. In a Bennett fracture, what tendon causes proximal migration of the thumb metacarpal?
   The Abductor pollicis longus.
3. In a Bennett fracture, the small fracture fragment is attached to the trapezium via what ligament?
   The Anterior oblique ligament or volar beak ligament.
4. What are the deforming forces in a proximal phalanx fracture?
   The proximal fragment is brought into flexion by the interossei and the distal fragment is brought into extension by the central slip.
5. Dorsal PIPJ fracture-dislocations often have what associated osseous injury?
   Fracture of the volar lip of the middle phalanx.

Recommended Readings
1. Haase SC, Chung KC. Current concepts in treatment of fracture-dislocations of the proximal interphalangeal joint. *Plast Reconstr Surg.* 2014;134(6):1246-1257.
2. Henry MH. Fractures of the proximal phalanx and metacarpals in the hand: preferred methods of stabilization. *J Am Acad Ortho Surg.* 2008;16:586-595.
3. Jones NF, Jupiter JB, Lalonde DH. Common fractures and dislocations of the hand. *Plast Reconstr Surg.* 2012;130(5):722e-736e.
4. Page SM, Stern PJ. Complications and range of motion following plate fixation of metacarpal and phalangeal fractures. *J Hand Surg Am.* 1998;23(5):827-832.
5. Wolfe SW, Hotchkiss RN, Pederson WC, Kozin SH. *Green's Operative Hand Surgery.* 6th ed. Elsevier; 2011.

36 Traumatic Amputation Injuries

Evangeline F. Kobayashi and Matthew T. Rasmussen

OVERVIEW

INITIAL ASSESSMENT

- Patient age. (Children heal more quickly and adapt more easily to changes in form and function.)
- Mechanism of injury (crush vs sharp, degloving), zone of injury (**see Chapter 38: Tendon Injuries and Tendonitis**).
- Hand dominance, occupation.
- Nicotine use, vascular disease, diabetes, other relevant past medical history.
- Determine perception of hand image vs function.
- Assess for other injuries.
- X-ray.
- Determine treatment with revision amputation vs replantation. Manage patient expectation from the start.

GOALS OF PRIMARY AND REVISION AMPUTATION

- Preserve functional length
- Create a durable amputation site/stump
- Preserve sensation; prevent neuromas
- Prevent adjacent joint contractures
- Early return to work and activity

DISTAL FINGER AMPUTATIONS

ASSESSMENT

- Dorsal vs volar fingertip injury
- Angle of injury
- Involvement of nail/nail bed (see Chapter 37: Fingertip and Nail Bed Injuries)
- Bone exposure

MANAGEMENT

- Goals: satisfactory appearance, preserve sensation and length, well-padded pulp, preserve nail bed, minimize time off work
- Reconstructive choice: consider location of the injury (palmar vs dorsal, radial vs ulnar), size of defect, and structures involved (skin, soft tissue, bone)
- **If No Bone Exposed**
  - **Healing by secondary intention**
    - Indication: ≤1 cm².
    - Gives the most sensate fingertip in most cases.

- Treat with semiocclusive (eg, Tegaderm) dressing changes and antibiotic ointment to keep moist and clean. Change every 7 days.
  - Cold intolerance is common.
- Primary closure
  - Loose closure is an option if tissue loss is minimal.
  - Tight closures can limit function, cause pain, and create hooked nail deformity.
- Skin grafts
  - Recovery of sensation is not as good as with secondary intention or primary closure.
  - If used, do a full-thickness skin graft. Best donor site options include the following:
    - Original skin (if salvageable)—aggressively trimmed of all fat and dermis as needed
    - Skin from ulnar/hypothenar aspect of hand, volar wrist, or antecubital region
  - Split-thickness skin grafts should only be used on noncritical areas (ie, ulnar side of index, middle, and ring fingers).
- **If Bone Exposed**
  - Revision amputation (bone shortening) with primary closure
    - Allows faster return to work than secondary intention or replantation
    - Best option for a patient unlikely or unwilling to do dressing changes
    - **Complications:** hook nail deformity if nail bed is pulled tightly into tip closure or with contraction of scar
  - Revision amputation with secondary intention
    - Patients are often skeptical about outcome initially: important to counsel patients on what to expect as normal.
    - Good option if a patient can tolerate dressing changes.
    - Often gives as good or better outcomes than flap repairs.
  - Fingertip flaps: many described surgical options; however, these procedures will not necessarily result in better outcomes or quicker recovery.

FLAP OPTIONS FOR FINGERTIP REPAIR

- The angle of injury or amputation, as well as individual surgeon experience, determines when and where to use a given technique.
- Advancement Flaps
  - Volar V-Y advancement flap (Atasoy-Kleinert flap) (Fig. 36-1)
    - Indication: dorsal oblique amputations
    - Triangular flap, with base no wider than nail bed
    - Skin incisions through the dermis; deep aspect dissected off phalanx

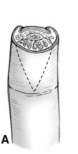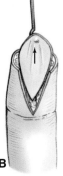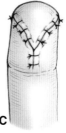

Figure 36-1 The Atasoy volar V-Y advancement flap. A–C: The Atasoy-Kleinert V-Y advancement flap. Note that the subcutaneous tissue has remained undisturbed to maintain blood supply. (Redrawn after Louis DS, Jebson PLJ, Graham TJ. Amputations. In: Green DP, Hotchkiss RN, Pederson WC, eds. *Operative Hand Surgery*. New York: Churchill Livingstone; 1999:48–94. *Master Techniques in Orthopaedic Surgery: Soft Tissue Surgery*. 2nd ed. Wolters Kluwer; 2017. Figure 3.11.)

A **B** **C**

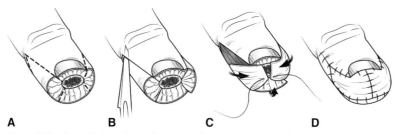

A **B** **C** **D**

Figure 36-2 **The Kutler lateral V-Y advancement flaps. A.** Advancement flaps are marked out on the midlateral aspects of the digit. **B.** The skin, subcutaneous tissue, and underlying septa are incised, and the flaps are elevated. The flaps are mobilized longitudinally over the fingertip (**C**) and secured using loose sutures (**D**). (Reproduced with permission from Lee DH, Mignemi ME, Crosby SN. Fingertip injuries: an update on management. *J Am Acad Orthop Surg.* 2013;21(12):756-766.)

- Advancement up to 10 mm possible
- Disadvantages: possible hypersensitivity or hook nail
  ○ **Lateral V-Y advancement flap (Kutler flap) (Fig. 36-2)**
    - Indication: transverse amputations.
    - Bilateral triangles: advanced and sutured to distal nail bed.
    - Can advance up to 5 mm if skin alone; 14 mm if a neurovascular flap is elevated down to the level of the periosteum.
    - Disadvantages: vascular supply sometimes unreliable; scar is at the tip, which may be painful or insensate.
  ○ **Volar neurovascular advancement flap (Moberg flap) (see Chapter 40: Thumb Reconstruction)**
- **Regional Flaps**
  ○ **Cross-finger flap (CFF) (Fig. 36-3)**
    - Indication: volar defect distal to proximal interphalangeal joint (PIPJ).
    - Dorsal skin from one digit is transferred to the injured area of an adjacent digit; can use for volar or dorsal amputations.
    - Pedicled flap with delayed division, usually in 2-3 weeks.
    - Donor site requires a skin graft.

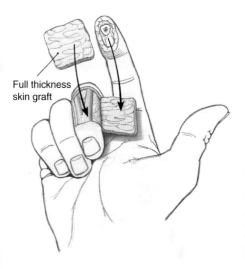

Full thickness skin graft

Figure 36-3 **The cross-finger flap.** Cross-finger flap from the dorsum of the middle finger is to be inset onto the amputated index tip. The full-thickness graft is placed to cover the defect over the dorsum of the donor area. (Used with permission of Mayo Foundation for Medical Education and Research, all rights reserved.)

- **Thenar flap**
  - Indication: large fingertip pulp loss >2 cm.
  - The digit injured is flexed and tucked into thenar area, and the palmar skin is used to cover the tip by raising dorsal and volar flaps—division at 2-3 weeks.
  - Advantage: no defect on adjacent fingers to injury.
  - Disadvantage: PIPJ flexion contracture of recipient finger, so mostly used in children who can resolve the contracture more easily than adults.
- **Neurovascular island transfer flap** (Littler flap)
  - Indication: insensate fingers following trauma to recreate sensibility in the tip.
  - Usually reserved for the thumb, index finger, or ulnar small finger.
  - Must balance recipient sensation restoration with donor site loss.
  - Flap pedicle is composed of digital vessels and nerve.
  - Typically raised from the ulnar aspect of the ring or middle finger; raised at level of flexor sheath.
  - Donor site is either closed primarily or either graft.
  - This flap is rarely used because of the high donor site morbidity incurred.
- **Reverse CFF**
  - Indication: dorsal skin defect from middistal phalanx to midproximal phalanx.
  - Dorsal subcutaneous tissue from donor digit is transferred to dorsal injured area of adjacent digit.
  - Pedicled flap with delayed division, usually in 2-3 weeks.
  - Recipient site requires a full-thickness skin graft; donor site skin is returned to donor site.

PROXIMAL FINGER AMPUTATIONS

AMPUTATIONS THROUGH DISTAL INTERPHALANGEAL JOINT (DIPJ)/PIPJ

- Bone: rongeur to smoothly contour the distal end by removing the condylar prominences and irregular bone spikes.
- Nerve: digital nerves must be sharply transected on tension and allowed to retract to prevent neuromas.
- Tendon: débride ends of tendons, but avoid suturing the ends together as this will limit excursion of both.
- Complications
  - **Quadriga effect**
    - If flexor digitorum profundus (FDP) tendon of injured digit is shortened and tethered, then the adjacent FDP cannot be fully contracted.
    - Leads to active flexion lag in adjacent fingers.
  - **Lumbrical plus deformity**
    - If FDP is severed from its insertion and migrates proximally, it pulls on the lumbrical.
    - Attempted flexion causes PIPJ extension (from FDP pull on lumbricals tendon pulling on extensor mechanism).
    - Treatment: sectioning of the lumbrical tendon.

MIDDLE AND PROXIMAL PHALANX AMPUTATIONS

- "Fish mouth" closure utilized with the incision oriented transversely across the end of the stump.
- If preserved, tendons are secured to their insertion on the phalanx.
  - If an amputation occurs too proximally along the middle phalanx to allow re-insertion of the tendon to bone, then use of the next joint will be limited.
  - Length preservation remains preferable, even if the joint is nonfunctional—joint should be fused.

METACARPAL AND CARPAL AMPUTATIONS

RAY AMPUTATIONS

- Injuries at or near the level of metacarpophalangeal joint (MCPJ) usually benefit from removal of most of the bone and closure of the space between remaining digits.
  - ○ Index finger: leaves a stump that can interfere with thumb use and creates a bulky web space
  - ○ Central rays: residual stump interferes with small object manipulation
- The overall appearance of the hand is better if the stump is removed and any gap closed, although the palm is made narrower in the process.
- Generally carried out electively after the wound has healed.

CARPAL AMPUTATIONS

- Initial treatment is tissue preservation.
- Anchor wrist flexor/extensor tendons to carpus.
- Functional recovery is poor, so some patients may opt for more proximal amputation, followed by fitting with a hand prosthesis.
- Alternatively, the tissue at the hand base can be preserved and used to anchor a nonfunctional cosmetic appliance.

AMPUTATIONS AT AND PROXIMAL TO THE WRIST

- **Wrist Disarticulation**
  - ○ Once felt to be inferior to a long below-elbow amputation, but now utilized more with prosthesis design improvements.
  - ○ Requires intact distal radial ulnar joint (DRUJ).
  - ○ Preserving the radioulnar joint allows for a full range of pronation and supination.
  - ○ "Fish mouth" skin closure (with a longer skin flap on the palmar side) is utilized.
- **Below-Elbow Amputation**
  - ○ Goal is length preservation—middle third of the forearm maintains length and is ideal.
  - ○ *More length preservation of the radius and ulna means greater pronation/supination; ideally, 5-10 cm of length should be preserved for maximal function.
- **Elbow Disarticulation and Above-Elbow Amputations**
  - ○ Humeral condyle preservation allows translation of rotation to the prosthesis; thus, an elbow disarticulation is an adequate level of amputation.
  - ○ In above-elbow amputations, length preservation is key.
    - ■ *At least 5-7 cm of residual length needed for glenohumeral mechanics.
    - ■ Amputations at or above the axillary fold have no real advantage vs shoulder disarticulations.

REPLANTATION

INITIAL EVALUATION

- "Life before limb"—patients may have other serious injuries, which must be addressed prior to any attempt at replantation.
- Additional information needed when considering replantation.
  - ○ Overall patient health and comorbidities.
  - ○ Social history including smoking and work history.
  - ○ Prior injuries to the extremity.
  - ○ Determine if patient would be compliant with post-op rehabilitation and able to tolerate lengthy time off work (average return to work is 7 months) with possible future reoperations.
- Obtain x-rays of both the hand and the amputated part.
- Ensure that tetanus is up-to-date and appropriate antibiotics given.
- Check hematocrit and perform fluid resuscitation.

- Assess injury, as outlined above in the "Amputation" section.
  - Sharp amputations do better than avulsion or crush amputations.
  - A "corkscrew" appearance of the arteries suggests traumatic stretch from an avulsion, which is an ominous sign, suggesting vein grafting would be necessary with worse chance of success.
  - Bruising of the neurovascular bundle also suggests avulsion or traction injury.
- **Length of ischemia time of part is critical.**
  - *Digits can tolerate up to 12 hours of warm and 24 hours of cold ischemia time.
  - *More proximal amputations (wrist and proximal) tolerate only 6 hours of warm ischemia and 12 hours of cold ischemia time.

INDICATIONS FOR REPLANTATION

- Thumb amputation at any level
  - Contributes to 40% of hand function.
  - Consider heterotopic pollicization when thumb is not salvageable.
  - Electively, a toe-to-thumb transfer can be offered.
  - Avulsions at the interphalangeal joint deserve replantation with fusion as infection rate for replanting extensor pollicis longus (EPL) and flexor pollicis longus (FPL) is high.
- Multiple finger amputations
- Any amputation in a child
- Amputation at the palm, wrist, or forearm level
- Single digit injury distal to flexor digitorum superficialis (FDS) insertion (zone I)

CONTRAINDICATIONS

- **Absolute Contraindications**
  - Life-threatening injuries
  - Prolonged ischemia time of amputated part, especially with large muscle content
  - Amputated part in multiple pieces (transected at more than one level)
  - Mangled limb or crush injury
- **Relative Contraindications**
  - Single digit proximal to FDS insertion (zone II)
  - Severe preexisting illness: diabetes mellitus, heart disease/atherosclerosis, recent stroke/myocardial infarction, psychiatric disorders
  - Gross contamination of site
  - Prior surgery/trauma to amputated part
  - Smoking history

PREOPERATIVE CARE

- *Care of Amputated Part: the part should be gently cleaned, wrapped in saline-moistened gauze, and placed in a sealed plastic bag.
  - *Bag placed in ice WITH saline bath will maintain the proper temperature for transport (~4 °C).
  - Do NOT place the finger directly on ice—freezing worse than warm ischemia.
- Consent: obtain surgical consent for replant attempts.
  - Detailed explanation of extensive recovery time, the need for significant rehabilitation, and the likely amount of optimal function.
  - The possibility of long hospitalizations, multiple reoperations, heparinization, and blood transfusions must be recognized.
  - The significant chance of failure must also be addressed. **Must inform the patient that further reconstruction may be needed, including possible revision amputation.**

OPERATIVE TECHNIQUES

- Operative Overview
  - Replant sequence
    - Prepare distal and proximal amputation sites and identify arteries, veins, nerves, and tendons. Place tagging sutures. General sequence is then: bony fixation, tendon repair, and arteries, veins, nerves, and soft tissue coverage.

- Finger order
  - Thumb (first), long, ring, small, index (last)
- When multiple digits involved, a "part-by-part" approach is usually preferred to "digit-by-digit" when all replantable parts are in equal condition (digit-by-digit takes the most time).
  - In parts with significant muscle, the risk of prolonged ischemia and subsequent reperfusion injury is high. In this case, arteries should be repaired first, followed by nerves, and finally veins.
- **Amputated Part (Fig. 36-4)**
  - Prepare the amputated part on the "back table" prior to patient arrival.
  - Carefully expose the vessels and nerves and tag their ends.
    - For fingers, use midaxial longitudinal incisions.
    - Corkscrew (avulsed) vessels need to be excised prior to replantation.
  - Preservation of "spare parts" may optimize outcome.
    - Heterotopic replants transfer tissue from one site to another (ie, thumb restoration with another amputated digit when the thumb is lost or unsalvageable).
    - Use of components from an unsalvageable amputated part for another part's replant is economical (ie, digital nerves from another amputated finger that cannot be replanted).
  - When the amputation is more proximal, it contains muscle and will swell after reperfusion.
    - Any fascial compartments in the part must be released.
- **Bone Fixation**
  - Bone should be débrided to decrease tension on anastomoses and skin closures.
  - Fixation can be achieved via

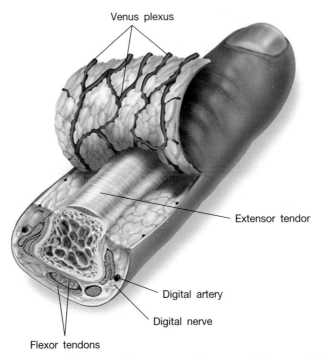

Venus plexus

Extensor tendor

Digital artery

Digital nerve

Flexor tendons

Figure 36-4 Anatomy of the amputated finger. Knowing the anatomy of the amputated digit will make replantation faster.

Section III: Upper Extremity

- Kirschner wires: simple. Can be placed retrograde in amputated part first for fixation
- Interosseous wires: can be used to augment K-wire fixation
- Plate fixation: useful for unstable fracture patterns in phalanges and amputations at or proximal to metacarpals
- External fixation: may be useful for forearm replants
- **Tendon/Muscle Repair**
    - Clean the tendon edges, but do not shorten excessively.
    - Extensor tendons are repaired first, with two or three horizontal mattress sutures using 4-0 braided polyester.
    - Flexor tendons repaired with a core suture technique, such as a modified Kessler or Tajima repair (**see Chapter 38: Tendon Injuries and Tendonitis**).
- **Vessel Anastomoses**
    - **Arterial repair**
        - The artery must be trimmed to healthy intima.
        - Vein grafts of the appropriate size may be found in the volar forearm, in the dorsal foot, or in "spare" amputated parts.
        - Papaverine and/or lidocaine are used to minimize vasospasm.
        - Repair of two arteries to a digit yields a higher successful replantation rate vs repair of a single artery, but one good anastomosis is adequate.
    - **Venous repair**
        - Two vein repairs per artery are preferred.
        - Tension on venous repair must be minimal to prevent congestion.
- **Nerve Coaptation**
    - Trim the nerves to undamaged areas.
    - Realign fascicles, when possible, to maximize the return of sensibility.
- **Closure or Coverage**
    - Skin is closed loosely over repaired vessels as a tight closure will restrict venous outflow.
    - Split-thickness skin grafts are used as needed.
    - Nail removed to assess for bleeding and allow leech attachment if congestion occurs.
    - For more proximal replants, local or free muscle flaps are used to cover the operative site and protect the anastomoses.
    - A well-padded splint (NO circumferential pressure) should be made to protect the replantation site.
        - Blood oozing often causes padding to become saturated, clotted, and restrictive, so it must be monitored carefully.

POSTOPERATIVE CARE

- Acute Care
    - Aggressive hydration to keep vessels patent.
    - Avoid ANY vasoconstrictors for 1 month or more post-op, including caffeine, chocolate, and nicotine.
    - Appropriate analgesia is important to minimize catecholamine release.
    - Keep replanted extremity warm (warm room, blankets, Bair Hugger).
    - Medical therapies used to diminish complication rates.
        - Systemic heparinization should be considered in cases of wide vessel damage such as in crush amputations—should be initiated intraoperatively for best results.
        - Daily aspirin to minimize platelet aggregation.
        - Other agents are advocated by some authors, including chlorpromazine (Thorazine), dipyridamole (Persantine), and calcium channel blockers.
- Frequent evaluation by the surgeon and staff for color and capillary refill (subjective monitoring) is essential.

- **Failing Replant**
  - In the acute setting, the problem is usually vascular (inflow or outflow).
  - **Arterial insufficiency**
    - Cool, pale replant; no capillary refill; pin prick produces little or no bleeding.
    - Thrombosis due to vasospasm is most common cause of early replant failure (within 12 hours).
    - Treat by releasing constrictive bandages, placing extremity in dependent position, consider medical therapies (heparin, Thorazine, etc.). Ensure patient is not hypovolemic.
    - Early surgical exploration if conservative management unsuccessful.
  - **Venous insufficiency**
    - Congested replant; increased tissue turgor; pin prick yields copious bleeding with dark blood.
    - Treat by elevating extremity or leech vs heparin-soaked pledgets.
      - Leeches secrete hirudin (potent anticoagulant that remains localized).
      - *Leeches associated with Aeromonas hydrophila infection—prophylaxis with ciprofloxacin or trimethoprim/sulfamethoxazole (Bactrim).
  - Reexploration is the definitive treatment for vascular problems.
    - Functional outcomes are poorer in patients requiring reoperation.
    - Outcomes are best when reoperation is performed within 6 hours of loss of perfusion.

OUTCOMES

- With good patient selection, replant failure rate is low, on the order of 20%; however, viable replants are not always valuable/functional replants.
- *Mechanism of injury is the most important factor influencing digit survival rate.
- Functional outcome depends upon multiple factors.
  - Sharp amputations have better recovery of sensation and function than crush or avulsion amputations.
  - Children have better outcomes for any given level, but they are more problematic during rehabilitation due to noncompliance.
  - Thumb replants do best. Even if mobility is poor, the replant has value as a sensate post.
  - Zone I finger replants: regain an average of 82° of motion at the PIPJ.
  - Zone II finger replants: regain an average of 35° of motion at the PIPJ.
  - Average two-point discrimination in a finger replant is 11 mm.
- **Acute Complications**
  - Replant failure (above)
  - Myonecrosis: greater concern in major limb replant
  - Myoglobinuria: secondary to muscle necrosis in larger replants. May lead to renal failure
  - Reperfusion injury: thought to be related to ischemia-induced hypoxanthine conversion to xanthine
  - Infection
- **Late complications** diminish the value of a replantation.
  - ~50% loss of motion.
    - Due to tendon adhesions and joint contracture.
    - Most common secondary procedure is tenolysis (35% of all replants).
  - Decreased sensation is a function of injury mechanism, repair technique, and level of injury.
  - Loss of motor function is a problem in more proximal amputations, where the slow axonal regeneration limits muscle reinnervation.
  - Chronic pain, including chronic regional pain syndrome.
  - Cold intolerance may improve somewhat for 2 years, but some residual intolerance is very common.

PEARLS

1. With amputation injuries, it is important to perform a full assessment of the patient and injury site to determine appropriate treatment with revision amputation vs replantation.
2. The amputated part should be placed in saline-moistened gauze, sealed in a plastic bag, and placed in a saline-ice bath (and not placed directly on ice).
3. When discussing replantation, ensure that the patient is consented for additional reconstructive options and for possible revision amputation.
4. Venous congestion following replantation can be treated by removing the nail and placing heparin-soaked pledgets or leeches on the exposed nail bed.
5. If using leeches, make sure to give prophylaxis (ciprofloxacin or trimethoprim/ sulfamethoxazole) against *Aeromonas*.

QUESTIONS YOU WILL BE ASKED

1. What is the difference between a CFF and a reverse CFF?
   A CFF is for a volar defect using dorsal skin, whereas reverse CFF is for a dorsal defect using dorsal soft tissue.
2. What are the indications, relative contraindication, and absolute contraindication to replantation?
   Indications include thumb amputations, proximal phalangeal amputations, multiple digits, and amputations in children. Relative contraindications include the need to return to work quickly, medical comorbidities, age, and tobacco use. Absolute contraindications are life-threatening injuries or medical illness which would preclude prolonged operative times and hospitalizations.
3. When considering replantation, what are the warm and cold ischemia times for fingers vs more proximal amputations?
   Amputations with significant muscle mass (ie, forearm) only have a 6-hour warm and a 12-hour cold ischemia tolerance. Digits have been replanted with as much as a 42-hour cold ischemia time in case reports.
4. How do arterial inflow obstruction and venous outflow congestion present differently? What are the treatments for each?
   Inflow obstruction presents with a cold, pale digit. It is treated with revision arterial anastomosis. Venous congestion presents with a swollen, blue or purple digit that bleeds dark blood when poked. It can be treated with medicinal leeches or occasionally with a return to the operating room for additional venous anastomosis.

Recommended Readings
1. Chang J, Jones N. Twelve simple maneuvers to optimize digital replantation and revascularization. *Tech Hand Up Extrem Surg*. 2004;8(3):161-166.
2. Germann G, Rudolf K, Levin S, Hrabowski M. Fingertip and thumb tip wounds: changing algorithms for sensation, aesthetics, and function. *J Hand Surg*. 2017;42:274-284. doi:10.1016/j.jhsa.2017.01.022
3. Marchessault J, McKay P, Hammert W. Management of upper limb amputations. *J Hand Surg*. 2011;36:1718-1726.
4. Tintle SM, Baechler MF, Nanos GP III, Forsberg JA, Potter BK. Traumatic and trauma-related amputations: Part II: upper extremity and future directions. *J Bone Joint Surg Am*. 2010;92:2934-2945.
5. Yoshimura M. Indications and limits of digital replantation. *JMAJ*. 2003;46(10):460-467.

37 Fingertip and Nail Bed Injuries

Alexander N. Khouri

OVERVIEW

EPIDEMIOLOGY

- Fingertip and nail injuries account for 45% of all emergency department (ED) hand injuries.
- The middle finger is most commonly injured.

ANATOMY

- Fingertip: defined as the portion of the finger that is distal to the insertion of the flexor and extensor tendons
- Innervation: paired radial and ulnar proper digital nerves that trifurcate at the distal interphalangeal (DIP) joint with branches to the nail bed, finger pulp, and distal fingertip
  - Meissner corpuscles: tactile organs located in the dermal papillae that generate two-point sensation
  - Pacinian corpuscles: mechanoreceptors that sense deep pressure and vibration
- Blood Supply: radial and ulnar proper digital arteries that also trifurcate and communicate via two anastomotic arches over the lunula and free edge of the nail
- Finger Pulp: fibrofatty compartment on the volar aspect of the distal phalanx that is separated by fibrous vertical septae creating a connective tissue framework
- Nail Anatomy (**Fig. 37-1**)
  - Germinal matrix—proximal nail bed that is responsible for nail growth. The matrix begins 7-8 mm proximal to the nail fold
  - Sterile matrix—distal nail bed that is responsible for nail plate adherence
  - Lunula—white crescent of the proximal nail that separates the germinal and sterile matrix
  - Eponychium—skin fold at the proximal aspect of the nail
  - Hyponychium—skin distal to the nail bed
  - Paronychium—skin surrounding the lateral nail folds
  - Perionychium—entire nail unity which includes the nail bed (sterile and germinal matrices), the eponychium, the hyponychium, and the paronychium

INITIAL EVALUATION

- **Perform basic hand history and examination (see Chapter 29: Hand and Wrist Anatomy and Examination)**
- **Physical Exam:** characterize the injury
  - Wound (simple/stellate/crush/avulsion/bite), angle of injury (ie, volar/dorsal, oblique/transverse), defect size, involvement of skin/pulp/nail plate/nail bed, examine for exposed bone.
  - Observe the resting posture and digital cascade of the fingertip.
  - Examine the nail for growth abnormalities, ridging, and discoloration.
  - Assess active and passive distal interphalangeal (DIP) joint flexion and extension.
  - Assess for neurovascular injury, fingertip viability (including cap refill), and cold intolerance (prior to local anesthetic).
  - Perform an Allen test as needed (for future reconstructive considerations).

---

* Denotes common in-service examination topics

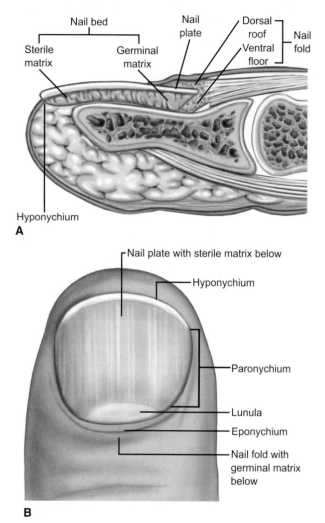

Figure 37-1 Fingertip (**A**) and nail bed anatomy (**B**). (From Hunt TR, Wiesel SW. *Operative Techniques in Hand, Wrist, and Elbow Surgery.* 2nd ed. Wolters Kluwer; 2017. Figure 138.1.)

- **X-ray** to assess for foreign body or bony abnormality
  - Prefer finger imaging to avoid overlapping digits.
  - Always radiograph any amputated parts.

NAIL BED INJURIES

SUBUNGAL HEMATOMA

- Presentation: severe, throbbing pain in the fingertip with a discolored nail bed
- Physical Exam: characteristic discolored nail bed; rule out associated nail plate injury, tendon injury, fracture, or neurovascular compromise

- X-ray to rule out underlying fracture
- Management
  - **If <50% of the nail bed is involved,** use an 18-gauge needle or handheld cautery to trephine a hole in the nail plate.
    - The collected blood will cool the cautery to prevent damage to underling nail bed.
    - Nondisplaced fractures with associated nail bed hematomas can also be managed with trephination. Splint with DIPJ in extension.
  - **If >50% of the nail bed is involved or there is an underlying displaced/unstable fracture,** remove the nail plate and repair nailbed laceration if present.
  - Hematomas managed with trephination or nail plate removal that have an associated distal phalanx fracture require antibiotic prophylaxis (converted to an open fracture).

NAIL BED LACERATION

- Presentation: after fingertip trauma, most commonly with nail intact and underlying subungual hematoma
- Physical exam with nail bed hematoma or nail abnormality with nail bed laceration; rule out associated nail plate injury, tendon injury, fracture, or neurovascular compromise
- X-ray to rule out underlying fracture
- Management
  - Nail bed repair with suture or 2-octylcyanoacrylate (skin glue)
  - Stent eponychial fold with either native nail plate or clean foil
- Special Considerations
  - Nail bed lacerations with associated distal phalanx fractures require antibiotic prophylaxis (as it is considered an open fracture).
  - Immobilize stable fractures. Consider operative fixation for unstable fractures to protect the nail bed repair (see fingertip fracture management in section below).

NAIL BED AVULSION

- Presentation: partial or complete removal of nail plate with nail bed damage
- Physical exam to assess for extent of soft tissue loss, nail bed laceration, tendon injury, fracture, or neurovascular compromise
- X-ray to rule out underlying fracture
- Management
  - **Partial avulsion:** realign in anatomical position similar to nail bed laceration repair.
  - **Complete avulsion with retained segment:** remove the nail plate and secure the avulsed segment as a composite graft using 7-0 chromic gut suture under loupe magnification then stent the eponychial fold.
  - Extensive damage to the nail bed may require skin grafting, advancement or rotational flap, or bilaminate neodermis placement.

COMMON COMPLICATIONS

- Untreated nail injuries can progress to nail deformity or partial/complete loss of the nail.
- **Hook Nail Deformity:** nail matrix grows without adequate bony support resulting in volar curving of the nail.
  - Nail bed must be shortened 2 mm proximal to the edge of the distal phalanx to prevent this deformity.
  - Requires surgical soft tissue or bony correction.
- **Split Nail:** scarring of the nail matrix to the eponychium (synechiae) that prevents nail growth.
  - Requires scar excision and nail bed repair (primary closure vs grafting)

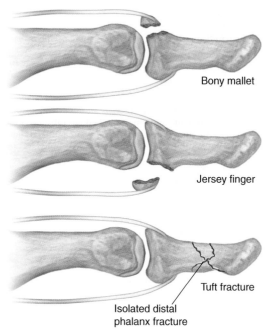

Figure 37-2 Types of distal phalanx fractures. A. Bony mallet fracture—dorsal base fracture with terminal extensor tendon disruption. **B.** Jersey finger—volar base fracture with avulsion of the flexor digitorum profundus. **C.** Distal phalanx shaft or tuft fracture. (From Chung KC, Disa JJ, Gosain A, et al., eds. *Operative Techniques in Plastic Surgery*. Wolters Kluwer; 2020. Figure 6.5.1.)

FINGER TIP FRACTURES

FINGERTIP FRACTURE

- Fractures of the distal phalanx are the most common fractures in the hand.
- The distal phalanx is divided into three anatomical zones: ungual tuberosity (tuft), diaphysis (waist), and epiphyseal (base) regions.
- Presents with pain and swelling of the fingertip after hand trauma, may be associated with nail bed hematoma or poor DIP joint ROM.
- Physical exam with tender and swollen fingertip; rule out associated nail plate injury or deformity, subungual hematoma, tendon injury, or neurovascular compromise.
- Finger x-ray to assess fracture pattern and rule out widened physis (**Fig. 37-2**).

TUFT FRACTURE

- Presentation: open or closed injury, commonly with subungual hematoma and nail bed laceration
- Associated with crush injuries
- Management
  - **If <50% bony involvement,** immobilize DIP joint 4 weeks.
    - May fail to unite but will be stabilized by fibrous union.
    - If nail plate remains intact, can consider splinting 1 week and then allowing the nail plate to act as a splint for the remainder of the period.
    - Do not immobilize the PIP joint to prevent unnecessary stiffness.

- If >50% bony involvement, consider CRPP (closed reduction percutaneous pinning) with K-wire.
- Associated subungual hematomas or nail bed lacerations should be treated (see nail bed injury section).
  - Removing or incising the nail converts a closed tuft fracture to an open fracture and requires antibiotics prophylaxis.

SHAFT FRACTURE

- Commonly transverse or longitudinal orientation.
  - Transverse fractures are at greater risk of displacement.
- Examine for proximal nail plate avulsion, which suggests an open shaft fracture.
- Management
  - **Nondisplaced fractures:** immobilize only DIP joint for 4 weeks
  - **Displaced, open, unstable, or short oblique fractures:** should be reduced and stabilized intraoperatively with CRPP to prevent nonunion and nail bed deformity

EPIPHYSEAL (BASE) FRACTURES

Mallet Finger (Table 37-1)
- Dorsal base fracture with disruption of the terminal extensor tendon distal to the DIP joint.
  - See Chapter 38: Tendon Injuries and Tendonitis for complete classification and management of zone I extensor tendon injuries.
  - Type IV zone I extensor injury is defined by an avulsed fracture at the dorsal base of the distal phalanx, known as a bony mallet.
- Presentation: after forcible flexion or axial loading to an extended digit with flexed, swollen, and tender DIP joint + loss of active DIP joint extension.
- X-ray to examine for bony fragment, joint congruity, and alignment.
- Management
  - Splint in extension for 6-8 weeks
  - **Surgical indications (CRPP through DIPJ)**
    - >1/3 articular surface involvement, type IIVB/C
    - Loss of congruity of DIP joint and an articular gap >2 mm
    - Volar subluxation of the distal phalanx
- Chronic mallet fingers >4 weeks since time of injury can be treated conservatively unless there is an extensor lag greater than 40 degrees or functional limitation.
- Untreated mallet fingers commonly progress to swan-neck deformity (see Chapter 38: Tendon Injuries and Tendonitis).

TABLE 37-1 Classification and Management of Bony Mallet Finger

Subtype	Description	Management
IVA	Transphyseal injury (pediatrics)	• DIP extension splinting continuously ×4 weeks • Keep PIP and MCP free to prevent stiffness, avoid splinting in hyperextension • Percutaneous pinning of DIP joint may rarely be indicated for children or poor adherence
IVB	Avulsion fracture involving 20%-50% of articular surface	• If no DIP joint subluxation or instability, consider DIP extension splinting ×4 weeks • >30% articular surface involvement or volar subluxation of distal phalanx requires ORIF vs CRPP (consider extension block technique)
IVC	Avulsion fracture involving >50% articular surface	• Must be treated surgically (ORIF vs CRPP) to prevent a mallet deformity or progression to swan-neck deformity

Jersey Finger
- Volar base fracture with disruption of the FDP insertion distal to the DIP joint
  - See **Chapter 38: Tendon Injuries and Tendonitis** for complete classification and management of zone I flexor tendon injuries.
  - Type III, IV, and V zone I jersey finger injury is defined by an avulsed fracture at the volar base of the distal phalanx, in addition to FDP injury.
- Presentation: after forcible extension or axial loading to a flexed digit with extended, swollen, and tender DIP joint and loss of active DIP joint flexion.
- X-ray to examine for bony fragment, joint congruity, and alignment.
- Management
  - Flexor tendon injury with associated volar fracture requires ORIF vs CRPP and tendon repair.

*Seymour Fracture
- Displaced physeal fracture with associated nail bed injury in pediatric patients
  - Interposition of the germinal matrix in the fracture site prevents adequate reduction.
- Presentation: crush injury in pediatric patient with finger flexed at the DIP joint
  - Flexor digitorum profundus (FDP) tendon inserts into the metaphysis, whereas extensor tendon inserts on the epiphysis. This injury results in flexed resting posture (mallet deformity).
  - Similar in presentation to a mallet finger; however, the extensor tendon insertion remains intact and the fracture does not enter the DIP joint.
- High suspicion in pediatric patients who present with a subungual hematoma, eponychial fold laceration, elongated nail bed, nail plate avulsion, or the nail plate lying superficial to the eponychium
- X-ray identifies a Salter-Harris I or II fracture, may show a widened physis
- Management
  - Isolated closed reduction in the emergency department is contraindicated.
  - Operative I&D, removal of interposed germinal matrix to ensure adequate reduction, nail bed laceration repair, CRPP with DIP joint in slight hyperextension.
  - High risk of osteomyelitis or septic arthritis if not accurately diagnosed and managed.

PEARLS

1. Do not confuse paronychium (sides of nail bed) with perionychium (entire nail unit) and paronychia (abscess of the nail fold).
2. Half of nail bed injuries are associated with distal phalanx fractures.
3. Seymour fractures require operative intervention, and there is a high risk of osteomyelitis and septic arthritis if they are missed.
4. Distal phalanx fractures with overlying nail plate avulsion or exposed nail bed injury are open fractures and need to be managed as such.

QUESTIONS YOU WILL BE ASKED

1. What is the location of arteries relative to nerves in the digits and in the palm? Arteries are dorsal to the nerves in the digits, volar to the nerves in the palm.

Recommended Readings
1. Chung KC. Chapter 8a: Seymour fractures and nail bed repair. *Operative Techniques: Hand and Wrist Surgery*. 4th ed. Elsevier Health Sciences; 2021.
2. Rozmaryn LM, ed. *Fingertip Injuries Diagnosis, Management and Reconstruction*. 1st ed. 2015.

38 Tendon Injuries and Tendonitis

Alexander N. Khouri and Lauren Bruce

OVERVIEW

TENDON PRINCIPLES

- **Tendon Healing**
  - Intrinsic healing occurs via tenocyte proliferation within the synovial fluid, does not form adhesions.
  - Extrinsic healing occurs via proliferation of fibroblasts surrounding the sheath and synovium, results in adhesion formation.
  - Phases of tendon healing (Table 38-1).
- **Tendon Types**
  - Unsheathed tendons are covered in paratenon and have a rich vascular supply that allows them to heal quickly via intrinsic healing.
  - Sheathed tendons (including hand flexor tendons) receive blood supply from the vincula system and undergo intrinsic and extrinsic wound healing.

TENDON INJURY HISTORY

- **History of Present Illness:** age, gender, hand dominance, mechanism of injury, timing of injury, history of previous hand trauma or surgery
- **Past Medical History:** diabetes mellitus, HIV/immunocompromised state, IV drug use, steroids, vascular disease, gout, tetanus status, smoking status
- **Social Determinants of Health:** baseline level of activity, avocation, occupation, and ability to participate in therapy

FLEXOR TENDON INJURIES

- **Epidemiology**
  - Incidence: 7 per 100 000 person-years
  - More common in men than women, highest incidence occurring at 20-30 years of age
- **Flexor Tendon Anatomy**
  - See Chapter 29: Hand and Wrist Anatomy and Examination for tendon anatomy, actions, and the pulley system.

EVALUATION

- **History:** see Tendon Injury History section above
- **Physical Exam**

TABLE 38-1 Phases of Tendon Healing

Inflammatory	Injured tendon bathed in exudative neutrophils and debrided by macrophages, tenocyte proliferation	Week 1
Proliferative	Angiogenesis and collagen production	Weeks 2-6
Remodeling	Longitudinal organization of collagen fibers in line with stress, scar continues to mature for up to a year after injury	Week 6-1 year

- ○ Assess for lacerations or open wounds.
- ○ Observe the resting posture and digital cascade of the hand.
  - ▪ Malalignment, malrotation, scissoring may indicate underlying fracture.
  - ▪ Level of skin injury may not correlate with level of tendon injury (ie, lacerations that occur with the finger in flexion will result in tendon injury more distally than the skin defect).
- ○ Assess tenodesis (extension of the digits in wrist flexion and flexion of the digits in wrist extension), consider in unconscious patients.
- ○ Assess active and passive PIPJ and DIPJ flexion and extension for each digit.
  - ▪ Suspect partial laceration if full range of motion, but patient has pain or weakness during resisted flexion.
- ○ Assess for neurovascular injury (prior to local anesthetic).
- • Diagnostics
  - ○ PA, lateral, and oblique radiographs to rule out underlying fracture.
  - ○ Consider ultrasound or MRI for suspected closed tendon rupture.
- • Flexor tendon injuries are divided into 5 zones (Chapter 29: Hand and Wrist Anatomy and Examination, Fig. 29-6).

TREATMENT OF FLEXOR TENDON INJURIES

- • Nonoperative Management
  - ○ Partial lacerations <50% do not require repair
    - ▪ Consider trimming frayed edges to prevent triggering.
  - ○ Local wound care, elevation, and early range of motion
- • Operative Management
  - ○ Repair laceration if >70% or >50-60% with triggering to prevent entrapment, late rupture, and adhesion formation.
    - ▪ Injured flexor tendons have a propensity to retract and can be associated with neurovascular injury, thus all flexor tendon repairs should be done intraoperatively under loupe magnification.
    - ▪ Direct end to end repair preferred.
  - ○ Performed emergently only for poorly vascularized digits.
  - ○ See Tables 38-2 and 38-3 for further management by zone.

Tendon Repair

- ○ **Core suture**: Strength of repair is proportional to the caliber and number of strands crossing repair.
  - ▪ Larger caliber suture increases strength of repair (synthetic braided nonabsorbable 3-0 or 4-0 suture).
  - ▪ Locking sutures provide better repair strength than grasping sutures.
  - ▪ Dorsal sutures are stronger than volar.
  - ▪ A minimum of 4+ core sutures is preferred (typically 4-6 needed for an early active motion rehabilitation protocol).
    - □ Additional core sutures will increase bulk and prevent proper tendon gliding.
  - ▪ Ideal suture purchase is 10 mm from the laceration site.
  - ▪ Knots buried in the repair site assist in smooth gliding.
  - ▪ (Fig. 38-1) Popular core suture techniques.
- ○ **Epitendinous suture**: peripheral suture that augments core suture
  - ▪ Continuous circumferential stitch with 5-0 or 6-0 monofilament polypropylene
  - ▪ Increases strength by 10%-50% and improves gliding within the tendon sheath
- • Primary Repair (<24 hours)
  - ○ Indications
    - ▪ Poorly vascularized digit/in conjunction with revascularization or replantation
    - ▪ If there is an associated phalangeal shaft fracture or other injury that requires operative fixation

TABLE 38-2 Management of Flexor Tendon Injuries by Zone

Zone	Possible injured structures	Considerations	Management
I Middle of middle phalanx to fingertip "Jersey finger"	FDP	• **Presents with inability to actively flex DIP joint** • Secondary to laceration or FDP avulsion from forced extension of an actively flexed finger • **Most injuries require repair to prevent hyperextensible DIP and decreased grip/pinch strength**	• **Direct end to end repair** • If distal end is too short for primary repair <1 cm, pull-out suture over dorsal button or suture anchor can attach proximal end directly to bone • For chronic injuries (>3 month): consider two-staged tendon grafting, DIPJ arthrodesis, or tendon reconstruction • Avoid advancing FDP >1 cm to prevent quadriga • **Splint the IP joints in neutral position postoperatively, to prevent flexion contracture** • For FDP avulsion, see Table 38-3
II Proximal A1 pulley to FDS insertion	FDS, FDP, digital nerves	• Loss of active DIP and PIP flexion • FDS and FDP often injured together due to shared synovial sheath • **Highest risk of adhesions in this zone**	• **Primary end to end repair** • Repair both tendons, if possible, to add strength to finger, prevent hyperextension deformity at PIP, and improve gliding of FDP • Explore and repair any lacerated digital nerves • **Early controlled ROM improves outcomes**
III Distal carpal tunnel to proximal A1 pulley	FDS, FDP, common digital nerves, proximal palmar nerve	Examine for "lumbrical-plus" deformity to differentiate FDP injury from FDS injury	• **Primary end to end repair** • May require A1 pulley release to avoid impingement of the repaired tendon on pulley • Proximal zone III injuries may require carpal tunnel release to retrieve retracted tendon
IV Within carpal tunnel	Transverse carpal ligament, flexor tendons, median/ulnar nerve	Isolated tendon injury is rare because of protective effects of flexor retinaculum	• **Primary end to end repair** • Transverse carpal ligament should be repaired in lengthwise fashion with wrist splinted in neutral position to prevent bowstringing
V Musculotendinous junction to forearm	Any carpal tunnel or forearm structure	Often presents with multiple tendon lacerations and neurovascular injury	• **Primary end to end repair** • Repairs may be done without epitendinous suturing
Thumb TI: FPL insertion to A2 pulley TII: IPJ/A2 pulley to distal A1 pulley TIII: distal A1 pulley to carpal tunnel (thenar prominence)	FPL	Oblique and A1 pulleys are the most important to preserve to prevent bowstringing	• **Primary end to end repair** • Avoid zone III to prevent injury to recurrent motor branch of median nerve • If proximal FPL has retracted into thenar muscles, a separate incision may be required • Early motion protocols do not improve long-term results and repairs have high rupture rates in the thumb

TABLE 38-3 Classification and Management of Zone I Jersey Finger Injury

Subtype	Description and considerations	Management
I	**FDP retracts into palm** (proximal to synovial sheath so tendon is devoid of nutrition) due to vincula disruption ± palpable tender mass in palm Worse prognosis of all zone I injuries	**Requires repair within 7-10 days** to avoid tendon contracture and necrosis
II	FDP retracts to level of PIP joint/A3 pulley Tendon sheath and vincula remain intact and muscle contracture does not readily occur Most common type of zone I injury	Repair within 3 weeks of injury for optimal results Repair is possible for up to 3 months after injury
III	**FDP attached to bony avulsion fracture,** prevents tendon retracting past the distal edge of A4 pulley Bony fragment often seen proximal to DIP on XR	Direct repair possible for up to 6 weeks, ideally within several weeks of injury Bony fixation using a K-wire or screw if fragment is large enough
IV/V	Bony avulsion fracture and **FDP tendon avulsed from bony fragment** (± concomitant distal phalanx fracture) **Tendon retracts beyond middle phalanx, possibly into palm**	**Requires ORIF of fracture(s),** followed by repair of tendon Repair within 7-10 days After 7-10 days, it becomes difficult to retrieve and reattach a tendon that has retracted into palm

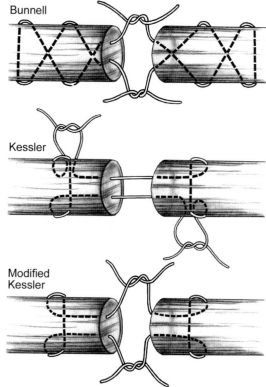

Bunnell

Kessler

Modified Kessler

Figure 38-1 Common core suture techniques. Generally modified Kessler is favored among contemporary surgeons. (From Berger RA, Weiss AC, eds. *Hand Surgery.* Lippincott Williams & Wilkins; 2004.)

- ○ Contraindications: lack of soft tissue coverage, wound contamination, infection, destruction of annular pulleys, or lengthy tendon defects
- ○ Considerations
  - ▪ Primary repair is rarely performed as outcomes are similar to delayed repair.
  - ▪ Minimize tendon handling to reduce adhesion formation.
- **Delayed Primary Repair (1-14 days)**
  - ○ Indications
    - ▪ Flexor sheath and pulleys are intact, stable soft tissue coverage, and full passive range of motion
    - ▪ Requires original tendon length
  - ○ Contraindications
    - ▪ Bony injuries involving joint or extensive soft tissue loss
    - ▪ Contaminated wound or active infection
    - ▪ Destruction of annular pulleys and lengthy tendon defects
  - ○ Consideration: increased adhesion formation with delays greater than 1 week
- **Primary Tendon Grafting (Secondary Repair)**
  - ○ Indications
    - ▪ Segmental loss of tendon (>1 cm)
    - ▪ Inability to perform primary repair due to contamination, infection, extensive damage, delayed presentation, or retraction of tendon
    - ▪ Rupture of tendon repair at primary or delayed primary stages
  - ○ Contraindications
    - ▪ Passive joint motion is very limited and extensive scarring present.
    - ▪ Open wounds or fractures are not well healed.
  - ○ General considerations
    - ▪ Need stable soft tissue coverage, full PROM, and intact flexor sheath and pulleys.
    - ▪ Secondary repair should be performed before significant muscle shortening (after about 3 weeks).
    - ▪ Independent muscles (ie, EPL) require earlier repair because they will retract faster than tendons with shared muscle bellies.
    - ▪ Decision for one-stage tendon graft or staged recon may need to be decided intraoperatively based on amount of scarring and destruction.
    - ▪ Donor tendons include ipsilateral palmaris longus, plantaris, or long toe extensor.
- **Two-Staged Tendon Reconstruction**
  - ○ Indications
    - ▪ Inadequate flexor sheath or damaged pulleys.
    - ▪ Severe soft tissue contracture or extensive scarring.
    - ▪ Previous repair attempts have been complicated by rupture, infection, bad scarring in tendon bed, or other soft tissue problems.
  - ○ **First stage**
    - ▪ Native tendon excised and temporary silicone implant (Hunter rod) is sutured to distal tendon stump.
    - ▪ Hunter rod encourages the formation of a pseudo-sheath.
    - ▪ Pulley reconstruction, tenolysis, correction of joint contractures, soft tissue reconstruction, or nerve or artery repair is performed.
  - ○ **Second stage**
    - ▪ After 2-3 months, the Hunter rod is exchanged for a tendon graft.
    - ▪ Donor tendons include ipsilateral palmaris longus, plantaris, or long toe extensor.
- **Tenolysis**
  - ○ Indications
    - ▪ Adhesions limiting active tendon excursion and digit range of motion.
    - ▪ Passive digital ROM exceeds active ROM.

- Desired ROM has not been achieved after at least 3 months of aggressive hand therapy.
- Patient is at least 6 months out from previous repair and the soft tissue is stable.
  ○ Contraindication
    - Joint contracture
    - Unable to initiate immediate postoperative motion protocol
  ○ General considerations
    - If intraoperative findings are not compatible with tenolysis (severe destruction of pulleys or lengthy lysed tendon), may need to proceed with first step of staged reconstruction intraoperatively.
    - Immediate postop ROM exercises are critical to success and should continue for 4-6 weeks postoperatively.

MANAGEMENT OF FLEXOR TENDON INJURY BY ZONE
- **Table 38-2**
- **Table 38-3**

POSTOPERATIVE CARE
- Flexor tendon rehabilitation protocols can be divided into delayed mobilization, early passive motion, and early active motion protocols.
- Early motion protocols require a motivated, adherent patient.
- Requires 12 weeks to regain enough tensile strength for normal activity.
- All protocols increase to heavy, weighted resistance after 14-16 weeks.
- **Delayed Mobilization Protocol**
  ○ Indications: no primary repair, children and nonadherent patients
  ○ Timing: 3-4 weeks of casting or fulltime orthosis
- **Early Passive ROM Protocols**
  ○ Examples: modified Kleinert or modified Duran program
  ○ Indications: primary repair, early active mobilization not indicated
  ○ Timing: begins postop day 3, progress to active motion week 3-4, strengthening begins week 8
- **Early Active Motion Protocols**
  ○ Example: Indiana Program
  ○ Indications: tendon primarily repaired with at least 4 core sutures, edema is well controlled (significant edema increases tendon drag and likelihood of rupture)
  ○ Timing: begins post-op day 3-5, strengthening begins week 8

COMPLICATIONS
- **Rupture**
  ○ Most common 7-10 days after primary repair.
  ○ Associated with gaps >3 mm.
  ○ Causes: poor suture material or surgical technique, overly aggressive therapy, poor patient compliance.
  ○ Treatment: prompt exploration and repair. For recurrent rupture or a collapsed flexor tendon sheath, consider tendon graft, tendon transfer, or arthrodesis.
- **Adhesions**
  ○ Presents as passive digital ROM > AROM.
  ○ The most effective prevention strategy is meticulous surgery with atraumatic handling of tendons and early postoperative motion.

○ Treatment: aggressive physical rehabilitation for at least 6 months postoperatively prior to considering tenolysis.

- **Quadriga**
  - ○ Flexion lag of adjacent digits following repair of FDP tendon of the middle, ring, or small finger due to their common muscle belly. The shortened tendon achieves full excursion too early, leaving the unaffected digits incompletely flexed.
  - ○ Often results from over advancing the FDP tendon > 1 cm during repair, a "too short" tendon graft, or scarring of the FDP tendon after amputation.
  - ○ Treatment: observation if minimally symptomatic, otherwise may require tenotomy, tenolysis, or tendon lengthening.
- **Lumbrical Plus**
  - ○ Paradoxical extension of IP joints of affected digit while attempting to flex the fingers into a fist.
  - ○ Causes include damage to FDP distal to lumbrical origin, a "too long" tendon graft, or DIP amputation.
  - ○ Treatment: observed if minimally symptomatic, otherwise tenodesis of FDP to terminal tendon or lumbrical release.
- **Flexion Contractures at PIP or DIP Joints**
  - ○ Late complication following early postoperative mobilization.
  - ○ Requires prompt recognition, modification of motion program to permit greater extension, and judicious use of static and dynamic splints. If no improvement after several months, may require tenolysis.

EXTENSOR TENDON INJURIES

- Epidemiology
  - ○ Incidence: 14 per 100 000 person-years.
  - ○ Extensor injuries occur most frequently in the dominant hand and are more common in men than women.
- Extensor Tendon Anatomy (**Fig. 38-2**)
  - ○ **See Chapter 29: Hand and Wrist Anatomy and Examination** for tendon anatomy and actions.

EVALUATION

- **History: See Tendon Injury History in Overview Section**
- **Physical Exam and Exam Findings**
  - ○ Assess for lacerations or open wounds.
  - ○ Observe resting posture and digital cascade.
  - ○ Assess strength and test for subluxation vs laceration.
  - ○ Assess for neurovascular injury (prior to local anesthetic).
  - ○ **Assess for EPL injury.**
    - ▪ Place hand flat on table and ask patient to lift thumb (retropulsion).
    - ▪ Extension of IP joint is an unreliable test, as EPB tendon inserts at varying levels and may be extend the IPJ in some people.
  - ○ **Perform Elson test for central slip evaluation.**
    - ▪ With PIP in 90° flexion, assess PIP and DIPJ extension.
    - ▪ DIPJ will remain floppy with an intact central slip; however, it will remain stiff in hyperextension if central slip is damaged.
    - ▪ **Figure 38-3.**
  - ○ Injury may be masked by the juncturae tendinum or mimicked by an MCP subluxation or PIN nerve palsy.

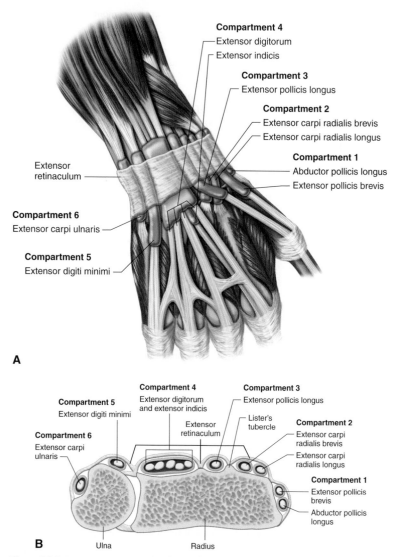

Figure 38-2 Extensor compartments of the wrist. A. Dorsal view. The extensor tendons lie in six compartments. Each compartment contains a synovial sheath for the tendon(s) it contains. The sheaths extend proximal and distal to the extensor retinaculum. The tendons of compartments two and six insert on the bases of the second/third and fifth metacarpals, respectively. Intertendinous connections are visible on the dorsum of the hand. **B.** Axial view. The extensor compartments are numbered from the radial to the ulnar side. Lister tubercle is the bony landmark that separates compartments two and three. (Adapted from Netter FH, Woodburne RT, Crelin ES, et al. Upper limb, wrist and hand. In: Musculoskeletal System, Part 1: Anatomy, Physiology and Metabolic Disorders. Ciba-Geigy; 1987:55-73. In: Beggs I. *Musculoskeletal Ultrasound*. Wolters Kluwer; 2014. Figure 5.2AB.)

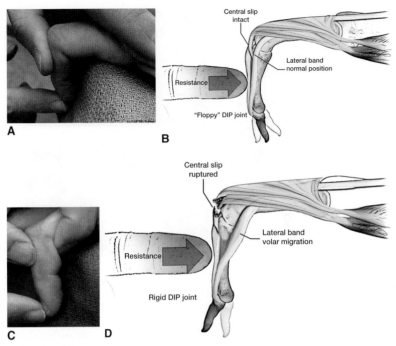

Figure 38-3 Elson slip test. The Elson test is used to diagnose incompetence of the central slip. The finger is positioned at 90° of flexion, and the examiner is asked to actively extend the PIP joint against resistance applied by the examiner to the middle phalanx. A, B. When the central slip is intact (negative Elson test), the PIP joint can be actively extended, and the DIP joint will be "floppy." C, D. When the central slip is incompetent (positive Elson test), the PIP joint may be weakly extended, but the patient will extend the distal phalanx through the attachment of the lateral bands, and thus the DIP joint will become rigid in extension. (From Wiesel SW, Albert T, eds. *Operative Techniques in Orthopaedic Surgery*. 3rd ed. Wolters Kluwer; 2022. Figure 6.52.4.)

- **Extensor Tendon Injuries Are Divided Into 9 Zones**
  - **Figure 38-4**
  - Odd zones are over joints, even zones are in-between
- **Diagnostics**
  - Clinical diagnosis
  - Radiographs to rule out underlying fracture, subluxed joint, or physis injury in a pediatric patient

MANAGEMENT OF EXTENSOR TENDON INJURIES BY ZONE

- **Table 38-4**
- **Table 38-5**

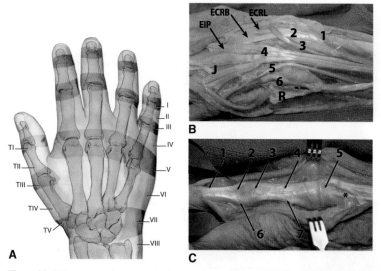

Figure 38-4 Extensor tendon zones. A. Extensor zones of injury. **B, C.** The digits are to the left and the wrist is to the right. **B.** The top of the figure is radial and the bottom is ulnar. Wrist and hand extensor tendon anatomy, with numbers (1-6) to identify the extensor tendon compartments. R is the reflected extensor retinaculum and J is a juncturae tendinum. Note the combined EDC tendon to the ring and small fingers. In the fourth compartment, the extensor indicis proprius (EIP) tendon is deep to the EDC tendons and has more distal muscle fibers. In the hand, it is just deep and ulnar to the index EDC tendon. **C.** The digital extensor mechanism: terminal tendon (1); triangular ligament (2); PIP joint (3); central slip tendon (4); sagittal band (5); lateral band, which will become the terminal tendon distally (6); and conjoined lateral band, with fibers to the base of the middle phalanx and to the lateral band (7). This patient has an unusual proprius tendon to the long finger (asterisk), passing under the ulnar to the EDC tendon and beneath the junctura. ECRB, extensor carpi radialis brevis; ECRL, extensor carpi radialis longus. (From Wiesel SW, Albert T, eds. *Operative Techniques in Orthopaedic Surgery.* 3rd ed. Wolters Kluwer; 2022. Figure 6.53.1.)

POSTOPERATIVE CARE

- **Basic Tenets of Extensor Tendon Rehabilitation**
  - Early motion decreases adhesion formation but can increase risk of rupture and gapping.
  - The greater the normal amount of tendon excursion within a zone, the more important early motion is to prevent excursion limiting adhesions.
  - Most protocols follow the same outline: splint controlled passive or active motion during the first 3-4 weeks postoperatively, followed by progressive out-of-splint active motion exercises.
  - The first 3 weeks of any rehabilitation program should include antiedema management.
  - Do not progress to next stage of rehabilitation protocol if significant extensor lag is present.

TABLE 38-4 Management of Extensor Tendon Injuries by Zone

Zone	Symptoms and considerations	Management
I Digit DIP joint, thumb IP joint "mallet finger"	Forced flexion of an extended DIP joint Painful, edematous DIP joint and loss of active DIP extension **Can progress to swan neck deformity**	**Nonoperative:** closed injuries, nondisplaced fractures, and chronic mallet injuries with supple joints **Operative:** open injury, unstable DIP joint, or large nonreducible avulsion fractures
II Digit middle phalanx, thumb proximal phalanx	Injury often due to laceration or crush injury Phalangeal extension should always be tested against resistance	**Nonoperative:** <50% tendon involvement, no extensor lag, and active digit extension **Operative:** primary repair for lacerations >50% tendon width or loss of active extension
III Digit PIP joint, thumb MCP joint	Presents with painful, edematous PIP, mild extension lag at PIP joint and weak active/resisted PIP extension Perform Elson test to assess central slip integrity Commonly missed diagnosis in the ED and misdiagnosed as jammed fingers **Can progress to boutonniere deformity**	**Nonoperative:** closed injuries treated with splinting. Transarticular K-wire fixation of PIP joint alternatively **Operative:** indicated for open injuries, displaced avulsion fractures of middle phalanx, PIP instability with loss of active or passive extension, and failed nonsurgical treatment. May include primary tendon repair, suture anchor repair for avulsions or distal central slip injuries, or central slip reconstruction followed by PIP extension splinting vs transarticular K-wire
IV Digit proximal phalanx, thumb metacarpal	Partial lacerations are common as tendons in this zone are broad and flat Associated with proximal phalanx fractures	Management similar to zone II injury Obtain rigid fixation of an associated phalanx fracture to allow early active ROM
V Digit MCP joint, thumb CMC joint "Fight bite"	**Always suspect human bite wound** Juncturae tendinum may mask injury Rule out sagittal band injury and subluxation of tendons. Patient will be able to maintain MCP extension when passively extended if subluxed Thumb zone V injuries often involve the APL and EPB tendons	**Nonoperative:** treat closed injuries with splinting and rehabilitation. Chronic injuries may require repair if extensor mechanism remains mispositioned **Operative** **Acute, open injury:** irrigate and debride aggressively in the OR, repair tendon, and leave wound open. If confirmed fight bite, give broad-spectrum IV antibiotics Sagittal band lacerations must be repaired to prevent extensor subluxation Explore thumb lacerations and repair the superficial radial sensory nerve if indicated **Old, open injury:** may require delayed treatment of tendon, until infection is controlled, and soft tissue is in equilibrium

(continued)

TABLE 38-4 Management of Extensor Tendon Injuries by Zone (*Continued*)

Zone	Symptoms and considerations	Management
VI Digit metacarpals	Extensor tendon injury may be masked by EIP, EDM, or juncturae tendinum Evaluate MCP extension against resistance	Repair in the ED if tendons are easily retrievable, otherwise repair in the OR
VII Wrist/dorsal retinaculum	Tendons may retract into forearm Evaluate for injury to sensory branches of radial and ulnar nerves	Repair tendons ± repair extensor retinaculum to prevent bowstringing Increased tendon thickness makes core sutures possible in this zone, 4-6 core sutures is preferred Chronic tear or ruptures: tendon transfer or grafting
VIII Distal forearm	Associated neurovascular injury is common	Primary tendon repair followed by immobilization with elbow in flexion and wrist in extension Tendon transfers may be required
IX Muscles of mid and proximal forearm	Secondary to penetrating trauma	Repair of muscle bellies is difficult and requires multiple figure-of-8 sutures using large bites Tendon transfers may be required

COMPLICATIONS

- Adhesions
- Tendon Rupture
- Swan Neck Deformity (DIP Flexion and PIP Hyperextension)
  - Figure 38-5
  - Associated with mallet finger (zone 1) injury

TABLE 38-5 Classification and Management of Zone I Extensor Injuries

Subtype	Description	Management
I	**Closed rupture** at tendon insertion, with or without small bone fragment	DIP extension splinting continuously for 6-8 weeks Keep PIP and MCP free to prevent stiffness Percutaneous pinning of DIP joint may rarely be indicated for children or poor adherence
II	**Open injury** or laceration at, or just proximal to the DIP joint	Treat with CRPP and primary tendon repair Repair with a single nonabsorbable suture passed tendon and skin, known as dermo to tenodesis
III	Open injury with **significant soft tissue loss**	Treat with CRPP and soft tissue coverage if necessary (skin graft, integra placement or local skin flap such as reverse cross finger flap)
IV	Avulsion fracture (bony mallet)	Subtypes based on extent of articular surface involvement CRPP and repair of terminal tendon with or without tendon graft May be treated conservatively if there is no DIP joint instability or subluxation

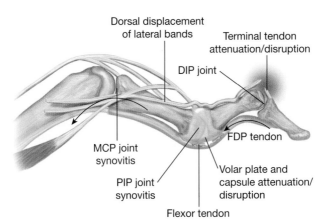

Figure 38-5 Swan neck deformity. (From Chung KC, ed. *Operative Techniques in Hand and Wrist Surgery*. Wolters Kluwer; 2020. Figure 24.6A.)

- Lateral band dorsal subluxation with oblique fibers and transverse retinacular ligament laxity and triangular ligament contracture
- Treatment
  - Splinting to limit PIP hyperextension may suffice for mild cases.
  - Operative treatment includes a Fowler central slip tenotomy, spiral oblique ligament reconstruction, or volar plate advancement with FDS tenodesis.
- **Boutonniere Deformity (DIP Hyperextension)**
  - **Figure 38-6.**
  - Central slip disruption with oblique fiber and transverse retinacular ligament contraction and triangular ligament rupture.
  - Perform Elson test for central slip evaluation.
  - Treatment: first-line treatment includes dynamic extension splinting (PIP extended and DIP free) for maximal passive motion.

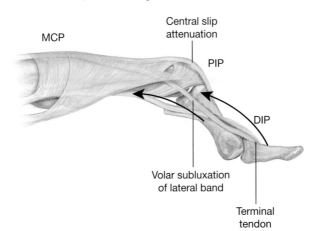

Figure 38-6 Boutonniere deformity. (From Chung KC, ed. *Operative Techniques in Hand and Wrist Surgery*. Wolters Kluwer; 2020. Figure 24.7A.)

TENDINITIS

- **Etiology**
  - Tendon becomes inflamed causing the synovium to swell and prevents proper tendon gliding.
  - Often associated with repetitive hand or wrist movements.
- **Evaluation and Treatment**
  - See Table 38-6 for classic signs, symptoms, exacerbating activities, and management recommendations for common tendinitis conditions.
  - Treatment often begins with conservative management, which includes **splinting, NSAIDs, activity modification, and steroid injections.**
  - Table 38-6.

TABLE 38-6 Tendinitis Diagnosis and Management

Name	Tendon(s) involved	Definition, signs, and symptoms	Management
Trigger finger (stenosing tenosynovitis)	FDS, FDP	**Signs/symptoms:** (1) catching, sticking, or locking of fingers in a flexed or extended position; (2) pain in distal palm with palpable palmar nodule; (3) worse in the morning **A1 pulley** and the **thumb** are most commonly affected	**Nighttime extension splinting** of the affected digits (*low success rate*) **Steroid injections** into tendon sheath (*50-90% success rate, but high recurrence*) Injections are less successful in patients with diabetes, chronic cases, and diffuse rather than nodular tenosynovitis, as seen with RA **Trigger finger release** is indicated for long-standing symptoms or failed conservative treatment **Percutaneous release** may be performed but is contraindicated in the thumb and index finger due to risk of digital nerve injury
De Quervain tenosynovitis	APL, EBL	**Signs/Symptoms:** 1) radial-sided wrist pain with thumb use; 2) tenderness over the first dorsal compartment/radial styloid Positive Finkelstein's test à pain with brisk thumb adduction Positive Eichoff test à pain with thumb tuck and wrist ulnar deviation **Rule out CMC joint arthritis** with normal axial grind test	Conservative management with forearm-based thumb spica splint **Steroid injection** into distal end of first dorsal compartment (*limited success due to 2-4 slips of the APL separated by multiple subcompartments*) **Surgery (tenosynovectomy)** if conservative treatment fails Avoid damage to the superficial radial nerve during dissection

TABLE 38-6 Tendinitis Diagnosis and Management (*Continued*)

Name	Tendon(s) involved	Definition, signs, and symptoms	Management
Intersection syndrome	APL/EBL and ECRL/ECRB	**Tenosynovitis at the junction of 1st and 2nd extensor compartments** Signs/symptoms: (1) swelling and tenderness where tendons intersect, ~4-6 cm proximal to Lister tubercle; (2) crepitus with wrist or thumb extension Seen with activities such as **rowing, skiing, and racquet sports,** due to repetitive wrist movements	Conservative management with forearm-based thumb spica splint **Surgery to release the second compartment for refractory cases** (*rarely required*)
Flexor carpi radialis tendonitis	FCR	Signs/symptoms: (1) pain and tenderness along FCR with resisted wrist flexion and radial deviation **Rule out Linburg-Comstock syndrome**—tenosynovitis due to tendinous connection between FPL and FDP to index finger	Conservative management **Surgery** to release FCR if conservative measured fail (*rarely required*) Avoid injury to palmar cutaneous branch of median nerve during dissection
Flexor carpi ulnaris tendonitis	FCU	Signs and symptoms: (1) pain and tenderness along FCU with resisted wrist flexion and ulnar deviation **Rule out pisotriquetral arthritis** with normal pisotriquetral grind test	Conservative management **Surgery** to release FCU if conservative measures fail (*rarely required*) Avoid injury to palmar cutaneous branch of ulnar nerve during dissection
Extensor carpi ulnaris tendonitis	ECU	Signs and symptoms: (1) pain and tenderness on ulnar side of wrist with resistant wrist flexion and extension, particularly in supination Associated with **racquet sports, golf, rugby, and basketball** Tendon subluxation may be associated with triangular fibrocartilage complex (TFC) tears	Conservative management **Consider imaging with US or MRI or arthroscopic evaluation** to assess for TFC or ligament injuries if atypical features or conservative treatment fails Consider tenosynovectomy with sheath release if necessary
Other	EIP, EDC, EPL	Extensor tenosynovitis (EIP or EDC) or drummer's tendonitis (EPL)	Conservative management Consider surgery for EPL tendinitis to prevent rupture

PEARLS

1. Open extensor tendon injuries with >50% tendon involvement can be repaired in the ED, whereas flexor tendon injuries are treated in the OR under loupe magnification.
2. The skin laceration does not always correlate with the level of tendon injury.

3. Flexor tendon repair requires balance between increasing the strength of the repair and limiting bulk that can prevent proper tendon gliding through the sheath and pulley system.
4. Successful postoperative outcomes after tendon repair are a result of motivated patients working with well-trained hand therapists.

QUESTIONS YOU WILL BE ASKED

1. Describe the flexor and extensor zones.
   See Figures 38-1 and 38-5.
2. Describe the location of the pulleys and identify which ones are most important to preserve to prevent bowstringing.
   Most important digital pulleys are A2 (over proximal phalanx) and A4 (over middle phalanx). Most important thumb pulley is the oblique pulley.
3. Describe the classification of a "jersey finger" injury.
   Subtype I: FDP retracts into palm
   Subtype II: FDP retracts to level of PIP/A3 pulley
   Subtype III: FDP attached to bony avulsion fracture, prevents tendon retracting past the distal edge of A4 pulley
   Subtype IV: FDP tendon avulsed from bony fragment and tendon retracts beyond middle phalanx, possibly into palm
   Subtype V: Same as type IV + concomitant distal phalanx fracture
4. When is the most common time for tendon rupture after primary repair?
   Post-op day 10 is the most common time for rupture after primary repair (tendon is weakest 7-10 days after repair).
5. What is the "quadriga effect"?
   The "quadriga effect" refers to limited excursion of the middle, ring, and small fingers due to tethering connections between the profundus tendons due to a common muscle belly. It can be from scarring of an FDP tendon or iatrogenic from an overly tight tendon repair or suturing of the FDP to the extensor.

Recommended Readings
1. Howell JW, Peck F. Rehabilitation of flexor and extensor tendon injuries in the hand: current updates. *Injury.* 2013;44(3):397-402. doi:10.1016/j.injury.2013.01.022
2. Ruchelsman DE, Christoforou D, Wasserman B, Lee SK, Rettig ME. Avulsion injuries of the flexor digitorum profundus tendon. *J Am Acad Orthop Surg.* 2011;19(3):152-162. doi:10.5435/00124635-201103000-00004
3. Tang JB. Flexor tendon injuries. *Clin Plast Surg.* 2019;46(3):295-306. doi:10.1016/j.cps.2019.02.003
4. Yoon AP, Chung KC. Management of acute extensor tendon injuries. *Clin Plast Surg.* 2019;46(3):383-391. doi:10.1016/j.cps.2019.03.004

39 Tendon Transfers

Widya Adidharma

OVERVIEW

- **Tendon Transfer (TT):** the relocation of a tendon from a functioning muscle to replace an injured or nonfunctional muscle-tendon unit
  - Concept of "muscle balance operation": tendon transfer (TT) is a redistribution of power units from areas of lesser functional need to areas of greater functional need
  - Developed in the late 1800s as a way to reconstruct the longstanding effects of polio
- **Tenets of TT**
  - Joints affected need to have a good passive range of motion; joint contractures need to be either prevented or repaired
  - Soft tissue coverage has to be supple and stable. TTs through scar tissue do poorly and any soft tissue reconstruction should be done prior to TT
  - Never introduce more than one change of direction in a tendon
  - Each transfer should have the goal of one function
  - Use an expendable donor with adequate strength and excursion
- Indications
  - Nerve injury: the most common indication. TT is often needed when nerve injuries are devastating or proximal, as reinnervation will not occur in time to salvage motor units (motor end plates are irreversibly damaged 18-24 months after denervation).
    - Loss of a single major nerve (ie, ulnar/median/radial) is more amenable to TT; if two or three nerves are damaged, severe extremity impairment is inevitable
  - Muscle/tendon destruction: trauma or disease processes such as rheumatoid arthritis.
  - Spastic disorders: TT can decrease spasticity and ease hand positioning and hygiene.

PREOPERATIVE PLANNING

Please refer to **Chapter 29** for hand anatomy and end of chapter for abbreviations

EVALUATION

- Establish patient goals/needs.
- Rank priority of the functions desired.
- Verify motivation and ability to follow through with rehabilitation.
- In nerve injury, distinguish between high and low injury (determines TT's chosen).
- **Wound site factors must be addressed before a TT**
  - The bony skeleton must be stabilized.
  - The wound surface must be healed or closed.
  - Scars must be soft or must be excised.

---

*Denotes common in-service examination topics.

- ○ Adequate soft tissue must be present to protect the TT
- ○ Joint mobility must be maximized for the best result

TIMING

- **Immediate TT:** only done if there is no chance of nerve functional recovery, that is, the muscle is destroyed or large section of the nerve is missing and repair/regrowth is not feasible.
- **Delayed TT:** usually performed 9-12 months following injury to allow for potential regrowth of the nerve before proceeding with TT. The higher the nerve injury, the longer regrowth will take.

DONOR TENDON AND MUSCLE ASSESSMENT

- **Donor Muscle Assessment:** inventory all muscles and rate their power. Only donor muscles with British Medical Research Council (MRC) power grades of 4 or 5 should be used for TT.
  - ○ 0: No active movement
  - ○ 1: Visible muscle movement but not at joint
  - ○ 2: Can create motion at joint, but against gravity
  - ○ 3: Can overcome gravity, but not added resistance
  - ○ 4: Can overcome resistance, but weaker than "normal"
  - ○ 5: Normal strength
- **Control:** tendons to be transferred should have independent power (eg, the flexor digitorum profundus [FDP] tendon slips do not have independent function and therefore are poor donor choices)
- **Excursion** (amplitude)
  - ○ Specific excursions
    - Finger flexors—70 mm
    - Finger extensors, FPL, EPL—50 mm
    - Wrist flexors and extensors—30 mm
  - ○ Tenodesis can increase excursion by ~25 mm
  - ○ Need to match the donor being transferred with the amount of excursion needed (eg, a wrist flexor will not work as digit extensor)
- **Need to match strength** (eg, FCU too strong for use as motor for APB). Therapy can improve muscle strength, but not excursion (**Table 39-1**).
- **Location:** reroute the donor tendon in as direct line as possible; do not change direction of tendon more than once.
- **Synergism:** if possible, use muscles that naturally work together (ie, wrist extensors and finger flexors); this makes postop rehabilitation easier.
- **Expendability:** is tendon function worth giving up for the benefit gained at its new location?

TABLE 39-1 Relative Strength of Tendons

Muscle	Relative strength
BR, FCU	2
Wrist extensors (ECRL, ECU), PT	1
Digital flexors (FPL, FDS, FDP)	1
Digital extensors (EDC, EIP, EDM)	0.5
APL, EPB, EPL, PL	0.1

TENDON TRANSFERS FOR SPECIFIC NERVE PALSIES

RADIAL NERVE PALSY

- High vs Low Palsy: whether lesion is proximal or distal to the elbow, respectively
- *High Radial Nerve Paralysis: wrist, thumb, and digit extension are lost producing a wrist drop deformity. Loss of wrist extension weakens power grip strength. Over time, patients develop an adaptive functional pattern:
    ○ Patients use wrist flexion to assist with finger extension, aka the "tenodesis effect"
    ○ Maladaptive wrist flexion may be difficult to overcome later with TTs
    ○ Splints should be worn to force wrist extension and assist with finger extension; splints are cumbersome and often tolerated only at night, but critical to eventual outcome
    ○ Alternatively, some surgeons advocate doing an end to side TT of PT to ECRB to facilitate grip strength during nerve recovery, termed an "internal splint" procedure
- **Low Radial Nerve Injury:** wrist extension preserved due to intact ECRL. Greater radial wrist deviation than higher level injury due to unopposed ECRL function with loss of other extensors
- *Common TTs for Radial Nerve Paralysis (Table 39-2)
    ○ Goal: correct wrist drop (high palsy), restore thumb extension, and restore finger extension. Therefore, require one tendon each for wrist, digit, and thumb extension.
- **Common transfers:** Brand, Jones, Boyes. Differ in tendons used for reconstructing finger and thumb extension

TABLE 39-2 Tendon Transfers for Radial Nerve Paralysis

Desired function	Tendon transfer	Comments
Wrist extension (high nerve palsies)	PT to ECRB (Brand, Jones, and Boyes)	PT is the optimal donor for wrist extension. It may not be needed if the injury is below the level of ECRB innervation
Wrist lateral deviation (low palsies)	ECRL to ECRB or ECU	Minimizes radial wrist deviation
Digit extension (low and high palsies)	FCR to EDC (Brand) FCU to EDC (Jones)	FCR is favored, as ulnar deviation is preserved FCU has twice the force of FCR but less excursion No independent digit extension is allowed with these TTs
	FDS-III to EDC (Boyes)	For independent motion
Thumb extension (low and high palsies)	PL to EPL (Brand and Jones)	PL is present in 80% of patients
	FDS-IV to EPL (Boyes)	FDS can be used if PL is not present
	BR to APL	APL tenodesis at the BR insertion at the radial styloid prevents flexion-adduction of the thumb metacarpal and compensatory MCP hyperextension and IP flexion

MEDIAN NERVE PALSY

- High vs Low Palsy: whether lesion is proximal or distal to origin of AIN
- **Low Median Nerve Palsy:** loss of nerve function at level of the wrist
  - *Loss of thumb opposition from paralysis of APB, OP, and superficial head of the FPB
  - Deep head of FPB and adductor pollicis are innervated by ulnar nerve and may provide adequate opposition
  - Loss of the lumbricals to the index and middle fingers
- **High Median Nerve Palsy**
  - *In addition to the low median nerve muscle losses, AIN is affected. Patients lose FPL, PQ, and FDP to index and middle fingers, resulting in loss of thumb and index flexion, in addition to the loss of thumb opposition.
  - Higher level injuries will damage FCR and PT function, but these losses do not require TTs.
- **Common TTs for Median Nerve Paralysis (Table 39-3)**
  - Goal: restore thumb opposition (and in high palsy also restore thumb and index finger flexion)

ULNAR NERVE PALSY

- High vs Low Classification: whether lesion is proximal or distal to origin of motor branches to FCU
- **Low Ulnar Nerve Palsy**
  - Paralysis of AP, the deep head of FPB, all interossei, hypothenar muscles, and the lumbricals to ring and little fingers.
  - *Clawing of the hand: specifically, MP hyperextension and IP flexion in the ring and little fingers due to loss of intrinsic musculature in the setting of intact extrinsic function.
  - **Weak key pinch:** due to denervation of the first dorsal interosseous and AP muscles. To compensate, patients use FPL flexion to stabilize the thumb and EPL to adduct the thumb. Exaggerated thumb IP flexion during key pinch is termed **Froment sign.**

TABLE 39-3 Transfers for Median Nerve Paralysis

Desired function	Tendon transfer	Comments
Thumb opposition (low and high palsies)	EIP to APB	EIP is usually preferred to avoid using a tendon from potentially scarred volar area
	ADM to APB	The **Huber procedure.** Also used for thumb hypoplasia, combined nerve palsies and trauma
Thumb opposition (low palsy)	FDS (RF) to APB	FDS (RF) is routed through a loop of FCU at the wrist to approach the APB at the proper angle
	PL to APB	The **Camitz procedure.** Used after long-standing CTS and can be performed at the time of CTR
Thumb flexion (high palsy)	BR to FPL	Allows thumb IP flexion
Index flexion (high palsy)	FDP (LF, RF) to FDP (MF, IF)	Tenorrhaphy (not transfer) allows DIP flexion of MF and IF
	ECRL to FDP (IF)	Provides strength to index flexion

- o Little finger ulnar deviation occurs due to unbalanced extensors (EDC and EDM) to that digit (Wartenberg sign)
- **High Ulnar Nerve Palsy**
  - o **Less clawing than with low ulnar palsies,** as the paralysis of the FCU and FDP to ring and little fingers decreases the deforming force.
  - o Reconstruction can improve the function of the hand, but normal function usually cannot be restored.
- *Common TTs for Ulnar Nerve Paralysis (Table 39-4). Goals: improve clawing and strengthen key pinch.

TABLE 39-4 Transfers for Ulnar Nerve Paralysis

Desired function	Tendon transfer	Comments
Thumb key pinch (low and high palsies)	ECRB or BR to abductor tubercle of the first metacarpal	Adductoplasty through the second intermetacarpal space to attach to the abductor tubercle. A PL tendon graft is usually required
	FDS (RF) to abductor tubercle of the first metacarpal	Adductoplasty. Use only radial half of the RF FDS tendon. Palmar fascia acts as pulley. No tendon graft is needed
Clawing (low palsy)	FDS (MF or RF) to LF, RF	Tendons are split and then sutured to lateral bands or to the proximal phalanx
	FDS "lasso" to LF, RF A2 pulley	FDS (RF or MF) is divided and looped through the A2 pulley and then sutured to itself, with half going to LF and half going to the RF
	EDC or BR to LF, RF lateral bands	Attached to the lateral bands. Stabilizes finger but does not aid in power flexion
	EIP or EDC (LF) to LF, RF LBs	Attached to the lateral bands through the intermetacarpal space
Clawing (high palsy)	FDP (MF) to FDP (LF, RF)	Side to side tenorrhaphy
Index abduction for key pinch (low and high palsies)	Slip of APL to first dorsal interosseous	Main part of the APL remains attached to thumb; may use tendon graft to augment
	EIP or EPB to first dorsal interosseous	Alternatives used to restore IF abduction. Many variations, but all attach to the first interosseous
Power digit flexion (low and high palsy)	ECRL to digits	Tendon grafts are used to extend the ERCL in two to four tails, which go under the TCL to attach to the digital lateral bands or to the A2 pulleys
Little finger adduction (low palsy)	EDM to LF	Ulnar half of EDM is passed through the metacarpal space to attach to either bone or the A2 pulley
Wrist flexion (high palsy)	FCR to FCU	Restores FCU function. Some authors feel this is not necessary

STATIC BLOCK PROCEDURES

- Can be done to prevent MCP hyperextension, including MCP arthrodesis, MCP joint capsulodeses, or bone blocks on the dorsum of the MCP head.
- These procedures can be used alone or in concert with TTs.

PEARLS

1. When evaluating for tendon transfers, it is absolutely necessary to accurately document all motor and sensory deficits, as well as normal findings on neuromuscular examination.
2. No functional recovery is expected if motor end plates are not reinnervated within 18-24 months due to muscle atrophy. (Slightly longer time frame in children, shorter in older adults.)
3. Supple joints, adequate soft tissue, and compliance with hand therapy are essential for successful tendon transfer.
4. Choice of transfer depends on expendability of the donor tendon and the strength, excursion, and location.

QUESTIONS YOU WILL BE ASKED

1. Is it better to do nerve transfers or tendon transfers for a given deficit?
   There is no clear answer, and each case is individualized based on expectations, surgeon preference, and experience.
2. Possible tendon transfers for a specific nerve palsy.
   Possible tendon transfers for nerve injuries listed in Tables 39-2 to 39-4. Alternatively, think of possibilities based upon expendability, strength, excursion, and location.

Recommended Readings
1. Sammer DM, Chung KC. Tendon transfers: part I. Principles of transfer and transfers for radial nerve palsy. *Plast Reconstr Surg.* 2009;123(5):169e-177e.
2. Sammer DM, Chung KC. Tendon transfers: Part II. Transfers for ulnar nerve palsy and median nerve palsy. *Plast Reconstr Surg.* 2009;124(3):212e-221e.

Thumb Reconstruction

Ryan O. Davenport and Shahan Saleem

OVERVIEW

GENERAL CONSIDERATIONS

- **Epidemiology**
  - Thumb amputation is most common in working age males.
  - Approximately 70% of traumatic injuries are related to machine injuries.
  - Other, less common etiologies include tumor or infection.
- **Relevant Anatomy**
  - Muscles by insertion
    - Distal phalanx—extensor pollicis longus, flexor pollicis longus
    - Proximal phalanx—extensor pollicis brevis, flexor pollicis brevis, abductor pollicis brevis, adductor pollicis
    - Metacarpal—abductor pollicis longus, opponens pollicis
  - Amputations at the level of the interphalangeal joint or distal aspect of the proximal phalanx may result in relatively well-maintained function due to muscular insertions at the base of the proximal phalanx.
- **Thumb Function**
  - *Thumb contributes 40% of the hand function.
  - Essential for prehensile hand function—precision and power grip.
  - Requires contact between the index and the thumb pulp to achieve tripod pinch, fine motor dexterity, and cylinder grasp.
- **Reconstructive Goals**
  - **Adequate length** for opposition
  - **Mobility and stability** for opposition, flexion, and pinch
    - Carpometacarpal (CMC) mobility is essential for normal function. If this cannot be achieved, CMC arthrodesis in full abduction-opposition is best.
    - Interphalangeal (IP) and metacarpophalangeal (MP) joint contribute less to overall function.
  - **Sensation**
    - Protective
    - Pain free: a painful digit will be avoided
  - **Durable** soft tissue coverage for regular use
  - **Aesthetic appearance**

EVALUATION

- **Patient Assessment**
  - Age: pediatric patients have greater neural plasticity compared with adults
  - Hand dominance
  - Health and comorbid conditions
  - Occupation, activities, and commitment to postoperative care
  - Associated injuries: particularly ipsilateral hand/digit or toe injuries
- **Injury Assessment**
  - Mechanism and timing of the injury
  - Level of injury, Lister Classification (**Table 40-1**)

---

*Denotes common in-service examination topics.

TABLE 40-1 Summary of Thumb Reconstructive Options By Amputation Level

Level of injury	Goals	Options	
Bony amputation at or distal to DIP; soft tissue loss with adequate length (2 cm proximal phalanx intact)	(1) Bone length is acceptable (2) Chief goal is soft tissue coverage of bone and length preservation	Local	Revision amputation with first web space narrowing, healing via secondary intention, skin graft Exposed bone/tendon: Moberg flap, V-Y advancement, lateral advancement flaps, FDMA flap, neurovascular (Littler) island flap, cross-finger flap
		Regional	Pedicled groin or thoracoepigastric flap
		Distant	Free great toe wraparound flap, free toe-pulp transfer
Bony amputation at or distal to PIP; subtotal amputation with questionable length and soft tissue deficit	Both restoration of bone length along with soft tissue coverage	Local	Phalangization. Metacarpal lengthening (distraction), heterotopic replantation
		Regional	Osteoplastic reconstruction: bone grafting with fasciocutaneous flap coverage (RF, PIA, or groin flaps)
		Distant	Great or second toe transfer, trimmed toe transfer, wrap-around toe flap, on-top plasty
Total amputation with intact basal joint	(1) Entire thumb restoration required (extensive bony and soft tissue reconstruction) (2) Thenar muscle integrity should be assessed and restored (opponens pollicis, abductor pollicis) (3) Web space reconstruction with soft tissue coverage (if damaged)	Local	Pollicization, metacarpal lengthening, heterotopic replantation, on-top plasty, web space deepening
		Regional	Osteoplastic reconstruction: bone grafting with fasciocutaneous flap coverage (RF, PIA, or groin flaps)
		Distant	Great or second toe transfer
Total amputation with loss of basal joint	(1) Stable post with appropriate position relative to other fingers (2) Web space reconstruction with soft tissue coverage (if damaged)	Local	Pollicization
		Distant	Great or second toe transfer with TMJ fusion

IP, interphalangeal; FDMA, first dorsal metacarpal artery; RF, radial forearm; PIA, posterior interosseous artery.

- Presence of other digit amputations: specific digit and level
- Presence of web space contracture, if secondary reconstruction
- Radiographs: three views (lateral, anteroposterior, and oblique) incorporating the CMC joint

TREATMENT

INDICATIONS FOR RECONSTRUCTION

- Reconstruction should be considered secondary to replantation when the replantation is not achievable. **See Chapter 36: Traumatic Amputation Injuries** for amputation and replantation.
- Restoration of "acceptable hand."
  - Functional thumb with three fingers of normal length and sensation

SOFT TISSUE LOSS WITH ADEQUATE LENGTH

- **General Principles**
  - Goal: preserve length, but not as the expense of stable coverage.
  - Reconstructive options are dictated by the size of the defect.
- **Small Defects:** <1 cm^2
  - **Healing by secondary intention**
    - Preserves sensation with minimal resultant defect
    - May require painful and prolonged wound care
  - **Local flaps**
    - VY advancement
    - Lateral advancement
  - **Skin grafts**
    - More rapid healing, but insensate
- **Larger Defects:** >1 cm^2, >50% of volar pad, exposed periosteum, bone, and tendon
  - **Palmar advancement** ("Moberg" flap) (**Fig. 40-1**)
    - Sensate flap that is ideal for defects 1-2 cm^2 of the volar pad.
    - Advances a palmar flap containing both neurovascular bundles.
    - May require up to 45° of IP joint flexion to achieve coverage, which may lead to long-term flexion contracture.
    - Defects that require more than 1.5 cm of advancement or to minimize IP flexion can be covered using a proximal releasing incision—still limited by neurovascular bundles.
  - **Heterodigital flaps:** indicated for defects >2.5 cm^2 or for loss of the entire volar pad
    - **Cross-finger flap**
      - See Chapter 36: Traumatic Amputation Injuries
    - **First dorsal metacarpal artery (FDMA) flap** (**Fig. 40-2**)
      - *An innervated, pedicled island flap transferring the FDMA, subcutaneous veins, dorsal branch of the radial sensory nerve, and skin from the index finger.
      - Pedicle runs under the first dorsal interosseous fascia and sometimes within the muscle.
      - First dorsal metacarpal artery is usually branch off of the radial artery.
      - Donor site is covered with a full-thickness skin graft.
      - Can cover both dorsal and palmar defects.
    - **Neurovascular island flap** ("Littler flap")
      - Pedicled, island flap that transfers the ulnar neurovascular bundle from the middle finger (requires sacrifice of radial neurovascular bundle to ring finger).
      - The ring finger can be used if median nerve is not intact.
      - Greater morbidity due to loss of palmar sensation along the ulnar aspect of the donor digit, as well as scarring and stiffness of the donor digit.
  - **Regional flaps**
    - Thoracoepigastric flap.
    - Groin flaps provide a large area of robust soft tissue coverage.
      - Disadvantages include need for multiple surgeries, patient convenience, failure in uncooperative patients, and graft bulk.

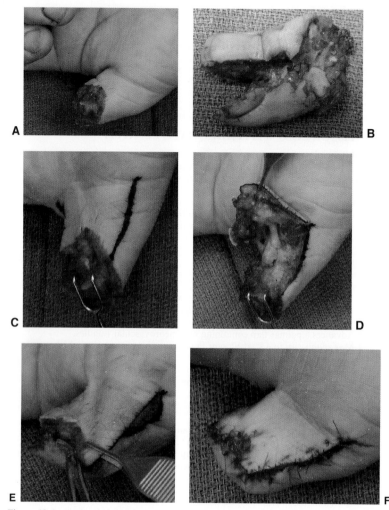

Figure 40-1 **A.** Thumb defect at distal aspect of proximal phalanx. **B.** Nonreplantable thumb tip. **C.** Longitudinal incision dorsal to radial and ulnar digital neurovascular bundles. **D.** Elevation of flap, including neurovascular bundles, from flexor tendon sheath. **E.** Testing mobility of elevated flap. **F.** Closure of defect without tension. (From Hunt TR, Weisel SW, ed. *Operative Techniques in Hand, Wrist and Elbow Surgery.* 2nd ed. Wolters Kluwer; 2016. Tech Figure 139.2.)

- ○ Free tissue transfer
  - Wraparound great toe transfer includes transfer of only the nail and great toe soft tissue. This can be used in degloving injuries or with conventional osteoplastic reconstruction (see below).
  - Toe-pulp transfer is typically from lateral great toe and provides sensate coverage.

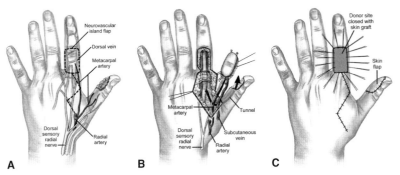

A   B   C

Figure 40-2 The first dorsal metacarpal artery flap is elevated off the dorsum of the index proximal phalanx and can provide coverage for the volar and dorsal thumb. The donor site is skin grafted. **A.** The skin is marked to incorporate the vascular supply of the first dorsal metacarpal artery flap. **B.** The flap is raised, elevating the first dorsal metacarpal artery and the dorsal veins. **C.** The flap is transposed to the thumb defect through a subcutaneous tunnel and the index finger defect is closed with a skin graft. (From Berger RA, Weiss AC, ed. *Hand Surgery*. Lippincott Williams & Wilkins; 2004.)

Section III: Upper Extremity

- ○ Revision amputation
  - ▪ Indicated only when stability and durable sensate coverage are not feasible.
  - ▪ *Functional length is well maintained when 2 cm of the proximal phalanx remains.

SUBTOTAL AMPUTATION WITH QUESTIONABLE LENGTH

- General Principles
  - ○ Proximal amputations result in diminished hand span, poor grasp, and decreased pinch dexterity.
  - ○ Injuries proximal to the midportion of the proximal phalanx may not achieve adequate length through phalangization procedures, and techniques to reconstruct an opposable thumb described in the next section may also be indicated.
- "Phalangization": to deepen first web space
  - ○ Z-plasty techniques
    - ▪ Requires at least one-half of the proximal phalanx intact, minimal soft tissue scarring, a mobile first metacarpal, and no muscle contracture.
    - ▪ Options include two-flap (60° angle), four-flap, or five-flap Z-plasty techniques.
  - ○ Dorsal rotational flap
    - ▪ Ideal in cases with extensive scarring.
    - ▪ Full-thickness skin grafting provides donor site coverage.
    - ▪ May use external fixator or supplemental K wires to hold the first web space in abduction during healing.
  - ○ Regional flap coverage
    - ▪ **Distally based posterior interosseous artery (PIA) flap**
      - ▫ PIA is usually a branch of the common interosseous artery and occasionally direct branch of ulnar artery.
      - ▫ In its proximal third, PIA lies deep to septum on the abductor pollicis longus with posterior interosseous nerve.
      - ▫ PIA pierces interosseous membrane 1/3 way down from elbow at junction of middle and proximal 1/3.

□ PIA pierces supinator and runs between EDQ and ECU.
□ Gives off large perforator in its middle third, which should be included in flap.
□ Flap centered over line between humeral lateral epicondyle and distal radioulnar joint when arm is flexed 90°. Place skin paddle at middle and distal 1/3 of this line.
- **Reverse radial forearm flap**
  □ Can be soft tissue only or composite of soft tissue and bone
  □ Requires sacrifice of radial artery thus not possibility if compromised ulnar artery

TOTAL AMPUTATION WITH PRESERVATION OF THE BASAL JOINT

- **Toe to hand transfer**
  - *Ideal if the metacarpal phalangeal joint is intact.
  - The great toe or second toe can be transferred to the thumb position and there is controversy among authors regarding preference.
    - Great toe is bulkier than the thumb. This leads to good strength, but more donor site morbidity. Size may be adjusted with a trimmed toe transfer.
    - Second toe is smaller than the thumb, but minimal donor site morbidity.
  - Anatomy can be variable: in general, the **first dorsal metatarsal artery (FDMA) supplies the great and second toe;** venous drainage provided by superficial dorsal veins to the saphenous vein; nerve supply from the plantar digital nerves from the medial plantar nerve.
- **Osteoplastic Reconstruction**
  - Bone grafting (eg, tricortical iliac crest) with fasciocutaneous flap coverage (eg, FDMA, radial forearm flap, and groin flap)
  - Requires stable CMC joint with good mobility
  - Difficult to achieve sensory reinnervation and bony resorption common
- **Distraction Lengthening**
  - Osteotomy is created at the base of the metacarpal and lengthening at 1.0-1.5 mm per day.
  - Can achieve up to 4 cm in length.
  - May require additional Z plasty soft-tissue release.
- **Pollicization**
  - Can transfer the index, middle, or ring finger to the thumb position as an island flap based on the digital neurovascular bundle.
  - The metacarpal is shortened, and the digit is pronated 120°-130° and abducted palmarly to create adequate opposition.
  - *The index finger is most commonly substituted.
    - Extensor indicis → extensor pollicis longus
    - Extensor digitorum communis → abductor pollicis longus
    - First palmar interosseous → adductor pollicis
    - First dorsal interosseous → abductor pollicis brevis
- **Heterodigital Replantation**
  - "Spare parts" approach to transfer an injured ray or digit to the thumb position for immediate reconstruction.
  - Reduced morbidity of secondary donor site such as toe.
  - Most appropriate in situations of index + thumb amputation.
  - Less appropriate in cases of multiple finger amputations.

TOTAL LOSS WITH DESTRUCTION OF THE BASAL JOINT

- Pollicization, see above
- Free digit transfer (eg, ring finger) with arthrodesis of the basal joint in opposition

POSTOPERATIVE CARE

- **General**
  - Catered to specific type of reconstruction (eg, primary closure, regional flap, toe transfer, etc.)
  - Toe transfers—care is similar to replantation (see **Chapter 36: Traumatic Amputation Injuries**)
- **Rehabilitation**
  - Motor—early mobilization may be beneficial to reduce swelling and minimize joint stiffness
  - Sensory
    - Reeducation training for toe transfer
    - Desensitization if development of painful neuroma
- **Complications**
  - Pain: potentially related to neuroma, scar formation
  - Loss of function: decrease in mobility or range of motion
  - Wound complications
  - Aesthetic appearance

PEARLS

1. Preoperative discussion and goals tailored to patient's needs are critical for successful reconstruction. Important considerations include vocation, time/motivation for rehabilitation, and discussion of realistic expectations.
2. Toe transfer procedures are technically demanding, but often suitable reconstructive options for a variety of injuries.
3. When toe transfers are undesired due to patient preference or not an option, pollicization may offer a functional result.

QUESTIONS YOU WILL BE ASKED

1. What types of soft tissue coverage options exist based on the size of the defect when there is adequate length?
   a. Defects < 1 cm²: revision amputation, VY flap
   b. Defects 1-2.5 cm²: Moberg advancement
   c. Defects > 2.5 cm²: heterodigital flaps (FDMA, neurovascular island, etc.)
2. What are commonly utilized local and regional flaps for thumb soft tissue coverage, including the anatomic course of their arterial supply?
   a. First dorsal metacarpal artery: branch of the radial artery distal to EPL tendon
   b. Radial forearm flap: perforator flap supplied by radial artery at the forearm
   c. Posterior interosseous artery: branch of common interosseous nerve, within floor of fourth extensor compartment
3. What are the differences between phalangization and pollicization?
   Phalangization includes soft tissue rearrangements to make the existing bony length functionally longer by deepening the first web space. Pollicization is utilized in situations of more severe loss of length, where another digit is sacrificed to create a thumb of adequate length.

Recommended Readings
1. Del Piñal F. Extreme thumb losses: reconstructive strategies. *Plast Reconstr Surg*. 2019;144(3):665-677.
2. Del Piñal F, Pennazzato D, Urrutia E. Primary thumb reconstruction in a mutilated hand. *Hand Clin*. 2016;32(4):519-531.
3. Graham D, Bhardwaj P, Sabapathy SR. Secondary thumb reconstruction in a mutilated hand. *Hand Clin*. 2016;32(4):533-547.

41

Soft Tissue Coverage of the Upper Extremity

Connor Mullen and Katherine L. Burke

GENERAL CONSIDERATIONS

GOALS

- Life, limb, function preservation, and then functional reconstruction
- Reconstructive priorities for the upper extremity: function, contour, stability
  - Thumb: accounts for 40%-50% of hand function.
  - One, ideally two, digits opposing the thumb so patient can perform tripod pinch.
  - Ring and little finger serve to aid power grip function.
  - Always reconstruct children.

EVALUATION

- See **Chapter 29: Hand and Wrist Anatomy and Examination**
- Additional Evaluation Aspects
  - Greater than 6 hours of warm ischemia leads to muscle death.
    - Can establish blood flow with vein graft or temporary shunt as bridge to formal revascularization.
    - Ischemia > 6 hours requires prophylactic fasciotomy.
    - The *critical* time for reperfusion for the upper extremity (arm, forearm) is 8-10 hours, longer than lower extremity (~6 hours).
  - Tourniquets can be applied when significant bleeding is present, but direct pressure is preferred. Tourniquet time should be limited to 2 hours and the tourniquet should be fully inflated when applied.
  - Nonspecific clamping of an arterial bleed can traumatize critical adjacent structures (ie, nerves) and should be avoided.
  - Broad-spectrum antibiotics should be initiated within 24 hours for all open fractures. Long antibiotic use postoperatively is not necessary because of judicious debridement efforts.
  - An understanding of intact vasculature is critical for reconstructive planning, that is, patients must have an intact palmar arch for regional flaps based on the ulnar or radial artery.

TREATMENT OVERVIEW

- Surgical treatment is based upon aggressive debridement, identification and repair of remaining structures, and coverage.
- Indications for Reconstruction
  - Clear understanding from patient and family of extensive rehabilitation requirements.
  - Patient's goals, expectations, and social support are consistent with reconstructive choice.
- Aggressive Debridement and Structured Inventory
  - List structures from superficial to deep, radial to ulnar, tag structures.
  - Scrub end of bones to remove contamination.
  - Copious irrigation under gravity. Pulse irrigation is more traumatic and possibly drives contaminants into compartments.

---

*Denotes common in-service examination topics.

- o Stabilize bone to reestablish the foundation.
- o If contaminated after debridement, stabilize skeleton and delay repair of other structures.
- o Can return for second debridement in 24-48 hours.
- Tendon and Muscle Repair
  - o **See Chapters 38: Tendon Injuries and Tendonitis and Chapter 39: Tendon Transfers.**
  - o Secondary surgeries are common: tendon and ligament reconstruction, tenolysis, joint surgery.
- Vascular and Nerve Repair
  - o Vascular injury takes precedence after stabilizing bone and may require vein grafts.
  - o Nerve injury occurs in about 3% of all upper extremity trauma.
- Soft Tissue Coverage
  - o Mandatory to cover tendon, nerve, bone ("white structures"), and vasculature.
  - o Higher rate of success with earlier free flap.
  - o Fasciocutaneous flaps are preferred; tendons glide better under fat and fascial plane.
  - o Important to understand a flap can be pedicled or free depending on indication and defect.
- Indications for Amputation
  - o Life-threatening complication
  - o Severe contamination
  - o Significant patient comorbid conditions
  - o Not fit or amenable to extensive rehabilitation required of complex surgery
- Overview of Forearm and Wrist Reconstruction
  - o Soft tissue reconstruction follows the reconstructive ladder.
  - o Following radical debridement, the wound is often much larger and deeper than anticipated, and the microvascular anastomoses must be placed well out of the zone of injury.
  - o Flaps can be combined with bone, include additional muscle, to meet the defect demands.
  - o Forearm and wrist injury
    - ▪ Superficial defects without exposed vasculature or "white structures" can be skin grafted.
    - ▪ Small/medium defects can be repaired with local transposition flaps.

SPECIFIC SOFT TISSUE RECONSTRUCTION OPTIONS

LOCAL FLAPS FOR FINGER RECONSTRUCTION

- For thumb reconstruction, see **Chapter 40: Thumb Reconstruction.**
- **Atasoy V-Y advancement flap**
  - o Indications: dorsal oblique and transverse fingertip amputation with exposed bone
  - o Contraindications: volar oblique injury, amputation injury proximal to lunula
  - o Preserves finger length, sensation, and function
- **Cross-finger flap**
  - o Indications: volar oblique injuries with exposed bone or tendon at middle or distal phalanx
  - o Contraindications: involvement of adjacent fingers
  - o Division at 8-10 days
- **Thenar flap**
  - o Indications: volar oblique injuries with exposed bone or tendon and extensive pulp loss of the index, middle, and ring finger
  - o Contraindications: conditions that preclude prolonged finger flexion (ie, rheumatoid arthritis, Dupuytren disease), extensive volar and dorsal tissue loss of the digit, high risk of flexion contracture in patients with concomitant PIP joint injury
  - o Division at 10-14 days

- **First dorsal metacarpal artery flap**
  - Indications: extensive volar or ulnar defect of the thumb, dorsal or radial defect of the thumb with exposed tendon or bone
  - Contraindications: extensive dorsal skin loss, injury to dorsal carpal circulation
  - Pedicle: first dorsal metacarpal artery
  - Flap pearls:
    - Includes terminal branch of superficial radial nerve to provide protective sensation
    - Requires cortical relearning and skin grafting of donor site

LOCAL AND REGIONAL FLAPS FOR HAND, WRIST, AND FOREARM RECONSTRUCTION

- **Digital fillet flap:** utilizes soft tissue from digits with intact vasculature with unsalvageable bony loss to cover palmar defects
- **Reverse radial forearm flap**
  - Indications: volar and dorsal hand defects, first web space reconstruction.
  - Contraindications: abnormal Allen test.
  - *Pedicle: radial artery identified between flexor carpi radialis (FCR) and brachioradialis (BR).
  - Flap design pearls: the reverse radial forearm flap should not be designed over the more distal forearm, can expose tendons, and make it difficult to close the donor side with a skin graft.
- **Posterior interosseous artery (PIA) flap**
  - Indications: proximal dorsal hand defects, first web space
  - Contraindications: near zone of injury
  - Pedicle: PIA identified between extensor carpi ulnaris and extensor digiti minimi tendons
  - Flap design pearls
    - Draw a line from lateral epicondyle to ulnar styloid. PIA arises at junction of proximal and middle third of this line. Pivot point ~2 cm proximal to ulnar styloid.
    - Venous congestion is not an uncommon complication.
- **Groin flap**
  - Indications: to preserve future options and in cases with large areas of soft tissue loss
  - Pedicle: perforators from superficial circumflex iliac artery
  - Flap design pearls
    - Maximum size: 10 × 25 cm long.
    - Flap design centered 2 finger breadths below the inguinal ligament. Beyond ASIS, the blood supply is random.
    - Flap is raised lateral to medial. When lateral sartorius encountered, dissection goes deep to muscle fascia to include superficial circumflex iliac artery perforators.
    - Flap division after 2-3 weeks.

ELBOW WOUND COVERAGE

- **Flexor carpi ulnaris pedicled muscle flap**
  - Indications: small anterior or posterior elbow defects
  - Contraindications: manual laborers—major wrist flexor and ulnar deviator, risk for adjacent ulnar nerve injury
  - Pedicle: ulnar artery, posterior ulnar recurrent artery
  - Flap pearls
    - Better overall cosmesis compared to radial forearm flap.
    - Flexor carpi ulnaris muscle has 2 heads—humeral head originates from the medial epicondyle while its ulnar head originates from the posterior border of the proximal ulna and medial side of olecranon.

- **Reverse lateral arm fasciocutaneous flap**
  - Indications: posterior elbow defects
  - Contraindications: overweight or obese patients (excessively bulky flap), epicondylitis
  - Blood supply: radial recurrent artery
  - Flap pearls: include skin over lateral epicondyle to preserve vascular network to distally based flap
- **Radial forearm fasciocutaneous flap**
  - Indications: elbow defects
  - Contraindications: abnormal Allen test, prior injury to radial artery
  - Pedicle: radial artery identified between FCR and BR
  - Flap pearls
    - Elevate flap ulnar to radial toward FCR above muscular fascia. Leave paratenon.
    - Preserve superficial branch of radial nerve. Can include LABC for neurotization.

COMMON FREE FLAP RECONSTRUCTION

- **Anterolateral thigh flap**
  - Versatile—can be harvested as a fascial, fasciocutaneous, or musculocutaneous flap (tensor fascia latae or vastus lateralis); can be large or small, thick or thin (as thin as 3 mm)
  - Indications
    - Forearm: extensive volar side defect with tendon exposure. May preserve subcutaneous tissue, which facilitates future procedure of tendon transfers.
    - Wrist, hand, and thenar web: traumatic or congenital anomalies. Often used for coverage after release of contracture. For thenar web, proper volume can be preserved at its central portion to offer a better aesthetic result.
  - Blood supply: descending branch of the lateral femoral circumflex
  - Innervation: lateral femoral cutaneous sensory nerve
- **Gracilis free functioning muscle flap**
  - Type II flap
  - Blood supply: medial femoral circumflex. Enters lateral/deep to gracilis ~7-8 cm inferior to pubic tubercle, passing between adductor longus and adductor brevis
  - Innervation: obturator nerve

PERFORATOR FLAPS

Detailed in **Chapter 3: Flaps**

POSTOPERATIVE CONSIDERATIONS

- Early mobilization remains a crucial component, particularly with tendon involvement.
- Volar injuries involving flexor tendons are managed with initial passive flexion with active extension technique.

PEARLS

1. Violent clamping of an arterial bleed can traumatize uninjured nerves essential for recovery of sensory and motor functions
2. Antibiotics should be initiated within 24 hours of an open fracture. Long antibiotic use is not necessary because of the judicious and aggressive debridement efforts
3. Complex upper extremity reconstruction begins with aggressive debridement and identification of remaining structures. Reconstructive options follow the basic principles of the reconstructive ladder.

QUESTIONS YOU WILL BE ASKED

1. Mathes–Nahai flap classification of flap types (know dominant and minor vessels).
   See Chapter 4: Vascularized Composite Allotransplantation, Tables 4-2 and 4-3
2. What the most commonly described muscle for use as a free functioning muscle in reconstruction of upper extremity function?
   The gracilis muscle is the most commonly described muscle for use as a free functioning muscle in reconstruction of upper extremity function. The gracilis muscle has good excursion, size, and length, but does lack strength compared with some other muscle options.
3. What is the blood supply of the revere lateral forearm flap?
   The radial recurrent vessels provide inflow to the reverse lateral arm flap
4. The vascular pedicle for the radial forearm flap passes between which tendons?
   Brachioradialis and flexor carpi radialis

Recommended Readings
1. Dibbs R, Grome L, Pederson WC. Free tissue transfer for upper extremity reconstruction. *Semin Plast Surg.* 2019;33(1):17-23. doi:10.1055/s-0039-1677702
2. Miller EA, Friedrich J. Soft tissue coverage of the hand and upper extremity: the reconstructive elevator. *J Hand Surg Am.* 2016;41(7):782-792. doi:10.1016/j.jhsa.2016.04.020
3. Miller EA, Iannuzzi NP, Kennedy SA. Management of the mangled upper extremity: a critical analysis review. *Plast Reconstr Surg.* 2018;6(4):e11. doi:10.2106/JBJS.RVW.17.00131
4. Saint-Cyr M, Gupta A. Indications and selection of free flaps for soft tissue coverage of the upper extremity. *Hand Clin.* 2007;23(1):37-48. doi:10.1016/j.hcl.2007.02.007

42 Hand Infections

Alexander N. Khouri and Meera Kattapuram

GENERAL CONSIDERATIONS

- **Initial Evaluation**
  - History of recent trauma: laceration, abrasion, bite, foreign body, hand surgery
  - Associated symptoms: onset, progression, pain, erythema, swelling, warmth, systemic symptoms
  - Past medical history: diabetes mellitus, HIV/immunocompromised state, IV drug use, steroids, vascular disease, tetanus status, smoking status
  - Social determinants of health: occupation
  - Physical examination: hand posture, tenderness, erythema, edema, warmth, range of motion, neurovascular examination, fluctuance, drainage, lymphadenopathy
  - X-ray to assess for foreign body, subcutaneous gas formation, joint space irregularity, osteomyelitis, or bony abnormality. Consider ultrasound to evaluate for abscess or fluid in tendon sheath
  - Cultures: aerobic/anaerobic + Gram stain, may need Lowenstein-Jensen culture medium or Ziehl-Neelsen stain for mycobacterium, KOH prep for fungal, cell count and crystal examination for gout
- **Microbiology (Table 42-1)**
  - Often start with broad-spectrum IV antibiotics. Antibiotics are often narrowed to cover specific organisms after cultures and sensitivities are determined. Consider ID consult if patient does not demonstrate clinical improvement with treatment.

NECROTIZING FASCIITIS

Life-threatening bacterial soft tissue infection with liquefactive necrosis of the fascia and selective spread along fascial planes.
- **Evaluation**
  - Risk factors: age >50, immunosuppression, peripheral vascular disease, diabetes mellitus (most common comorbidity), chronic liver disease, IV drug use
  - Physical examination: hemodynamic instability, pain out of proportion, tenderness extending beyond erythema, skin necrosis, bullae, crepitus (subcutaneous emphysema), nonpitting edema
    - Classic examination findings only present in 25% of cases.
    - Initial presentation can be similar to cellulitis.
  - X-ray with subcutaneous gas
  - Labs: sodium <135 (hyponatremia), WBC > 15 000, CRP > 150
    - Can calculate a LRINIC score to screen for necrotizing fasciitis
- **Treatment**
  - Surgical emergency requiring operative débridement
    - Higher mortality is associated with advanced age, delay in surgery >24 hours, and 2+ comorbidities.
    - Operative findings: foul-smelling dishwater fluid and liquefied subcutaneous fat.
  - Systemic resuscitation if patient in shock
  - Broad-spectrum IV antibiotics

---

*Denotes common in-service examination topics.

TABLE 42-1 Common Risk Factors and Pharmacologic Therapy

Common risk factors/injuries	Consider coverage for	Empiric treatment
Prolonged hospitalization, chronic illness, IV drug use, homeless, prison	MRSA	IV: Vancomycin PO: Bactrim, doxycycline, linezolid
Immunocompromised	Fungal	IV fluconazole
Punch to teeth	*Actinomyces israelii*	Penicillin
Human bite	*Eikenella corrodens*	Amoxicillin and clavulanic acid

- Broad spectrum: Zosyn and vancomycin, consider cefepime/Flagyl with penicillin allergy.
- Clindamycin has antitoxin effects against GAS and *Clostridia* species.

PYOGENIC FLEXOR TENOSYNOVITIS

Infection of the synovial sheath surrounding the flexor tendon.
- **Evaluation**
  - Risk factors: recent puncture wound (violation of tendon sheath) or gonococcal infection (hematogenous spread), hand space infection (contiguous spread), diabetes, immunocompromised, IV drug use.
  - Labs: WBC, ESR, CRP may be elevated or normal.
  - *Physical examination: Kanavel signs (Fig. 42-1).
    - Intense pain on passive extension of finger (earliest and most sensitive sign).
    - Finger is uniformly swollen and red (fusiform digit swelling).
    - Finger is guarded and held in flexion.
    - Tenderness present along flexor sheath.
  - X-ray to rule out foreign body or underlying bony abnormality.
- **Treatment**
  - Conservative treatment if within 24 hours of symptom onset
    - Admit for broad-spectrum IV antibiotics (consider fluoroquinolone/ceftriaxone for *Neisseria gonorrhoeae*), serial examinations, and NPO status.
    - Will require surgical débridement if no improvement within 24 hours.

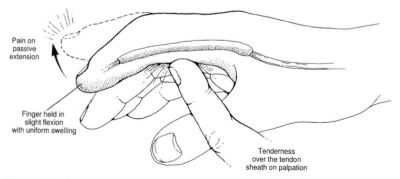

Pain on passive extension

Finger held in slight flexion with uniform swelling

Tenderness over the tendon sheath on palpation

Figure 42-1 Flexor tenosynovitis. The diagnosis is made by Kanavel four signs: the finger held in slight flexion, fusiform swelling of the finger, tenderness over the tendon sheath, and pain on passive extension. (From Lawrence PF. *Essentials of Surgical Specialties*. 3rd ed. Lippincott Williams & Wilkins; 2007.)

- o Operative washout
  - Indications: unresponsive to antibiotics after 24 hours of treatment, late/severe presentation
  - Multiple surgical approaches including angiocatheter irrigation through limited incisions at distal A5 and proximal A1 pulleys or open washout and débridement +/– release of A1 pulley
- o Complications: digital stiffness (most common) 2/2 flexor tendon adhesions and damage to sheath and pulley system, flexor tendon rupture, skin loss, amputation.
- o Predictors of poor outcomes include advanced age, multiple comorbidities, subcutaneous purulence, digital ischemia, and/or polymicrobial infections.

DEEP HAND SPACE INFECTIONS

Ten compartments of the hand: thenar, hypothenar, adductor pollicis, and interossei (four dorsal, three volar) compartments. Infection of the deep spaces of the hand includes thenar, hypothenar, and midpalmar space (**Fig. 42-2**).

- **Evaluation**
  - o Risk factors: recent trauma, bites, IV drug use
  - o Physical examination: pain spreading from finger to hand or forearm, edema, overlying erythema, palpable fluctuance
    - Thenar: pain with thumb flexion (most commonly infected deep space).
    - Hypothenar: pain with small finger flexion.
    - Midpalmar: pain with middle finger and ring finger flexion and loss of palmar concavity.
    - *Space of Parona (potential space between pronator quadratus and flexor tendons, and between flexor carpi ulnaris [FCU] and FPL; horseshoe abscess): pain with passive thumb and small finger flexion. May present as acute carpal tunnel syndrome or flexor tenosynovitis.

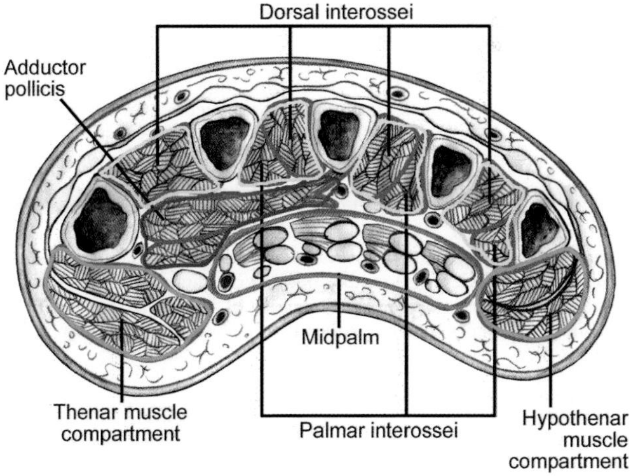

Figure 42-2 **Cross-sectional anatomy of the hand.** Each compartment is labeled and outlined. The volar compartments are the thenar, hypothenar, and carpal tunnel (midpalmar and adductor pollicis). The dorsal compartments consist of the four interossei compartments. (From Berger R, Weiss A-PC, eds. *Hand Surgery*. Lippincott Williams & Wilkins; 2003.)

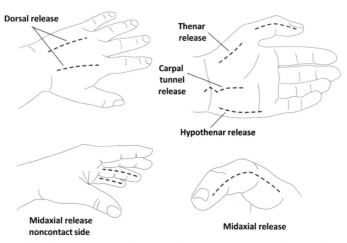

Figure 42-3 Incisions commonly used in the hand for both compartment syndrome and deep space infections. (From Wiener-Kronish JP, ed. *Critical Care Handbook of the Massachusetts General Hospital.* 6th ed. Wolters Kluwer; 2016. Figure 34.4.)

- Superficial dorsal subcutaneous and dorsal subaponeurotic spaces have similar presentations; however, superficial infections do not have well-defined anatomic borders.
- **Collar Button Abscess**
  - Infection of the interdigital web space between fingers
  - Separate dorsal and volar infections connected through a narrow stalk, which resembles the dumbbell shape of old collar buttons
  - Physical examination: abducted finger posture
- **Thenar Abscess**
  - Infection of the thenar space superficial to adductor pollicis and deep to flexor tendons, communicates web of the thumb and under flexor retinaculum
    - "Pantaloon" or dumbbell abscess results if infection spreads dorsally over adductor pollicis and the first dorsal interosseous
  - Physical examination: thumb held in abduction
- **Treatment**
  - Incision and débridement of infected space along with antibiotics
  - Incision considerations
    - Avoid web space incisions, which result in high rates of contracture.
    - Collar button abscess will require both a volar and dorsal surgical approach.
    - Watch out for the recurrent motor branch of the median nerve when designing volar curvilinear incisions for thenar abscess incision and drainage (**Fig. 42-3**).

SEPTIC ARTHRITIS

Infection of the joint
- **Evaluation**
  - Etiology: traumatic inoculation (penetrating trauma, bites), systemic bacteremia, contiguous spread (adjacent infection).

○ If unvaccinated and young, consider *Haemophilus influenzae*.
  ▪ If monoarticular and nontraumatic, consider *N. gonorrhea*.
  ▪ Commonly *Staphylococcus aureus* and group A *Streptococcus*.
○ Differential diagnosis includes gout, pseudogout, and inflammatory arthropathies.
○ Physical examination: erythema, edema, and warm joint, pain with ROM, pain on axial loading.

• **Diagnosis**: x-ray and wrist joint tap
  ○ X-ray: TFCC calcifications and SL widening suggest pseudogout.
  ○ Uric acid level.
  ○ Joint fluid analysis: send fluid for fluid cell count, cultures, crystals.
    ▪ Suggestive of septic arthritis: >50K WBC, >75% PMN, synovial glucose <60% fasting serum glucose, positive Gram stain or culture
    ▪ Wrist joint tap procedure tip: aim for area just distal and ulnar to Lister tubercle, between third and fourth extensor compartments

• **Treatment**
  ○ Admit for broad-spectrum IV antibiotics and serial examinations.
  ○ Patient will require operative washout if not improving clinically or positive arthrocentesis.

CELLULITIS

Infection of the dermis and subcutaneous tissue without accompanying abscess.
• **Evaluation**
  ○ Physical examination: proximal spread, erythema, induration, no palpable fluid collection
  ○ X-ray to rule out foreign body, osteomyelitis, or bony abnormality
• **Treatment**
  ○ Nonoperative management with antibiotics, splint for comfort, and elevation.
    ▪ Outpatient oral antibiotics ×5 days appropriate if hemodynamically stable
    ▪ Cover *S aureus* or group A *Streptococcus* (IV cefazolin or PO cefalexin)
    ▪ MRSA coverage if high risk (IV vancomycin or PO Bactrim/doxycycline)
  ○ Open wounds: can soak with hydrogen peroxide and normal saline (mixed 1:1) three times daily.
  ○ Mark area of erythema for serial examinations and monitoring.
  ○ If worsening symptoms, reevaluate antibiotic choice and examine for evolution to abscess formation, which requires I&D.

BITES

ANIMAL BITES

• **Evaluation**
  ○ Most commonly presents as cellulitis
  ○ History: tetanus status, animal vaccination status
    ▪ Cat bites: small, sharp teeth cause puncture wounds that close immediately resulting in high rates of infection including cellulitis, abscess, septic arthritis, and osteomyelitis.
    ▪ Animal bites are commonly *Pasteurella multocida* vs *Bartonella henselae* (catscratch disease).
  ○ Physical examination: puncture wounds, tenderness, erythema, swelling, neurovascular status, joint involvement, tendon sheath involvement, palpable fluid collection
  ○ X-ray to rule out foreign body or underlying fracture

- **Treatment**
  - Tetanus prophylaxis based on immunization status
  - Rabies vaccine and immunoglobulin if bite from unvaccinated dog, racoon, skunk, fox, bat
  - Incision and drainage if a fluid collection is present
  - If open wounds, hydrogen peroxide soaks—1:1 mix with normal saline up to three times daily
  - Antibiotics: duration ~10-14 days
    - Empiric IV amoxicillin-clavulanate (inpatient) or PO ampicillin-sulbactam (outpatient)
      - If β-lactam allergy: clindamycin + fluoroquinolone
- **Special Considerations**
  - *Capnocytophaga canimorsus* is associated with dog bites in immunocompromised patients and presents as sepsis, disseminated intravascular coagulopathy (DIC), renal failure, and endocarditis.
  - Monkey bites are associated with B virus (herpesvirus simiae) and present as fatal encephalitis. Treat with valacyclovir + acyclovir or ganciclovir.
  - Snake bites are treated with CroFab (used in rattle snakes and water moccasins) or antivenom.

HUMAN BITES

- Commonly group A *Streptococcus* vs *Eikenella corrodens*
- Associated with direct clenched-fist trauma from punching another individual and results in dorsal third or fourth metacarpal phalangeal joint injury
- Examine for extensor tendon injury or joint capsule violation
  - Extensor tendon injury may be proximal to soft tissue defect if injured with metacarpal phalangeal joint in flexed positioned (ie, a fist) and examined in extension

FINGERTIP INFECTIONS

FELON

Infection involving the finger pulp (fibrofatty compartment on the volar aspect of the distal phalanx) trapped by multiple fibrous septa and resulting in compartment syndrome of the distal phalangeal pulp

- **Evaluation**
  - Most commonly *S aureus*
  - Risk factor: penetrating trauma
  - Physical examination: swelling, erythema, and severe pain at fingertip
    - Will not extend proximal to DIP flexion crease.
    - Worsening fluctuance can compress vascular bed, which will result in tissue necrosis and progress to osteomyelitis.
- **Treatment**
  - Incision and drainage, antibiotics and warm water soaks (**Fig. 42-4**)

ACUTE PARONYCHIA

- Most common infection in the hand
  - Infection of the lateral or proximal nail fold and surrounding soft tissue due to disruption of the seal between the nail plate and fold resulting in bacterial inoculation
- **Evaluation**
  - Caused by *S aureus* in adults, mixed oropharyngeal flora in kids, and polymicrobial infection in diabetics
  - Risk factors: hangnails, manicures, nail biting, and penetrating trauma
  - Physical examination: erythema, swelling, tenderness +/− fluctuance

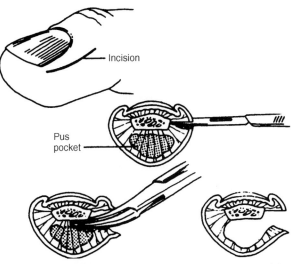

Figure 42-4 Drainage of a felon using a midlateral incision. Complete division of the vertical septae should be performed. (From Seiler JG III. *Essentials of Hand Surgery*. Lippincott Williams & Wilkins; 2002, with permission from American Society for Surgery of the Hand.)

- **Treatment**
  - Discourage nail biting
  - Incision and drainage (may need to do partial/total nail plate removal), warm hydrogen peroxide soaks (mixed 1:1 with saline), antibiotics × 7-10 days, and elevation

CHRONIC PARONYCHIA

- **Evaluation**
  - Symptoms present for at least 6 weeks
  - Caused most often by *Candida albicans* in patients with diabetes
  - Risk factors: prolonged water exposure (dishwashers, swimmers, health care professionals) and retroviral drugs (indinavir)
  - Physical examination: nail plate hypertrophy and transverse ridges, nonsuppurative
- **Treatment**
  - Discourage exposure to moist environments
  - Eponychial marsupialization, hydrogen peroxide soaks (mixed 1:1 with saline), oral antibiotics and topical antifungal (miconazole or 3% clioquinol in triamcinolone-nystatin mixture), and elevation

HERPETIC WHITLOW

- **Evaluation**
  - Intense throbbing and pain followed by the development of coalescing clear vesicles. May be associated with a viral prodrome
  - Commonly caused by herpes simplex virus type 1
  - Risk factors: oral saliva exposure (young children with herpetic gingivostomatitis and dental/health care workers)
    - Transmission occurs through direct contact with actively shedding infected individuals; recurrent infections occur from reactivation of latent virus.
  - Diagnosis: confirmed by multinucleated giant cells on Tzanck test. Often a clinical diagnosis

- **Treatment**
  - Self-limited condition.
  - Acyclovir/valacyclovir shortens duration of symptoms if started within 2-3 days of symptom onset.
  - Cover active lesions until epithelialization occurs to prevent transmission.
  - Avoid débridement to prevent a superimposed bacterial infection and viral spread.
    - Viral encephalitis has been reported after misdiagnosis and treatment of a herpetic infection as a felon.

OSTEOMYELITIS

- **Evaluation**
  - Most often caused by direct inoculation from penetrating trauma and involves the distal phalanx.
  - Commonly *S aureus* or *Streptococcus.*
    - Consider *Salmonella* in a child with a hemoglobinopathy
  - Physical examination: erythema, swelling, tenderness, warmth.
  - Labs: CRP may be elevated; however, inflammatory markers are often normal.
  - X-ray often normal, delayed findings including soft tissue swelling, osteolysis, periosteal thickening, and new bone apposition. MRI has marginally better sensitivity and specificity but can be useful in the diagnosis of early acute osteomyelitis.
  - Bone biopsy is the gold standard for diagnosis.
- **Treatment**
  - Bone biopsy and débridement
  - Culture-guided antibiotic therapy for 4-6 weeks duration

PEARLS

1. Hemodynamic instability and pain out of proportion on examination should raise concern for necrotizing fasciitis, a time-sensitive and life-threatening surgical emergency.
2. Pyogenic flexor tenosynovitis is a clinical diagnosis made using Kanavel signs.
3. Incision and drainage of hand infections often require large incisions and wide spreading to ensure complete loculation disruption and allow for proper wound care.
4. Dorsal hand wounds after a fight/punch usually have more serious and extensive underlying injury than evident on examination and require operative débridement.

QUESTIONS YOU WILL BE ASKED

1. What are Kanavel signs for pyogenic flexor tenosynovitis?
   a. Intense pain on passive extension of finger (earliest and most sensitive)
   b. Finger is uniformly swollen and red (fusiform swelling)
   c. Finger guarded and held in flexion
   d. Tenderness present along flexor sheath
2. What is the most common hand infection?
   Acute paronychia.

Recommended Readings
1. Al-Qattan MM, Helmi AA. Chronic hand infections. *J Hand Surg Am.* 2014;39(8):1636-1645. doi:10.1016/j.jhsa.2014.04.003
2. McDonald LS, Bavaro MF, Hofmeister EP, Kroonen LT. Hand infections. *J Hand Surg Am.* 2011;36(8):1403-1412. doi:10.1016/j.jhsa.2011.05.035
3. Osterman M, Draeger R, Stern P. Acute hand infections. *J Hand Surg Am.* 2014;39(8):1628-1635; quiz 1635. doi:10.1016/j.jhsa.2014.03.031

Compartment Syndrome and High-Pressure Injections

Alexandria Sherwood and Stacia M. Ruse

COMPARTMENT SYNDROME

OVERVIEW

- **Definition**
  - Elevation of hydrostatic pressure within a closed anatomic compartment that impairs oxygen delivery to tissues
- **Causes**
  - Blunt trauma, penetrating trauma, fractures, crush injury, vascular injury, reperfusion injury, injection injury, electrical injury, burns

COMPARTMENTS OF THE UPPER EXTREMITY

- **Arm**
  - Anterior
    - Muscles: biceps brachii, coracobrachialis, brachialis
    - Neurovascular: median nerve, brachial artery
  - Posterior
    - Muscles: triceps brachii
    - Neurovascular: ulnar nerve, radial nerve
- **Forearm (Fig. 43-1)**
  - Flexor compartment
    - Superficial
      - Muscles: flexor carpi radialis, palmaris longus, pronator teres, flexor carpi ulnaris (FCU), flexor digitorum superficialis (FDS)
    - Deep
      - Muscles: flexor digitorum profundus (FDP), flexor pollicis longus, pronator quadratus
      - Neurovascular: anterior interosseous artery, anterior interosseous nerve
  - Mobile wad compartment
    - Muscles: brachioradialis, extensor carpi radialis longus, extensor carpi radialis brevis
  - Extensor compartment
    - Muscles: supinator, abductor pollicis longus, extensor pollicis brevis, extensor pollicis longus, extensor digitorum communis, extensor indicis, extensor digiti minimi, extensor carpi ulnaris
    - Neurovascular: posterior interosseous nerve
- **Hand**
  - Thenar
    - Abductor pollicis brevis, opponens pollicis, flexor pollicis brevis
  - Hypothenar
    - Abductor digiti minimi, opponens digiti minimi, flexor digiti minimi
  - Adductor pollicis
  - Four dorsal interossei
  - Three volar interossei

*Denotes common in-service examination topics.

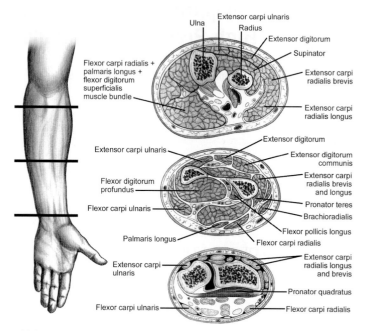

Figure 43-1 Cross-sectional anatomy of the forearm compartments. (From Berger RA, Weiss AC, eds. *Hand Surgery*. Lippincott Williams & Wilkins; 2004.)

DIAGNOSIS

- History
  - ○ Assess for etiology: trauma, fractures, casts, dressings, coagulopathy
  - ○ Pertinent comorbidities, other trauma
- Physical Examination
  - ○ *Six Ps
    - ▪ **Pain** out of proportion to injury
    - ▪ **Pain** on passive stretch of muscles in affected compartment
    - ▪ **Pallor** (uncommon finding)
    - ▪ **Paralysis**
    - ▪ **Paresthesias**
    - ▪ **Pulselessness** (last finding, usually a sign of irreversible muscle necrosis)
  - ○ Palpation: unreliable means of determining compartment pressures
  - ○ Measuring compartment pressures: can be a component of the examination and diagnosis
    - ▪ Stryker compartment pressure monitor.
    - ▪ Arterial line setup with manometer may be used otherwise.
    - ▪ Objective criteria
      - □ Compartment pressure >30 mm Hg
      - □ Difference between diastolic pressure and compartment pressure of <30 mm Hg
      - □ Important to follow the trend of compartment pressures, not one value in time only (when possible)

TREATMENT

- **Immediate surgical release** of affected compartments
- **Prophylactic fasciotomies** in certain cases

- ○ Obtunded patient with equivocal findings
- ○ Revascularized extremities after prolonged ischemia time
- ○ Electrocution
- ○ Circumferential burns—inelastic eschars
- • **Surgical Approaches**
  - ○ There are many different approaches. The goal is the same—release all compartments.
  - ○ **Forearm (Fig. 43-2)**
    - ▪ At our institution, we prefer two incision release.
    - ▪ Ulnar approach: can release volar compartment. To release deep volar, between FDS and FCU, releasing deep and superficial flexor compartments between FDS and FDP.
    - ▪ Radial approach: can release mobile wad and posterior compartment.
    - ▪ Pitfalls to avoid

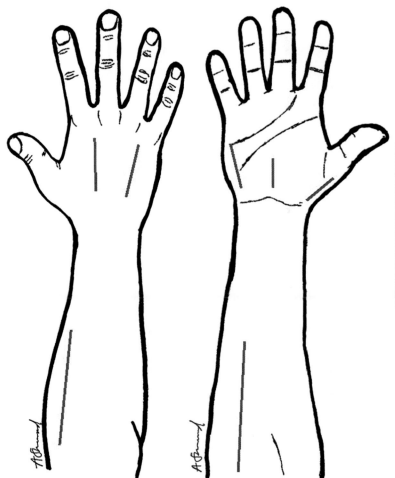

Figure 43-2 Volar and dorsal incisions for fasciotomy of the forearm.

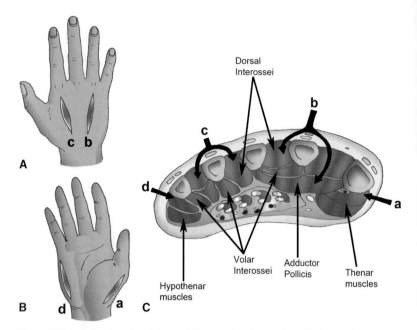

Figure 43-3 A-C. Fasciotomies of the hand. Cross section through the midpalm that demonstrates the pathways (*arrows*) that are used to release the dorsal interosseous, palmar interosseous, the adductor pollicis, thenar, carpal tunnel, and hypothenar compartments. The dorsal incisions, which are 3-4 cm in length, are centered over the midportion of the index and ring finger metacarpals.(From Galez MG, Chang J. Upper extremity arterial reconstruction and revascularization distal to the wrist. In: Mulholland M, ed. *Operative Techniques in Surgery*. Wolters Kluwer Health; 2015:1894-1901.)

- Inadequate release of compartments.
- Failure to explore deeper aspects of volar compartment.
- Poor flap planning can lead to exposure and desiccation of nerves and vessels.
  - **Hand (Fig. 43-3)**
    - Parallel longitudinal incisions over second and fourth metacarpals. Release all interossei and adductor pollicis
    - Thenar space: longitudinal incisions along first metacarpal
    - Hypothenar space: longitudinal incision along fifth metacarpal

UNTREATED COMPARTMENT SYNDROME

- **Muscle fibrosis and death:** Volkmann ischemic contracture usually takes 6-12 hours to develop. Most likely to affect deep compartment muscles such as FDP and FPL.
- **Nerve injury and dysfunction:** median nerve often affected more significantly than the ulnar nerve.
- **Typical posture of the involved hand and forearm**
  - Elbow flexion
  - Forearm pronation
  - Wrist flexion
  - Metacarpophalangeal extension
  - Interphalangeal flexion

- **Classification**

	Tsuge classification		
	Muscle involvement	Nerve involvement	Treatment
Mild	Only FDP	None	Nonsurgical, splinting
Moderate	FDP, FPL, PT, some FDS and FCU	Sensory neuropathy of median and ulnar	Flexor pronator slide, fractional lengthening, tendon transfers
Severe	All flexors, variable extensor involvement	Severe neurologic injury	Muscle débridement, neurolysis, tendon transfers, free muscle transfers, bony procedures

HIGH-PRESSURE INJECTION INJURIES

OVERVIEW

- **Mechanism:** paint guns, power washers, hydraulic hoses, grease guns all have the capability to inject large volumes under high pressures.
  - Results in rapid tissue necrosis from pressure.
  - Inflammation from trauma induces elevated pressure in compartment and vasospasm and worsens local swelling and ischemia.
- **Chemicals Frequently Introduced**
  - Paint, paint thinner
  - Cleaning solutions
  - Hydrocarbons
  - Water

PRESENTATION

- Innocuous wound or point of entry
- Relatively few symptoms including mild pain
- Often index finger of nondominant hand

HISTORY AND PHYSICAL EXAMINATION

- Agent injected
- Pounds per square inch of tool being operated
- Timing of injury
- Location of wounds
- Assessment of compartments

TREATMENT

- **Initiate broad-spectrum antibiotic coverage** (first- or third-generation cephalosporin, tetanus toxoid)
- **Water or air injections:** observation
- **Other Agents**
  - Decompress involved compartments.
  - Débride foreign material.
  - Repeat débridements may be needed every 48-72 hours to maximally remove the offending substance.
    - Region affected often larger than initially appreciated
    - **Time to surgery**
      - Organic solvent (paint, paint thinner, gasoline, oil, jet fuel) injections did better with earlier (<6 hours from injury) débridement with a 38% amputation rate.
      - Organic solvent injections débrided >6 hours after injury resulted in a 58% amputation rate.
    - **Overall amputation rate:** 48%

PEARLS

1. Diagnosing compartment syndrome requires an index of suspicion.
2. Prophylactic fasciotomies are reasonable in patients who are obtunded or have a high likelihood of developing compartment syndrome.
3. Injection injuries—particularly those with hydrophobic substances like oil-based paint—are often much worse than they appear at first presentation. Patients must be counseled on the of amputation.

Recommended Readings
Compartment Syndrome
1. Ouellette EA, Kelly R. Compartment syndromes of the hand. *J Bone Joint Surg Am.* 1996;78(10):1515-1522.
2. Prasarn ML, Ouellette EA. Acute compartment syndrome of the upper extremity. *J Am Acad Orthop Surg.* 2011;19(1):49-58. doi:10.5435/00124635-201101000-00006. Erratum in: *J Am Acad Orthop Surg.* 2011;19(5):50A.
3. Tsuge K. Treatment of established Volkmann's contracture of the forearm. *Nihon Seikeigeka Gakkai Zasshi.* 1967;40(13):1569-1584.

Injection Injuries
1. Cannon TA. High-pressure injection injuries of the hand. *Orthop Clin North Am.* 2016;47(3):617-624. doi:10.1016/j.ocl.2016.03.007
2. Hogan CJ, Ruland RT. High-pressure injection injuries to the upper extremity: a review of the literature. *J Orthop Trauma.* 2006;20(7):503-511.

Hand Tumors

Paul Gagnet

OVERVIEW

- **Benign Tumors**
  - Most tumors of the hand are benign (>90%).
  - Usually can be diagnosed clinically and requires no treatment.
  - If lesion suddenly changes in size, appearance, or aggressiveness, appropriate workup (ie, biopsy) must be done.
- **Malignant Tumors**
  - Squamous cell carcinoma is the most frequent primary malignancy of the hand.
  - Other malignancies are far less common
    - Malignant metastases to the bones of the hand are exceedingly rare. The most common metastasis to the hand originates in the lung.
    - A significant proportion of soft tissue sarcomas and melanomas occur in the upper extremity.
- **Examination**
  - Mass: size, mobility, firmness
  - Red flags for malignancy: large mass (>5 cm), rapid enlargement, venous/lymphatic obstruction
  - Examine lymph nodes: epitrochlear (around the medical epicondyle), axillary, and deltopectoral area along the cephalic vein
- **Imaging**
  - XR: assess bony involvement. For bone mass, assess for pathologic fractures.
  - U/S: can be used as an adjunct for soft tissue masses (cystic vs solid).
  - CT: offers anatomic details of bone tumor.
  - MRI: characterizes soft tissue tumors. Particularly important for soft tissue sarcoma.
  - May need to assess for metastasis (CT or PET).

BENIGN SOFT TISSUE TUMORS

GANGLION CYSTS

- **General**
  - 50%-70% of all hand tumors
    - Most common benign tumor of the hand. 3:1 female predilection
    - Most often occur in second to fourth decade of life, though can occur in children and the aged
    - Most often occur at the dorsal wrist (60%-70%), followed by volar wrist (10%-20%), flexor tendon sheath (volar retinacular), and distal interphalangeal (DIP) joint (mucous cyst)
  - Appearance
    - Mucin-filled cyst attached to the tendon, tendon sheath, or joint capsule
    - Transilluminates, often multilobulated
    - Can be associated with carpometacarpal bossing

---

*Denotes common in-service examination topics.

- **Dorsal Wrist Ganglion**
  - *Anatomy: usually over the scapholunate (SL) junction between the third and fourth extensor compartments. Approximately 75% connect by the stalk with the SL joint ligament.
  - **Presentation:** compressible, transilluminating, mobile, limited wrist dorsiflexion, aching discomfort.
  - **Diagnosis/workup:** clinical exam, ± diagnostic ultrasound (US) if unsure, magnetic resonance imaging (MRI) if diagnosis remains elusive.
  - **Treatment**
    - Observation: if not symptomatic or impairing. 50% resolve spontaneously
    - Supportive splinting/nonsteroidal anti-inflammatory drugs (NSAIDs)
    - Surgical excision: indicated for pain, impairment, and failure of conservative treatment. Usually open technique, transverse incision, dissect down to stalk and coagulate base
  - **Outcomes:** recurrence is very low if small cuff of normal tissue is taken with the cyst and stalk.
  - **Complications:** injury to radial sensory branches, wrist stiffness, SL dissociation
- **Volar Wrist Ganglion**
  - **Anatomy:** usually between the radial artery and the flexor carpi radialis tendon sheath. About 60% arise from the radioscaphoid joint and 30% from the scaphotrapezial joint.
  - **Presentation:** similar to dorsal ganglion. Possible median or ulnar nerve palsies with mass effect.
  - **Diagnosis/workup:** clinical exam. Requires imaging and additional workup if history of penetrating injury to volar forearm (check for bruits, Doppler US to rule out pseudoaneurysm), or symptoms of nerve palsy (US or MRI: extent of mass).
  - **Treatment**
    - Observation: if asymptomatic
    - Supportive splinting/NSAIDs
    - Surgical excision: similar indications as dorsal ganglion
  - **Outcomes:** similar to dorsal ganglions
  - **Complications**
    - Nerve injuries: palmar cutaneous median branch and lateral antebrachial cutaneous nerve
    - Radial artery injury
    - Wrist stiffness
- **Volar Retinacular Ganglion Cyst**
  - **Epidemiology:** 5%-10% of hand and wrist ganglions
  - **Anatomy:** arise from digital flexor sheath at A1 or A2 pulley, near proximal digital flexor crease or metacarpophalangeal (MCP) joint. No movement with flexor excursion. Propensity for middle finger.
  - **Presentation:** firm immobile "pealike" mass. Diminished sensation if it impinges on digital neurovascular bundle. Discomfort with forceful grip. May present with trigger finger.
  - **Diagnosis/workup:** clinical exam
  - **Treatment**
    - Observation: if asymptomatic
    - Aspiration: can be curative. Risk of injury to digital neurovascular bundle
    - Injection: can be curative; 1% lidocaine and methylprednisone into the cyst to rupture it
    - Surgical excision: if patient preference or conservative measures fail

- ○ **Outcomes:** recurrence is rare
- ○ **Complications:** digital neurovascular bundle injury
- **Degenerative Mucous Cysts**
  - ○ **Epidemiology:** predilection for middle aged and elderly. Associated with osteoarthritis at DIPJ
  - ○ ***Anatomy:** over dorsal DIP joint. Propensity for index and long fingers. Nail deformity common (due to pressure on the germinal matrix)
  - ○ **Presentation:** firm, minimally mobile, transilluminating, thinned skin over lesion. Drainage of cystic fluid if thinned skin ruptures. Soft tissue infection and septic arthritis possible with ruptured cyst. Can have nail abnormalities.
  - ○ **Diagnosis/workup:** clinical exam. Radiographs for degenerative changes of osteoarthritis
  - ○ **Treatment**
    - ▪ Observation: if asymptomatic and no perceived risk of rupture.
    - ▪ Aspiration: potential for recurrence, need for multiple treatments, risk of infection, and septic arthritis.
    - ▪ Surgical excision: highest success rate with low complications risk. Remove osteophyte when present.
  - ○ **Outcomes:** recurrence uncommon. Nail deformity may resolve after excision
  - ○ **Complications**
    - ▪ DIP joint extensor lag, stiffness, radial/ulnar deviation
    - ▪ Residual pain
    - ▪ Infection including septic arthritis
    - ▪ Nail plate deformity
  - ○ **Adjunctive procedures:** DIP joint arthrodesis if debilitating pain from osteoarthritis

EPIDERMAL INCLUSION CYSTS

- **Epidemiology**
  - ○ Often from trauma: epithelial cells introduced into subcutaneous tissue or bone. Unapparent for months to years following inciting event
  - ○ Third most common tumor of the hand, predilection for men
- **Anatomy:** propensity for the fingertip just beneath the skin. Fingertip cysts may erode into the bone causing lytic lesion
- **Presentation**
  - ○ Firm, well circumscribed, and slightly mobile
  - ○ Slow growing and present for months to years
  - ○ Does not transilluminate
- **Diagnosis/Workup:** clinical exam
- **Treatment:** excision
- **Outcomes:** recurrence is rare

GIANT CELL TUMOR OF TENDON SHEATH

- Also known as localized nodular synovitis, fibrous xanthoma, and pigmented villonodular tenosynovitis
- **Epidemiology**
  - ○ Second most common soft tissue tumor in the hand
  - ○ Fourth to sixth decade of life, slight predilection for women
- **Anatomy**
  - ○ Multilobular, well circumscribed
  - ○ Propensity for radial three digits specifically in the DIP joint region
  - ○ May displace or envelope neurovascular bundle
  - ○ Can be locally aggressive and involve bone

- **Presentation**
  - Slow growing, firm painless mass usually on the volar finger, does not transilluminate
  - Neuropathic symptoms with digital neurovascular bundle involvement
- **Diagnosis/Workup:** radiographs may show scalloping of adjacent bone
- **Treatment:** marginal excision
- **Outcomes:** recurrence can be as high as 50%

GLOMUS TUMORS

- Benign vascular tumor from arterial end of glomus body
- **Epidemiology:** consist of 1%-5% of benign tumors of the hand
- **Presentation:** painful, most commonly subungal lesion with a blue hue. Causes a triad of severe pain, hypersensitivity to cold, and pinpoint tenderness in the lesion
  - *Hildreth sign: cessation of pain with inflation of blood pressure cuff, tourniquet or elevation of the limb is a diagnostic exam maneuver
- Diagnosis/workup: clinical exam
- Treatment: excision

MALIGNANT SOFT TISSUE TUMORS

GENERAL CONSIDERATIONS

- Commonly presents as painless mass that may be rapidly enlarging
- Proper workup is key including plain radiographs, which may show soft tissue calcifications or bony erosions. MRI should be ordered with and without contrast to evaluate for soft tissue enhancement. If there is high suspicion for a sarcoma, the patient should be referred to a sarcoma center.
- Excisional biopsy may be performed for lesions <2 cm. Incisional biopsy or core needle biopsy should be used for larger lesions. Any biopsy performed should be in-line with future incisions so the tract may be excised at the time of resection.
- *After diagnosis, patients should be staged with a chest CT to evaluate for pulmonary metastasis. Angiosarcoma, clear cell sarcoma, epithelioid sarcoma, and rhabdomyosarcoma should all receive a sentinel lymph node biopsy to evaluate for metastasis.
- Adjuvant chemotherapy and XRT can be considered in lesions >5 cm that are high grade.
- The goal of resection should be to achieve negative margins with curative intent.
- Most common soft tissue sarcomas of the hand include epithelioid sarcoma, synovial cell sarcoma, myxofibrosarcoma, and rhabdomyosarcoma.

EPITHELIOID AND SYNOVIAL CELL SARCOMA

- **Epidemiology**
  - Only 4% of sarcomas present in the hand, the two most common sarcomas in hand being epithelioid and synovial cell (**Table 44-1**).
  - First to third decade with male preponderance.
- **Presentation**
  - Epithelioid: firm or ulcerating nodule, often in the hand. Can spread proximally along tendon.
  - Synovial: slow-growing painless mass. Occurs in tendons or bursa, usually close to joints.
- **Diagnosis/Workup**
  - May visualize soft tissue calcifications on plain radiographs in synovial sarcoma.
  - MRI with and without contrast.
  - Biopsy.
  - Staging with PET/CT and multidisciplinary discussion is critical.

TABLE 44-1 Common Types of Soft Tissue Sarcomas

Normal tissue correlate	Sarcoma type	Subtypes
Fat	Liposarcoma	Myxoid
		Round cell
		Pleomorphic
		Well differentiated
Nerve	Malignant peripheral nerve sheath tumor	—
Vascular	Angiosarcoma	—
Smooth muscle	Leiomyosarcoma	—
Striated muscle	Rhabdomyosarcoma	Alveolar
		Embryonal
Fibrous tissue	Fibrosarcoma	Storiform-pleomorphic
	Malignant fibrous histiocytoma	Giant cell
	Epithelioid sarcoma	Inflammatory
	Synovial sarcoma	Myxoid

- **Treatment Options**
  - Neoadjuvant radiation: depending on stage. When adjacent to vital structures.
  - *Epithelioid: limb-sparing wide or radical excision with sentinel node biopsy and adjuvant radiation. Some indications for adjuvant chemotherapy (depends on the size, grade, nodal, and metastatic status).
  - Synovial: limb-sparing wide or radical excision with adjuvant radiation and chemotherapy.
  - Amputation if wide excision is not possible.
- **Outcomes:** compared to similar type tumors in the extremities, hand tumors may have improved outcomes
- **Complications**
  - Recurrence
  - Impaired wound healing, usually due to XRT
- **Follow-up/Surveillance**
  - Local: physical examination, MRI
  - Systemic: chest imaging Q3-6 months for 3 years, then Q6 months for 4-5 years, then annually

BENIGN BONE AND CARTILAGE TUMORS

ENCHONDROMA

- **Epidemiology**
  - *Most common bone tumor of the hand. Approximately 90% of all hand bone tumors.
  - Multiple enchondromas: Ollier disease (enchondromatosis) and Maffucci syndrome (enchondromatosis and multiple hemangiomas)
  - Diagnosed in all ages. Patients with enchondromatosis present earlier.
  - Malignant transformation (to chondrosarcoma or osteosarcoma): rare but can occur roughly 25% of the time in Ollier disease or Maffucci syndrome.
- **Anatomy**
  - Proximal phalanges > metacarpals > middle phalanges
  - Intramedullary
- **Presentation**
  - Asymptomatic with local edema
  - *Sudden onset of pain, swelling, and edema = pathologic fracture
  - Rapid growth: concern for malignant degeneration
- **Diagnosis/Workup:** plain radiographs will show lytic lesion, may see punctate calcifications. Cortical expansion and thinning can be frequently seen.
- **Treatment**
  - Observation: acceptable for small asymptomatic tumors with no concerns for malignancy (discuss the potential for fracture).
  - Surgical treatment.
  - *If the patient presents with a pathologic fracture, first heal the fracture (with immobilization or pins as needed) and then resect the lesion.
- **Surgical Treatment**
  - Curettage of lesion.
  - Extend margins with burr if possible. May use adjuvants such as ethanol or phenol in the cavity.
  - To fill space, some surgeons perform cancellous bone grafting.
- **Outcomes**
  - Recurrence after curettage ranges from 2% to 15%
  - If recurrent: rule out malignancy
- **Complications:** infection, fracture, recurrence
- **Follow-up/Surveillance**
  - After curettage and grafting: radiographs and clinical exam at 6 months, 1 year, and 2 years
  - For observed patients: radiograph and 6 and 12 months to confirm stability

GIANT CELL TUMOR (GCT) OF THE BONE

- **Epidemiology**
  - Uncommon in the hand
  - >20 years of age. Predilection for women
  - Benign but locally aggressive; can rarely metastasize to lungs
  - Hand and wrist tumors: higher rates of local recurrence
- **Anatomy:** most common in the epiphyseal bone of the distal radius. Can occur in the carpus
- **Presentation:** pain and swelling. May present with pathologic fracture

- **Diagnosis/Workup**
  - Plain radiographs: lytic with cortical expansion and indistinct borders
  - MRI for treatment planning. Chest CT scan to evaluate for metastasis
  - Incisional biopsy
- **Treatment**
  - Denosumab may be used as an adjuvant to decrease the size of the bony defect.
  - Curettage with adjuvant treatments (phenol, high-speed endosteal burring, ethanol). Cavity packed with methyl methacrylate or bone graft.
  - If significant cortical breakthrough can consider wide en bloc excision with reconstruction.
  - Amputation may need to be considered in recurrent lesions.
- **Outcomes**: high rates of recurrence up to between 12% and 50%
- **Complications**
  - Stiffness, impaired range of motion, joint collapse
  - Infection
  - Neurapraxia
  - Recurrence
- **Follow-up:** for local and systemic disease with XR of the hand and chest. CT chest for patients presenting with recurrence

ANEURYSMAL BONE CYST

- **Epidemiology**
  - Uncommon in the hand, 5% of cases
  - 75% in patients <20 years. No gender predilection
  - Locally aggressive and destructive. No metastatic potential
- **Anatomy:** usually in metacarpals and proximal phalanges.
- **Presentation**
  - Slowly enlarging firm mass with or without pain
  - Significant edema and warmth may be present
  - May present with pathologic fracture
- **Diagnosis/Workup:** plain radiographs. MRI will show fluid-fluid levels.
- **Treatment**
  - Treatment is curettage and bone grafting, may need several tx
  - Adjuvant treatments: high-speed burring and ethanol
  - En bloc excision for aggressive tumors with no good bone stock
  - Amputation for destructive distal phalanx tumors
- **Outcomes:** up to 60% recurrence with curettage and no adjuvant treatment. Adjuvant treatments improve outcomes (come with complications).
- **Complications:** fracture (high-speed burring) and recurrence.

OSTEOID OSTEOMA/OSTEOBLASTOMA

- **Epidemiology**
  - 10% of all benign bone tumors; 5%-15% of all osteoid osteomas are in the hand/wrist
  - Second to third decade of life
  - 2:1 male predilection
- **Anatomy**
  - Predilection for carpus (scaphoid and capitate) and proximal phalanges
  - Propensity to be juxta-articular
  - Osteoid osteoma generally <2 cm in size and osteoblastoma is >2 cm in size
- **Presentation**
  - Significant focal dull ache, worse at night. Osteoid osteoma will have relief with NSAIDs. Osteoblastoma will see partial relief with NSAIDs.
  - Soft tissue edema and limited motion at nearest joints.
- **Diagnosis/Workup**

- ○ *Radiographs, small round lucency (the nidus), situated within the cortex, surrounded by sclerotic, reactive bone.
- ○ Thin-cut CT and bone scan have higher sensitivity than plain radiographs.
- **Treatment**
  - ○ Symptomatic treatment with NSAIDs for osteoid osteoma as it is generally self-limiting.
  - ○ Surgical treatment for osteoblastoma: curettage and grafting.
- **Outcomes:** recurrence ranges from 0% to 25%
- **Complications:** fracture and recurrence

MALIGNANT BONE AND CARTILAGE TUMORS

CHONDROSARCOMA

- **Epidemiology**
  - ○ *Most common primary malignant bone tumor of the hand
  - ○ Most likely malignant degeneration of preexisting lesion (enchondroma, osteochondroma, and fibrous dysplasia). Can occur in Maffucci syndrome or Ollier disease
  - ○ Fourth to sixth decade of life
- **Anatomy:** occurrence in proximal phalanx > metacarpals. Rare in carpus
- **Presentation**
  - ○ Slow growing, often painful
  - ○ Symptoms could be present >10 years
- **Diagnosis/Workup**
  - ○ Can be difficult to differentiate between benign and malignant lesions. XR shows mineralization within lytic lesion. Cortical expansion and destruction can be seen.
  - ○ MRI with and without contrast to evaluate for soft tissue involvement. If there is soft tissue extension need to have a high suspicion of malignancy.
  - ○ Core needle biopsy in area of planned incision.
  - ○ Staging chest CT after confirmation of chondrosarcoma.
- **Treatment:** for low-grade lesions can perform curettage and cementation. Higher grade lesions should be treated with digit or ray amputation. Wide resection can be performed if possible.
- **Outcomes**
  - ○ Most are low grade with lower potential of metastasis. Approximately 10% risk of metastasis, usually to the lung
  - ○ Good local control with amputation and ray resection
- **Complications:** recurrence
- **Follow-up/Surveillance:** monitor for local recurrence with MRI and pulmonary metastasis with CT scan

OSTEOSARCOMA

- **Epidemiology**
  - ○ <0.2% of all osteosarcomas are in the hand
  - ○ Can occur between ages of 10 and 30 but can also occur in middle age. No gender predilection
  - ○ Usually arise *de novo* from the bone. May be secondary to Paget disease and radiation exposure
  - ○ Metastasis from hand tumors less common than tumors elsewhere
- **Anatomy**
  - ○ Metacarpals and phalanges. Carpal tumors rare
  - ○ Propensity for metaphysis
- **Presentation**
  - ○ Rapidly enlarging mass, pain and swelling

- ○ May present with pathologic fracture
- ○ Average duration before presentation is 3 months
- **Diagnosis/Workup**
  - ○ Plain films of the entire bone involved, bone scan or FDG PET, and CT scan of the chest for staging
  - ○ Classic radiographic appearance: radial ossification ("sun burst" pattern), periosteal elevation with Codman triangles
  - ○ MRI of involved hand for surgical planning
  - ○ Core or incisional biopsy
- **Treatment**
  - ○ Neoadjuvant chemotherapy
  - ○ Limb-sparing wide en bloc excision and reconstruction or amputation
- **Outcomes**
  - ○ Overall 5-year survival is 70%. Osteosarcomas in the hand tend to have a lower predilection of being high grade compared to the rest of the upper extremity.
  - ○ Up to 80%-85% 5-year survival if >90% tumor necrosis with preoperative induction chemotherapy.
- **Complications:** wound healing difficulties, fracture, recurrence

EWING SARCOMA

- **Epidemiology**
  - ○ 1.4% of cases arise in the upper extremity
  - ○ Presents in children and adolescents
- **Anatomy:** metacarpals and phalanges
- **Presentation**
  - ○ Swelling, pain, and erythema; may present with fever; can mimic infection
  - ○ May show leukocytosis and elevated sedimentation rate (nonspecific)
- **Diagnosis/Workup**
  - ○ May be mistaken for an infection
  - ○ MRI
  - ○ Core or incisional biopsy
  - ○ Chest CT, bone scan, or PET, bone marrow aspirate for oncologic workup
- **Treatment Options**
  - ○ Neoadjuvant chemotherapy
  - ○ Wide en bloc resection and reconstruction
  - ○ Radiation
- **Outcomes:** up to 75% 5-year survival with adjuvant chemotherapy
- **Complications:** recurrence

GENERAL MANAGEMENT PRINCIPLES OF PATIENTS WITH UPPER EXTREMITY MALIGNANT TUMORS

- **Biopsy Considerations**
  - ○ Incisional (usually when >2 cm) vs excisional biopsy. Core biopsy can be performed under radiographic guidance. Any incisional or core biopsy should be made in the area of the planned surgical incision so the tract may be excised during the wide resection.
  - ○ Do not exsanguinate the extremity but may use a tourniquet (no Bier blocks).
  - ○ *Longitudinal incisions: can subsequently be incorporated into a limb salvage procedure or completely excised during an amputation (do not use transverse, zig-zag, or Bruner-type incisions).
  - ○ Limit skin flaps to minimize potential soft tissue contamination.
  - ○ Notify surgical pathologist in advance; discuss differential diagnosis and handling of specimen; and use frozen sections to determine if specimen is adequate (not to determine diagnosis).
  - ○ Culture every specimen for bacteria, tuberculosis, and fungus.

- **Types of Surgical Margins**
  - Intracapsular or intralesional (piecemeal): leave gross tumor behind
  - Marginal (shell out the tumor): passes through the pseudocapsule or reactive tissue surrounding the tumor
  - Wide (intracompartmental): lesion removed with normal adjacent tissue
  - Radical (extracompartmental): removes entire compartment of involved and noninvolved tissues
- **Surgical Management of a Malignant Tumor**
  - Function is secondary to eradication of tumor
  - Need a complete workup prior to final resection
  - Know the sensitivity of the tumor to XRT and chemotherapy
  - **Site-specific management**
    - **Distal phalanx**
      - Usually amputate through the DIP joint or distal middle phalanx
      - Usually ray amputation not necessary
    - **Middle/proximal phalanx:** ray amputation often provides better function and aesthetics than MCP disarticulation
    - **Thumb metacarpal**
      - If confined to bone, excise and bone graft
      - If soft tissues involved, perform a ray resection
      - To resect second metacarpal to obtain a clear margin, consider index pollicization
    - **Metacarpals 2-5:** may require resection of surrounding rays
    - **Wrist/distal forearm**
      - Should not be treated with local excision
      - Leaving nerve or tendon for function could result in a high rate of recurrence

PEARLS

1. Seemingly benign lesions can simply undergo excision for treatment and diagnosis.
2. Seemingly malignant lesions require further imaging—usually MRI—and tissue diagnosis with an incisional or core biopsy.
3. Always design biopsies or excisions longitudinally in the extremities. It allows positive margins to be more easily excised while sacrificing less normal tissue.
4. Glomus tumors: usually subungual. Presentation: intermittent extreme pain, cold sensitivity (love sign), tender to palpation. Diagnosis: MRI. Treatment: excision.
5. Neurilemmoma: usually in volar forearm. Presentation: painless nonadherent mass, Tinel sign present over mass, no neurologic deficit. Diagnosis: MRI. Treatment: nerve-sparing excision.
6. Greater than 90% of all hand tumors are benign.

QUESTIONS YOU WILL BE ASKED

1. What is the most common benign tumor?
   Ganglion cyst.
2. What is the most frequent primary malignancy of the hand?
   Squamous cell carcinoma.
3. What is classic triad associated with glomus tumor?
   Severe pain, cold sensitivity, and tenderness.
4. What is the most common primary bone tumor of the hand?
   Enchondroma.
5. What tumor presents with nocturnal pain that is typically relieved by aspirin or NSAIDs?
   Osteoid osteoma.

Recommended Readings
1. Chapman T, Athanasian E. Malignant tumors of the hand. *J Am Acad Orthop Surg.* 2020;28(23):953-962. doi:10.5435/JAAOS-D-20-00333
2. Gude W, Morelli V. Ganglion cysts of the wrist: pathophysiology, clinical picture, and management. *Curr Rev Musculoskelet Med.* 2008;1(3):205-211.
3. Lans J, Yue KC, Castelein RM, et al. Soft-tissue sarcoma of the hand: patient characteristics, treatment, and oncologic outcomes. *J Am Acad Orthop Surg.* 2021;29(6):e297-e307. doi:10.5435/JAAOS-D-20-00434
4. Plate AM, Lee SJ, Steiner G, Posner MA. Tumorlike lesions and benign tumors of the hand and wrist. *J Am Acad Orthop Surg.* 2003;11(2):129-141.

45 Nerve Injuries, Neuromas, and Compression Syndromes

Shelby Svientek

NERVE ANATOMY AND INJURY

PERIPHERAL NERVE ANATOMY (SEE FIG. 45-1)

- **Nerve Fiber Types:** motor, sensory, mixed sensorimotor, or autonomic
  - **Motor (efferent) nerve fibers**
    - Carry nerve signals away from the spinal cord and terminate on motor end plates within innervated muscle.
    - The large (multipolar) cell body resides within the ventral horn of the spinal cord, and the axon exits the cord via the ventral root.
  - **Sensory (afferent) nerve fibers**
    - Carry nerve signals from free nerve endings or target sensory end organs (eg, Pacinian corpuscles in skin, spindle cells in muscle tissue, etc.) to the spinal cord.
    - The small (pseudo unipolar) cell body is located within the dorsal root ganglion, entering the spinal cord via the dorsal root.
    - These fibers can terminate in the dorsal horn or ascend directly to the brainstem.
  - **Autonomic nerve fibers**
    - Regulate involuntary processes including heart rate, blood pressure, digestion, breathing, etc.
    - Consist of sympathetic, parasympathetic, and enteric divisions.
    - The large (multipolar) cell body lies within the sympathetic chain ganglion near the spinal cord or within/near the target organ itself for parasympathetic and enteric fibers (except for the four paired parasympathetic ganglia of the head and neck).
    - Preganglionic nerve fibers (white rami) are cholinergic and myelinated.
    - Postganglionic nerve fibers (grey rami) are unmyelinated and either cholinergic (parasympathetic) or adrenergic (sympathetic).
- **Peripheral Nerve Components**
  - **Nerve fiber axon**
    - Can be myelinated or unmyelinated.
    - Nerve conduction velocity increases with nerve fiber diameter independent of myelination (due to less resistance).
  - **Schwann cells**
    - Provides myelination to a single nerve fiber or can envelop multiple unmyelinated fibers.
    - Each Schwann cell covers approximately 1 mm of axonal length.
    - Gaps between Schwann cells are referred to as Nodes of Ranvier, which increase conduction velocity by allowing action potentials to jump from node to node—saltatory conduction.
  - **Connective tissue**
    - **Endoneurium**
      - Surrounds individual axons within a fascicle
      - Myelinated axon diameter: 3-20 μm
      - Unmyelinated axon diameter: 0.2-1.5 μm

---

*Denotes common in-service examination topics.

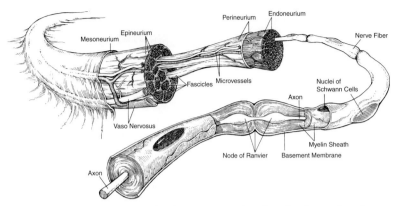

Figure 45-1 Nerve anatomy. A peripheral nerve consists of myelinated and unmyelinated axons organized into bundles of fascicles. This peripheral nerve tissue is surrounded and protected by four major connective tissue sheaths: the endoneurium, perineurium, epineurium, and mesomerism. (From Thorne CH, ed. *Grabb and Smith's Plastic Surgery*. 6th ed. Lippincott Williams & Wilkins; 2007.)

- **Perineurium**
  - □ Surrounds individual fascicles within the nerve.
  - □ Fascicles represent a group or arrangement of nerve fibers.
  - □ What is sutured together in fascicular repair
- **Epineurium**
  - □ Outer epineurium surrounds the nerve as a protective sheath.
  - □ Inner epineurium consists of loose connective tissue and acts as a cushion for fascicles during trauma.
  - □ What is sutured together in epineural repair
- **Mesoneurium**
  - □ Outermost layer of nerve connective tissue analogous to mesentery of the intestine, suspends the nerve within the surrounding connective tissue
  - □ Contains nerve blood supply and is continuous with the epineurium
  - ○ **Blood supply**
    - ■ Vasa nervorum are small segmental vessels arranged as longitudinal plexi within the epineurium and mesoneurium.
    - ■ Extrinsic vessels provide additional support.

CHRONOLOGY OF NERVE INJURY

- **Nerve Degeneration**
  - ○ Wallerian degeneration occurs at and distal to the site of nerve injury (may also involve up to 2 cm of the proximal stump).
  - ○ Macrophages invade and clear debris from the axonal tract.
  - ○ Neuronal cell body swells and increases protein synthesis to rebuild its injured axon.
  - ○ Chromatolysis, or dissolution of the Nissl bodies and peripheral migration of the nucleus, occurs in response to nerve injury or ischemia.
- **Nerve Regeneration**
  - ○ Injured peripheral nerve fibers can regenerate, provided continuity with the distal portion of the nerve is maintained or is reestablished surgically.
  - ○ Proliferation of Schwann cells and realignment of the remaining connective tissue into an endoneurial tube occurs (Bands of Büngner), which helps guide the regenerating axon.
  - ○ Within 24 hours postinjury, a growth cone is formed at the proximal nerve segment containing an abundance of axonal sprouts.

TABLE 45-1 Nerve Fiber Classification

Nerve fiber type	Function	Diameter	Myelinated	Conduction velocity
A alpha	Motor (extrafusal muscle fibers)	Large	Yes	High
A beta	Touch/pressure	Large	Yes	High
A gamma	Proprioception and motor (intrafusal muscle fibers)	Large	Yes	High
A delta	Pain/temperature	Medium	Yes—thin	Moderate—high
B	Preganglionic autonomic	Small	Yes—thin	Moderate
C	Pain/temperature	Small	No	Low

- ○ Neurotrophic growth factors and chemotactic agents guide the regenerating axons to either motor end plates or sensory end organs.
- ○ Regenerating axons demonstrate neurotropism, or an affinity for neural tissue with end-organ specificity.
- ○ If nerve disruption and/or scarring is severe, regenerating axons cannot cross the gap, and regeneration does not occur.

CLASSIFICATION OF NERVE INJURY (TABLES 45-1 AND 45-2)

- *Seddon: based on degree of nerve fiber damage
  - ○ **Neuropraxia:** local transient block in nerve conduction with minimal axonal damage
    - ▪ Anatomic continuity is preserved.
    - ▪ Wallerian degeneration does not occur.
    - ▪ Recovery is a few days or weeks.
  - ○ **Axonotmesis:** severe axonal damage occurs within the nerve
    - ▪ Anatomic continuity is preserved.
    - ▪ Wallerian degeneration occurs.
    - ▪ Recovery is a few months.
  - ○ **Neurotmesis:** nerve is transected
    - ▪ Anatomic continuity is lost.
    - ▪ Wallerian degeneration occurs.
    - ▪ Recovery is never complete, and best outcomes are achieved with nerve repair.

TABLE 45-2 Nerve Injury Classification

Sunderland	Seddon	Myelin	Axon	Endoneurium	Perineurium	Epineurium
I	Neuropraxia	+/−	−	−	−	−
II	Axonotmesis	+	+	−	−	−
III	Axonotmesis	+	+	+	−	−
IV	Axonotmesis	+	+	+	+	−
V	Neurotmesis	+	+	+	+	+
VI	Mixed	+/−	+/−	+/−	+/−	+/−

+, injured; −, not injured.

- *Sunderland (With Mackinnon Modification): expanded on Seddon and later modified by Mackinnon
  - **First-degree** injury: same as Seddon neuropraxia, injury is limited to myelin only.
  - **Second-degree** injury: same as Seddon axonotmesis.
  - **Third-degree** injury: myelin, axon, and endoneurium are disrupted, and recovery varies from almost complete to no recovery whatsoever.
  - **Fourth-degree** injury: perineurium is disrupted in addition to third-degree injury findings, and nerve regeneration is prevented by scar tissue at the site of injury. Also known as a neuroma-in-continuity.
  - **Fifth-degree** injury: same as Seddon neurotmesis, where the nerve is transected and no functional recovery is expected without repair.
  - **Sixth-degree** injury: nerve injury results in mixed recovery due to varying degrees of pathology along the length of the nerve and from fascicle to fascicle. Recovery is unpredictable.

DIAGNOSIS OF NERVE INJURY

- **Patient History**
  - Mechanism as well as time elapsed since injury can guide interventions (eg, injuries over 1.5-2 years out will see little to no benefit from nerve repair).
  - Description, location, and changes in symptoms over time.
  - Any prior interventions performed or preexisting neuromuscular/sensory deficits.
- **Neuromuscular Examination**
  - Thorough documentation of a complete motor and sensory exam (including normal findings) will allow for monitoring of recovery as well guide decision-making on whether to observe vs intervene.
  - **Motor**
    - Signs of motor deficit include loss of function, weakness, and muscular atrophy.
    - Muscle can tolerate some degree of permanent motor efferent axon loss through the process of terminal axonal sprouting (sprouting of intact axons to denervated tissue).
    - Often difficult to obtain in the obtunded or inebriated patient and, therefore, should be repeated as soon as the patient's mental status improves.
    - Be aware that certain anatomic anomalies can mask the site of nerve injury.
      - Martin-Gruber anomaly: motor connections from the median nerve cross over to the ulnar nerve in either the proximal forearm (from the median nerve) or the distal forearm (from the anterior interosseus nerve).
      - Riche-Cannieu anomaly: motor connections between the recurrent motor branch of the median nerve and the deep branch of the ulnar nerve in the palm.
  - **Sensory (Table 45-3)**
    - Signs of sensory deficit include loss of sensation, uncoordinated fine motor control due to loss of graded somatosensory feedback, and flattening of dermal ridges.

TABLE 45-3 Sensory Testing After Nerve Injury

Mechanical stimulus	Innervation threshold	Innervation density	Nerve fiber adaptivity
Static	Semmes-Weinstein monofilament (pressure)	Static 2PD	Slowly adapting
Moving	Tuning fork (vibration)	Moving 2PD	Rapidly adapting

2PD, two-point discrimination.

Section III: Upper Extremity

◻ Patients can also develop neuropathic pain: hyperalgesia (increased pain response to painful stimuli) and allodynia (pain response to nonpainful stimuli).

◻ Skin wrinkle test: submersion of digits in water will result in a lack of skin wrinkling in those affected (secondary to interruption of autonomic and thereby sensory fibers).

- **Cutaneous mechanoreceptors**
  ◻ Provide the senses of touch, pressure, and vibration.
  ◻ Merkel disks are present in hair-bearing and glabrous skin, respond to light touch, and are slow adapting.
  ◻ Meissner corpuscles are located in fingertips and eyelids, respond to fine touch and low-frequency vibrations, and are rapidly adapting.
  ◻ Ruffini endings are present in the deep layers of hair-bearing and glabrous skin, respond to stretch forces, and are slow adapting.
  ◻ Pacinian corpuscles are located in the deep layers of skin, respond to deep pressure and high-frequency vibrations, and are rapidly adapting.
  ◻ Also located in bone periosteum, joint capsules, and viscera.
- **Cutaneous thermoreceptors**
  ◻ Ruffini endings respond to warmth.
  ◻ Free nerve endings are lightly myelinated or unmyelinated and can respond to cold or warmth.
- **Tinel sign**
  ◻ Lightly percussing over the distal end of the proximal nerve segment elicits paresthesias that can radiate along the course of the nerve.
  ◻ Presence of Tinel sign indicates that growth cones are attempting regeneration. Advancing Tinel sign is an indicator of active nerve regeneration.
  ◻ Static Tinel sign could indicate the presence of neuroma.
- **Two-point discrimination (2PD)**
  ◻ A measurement of innervation density.
  ◻ Static 2PD is normal up to 6 mm.
  ◻ Moving 2PD is normal up to 3 mm.
- **Tuning fork (vibration)**
  ◻ A measurement of innervation threshold
  ◻ Use a 128-Hz tuning fork placed over a bony prominence
- **Semmes-Weinstein monofilaments (pressure)**
  ◻ A measurement of innervation threshold.
  ◻ The monofilament delivers a constant pressure directly proportional to its stiffness and is designed to bend at a predefined weight.

- **Electrodiagnostic Studies**
  ○ Evaluates the electrophysiological health of motor and sensory nerves and their effector organs (eg, muscle, sensory end organs)
  ○ Serves as a diagnostic adjunct to managing peripheral nerve injuries
  ○ **Nerve conduction studies**
    - An electrical stimulus is applied to the nerve proximal to the recording area of interest.
    - Compound muscle action potentials or sensory nerve action potentials are then recorded distally from muscle or terminal cutaneous sensory branches, respectively, and represent the sum of all action potentials produced in an individual motor or sensory nerve.
    - Amplitude of the action potential is a function of the number of axons that are intact and thus depolarized by the electrical stimulus.
    - Latency of the action potential is the delay or time between the onset of the electrical stimulus and the onset of the negative peak (eg, how long it takes muscle to fire after nerve is stimulated).

- Conduction velocity is the rate by which an action potential propagates down the nerve and is influenced by nerve diameter and myelination.
- Three pathologic mechanisms affect peripheral nerve injuries.
  □ Axonal degeneration manifests as reduced amplitude.
  □ Demyelination manifests as reduced conduction velocity and increased latency.
  □ Conduction block demonstrates no conduction across the region of abnormality, but normal conduction when nerve is stimulated distal to the injury.
  ○ Electromyography
    - Needle electrodes are inserted into muscle or surface electrodes are used on the skin overlying the muscle of interest to record electrical activity.
    - Note: correct placement of surface electrodes is key due to the risk of nearby muscle signal contamination.
    - Recordings are made at rest, with needle insertion, and with voluntary muscle contraction.
      □ Normal muscle is electrically silent at rest.
      □ Needle insertion produces a brief characteristic burst known as insertional activity.
      □ During voluntary muscle contraction, motor units fire repetitively with a frequency proportional to the amount of effort exerted.
    - A motor unit is a single A *alpha* neuron and all the muscle fibers innervated by it.
      □ The sum of all action potentials produced by the muscle fibers within a motor unit is known as the motor unit action potential (MUAP).
      □ The MUAP amplitude, duration, and firing pattern are typically recorded and correlate with overall muscle health.
    - Spontaneous firing of individual muscle fibers at rest is abnormal and represents denervation of the muscle.
      □ Fibrillations are spontaneous subclinical contractions of individual muscle fibers.
      □ Fasciculations are involuntary contractions of muscle fiber groups (fascicles) or of the entire muscle.
      □ Myotonia is the delayed relaxation of muscle after a contraction.
      □ While fibrillations can be detected on electromyography, both fasciculations and myotonia are clinically noted.
    - Clinical correlates
      □ Myopathic disease results in shorter duration and lower amplitude of MUAPs and a decrease in the number of motor units.
      □ Neuropathic disease demonstrates poor motor unit recruitment with increasing effort.
      □ Reinnervated muscle demonstrates MUAPs with higher amplitudes and longer durations due to an increased number of muscle fibers per motor unit.
      □ Denervated muscle will fibrillate with positive sharp waves that usually appear 2-3 weeks after axonal loss; MUAPs and motor unit recruitment will additionally decrease.
      □ Regenerating axons in nerve injury will produce nascent potentials in muscle before voluntary muscle movement is clinically evident. These potentials typically develop several months after the inciting injury.

NERVE REPAIR

TIMING OF NERVE REPAIR

- **Reconstruction of motor nerves** is performed when reinnervation is expected before complete muscle atrophy, and there is muscle present distally that is functionally suitable for reinnervation.

- o *Nerves regenerate at a maximal rate of 1 mm per day (1 inch per month).
- o Muscle atrophy begins immediately, and little recovery is expected if nerve repair occurs later than 18-24 months postinjury. Can "babysit" the muscle with sensory nerve to prevent atrophy.
- o There is no time limit for reinnervation of sensory end organs, but it is unlikely to return to baseline after prolonged periods.
- It is important to prioritize reconstruction in the case of multiple nerve injuries and proximal nerve injuries.
  - o Example: Recovery of meaningful intrinsic hand function after reconstruction of an adult brachial plexus injury is unlikely because of the time and distance required for reinnervation.
  - o Reconstruction should focus on reinnervating the proximal musculature to restore shoulder abduction and elbow flexion, as well as providing protective sensation to the ulnar aspect of the hand. Surgeons often focus on restoration of elbow function, but studies have shown patients often prefer having shoulder functionality.
- **Transected Nerve:** immediate primary repair of a sharply transected nerve is associated with the best functional recovery.
  - o *After 72 hours, the distal nerve segment will no longer respond to direct electrical stimulation secondary to depletion of neurotransmitters and can become exceedingly difficult to find intraoperatively.
- **Stretched, Crushed, Avulsed, or Blasted Nerve:** zone of injury often extends proximally and distally beyond the site of initial insult.
  - o Immediate primary repair should be avoided.
  - o In the acute setting, the proximal and distal nerve segments should be sutured together or secured as close as possible to prevent retraction.
  - o Once the wound is stable with no infection (~3 weeks), scarred tissue and affected nerve must be removed (this often results in a nerve gap not amenable to primary repair).
  - o Definitive reconstruction often requires use of a nerve graft.
- **Closed Nerve Injuries:** the patient should be followed closely for recovery of function.
  - o Electrodiagnostic studies should be obtained early to determine baseline values (within the first 4-6 weeks).
  - o Electrodiagnostic studies should then be repeated at 12 weeks.
    - If incomplete recovery, continue to observe patient with periodic electrodiagnostic studies and neuromuscular examinations.
    - If no clinical or electrical signs (absence of MUAPs) of recovery are evident, then nerve exploration is warranted.
    - Motor recovery is often the first to be lost and the last to recover (sympathetic activity and pain recover first typically).

PRIMARY NERVE REPAIR

- The procedure of choice when there is minimal to no nerve gap
- **Goals of Nerve Repair**
  - o Align the nerve ends, often guided by fascicular anatomy and vascular landmarks.
  - o Use the fewest number of sutures possible to minimize bulk and foreign body response.
  - o Sharply trim the nerve ends to remove scar, hemorrhage, and any protruding fascicles.
  - o Coapt the nerve ends with minimal tension and bunching at the repair site; high tension repairs can inhibit Schwann cell activation and regeneration.
  - o In some areas, the proximal and distal nerve segments can be mobilized to gain additional length to facilitate nerve repair and avoid nerve grafting (eg, up to 3 cm of length can be gained when the ulnar nerve is transposed anterior to the medial epicondyle).

TYPES OF NERVE REPAIR

- **Epineurial Repair**
  - Commonly used for digital nerves.
  - Advantages include shorter operative time, less traumatic with no violation of intraneural contents, and technically easier.
  - Disadvantages include may not ensure proper fascicular alignment and tension on repair site from tendency of nerve ends to retract.
- **Fascicular (Perineurial) Repair**
  - Commonly used for nerves with fewer than five fascicles and for nerve grafting.
  - Main advantage is maximal control over fascicular alignment.
  - Disadvantages include longer operative time, more traumatic, and technically demanding.
- **Group Fascicular Repair**
  - Indicated when the topography of the nerve is clearly defined and when motor and sensory branches are readily identifiable within the main trunk (eg, median nerve 5 cm proximal to the wrist, ulnar nerve 7-8 cm proximal to the wrist).
  - Intraoperative awake stimulation and histochemical evaluation of distal motor (acetylcholinesterase) and proximal sensory (carbonic anhydrase) axons can be performed to aid fascicular identification.
- The superiority of one nerve repair type over another has not been clearly established.

NERVE TRANSFER

- **Goal:** convert a proximal nerve injury into a distal nerve injury by sacrificing a less important or redundant nerve to reconstruct a more important nonfunctioning nerve close to its effector organ, thus promoting earlier reinnervation.
- **Indication:** brachial plexus injuries, proximal nerve injuries, delayed presentation, segmental loss, and scarred wound bed.
- If the distal nerve segment is unavailable, direct muscle implantation (neurotization) may allow for some return of motor function.
- General Principles
  - Donor nerve should be expendable, close to target. Synergistic transfers for motor nerve transfers.
  - Donor distal, recipient proximal.

NERVE GRAFTING

The procedure of choice when a nerve gap is present

TYPES OF NERVE GRAFTS

- **Autografts**
  - Gold standard; best choice for nerve gaps >3 cm. Functional recovery unlikely for graft >12 cm.
  - Indicated when primary nerve repair is not possible without producing tension at the repair site.
  - Provide a biologic scaffold containing neurotrophic factors and viable Schwann cells supporting axonal regeneration.
  - Vascularized autografts are preferred in scarred or radiated wound beds, or when extremely long donor nerves are required.
- **Allografts**
  - Similar to autografts, freshly harvested allografts provide a biologic scaffold that is eventually repopulated by host Schwann cells and axons.
  - Limiting factor: host immunosuppression; consequently, allografting is almost never performed.
  - Currently preferred immunosuppressive agent is tacrolimus (FK506) due to its neuroregenerative potential.

- **Acellular allografts**
  - Cadaveric nerves are harvested and enzymatically treated to remove cellular constituents while leaving the nerve architecture intact.
  - Meaningful recovery in nerve gaps up to 7 cm. Similar outcomes as autograft in gaps <3 cm and significantly better sensory recovery than conduit for gaps <2.5 cm.
- **Nerve conduits**
  - Consist of a variety of materials including biologic (veins and arteries) and synthetic degradable (caprolactone, PGA, collagen, chitin, etc.); synthetic nondegradable is associated with significant inflammation and is largely no longer used.
  - Can be used for nerve gaps <3 cm; larger nerves have a smaller gap threshold to achieve adequate outcomes (<1-2 cm).
  - Additionally utilized in primary nerve repair as a bolster to secure and approximate transected nerve endings for a "suture-free" repair.

COMMONLY USED DONOR NERVES

- Ideal donor nerves are long with minimal branching patterns, and the sensory deficit produced by their harvest should be limited to a noncritical region.
- Donor nerves with multiple branches should be reversed in orientation during inset to minimize loss of regenerating axons through the branches, thereby maximizing the number of regenerating axons that ultimately innervate the end organ.
- **Sural Nerve**
  - Provides 30-40 cm of nerve graft.
  - *Located immediately adjacent to the lesser saphenous vein 2 cm posterior to the lateral malleolus and approximately 1-2 cm proximal.
  - The nerve is composed of spinal nerve roots from S1 and S2 and is <u>formed from branches of both the common peroneal and posterior tibial nerves.</u>
  - In the posterior calf, the sural nerve emerges from between the two heads of the gastrocnemius muscle and runs with the small saphenous vein inferiorly to curve under the lateral malleolus.
  - In the area of the lateral malleolus, the nerve divides into several branches that run over the lateral foot. The branching pattern may be variable.
  - May be harvested as a vascularized nerve graft within the cutaneous paddle of a fibula free flap and is often identified during skin paddle dissection of the fibula flap.
  - Harvest results in loss of sensation along the dorsolateral foot; generally well tolerated, but painful neuromas form in 5% of patients.
- **Lateral Antebrachial Cutaneous Nerve**
  - Provides 5-8 cm of nerve graft.
  - Located adjacent to the cephalic vein at the junction of the lateral and middle thirds of the forearm.
  - Harvest results in loss of sensation along the lateral aspect of the forearm.
- **Anterior Division of the Medial Antebrachial Cutaneous Nerve**
  - Provides 10-20 cm of nerve graft.
  - Located adjacent to the basilic vein at the junction of the middle and medial thirds of the forearm.
  - Harvest results in loss of sensation along the medial aspect of the forearm.
- **Posterior Interosseus Nerve (Terminal Sensory Branch)**
  - Provides 2-5 cm of nerve graft
  - Located in the floor of the fourth extensor compartment
- Additional options for reducing a nerve gap and possibly avoiding the need for nerve grafting include nerve transposition, nerve mobilization, and bone shortening.

NEUROMA

PATHOPHYSIOLOGY OF NEUROMA FORMATION

- **End Neuroma**
- Consist of a disorganized mass of nerve fibers located at the distal end of a previously transected nerve.
  - ○ Classically found in patients with digit or extremity amputations.
  - ○ Results from a failure of the regenerating nerve cone to reach its distal target.
- Symptoms: pain and paresthesia typically occur in the location of the neuroma or along the nerve's course.
  - ○ *Tinel sign is typically noted immediately overlying the neuroma.
  - ○ These patients can additionally have allodynia (pain to nonpainful stimuli), hypersensitivity, and central sensitization to pain.
  - ○ Although neuromas and phantom limb pain can classically occur together, neuroma is not necessarily the cause of phantom limb pain.
- Diagnosis is clinical in nature and requires a history of nerve injury alongside presence of symptoms.
  - ○ Local anesthetic blocks: if a nerve block reduces/resolves symptoms, etiology is likely a neuroma.
  - ○ Imaging: can utilize ultrasound, CT, and MRI (compression of the neuroma with the ultrasound probe often produces paresthesias) though not required for diagnosis.
- **Neuroma-in-Continuity**
  - ○ Can occur when internal nerve fibers are damaged (direct trauma, stretch, compression, etc.), resulting in a loss of internal architecture while the external architecture remains in continuity; these damaged fibers then fail to regenerate properly secondary to internal scarring.
  - ○ Can cause pain symptoms like end-neuromas as well as a reduction/loss of distal motor function if motor fascicles are affected.
  - ○ Surgical exploration can reveal a seemingly normal exterior appearance, but EMG will display abnormalities consistent with nerve injury.
  - ○ Important to document full motor and sensory exam before any interventions.

NEUROMA TREATMENT

- **Nonsurgical Therapies**
  - ○ Medications
    - ▪ Chronic opiate use is not recommended; associated with adverse side effects with minimal long-term reduction in pain.
    - ▪ Medications such as ketamine, amitriptyline, pregabalin, and gabapentin are more effective with a safer side effect profile.
    - ▪ Topical medications such as lidocaine patches work at the level of the neuroma itself.
  - ○ Physical Therapy
    - ▪ Neural glide exercises can prevent scar tethering.
    - ▪ Massage and stretching can reduce some of the effects of scar tissue.
  - ○ Cognitive Therapy
    - ▪ Mirror therapy utilizes a mirror to project images of the intact extremity over the absent extremity; the predominance of visual pathways is used to override the abnormal nerve's central sensory input leading to central reorganization and normalization of these abnormal responses from the affected nerve.
    - ▪ Mental imagery therapy works similarly to mirror therapy, but the patient is asked to imagine using the affected extremity instead of relying on visual inputs from a mirror.
- **Neuromodulation:** spinal cord stimulation can reduce pain through the theory of gate control; repeated stimulation of the target nerve overwhelms non-nociceptive nerve fibers preventing transmission of pain along the nociceptive fibers.

- **Surgical Treatment**
  - Surgical resection of the neuroma alone can result in recurrence rates up to 50%.
  - Following resection of the neuroma end bulb, historically treatments included chemical/thermal ablation, nerve implantation into bone or muscle, nerve capping, and end to side neurorrhaphy.
  - Neuroma-in-continuity requires careful excision of the affected fascicles and subsequent nerve grafting; if the damage is extensive, excision of the entire affected nerve segment may be required.
    - Must counsel patients on the potential for permanent functional deficits
    - Important to determine if resection is worth risking function
  - The most successful methods of neuroma treatment rely on giving the nerve a "job" to do, that is, a reinnervation target.
- **Targeted Muscle Reinnervation (TMR)**
  - Following resection of a neuroma, the residual nerve ending is then grafted to a nearby donor motor nerve.
  - Instead of reforming a neuroma, these nerve fibers reinnervate the distal donor nerve segment as well as its distal muscle target.
  - This method requires sacrifice of a nearby motor nerve and significant fiber count mismatch can exist, increasing the risk of recurrent neuroma.
  - Can be used prophylactically or as a treatment modality.
  - The muscle reinnervation that occurs has been repurposed for myoelectric prosthetic control; these previously transected nerves now produce muscle contraction that can be detected with electrodes.
- **Regenerative Peripheral Nerve Interface (RPNI) (Fig. 45-2)**

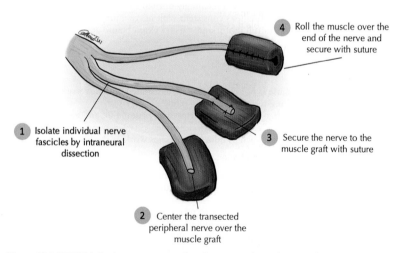

4 Roll the muscle over the end of the nerve and secure with suture

1 Isolate individual nerve fascicles by intraneural dissection

3 Secure the nerve to the muscle graft with suture

2 Center the transected peripheral nerve over the muscle graft

Figure 45-2 RPNI fabrication on a transected median nerve. The median nerve has been separated into individual fascicles with a corresponding segment of free muscle graft placed below. The epineurium of each fascicle is sutured to the interior portion of the muscle graft, which is then wrapped circumferentially around the nerve and secured in place with nonabsorbable sutures. (Courtesy of Catherine T. In: Kaye AD, Urman RD, eds. *Acute Pain Management Essentials*. Wolters Kluwer; 2023. Figure 30.1.)

○ Following neuroma resection, the residual nerve end is implanted into a segment of free muscle or dermal graft; this graft is wrapped around the implanted nerve and secured in place with suture.
  ▪ Muscle graft is typically harvested from the amputated extremity or from vastus lateralis.
  ▪ Dermal graft is typically harvested though an elliptical incision used for access to the nerve.
○ Over time, the graft revascularizes, regenerates, and becomes reinnervated by the contained nerve, providing targets for these previously purposeless axons.
○ This method has shown success both in prophylactic prevention of neuroma formation and treatment of existing neuroma and works with motor, sensory, and mixed sensorimotor nerves. RPNIs have been shown to significantly reduce phantom limb pain in addition to residual limb (ie, neuroma) pain.
○ RPNIs have shown considerable utility in control of myoelectric prosthetics as reinnervation of these muscle grafts produces visible muscle contraction upon activation of the contained nerve. Electrodes can be implanted into these RPNIs and used to produce fine motor control in advanced prosthetic devices.
• **Dermal Sensory Regenerative Peripheral Nerve Interface**
○ Similar to the RPNI, but the nerve end is instead implanted into a segment of free dermal graft.
○ Dermal sensory regenerative peripheral nerve interface theoretically could result in better outcomes for pure sensory nerves as dermis has more suitable sensory end organ targets for sensory nerves than muscle tissue.

COMPRESSION SYNDROMES

PATHOPHYSIOLOGY OF NERVE COMPRESSION

• **Mechanical Compression**
○ Acute nerve compression causes local ischemia that results in a focal conduction block; considered reversible if compression is brief.
○ Increasing pressure on the nerve leads to predictable changes in nerve dynamics.
  ▪ 20 mmHg: reduced epineurial blood flow
  ▪ 30 mmHg: impaired axonal transport
  ▪ 40 mmHg: paresthesias
  ▪ 50 mmHg: epineurial edema
  ▪ 60 mmHg: complete intraneural ischemia
○ Prolonged nerve compression eventually causes focal demyelination.
○ This is followed by subendoneurial and synovial edema, axonal damage, and finally nerve fibrosis.
○ Chronic nerve entrapment syndromes usually present with a mixed clinical picture of demyelinating and axonal patterns of injury.
• **Traction**
○ Entrapment can tether the nerve leading to limited excursion and reduced gliding.
○ Limb motion can further cause traction-induced conduction block.
• **Double-Crush Phenomenon**
○ A given foci of compression impairs axonal transport along the entire nerve.
○ The nerve is predisposed to develop a second foci of compression, generating associated symptoms (eg, thoracic outlet syndrome leading to development of carpal tunnel syndrome).
• **Systemic Conditions**
○ Can depress overall peripheral nerve function and tolerance for injury, reducing the threshold for development of symptoms. For example, diabetes mellitus, alcoholism, hypothyroidism, lysosomal storage diseases, polysaccharidoses, and exposure to industrial solvents.

MEDIAN NERVE (SEE FIG. 45-3A)

- **Carpal Tunnel Syndrome**
  - ○ **Epidemiology**
    - ▪ Most common mononeuropathy of the upper extremity.
    - ▪ Typically caused by mechanical compression of the median nerve in a fixed, rigid space due to idiopathic synovitis of the digital flexor tendons.

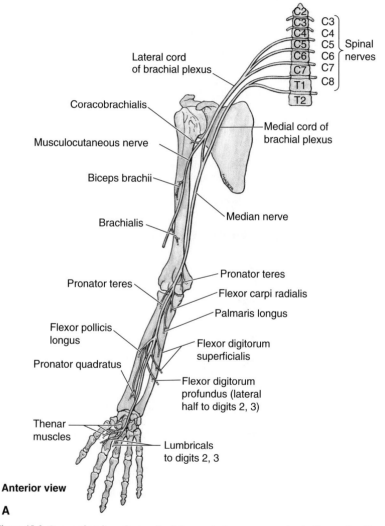

Anterior view

A

Figure 45-3 Course of median, ulnar, and radial nerves in the upper extremity. A. Course of median nerve. **B.** Course of ulnar nerve. **C.** Course of radial nerve. (From Dalley AF II, Agur AMR. *Moore's Clinically Oriented Anatomy.* 9th ed. Wolters Kluwer; 2023. Figure 3.48.)

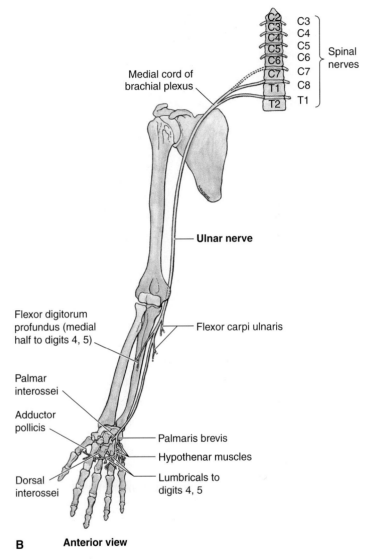

B   **Anterior view**

Figure 45-3 (*continued*)

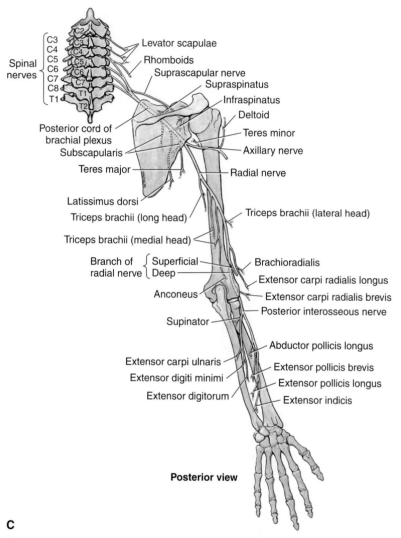

Spinal nerves
- C3
- C4
- C5
- C6
- C7
- C8
- T1

Levator scapulae
Rhomboids
Suprascapular nerve
Supraspinatus
Infraspinatus
Deltoid
Teres minor
Axillary nerve
Radial nerve

Posterior cord of brachial plexus
Subscapularis
Teres major

Latissimus dorsi
Triceps brachii (long head)
Triceps brachii (lateral head)
Triceps brachii (medial head)

Branch of radial nerve { Superficial / Deep }
Brachioradialis
Extensor carpi radialis longus
Anconeus
Extensor carpi radialis brevis
Posterior interosseous nerve
Supinator

Abductor pollicis longus
Extensor carpi ulnaris
Extensor pollicis brevis
Extensor digiti minimi
Extensor pollicis longus
Extensor digitorum
Extensor indicis

Posterior view

C

Figure 45-3 (*continued*)

- Less common causes include herniation of a ganglion cyst, hypertrophied lumbrical muscles, anomalous flexor pollicis longus muscle belly, amyloidosis, and persistent median artery.
- Intrinsic risk factors include female gender, pregnancy, diabetes mellitus, and rheumatoid arthritis.
- Controversial risk factors include repetitive or forceful tasks, mechanical stress, occupational posture, vibration, and temperature.

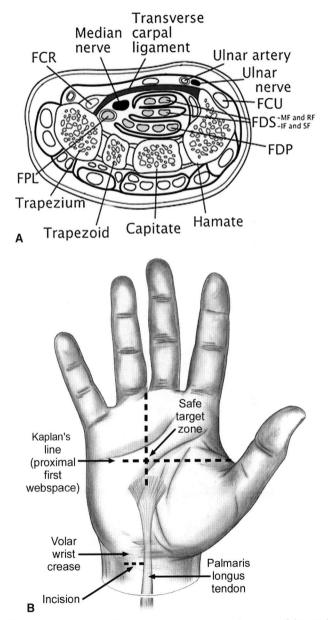

Figure 45-4 The carpal tunnel. A. Illustration of the cross-sectional anatomy of the carpal tunnel. **B.** Illustration of the "safe-zone" for a carpal tunnel release. Intersection of Kaplan line with ring finger is classically the location of the recurrent branch of the median nerve. (From Berger RA, Weiss AC, eds. *Hand Surgery.* Lippincott Williams & Wilkins; 2004.)

- An anatomically small carpal tunnel is not a risk factor.
- Fracture dislocations of the distal radius and carpal bones (eg, lunate dislocation) can cause acute carpal tunnel syndrome—this is a surgical emergency.
○ **Anatomy**
  ▪ **Carpal tunnel boundaries (Fig. 45-4)**
    ▫ Radial: scaphoid tuberosity and trapezium
    ▫ Ulnar: pisiform and hook of the hamate
    ▫ Roof: transverse carpal ligament
    ▫ Floor: carpal bones and volar interosseus ligaments
  ▪ **Carpal tunnel contents**
    ▫ One nerve: median nerve.
    ▫ Nine tendons: flexor pollicis longus (one), flexor digitorum superficialis (four), and flexor digitorum profundus (four).
    ▫ FDS tendons to the ring and middle fingers lie volar to the index and small finger tendons; FDP tendons are located deep to these.
  ▪ **Median nerve branches**
    ▫ *Palmar cutaneous branch: arises 4-5 cm proximal to the wrist and provides sensation to the thenar skin
    ▫ Recurrent motor branch: usually arises at or just beyond the distal edge of the transverse carpal ligament from the radiopalmar aspect of the nerve and supplies the thenar musculature and the radial two lumbricals
  ▪ **Kaplan cardinal line**
    ▫ Oblique line from the apex of the interdigital fold between the thumb and index finger toward the hook of hamate and parallel with the proximal palmar crease.
    ▫ Intersection of this line with the axis of the long finger localizes the recurrent motor branch.
○ **Diagnosis**
  ▪ **History and neuromuscular examination**
    ▫ Pain and paresthesias of the radiopalmar hand, often worse at night and with repetitive movements.
    ▫ The thenar skin is spared of sensory disturbances because it is innervated by the palmar cutaneous branch that arises proximal to the carpal tunnel.
    ▫ Advanced cases may demonstrate thenar wasting.
    ▫ **Phalen maneuver:** the wrist is palmar flexed to 90° and paresthesias are observed in the median nerve distribution of the affected hands within 60 seconds.
    ▫ **Tinel sign:** lightly percussing over the flexor retinaculum elicits paresthesias (less sensitive, but more specific than the Phalen maneuver)
  ▪ **Electrodiagnostic studies** (highly operator dependent)
    ▫ Motor latencies greater than 4.5 ms
    ▫ Sensory latencies greater than 3.5 ms
    ▫ Conduction velocities less than 50 m/s
○ **Nonoperative treatment** (first-line treatment)
  ▪ Splint the wrist in neutral position, and wear continuously or only at night depending on the severity of symptoms.
  ▪ Anti-inflammatory agents (eg, NSAIDs) to reduce inflammation.
  ▪ Optimize management of systemic conditions (eg, diabetes mellitus and rheumatoid arthritis).
  ▪ Steroid injections may offer transient relief in 80% of patients, with better results in milder cases.
    ▫ Often beneficial in pregnant patients with debilitating symptoms, or others with transient edema.
    ▫ Response to steroids is also prognostic, predictive of a good response to surgery.

- ○ **Operative treatment**
  - ■ Open carpal tunnel release
    - □ Complete release of the transverse carpal ligament through an incision ulnar and parallel to the thenar crease to avoid injury to the palmar cutaneous branch
    - □ Provides better exposure but leaves a longer scar
  - ■ Endoscopic-assisted carpal tunnel release
    - □ Leaves a shorter scar, but anatomic anomalies may be more difficult to recognize given impaired visualization relative to the open technique.
    - □ No superiority has been demonstrated over the open technique.
  - ■ Synovectomy is only indicated in cases of proliferative or invasive tenosynovitis.
  - ■ Internal neurolysis, epineurotomy, and decompression of Guyon canal are not indicated routinely in carpal tunnel syndrome.
- • **Pronator Syndrome**
  - ○ **Sites of compression** (from proximal to distal)
    - ■ Proximal ligamentous attachment or accessory origin of the humeral head of the pronator teres (ligament of Struthers)
    - ■ Bicipital aponeurosis (lacertus fibrosis)
    - ■ Between the humeral and ulnar heads of the pronator teres (most common)
    - ■ Proximal edge of the flexor digitorum superficialis arch
  - ○ **Diagnosis**
    - ■ *Pain in the proximal volar forearm with associated hypoesthesia/paresthesias in the median nerve distribution, including involvement of the palmar cutaneous branch (helps differentiate it from carpal tunnel syndrome and anterior interosseus syndrome).
    - ■ Reproducible symptoms with isolated, resisted contraction of the biceps, pronator teres, or flexor digitorum superficialis may indicate the site of compression.
    - ■ Electrodiagnostic studies are of limited benefit.
  - ○ **Treatment**
    - ■ Splinting and rest may resolve symptoms in up to 50% of patients.
    - ■ If conservative measures fail, then all potential sites of compression above and below the elbow must be explored and released.
- • **Anterior Interosseus Syndrome**
  - ○ **Etiology**
    - ■ Probably not a true compression neuropathy, but a shared clinical manifestation or constellation of symptoms among several different causes, including mechanical compression (eg, anatomic anomaly, forearm mass), inflammatory (eg, infection, idiopathic), and posttraumatic (eg, forearm fracture, hemorrhage into the deep musculature).
    - ■ Approximately one-third of cases occur spontaneously.
    - ■ The most common site of compression is between the humeral and ulnar heads of the pronator teres.
  - ○ **Diagnosis**
    - ■ Weakness or loss of function of the flexor pollicis longus, flexor digitorum profundus to the index and long fingers, and pronator quadratus.
    - ■ *Since the anterior interosseus nerve is purely motor, no sensory symptoms.
    - ■ If asked to make an "OK" sign, the patient will make a triangle instead of circle due to lack of flexion of the interphalangeal joint of the thumb and distal interphalangeal joint of the index finger (pinch deformity).
    - ■ Unlike the pronator syndrome, electrodiagnostic studies are a useful diagnostic adjunct.

○ Treatment
  ▪ Managed similar to a closed nerve injury with baseline electrodiagnostic studies obtained within 4-6 weeks.
  ▪ Repeat electrodiagnostic studies at 12 weeks and if recovery is still incomplete, continue to observe patient.
  ▪ If no clinical or electrical signs (absence of MUAPs) of recovery are evident at 12 weeks, then nerve decompression is warranted.

ULNAR NERVE (SEE FIG. 45-3B)

• Cubital Tunnel Syndrome
  ○ **Sites of compression** (from proximal to distal) (**Fig. 45-5**)
    ▪ Medial intermuscular septum of the brachium
    ▪ Thick fascial band between the medial head of the triceps and the medial intermuscular septum located 8 cm above the elbow (arcade of Struthers)
    ▪ Cubital tunnel
      □ Roof: aponeurotic expansion of the two heads of the flexor carpi ulnaris (Osborne ligament)
      □ Floor: ulnar collateral ligament of the elbow, joint capsule, and olecranon
    ▪ Fascia of the flexor carpi ulnaris
  ○ **Diagnosis**
    ▪ History and neuromuscular examination
      □ Hypoesthesia/paresthesias of the small and ulnar half of the ring fingers and dorsoulnar hand.
      □ Weakness of grip strength and intrinsic wasting in advanced cases.
      □ Positive Tinel sign over the medial elbow.
      □ Possible ulnar nerve subluxation with elbow flexion.
      □ Phalen analog: hypoesthesia/paresthesias in the ulnar nerve distribution within 60 seconds of full elbow flexion.
      □ Scratch collapse test (controversial): with palms facing one another, a patient attempts adduction resistance to an examiner's efforts. The examiner then scratches the skin over the potential site of compression and attempts to adduct the forearm—sudden, temporary weakness of that forearm is a positive response.
      □ Froment sign: patient is unable to pinch and hold a piece of paper between their fully extended thumb and index finger against an examiner's attempt to pull away the paper—this is due to weakness of the ulnar nerve-innervated adductor pollicis muscle.

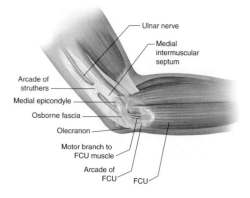

Figure 45-5 Anatomy of the cubital tunnel. FCU, flexor carpi ulnaris. (From Chung KC, Disa JJ, Gosain A, et al. *Operative Techniques in Plastic Surgery.* Wolters Kluwer; 2020. Figure 6.28.1.)

- Ancillary studies
  - □ Evidence of denervation in the first dorsal interosseus on electromyography (most common).
  - □ Abductor pollicis brevis should be normal (this excludes a C8/T1 nerve root or plexus lesion).
  - □ Obtain elbow plain films if history of trauma or abnormal range of motion.
  - ○ **Operative treatment**
    - *In situ* decompression: procedure of choice given similar outcomes with transposition techniques
    - Ulnar nerve transposition (subcutaneous, submuscular, or intramuscular): some centers advocate transposition with decompression as first line. Indicated in recurrent cases of cubital tunnel syndrome and patients with ulnar nerve subluxation
    - Medial epicondylectomy: useful in posttraumatic cases with bony deformity but carries the risk of damaging the ulnar collateral ligament leading to elbow instability
- **Ulnar Tunnel Syndrome** (compression of ulnar nerve in Guyon canal)
  - ○ **Etiology**
    - Ganglion cyst (most common)
    - Muscle anomalies
    - Thrombosis or pseudoaneurysm of the ulnar artery (hypothenar hammer syndrome)

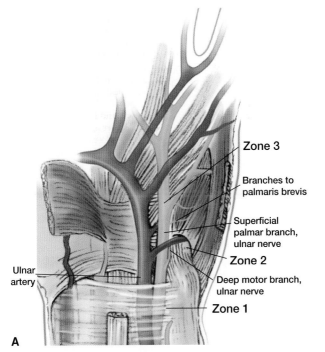

Zone 3

Branches to palmaris brevis

Superficial palmar branch, ulnar nerve

Zone 2

Ulnar artery

Deep motor branch, ulnar nerve

Zone 1

A

Figure 45-6 A-C. Anatomy of Guyon canal at the wrist. (From Wiesel SW, Albert T. *Operative Techniques in Orthopaedic Surgery*. 3rd ed. Wolters Kluwer; 2022. Figure 6.62.1.)

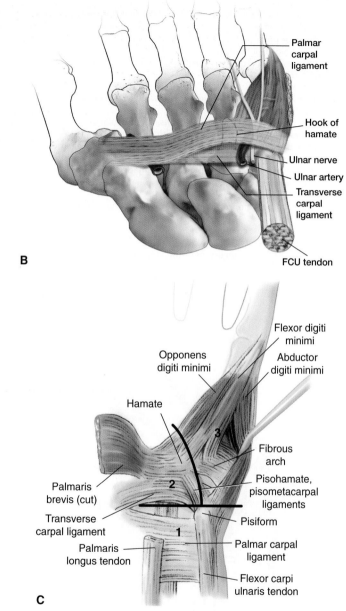

B

Palmar carpal ligament

Hook of hamate

Ulnar nerve

Ulnar artery

Transverse carpal ligament

FCU tendon

Flexor digiti minimi

Opponens digiti minimi

Abductor digiti minimi

Hamate

Fibrous arch

Pisohamate, pisometacarpal ligaments

Palmaris brevis (cut)

Transverse carpal ligament

Pisiform

Palmaris longus tendon

Palmar carpal ligament

Flexor carpi ulnaris tendon

C

Figure 45-6 (*continued*)

- Hook of the hamate fracture
- Edema/scarring from burns
- Inflammatory arthropathy

○ Anatomy (Fig. 45-6)
- **Guyon canal boundaries**
  - Radial: hook of the hamate
  - Ulnar: pisiform
  - Roof: volar carpal and pisohamate ligaments
  - Floor: transverse carpal ligament
- **Guyon canal contents**
  - One artery: ulnar artery.
  - One nerve: ulnar nerve.
  - The ulnar nerve is located ulnar to the ulnar artery.
- **Guyon canal zones**
  - Zone 1: proximal to the ulnar nerve bifurcation
  - Zone 2: contains the deep motor branch of the ulnar nerve
  - Zone 3: contains the superficial sensory branch of the ulnar nerve
- **Ulnar nerve branches**
  - *Dorsal sensory branch: arises 4-5 cm proximal to the pisiform and provides sensation to the dorsoulnar hand
  - Deep motor branch: arises within Guyon canal (more radial) and supplies the intrinsic musculature
  - Superficial sensory branch: arises within Guyon canal (more ulnar) and provides sensation to the small and ulnar half of the ring fingers

○ Diagnosis
- Pain in the ulnar wrist with hypoesthesia/paresthesias in the small and ulnar half of the ring fingers.
- *The dorsoulnar hand is spared of sensory disturbances because it is innervated by the dorsal sensory branch.
- Positive Tinel sign over Guyon canal.
- Symptoms are exacerbated by sustained hyperextension or hyperflexion of the wrist.
- Ulnar "Paradox": more likely to get clawing with distal compared to proximal ulnar nerve compression due to sparing of the flexor digitorum profundus.
- A bruit may be present.
- Electrodiagnostic studies are a useful diagnostic adjunct.

○ Nonoperative treatment
- Indicated if no identifiable lesion is present
- Splint the wrist in neutral position
- Anti-inflammatory agents (eg, NSAIDs) to reduce inflammation
- Activity modifications

○ Operative treatment
- Indicated if an identifiable lesion is present or failure of conservative measures
- Open ulnar tunnel release
  - Complete release of the volar carpal and pisohamate ligaments.
  - Divide the fibrous arch near the origin of the hypothenar musculature.
  - Explore the floor of Guyon canal for masses and fractures.
  - Examine the ulnar artery with the tourniquet up and then down.

RADIAL NERVE (SEE FIG. 45-3C)

- **Posterior Interosseus Syndrome**
  ○ Sites of compression (from proximal to distal)
  - Thickened fascial tissue superficial to the radiocapitellar joint
  - Recurrent vessels of the radial artery (leash of Henry)

- Fibrous bands within the extensor carpi radialis brevis
- Proximal edge of the supinator (arcade of Frohse, most common)
- Distal edge of the supinator
  - ○ **Diagnosis**
    - History and neuromuscular examination
      - □ Gradual weakness of finger and wrist extensors.
      - □ Similar to anterior interosseus syndrome where motor deficit is the primary issue with lack of sensory complaints.
      - □ Acute onset after trauma.
      - □ Rheumatoid disease at the elbow can mimic symptoms.
      - □ *Incomplete syndrome may be confused for tendon rupture (check for tenodesis).
    - Ancillary studies
      - □ Electrodiagnostic studies are a useful diagnostic adjunct.
      - □ Elbow plain films to rule out radial head dislocation or fracture.
      - □ Magnetic resonance imaging or ultrasound if there is concern for a soft tissue mass.
  - ○ **Treatment**
    - Managed similar to a closed nerve injury with baseline electrodiagnostic studies obtained within 4-6 weeks.
    - Repeat electrodiagnostic studies at 12 weeks and if recovery is still incomplete, continue to observe patient.
    - If no clinical or electrical signs (absence of MUAPs) of recovery are evident at 12 weeks, then nerve exploration is warranted.
    - Other indications for nerve exploration include posttraumatic (eg, proximal radius fracture) or if an identifiable lesion is present.
    - Steroid injections may be of some benefit in patients with rheumatoid disease.
- **Radial Tunnel Syndrome**
  - ○ **Anatomy**
    - **Radial tunnel boundaries**
      - □ Roof: extensor carpi radialis longus and brevis
      - □ Floor: radiocapitellar joint capsule proximally, and the biceps tendon and deep head of the supinator distally
    - Radial tunnel contents
      - □ One nerve: radial nerve
      - □ It runs approximately 5 cm in length from the radiocapitellar joint to the distal edge of the supinator
    - **Radial nerve branches**
      - □ Superficial branch: provides sensation to the dorsoradial hand
      - □ Deep branch: supplies motor innervation to the finger and wrist extensors
  - ○ **Diagnosis**
    - *Patients primarily complain of pain (weakness is secondary).
    - Pain is located at the lateral elbow and is exacerbated by resisted supination.
    - Often related to a work setting consisting of repetitive forceful elbow extension and forearm rotation.
    - Must differentiate from lateral epicondylitis (tenderness is more distal in radial tunnel syndrome).
    - Middle finger test: resisted middle finger extension produces pain in the proximal forearm.
    - Electrodiagnostic studies are of limited benefit.
    - Steroid injections are both diagnostic and prognostic, predictive of a good response to surgery.
  - ○ **Treatment**
    - Conservative measures are the mainstay of treatment including rest, splinting, steroid injections, and anti-inflammatory agents (eg, NSAIDs).

- Nerve exploration is only indicated if conservative measures fail.
- No progression to muscle palsy has ever been documented.

- **Wartenberg Syndrome**
  - **Definition:** compression of the superficial branch of the radial nerve
  - **Etiology**
    - *The superficial branch of the radial nerve becomes subcutaneous 9 cm proximal to the radial styloid between the brachioradialis and extensor carpi radialis longus tendons.
    - Many different causes of compression including external (eg, watch, handcuffs), overuse/repetitive activity (eg, using a screwdriver), posttraumatic (eg, wrist contusion), and scissoring of the brachioradialis and extensor carpi radialis longus tendons.
  - **Diagnosis**
    - *Pain and paresthesias over the dorsoradial hand that is exacerbated by wrist movement, index-thumb pinch, or forceful pronation of the forearm.
    - May get a false-positive with Finkelstein test (pain with ulnar deviation of the wrist with the thumb grasped in the palm).
    - Diagnosis can be confirmed by tracing Tinel sign or performing a diagnostic nerve block.
    - Electrodiagnostic studies are of limited benefit.
  - **Treatment**
    - Conservative measures are the mainstay of treatment including rest, splinting, steroid injections, and anti-inflammatory agents (eg, NSAIDs).
    - Nerve exploration is only indicated if conservative measures fail.

THORACIC OUTLET SYNDROME

- **Epidemiology**
  - Represents a common clinical manifestation or constellation of symptoms among several different causes
    - Neurologic: 95% (eg, brachial plexus)
    - Venous: 3%-4% (eg, subclavian vein)
    - Arterial: 1%-2% (eg, subclavian artery)
  - Three times more common in women than in men
  - Usually arises between the third and sixth decades of life
  - May be associated with occupations that involve awkward or static arm positioning at or above the shoulder level (eg, painters and nurses)
  - Paget-Schroetter disease: sudden, effort-induced thrombosis of the upper extremity deep venous system
- **Sites of Compression**
  - Interscalene triangle: between the anterior and middle scalene and the first rib
  - Costoclavicular triangle: between the clavicle and the first rib
  - Congenital fibromuscular bands: more common in neurologic cases
  - Cervical ribs: present in 0.5% of the general population and more common in arterial cases (50%-80% are bilateral)
- **Diagnosis**
  - **History and neuromuscular examination**
    - Pain or dull ache of insidious onset in the shoulder, upper back, and neck (easy fatigability and nighttime pain are common).
    - If neurologic involvement, may have paresthesias.
    - If venous involvement, may have visible engorged collateral veins.
    - If arterial involvement, may have claudication symptoms.
  - **Provocative tests**
    - Positive response is if the symptoms are reproduced or there is loss of the radial pulse.
    - All provocative tests lack sufficient sensitivity and specificity to make the diagnosis with any degree of certainty.

- Adson test: with the affected arm in the dependent position, turn the head to the ipsilateral shoulder, hyperextend the neck, and breathe deeply.
- Halstead (costoclavicular) test: with the affected arm in the dependent position, move the shoulder down and back with the chest out.
- Wright (hyperabduction) test: with the affected arm externally rotated and abducted 180°, breathe deeply.
- Cervical rotation lateral flexion test: rotate the head away from the affected arm, then flex the head toward the affected arm (positive response is bone blocking lateral flexion).
  - Ancillary studies
    - Cervical and chest plain films looking for bony abnormalities, cervical ribs, and lung masses (Pancoast tumor).
    - Vascular studies including Doppler, CTA, or arteriogram/venogram (gold standard, but invasive).
    - Magnetic resonance imaging and electrodiagnostic studies are of limited benefit.
    - Attempt diagnostic nerve block with injection into the scalenes.
- Treatment
  - Conservative measures should be attempted first including postural training, stretching/strengthening exercises, activity modification, and anti-inflammatory agents (eg, NSAIDs).
  - Indications for operative intervention include failure of conservative measures, intractable pain, significant neurologic deficit, and impending or acute vascular catastrophe.
  - Operative treatment focuses on removing any potential sites of compression (eg, cervical rib, release or excision of anterior and middle scalenes, neurolysis of the brachial plexus as indicated).
  - If venous obstruction, consider thrombectomy.
  - If arterial obstruction, consider thromboendarterectomy, resection and interpositional graft, or bypass.
  - Complications include brachial plexus injury, hemothorax, pneumothorax, chylothorax, and causalgia.

PEARLS

1. Assessment of pressure and vibratory sensation measure innervation threshold, whereas two-point discrimination measures innervation density.
2. In EMG, compound muscle action potentials reflect the number of functional axons and are reduced in the setting of axonal damage.
3. Little to no functional gains are expected in repairs of nerve injuries after 18-24 months secondary to atrophy of distal muscle targets.
4. In the setting of nerve transection injury, the distal nerve segments neurotransmitters are depleted after 72 hours and no longer respond to electrical stimulation, making surgical repair less effective.
5. The most successful treatments for neuroma appear to be methods that return function to the purposeless axons (eg, RPNI).
6. Paresthesias or numbness in the radiopalmar hand in the setting of wrist/carpal fracture should raise concern for an acute carpal tunnel syndrome.
7. Anterior and posterior interosseus syndromes produce motor deficits without sensory deficits.
8. Proximal and distal median and ulnar nerve compressions can be differentiated based on the presence or absence of sensory deficits at the radiopalmar or dorsulnar hand.

QUESTIONS YOU WILL BE ASKED

1. In the setting of significant extremity trauma with a resultant nerve injury with a 10 cm gap, is it better to use autologous nerve graft, conduit, or cadaveric allograft?
   In gaps over 3-5 cm, nerve autografts have shown superior recovery of functional and sensory deficits over the other choices.
2. In the setting of a nerve laceration, how long can the distal segment be electrically stimulated in the OR, producing visible muscle contraction?
   Approximately 72 hours.
3. Diagnostic electrical studies will show what findings in the setting of peripheral nerve injury and later recovery?
   After nerve injury, decreased motor unit potential amplitude, fibrillation potentials, positive sharp waves, and decreased motor unit recruitment will be seen. Nascent potentials occur months after injury and are the only finding specific to recovery.

Recommended Readings
1. Dvali L, Mackinnon S. Nerve repair, grafting, and nerve transfers. *Clin Plast Surg.* 2003;30(2):203-221.
2. Kubiak CA, Kemp SWP, Cederna PS. Regenerative peripheral nerve interface for management of postamputation neuroma. *JAMA Surg.* 2018;153(7):681-682. doi:10.1001/jamasurg.2018.0864
3. Maggi SP, Lowe JB III, Mackinnon SE. Pathophysiology of nerve injury. *Clin Plast Surg.* 2003;30(2):109-126.
4. Neal S, Fields KB. Peripheral nerve entrapment and injury in the upper extremity. *Am Fam Physician.* 2010;81(2):147-155.

46

Rheumatoid Arthritis, Osteoarthritis, and Dupuytren Contracture

Stacia M. Ruse and Alexandria Sherwood

RHEUMATOID ARTHRITIS (RA)

OVERVIEW

- **Definition:** chronic systemic disease caused by autoimmune response against soft tissue, cartilage, and bone. Characterized by morning stiffness, subcutaneous nodules, polyarthropathy, with progressive deformity of the hand and wrist
- Affects 3% of women and 1% of men
- **Diagnosis (Table 46-1)**
- **Pathophysiology**
  - Inflamed synovium (pannus) invades and destroys articular cartilage as well as tendons.
  - Reactive synovium leads to articular cartilage damage, joint laxity, joint destruction, and destruction of tendons.
- **Wrightington Classification for Rheumatoid Arthritis of the Wrist**
  - Grade I: wrist architecture preserved, mild RSS, periarticular osteoporosis, early cyst formation
  - Grade II: ulnar translocation, lunate volar flexed, flexed scaphoid, radiolunate destruction (RS and midcarpal preserved)
  - Grade III: intercarpal joints arthritic, radioscaphoid eroded, volar subluxation of carpus (gross bony architecture preserved)
  - Grade IV: loss of large amount of bone stock from distal radius, gross erosion of ulnar side of radius

PREOPERATIVE EVALUATION

- **Physical Examination Findings (Fig. 46-1)**
  - Digital findings
    - Swan-neck and boutonnière deformities
    - Tendon ruptures
    - Thumb deformities

TABLE 46-1 Criteria for Rheumatoid Arthritis Diagnosis

Criteria established by the American College of Rheumatology for diagnosing rheumatoid arthritis (RA) → have ≥4 of the 7 criteria for a 6-week period
• Morning stiffness lasting at least 1 hour
• Swelling of three or more joint areas
• Arthritis of hand joints including wrist, MCP, and PIP joints
• Symmetric arthritis of the same joint on both sides of the body
• Rheumatoid nodules
• Sero-positive RF
• Radiographic changes consistent with RA

---

*Denotes common in-service examination topics.

- Rheumatoid nodules (strong association with positive serum rheumatoid factor (RF))
    - Arthritis mutilans
  - Hand findings
    - Ulnar drift at MP joint
    - Radial sagittal band failure
  - Wrist findings
    - Caput ulna
    - Radiocarpal collapse
  - Rheumatoid elbow
- **X-ray Changes:** periarticular erosions and osteopenia
- **Laboratory Values**
  - Anti-CCP (most sensitive and specific test)
  - Anti-MCV
  - Elevated ESR/CRP
  - Positive RF titer (most commonly IgM) → elevated in 75%-80% of patients with RA

TREATMENT

- **Treatment Goals:** pain control, control synovitis, maintain joint function, and prevent deformity
- **Priorities for Hand Surgery in Rheumatoid Patients**
  - **Alleviation of pain:** alleviation of medically refractory pain is the primary indication for surgery
  - **Improvement of function**
    - Loss of function is not synonymous with deformity.
    - Surgery cannot restore full function and may further weaken the hand.
    - Reconstruction before onset of severe deformity may offer better results.
  - **Halt progression**
    - Earlier reconstruction/procedure with more predictable outcome is preferable.
    - Tenosynovectomy may prevent tendon rupture.
    - Wrist stabilization and distal ulna excision to prevent wrist collapse.
  - **Improvement of appearance:** surgery to correct deformity should be avoided in patients with minimal functional loss or pain
- **Maximize medical management:** the patient should usually be under the care of a rheumatologist for at least 6 months before considering an operation.
  - Pharmacologic treatment is the mainstay.

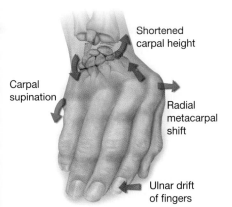

Shortened carpal height

Carpal supination

Radial metacarpal shift

Ulnar drift of fingers

Figure 46-1 Rheumatoid arthritis changes at the wrist. Volar and ulnar translation of the wrist with progressive supination occurs as the restraining ligaments are successively disrupted.

- Significant advances in medical management (DMARDs) have dramatically changed the prognosis of the disease. This had led to a drastic decrease in surgical intervention.
- Surgery
  - Need to coordinate timing with the rheumatologist; maximize medical control
  - Preoperative cervical spine evaluation is essential
  - *Generally, address joints from proximal to distal
  - Can be prophylactic, not just for late complications
  - Early disease—synovectomy, tenosynovectomy, tendon reconstructive surgery
  - Advanced disease—arthroplasty, arthrodesis (goal is to improve pain, deformity, and arc of motion)

TENOSYNOVITIS

- **Background**
  - Tenosynovitis is common with 50%-70% of RA patients developing tendon sheath inflammation.
  - May occur before joint involvement. May lead to pain, tendon dysfunction, compressive neuropathy, and tendon rupture.
  - Common sites of involvement are dorsal wrist, volar wrist, and volar aspect of digits.
- **Dorsal Wrist Tenosynovitis**
  - Painless dorsal wrist swelling. May involve one, some, or all tendons in all compartments.
  - Tendon ruptures frequent from invasion by hypertrophic synovium and attrition.
  - Although remission may occur from conservative therapy (rest, steroid injection, and antirheumatoid agents), early dorsal tenosynovectomy is suggested for focal synovitis.
- **Volar Wrist Tenosynovitis**
  - Usually leads to restriction of flexor tendons leading to restricted active and passive motion.
  - Compression of median nerve may occur.
  - Again, early surgical treatment is indicated to prevent permanent damage.
  - Volar tenosynovectomy with carpal tunnel decompression is treatment of choice.
- **Digital Tenosynovitis**
  - Mild synovial hypertrophy can affect function as tendons travel in a tight fibro-osseous canal.
  - Rheumatoid nodule in digital tendons can cause trigger finger.
  - Prolonged tenosynovitis may lead to tendon rupture.
  - Flexor tenosynovectomy and excision of flexor tendon nodules are indicated.

SWAN-NECK DEFORMITY

- Hyperextension of proximal interphalangeal joint (PIPJ) with distal interphalangeal joint (DIPJ) flexion (**Fig. 46-2**)
- *Mechanism of Deformity
  - Synovitis of the DIPJ leads to terminal tendon rupture → DIP flexion.
  - Synovitis leads to FDS, volar plate, and collateral ligament attenuation → decreased volar support of the PIPJ → PIPJ hyperextension deformity.
  - Lateral bands subluxate dorsal to the PIP axis of rotation.
  - Contracture of the triangular ligament and attenuation of the transverse retinacular ligament.
- Goals: correct PIPJ hyperextension, improve PIPJ ROM, correct DIPJ and MCPJ flexion deformity
- **Correction of Deformity Depends on PIPJ Mobility**
  - If full PIPJ active flexion, but "snapping" when flexing → do lateral band relocation
  - If PIPJ passively correctable in all metacarpophalangeal joint (MPJ) positions, capsular restriction at PIPJ is suggested → release of PIPJ

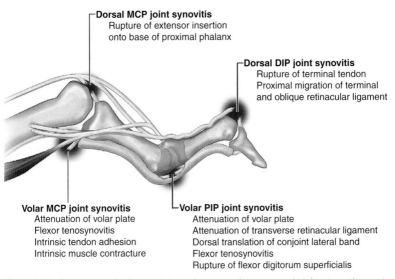

Dorsal MCP joint synovitis
Rupture of extensor insertion
onto base of proximal phalanx

Dorsal DIP joint synovitis
Rupture of terminal tendon
Proximal migration of terminal
and oblique retinacular ligament

Volar MCP joint synovitis
Attenuation of volar plate
Flexor tenosynovitis
Intrinsic tendon adhesion
Intrinsic muscle contracture

Volar PIP joint synovitis
Attenuation of volar plate
Attenuation of transverse retinacular ligament
Dorsal translation of conjoint lateral band
Flexor tenosynovitis
Rupture of flexor digitorum superficialis

Figure 46-2 Illustration of the characteristic configuration of the swan-neck deformity with synovitis of the flexor tendon sheath, flexion at the metacarpophalangeal joint, hyperextension at the proximal interphalangeal joint, and flexion at the distal interphalangeal joint. (From Kelley BP, Chung KC. Correction of swan-neck deformity. In: Chung KC, ed. *Operative Techniques in Hand and Wrist Surgery*. 3rd ed. Elsevier; 2018:350.)

- ○ If PIPJ flexion changes with MPJ position (motion increases with MCP flexed) → fix MPJ subluxation or release tight intrinsics
- ○ If there is a fixed flexion deformity without joint destruction → lateral band mobilization, fix underlying deforming force
- ○ If there is a fixed flexion deformity with joint destruction → arthrodesis vs silicone arthroplasty of PIPJ
  - ▪ Fuse joints where stability is most important.
    - ▫ Index (to maintain pinch): fuse at 30°
    - ▫ When necessary, can fuse middle finger at 35°, ring at 40°, and small at 45°
  - ▪ Replace joints where motion is important: typically middle, ring, and small fingers (to maintain power grip).

BOUTONNIÈRE DEFORMITY

- Flexion at PIPJ with hyperextension at DIPJ and MPJ (**Fig. 46-3**)
- *Mechanism of Deformity
  - ○ Synovitis at PIPJ → attenuation of central slip and dorsal capsule → flexion at PIPJ → volar subluxation of lateral bands
  - ○ Oblique retinacular ligament contracture → DIPJ hyperextension
  - ○ Compensatory MPJ hyperextension
- Correction of Deformity
  - ○ If passively correctable with mild deformity: synovectomy and splinting ± tenotomy of terminal tendon
  - ○ If passively correctable with moderate deformity: synovectomy with central slip/lateral band reconstruction ± tenotomy of terminal tendon
  - ○ If there is a fixed flexion deformity: arthrodesis vs arthroplasty of PIPJ as above (see section "Swan-Neck Deformity")

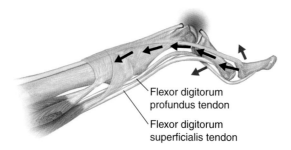

Flexor digitorum profundus tendon

Flexor digitorum superficialis tendon

Figure 46-3 Characteristic configuration of rheumatoid boutonnière deformity with metacarpophalangeal joint hyperextension, proximal interphalangeal joint flexion, and distal interphalangeal joint hyperextension, with florid synovitis depicted over the proximal interphalangeal joint. (From Chung KC. *Grabb and Smith's Plastic Surgery*. 8th ed. Wolters Kluwer; 2020. Figure 92.10B.)

TENDON RUPTURES (TABLE 46-2)

- It is important to differentiate the cause of a sudden inability to extend a finger (Table 46-3)
- Extensor Tendon Rupture
  - EDM is the most common extensor tendon to rupture (frequency EDM > EDC (ring) > EDC (small) > EPL)
  - **Vaughan-Jackson syndrome:** rupture of digital extensor tendons from ulnar to radial due to prominent ulnar head
    - Pathoanatomy: DRUJ instability + volar carpal subluxation → dorsal ulnar head prominence → attritional rupture of extensor tendons
    - EDM is the first that ruptures
  - *Treatment: tenosynovectomy, address caput ulna (with Darrach procedure), tendon transfers
    - EPL rupture: transfer EIP, EDM, or extensor pollicis brevis
    - EDM rupture: transfer EIP if necessary
    - Single EDC rupture (usually SF): cross-link to adjacent EDC (usually RF)
    - 2 EDC ruptures: transfer EIP

TABLE 46-2 Treatment for Different Types of Tendon Ruptures

Type of rupture	Treatment
Ruptures—all	Dorsal tenosynovectomy Removal of bone spikes Retinacular relocation to cover bone Ulnar head resection as needed
Single rupture	Primary repair Intercalated graft Adjacent suture
Double rupture—usually EDC (ring and small), EDQ	As for single rupture, plus extensor indicis proprius (EIP) transfer
Triple rupture	As for double rupture, plus FDS (middle) transfer Wrist extensor transfer (wrist fusion) EPL transfer (MP fusion)
Quadruple rupture	As for triple rupture, plus an additional FDS

TABLE 46-3 Tendon Ruptures vs Extensions

	Active extension	Maintenance of extension	Tenodesis effect
Extensor tendon rupture from attrition	−	+	+
Ulnar subluxation of extensor tendon at MPJ	−	+	+
PIN palsy at elbow from synovitis	−	−	+

- *Flexor Pollicis Longus (FPL) Rupture (Mannerfelt Syndrome): most common flexor tendon rupture
  - Inability to flex the thumb IPJ, caused by scaphoid spur and synovitis
  - Treatment is synovectomy, osteophyte resection, and tendon graft or transfer
- **Radial Sagittal Band Failure**
  - Extensor tendons migrate into the ulnar gutter and volar to the center of rotation of the MCP joint.
  - Exam: loss of active extension. Patient can maintain extension if MCP placed in extension.
  - Treatment: sagittal band reconstruction (extensor hood reconstruction).

RHEUMATOID NODULES

- **Most Common extra-articular manifestation of RA:** seen in 25% of patients with RA
  - An extra-articular process found over the IP joints, olecranon, and ulnar border of the forearm
- Associated with aggressive disease and poor prognosis. Erosion through skin may lead to sinus tract formation
- Treatment
  - Nonoperative: steroid injection
  - Operative: surgical excision for pain relief, cosmesis, and/or diagnostic biopsy

ULNAR DRIFT AT MP JOINT

- **Mechanism of Deformity**
  - Condylar joints (biplanar movements) inherently less stable.
  - Synovitis at the MP joint causes capsule, ligament, and volar plate laxity.
  - Radial sagittal band laxity causes ulnar deviation of the extensor tendons.
  - Contraction of the ulnar intrinsics.
- **Treatment Depends on Degree of MPJ Destruction**
  - Address the wrist first
  - **If no joint destruction:** cross intrinsic tendon transfer, synovectomy, and ulnar intrinsic release
    - Indicated for persistent synovitis with early volar subluxation and ulnar drift or young patients with slowly progressing disease
    - Extensor relocation indicated with ulnar subluxation of extensor tendon
  - **If joint destruction (cannot correct passively):** silicone MP arthroplasty (SMPA)
    - Indicated for severe disease with MP dislocation, ulnar drift, and articular involvement
    - Contraindications: inadequate skin coverage, active infection, excessive destruction of periarticular bone (increased rates of implant dislocation)
    - Provides durable deformity correction and pain relief
    - Arthrodesis considered if not SMPA candidate. Typically limited to thumb, avoid in IF

CAPUT ULNA

- **Mechanism of Deformity**
  - DRUJ synovitis and capsule stretch (piano key sign) → supination of carpal row with volar and ulnar translocation + dorsal subluxation of the ulnar head
- **Nonoperative Treatment:** optimize medical management, splinting, local steroid injection
- **Operative treatment is indicated for pain relief with motion.** These approaches require that the hand be under minimal load-bearing demands.
  - Synovectomy of the DRUJ
  - Distal ulnar resection for unstable ulna (**Darrach procedure**)
    - Extensor retinaculum flap over distal ulna to decrease future tendon erosion
    - Can stabilize ulna with ECU, FCU, or PQ
  - Distal ulnar pseudarthrosis (**Sauve-Kapandji procedure**)
    - Indication: younger patients because preserves TFCC
    - Contraindication: prior radial head resection, insufficient/deformed distal ulna
  - Hemiresection arthroplasty of DRUJ: may be considered for symptomatic stump instability after prior distal ulna procedures

RADIOCARPAL DESTRUCTION

- **Pathoanatomy**
  - Synovitis and capsular distension → supination, radial deviation of the carpus
  - Ulnar and volar translocation of the carpus on the radius
  - Scaphoid flexion, radiolunate widening, lunate translocation
  - Secondary radioscaphoid arthrosis
  - Ulnar deviation of the fingers at the MP joints creates a classic zigzag deformity
- **Treatment**
  - Synovectomy
    - Indications: early disease
    - Technique: transfer ECRL to ECU (diminishes deforming forces—Clayton procedure)
  - Radiolunate fusion or RSL fusion
    - Indications: preserved midcarpal joint
  - Wrist fusion
    - Indications: advanced disease and poor bone stock
    - Remains gold standard and is often combined with Darrach
  - Total wrist arthroplasty
    - Indications: sedentary patients with good bone stock
    - Advantages: better motion than wrist fusion

RHEUMATOID ELBOW

- **Nonoperative:** rheumatoid elbow is mainly managed with medical treatment and cortisone injections
- **Operative:**
  - Arthroscopic or open synovectomy
    - Indications: pain without instability. No significant loss of ROM
  - Synovectomy and radial head excision
    - Indications: degeneration is mainly in radiohumeral joint. PIN compression secondary to radial head synovitis
    - Technique: lateral approach to the elbow
  - Interposition arthroplasty
    - Indications: young patients who are not candidates for Total elbow athroplasty (TEA)
    - Results are less predictable than TEA but avoids prosthetic complications
  - TEA

- Indications: pain, loss of motion, instability
- Technique: semi-constrained devices have the best results
- Outcomes: reliable procedure for advanced RA of the elbow

OSTEOARTHRITIS

GENERAL CONSIDERATIONS

- **Osteoarthritis (OA)** is a noninflammatory primary cartilage disease that is characterized by progressive articular cartilage deterioration and reactive new bone formation.
- Most common form of arthritis: clinically affects 3%-7% of adults.
- Cartilage changes are manifested by joint enlargement, pain, stiffness, contracture, and angular deformity. In contrast to RA, OA has less inflammatory reaction in the joints.
- Females > males, usually over 40 years of age, possible genetic predisposition.
- Incidence: DIP (most common in the hand) > thumb CMC > PIP > MCP.
- Nonoperative therapy is the mainstay of treatment, though there are surgical options for recalcitrant cases.

HISTORY AND EVALUATION

- Most common complaint is an insidious onset of joint pain and stiffness that interferes with function of the hand. **Pain is usually activity related.**
- **Examination**
  - Joint swelling and occasional tenderness.
  - Periarticular enlargement (**Heberden nodes at distal interphalangeal [DIP] and Bouchard nodes at proximal interphalangeal [PIP]**).
  - Mucous cysts can be present at the DIP and cause nail deformities.
  - Crepitus with joint passive range of motion and positive "grind test."
- **X-rays**
  - Dedicated three-view radiographs are generally all that is needed to confirm the diagnosis of an osteoarthritic joint.
  - Findings include osteophytes, narrowed joint space, eburnation (bony sclerosis), and subchondral cysts.

NONOPERATIVE TREATMENT

- **No medical treatment** is available for the underlying disease process in OA.
- **Treatment goal is symptomatic control**: activity modification, splints, NSAIDs, injection (steroids, hyaluronic acid).

SURGICAL TREATMENT

- **DIPJ**
  - **Mucous cyst excision: see Chapter 44: Hand Tumors**
  - Arthrodesis
    - Can be done with longitudinal K-wires or Acutrak or Herbert screw
    - Usually done with 5°-10° of flexion
- **PIPJ**
  - **Arthrodesis**
    - Indicated for pain relief but loss of range of motion is less than ideal, particularly in the ulnar digits for power grip
    - Headless screw fixation has highest fusion rates
    - Goal is to recreate normal cascade of the fingers/PIPJ flexion angles
      - Index—30°
      - Long—35°
      - Ring—40°
      - Small—45°

- Silicone arthroplasty for middle and ring PIPJ
  - Radial collateral ligament should be intact to tolerate pinch grip
  - Indications: central digits with good bone stock. No angulation or deformity
  - Outcomes: volar better than dorsal approach (lower revision rate)
- Collateral ligament excision, volar plate release, osteophyte excision
  - Predominant contracture with minimal joint involvement
  - MCP Joint: pyrocarbon arthroplasty is a good option at this joint

THUMB CMC JOINT ARTHRITIS

- **Findings**
  - Early symptoms: pain, swelling, crepitus, and weak pinch
  - Late symptoms: metacarpal adduction and web contracture
  - Signs: positive grind test (pain with axial loading of thumb CMC). Concomitant carpal tunnel syndrome in up to 50%
- **Imaging:** AP, lateral, and Roberts view (XR beam centered on trapezium and metacarpal with thumb flat and hyperpronated on cassette)
- **Incidence:** seen in 25% of men and 40% of women >75 years of age
- **Mechanism of Deformity:** volar carpal (beak) ligament from volar-ulnar base of the first metacarpal to the trapezium degenerates → destabilizes the thumb CMC → joint wear
  - Anterior oblique (volar beak) ligament is the primary stabilizing static restraint to subluxation of the CMC joint
- Eaton and Littler Classification
  - Stage I: slight joint space widening (prearthritis)
  - Stage II: slight narrowing of CMC, sclerosis, osteophytes <2 mm
  - Stage III: marked narrowing of CMC, sclerosis, osteophytes >2 mm
  - Stage IV: pantrapezial arthritis (STT involvement)
- Nonsurgical Options
  - NSAIDs, thumb spica bracing (first line)
  - Injections → second line for mild to moderate disease
    - Good evidence to support steroid injections
    - Hyaluronic acid injections NOT indicated (no difference for relief of pain and improvement in function when compared to placebo and steroids)
- **Surgical Options**
  - **Arthrodesis**
    - Fuse at 30°-40° palmar abduction, 30° radial abduction, and 15° pronation.
    - Nonunion is a frequent complication.
  - **Trapeziectomy with/without ligament reconstruction**
    - Multiple techniques (none showing clear benefit over others). All trades pain relief for some residual weakness
      - Trapeziectomy + ligament reconstruction and tendon interposition (most common)
      - Trapeziectomy alone
      - Trapeziectomy + suture suspension with APL to FCR
      - Volar ligament reconstruction with FCR
      - Excision of proximal third of trapezoid
    - Subsidence occurs with all surgical options
  - **CMC arthroscopic debridement:** for early disease
  - **First metacarpal osteotomy:** early stage I-II disease. Contraindicated with hypermobility or fixed subluxation of the CMC

DUPUYTREN DISEASE

GENERAL

- Benign proliferative disorder characterized by contractures and painful fascial nodules leading to decreased hand function

- **Major Clinical Features**
  - Painful nodules and cords, which can result in digital contractures.
  - Progression is neither linear nor homogeneous.
- Histologically, there is uncontrolled tissue proliferation, myofibroblast, and increased extracellular matrix synthesis.
- Pathogenesis remains controversial. Underlying cause is unknown; not occupational or traumatic.

EPIDEMIOLOGY

- **Demographics**
  - Almost exclusively a disease of Caucasians—most commonly, people of Northern European ancestry (rare in South America, Africa, China)
  - 2:1 male to female ratio (more severe disease in men)
  - Incidence peaks between the fifth and seventh decade of life (usually presents earlier in men)
  - Autosomal-dominant inheritance with variable penetrance
- **Location**
  - Dupuytren disease affects the palm and most commonly the ring and small fingers.
  - Radial side involvement is more common in diabetics.
- **Pathophysiology**
  - Occurs in the fibrofatty subcutaneous layer of the volar hand (palmar fascia). Myofibroblast is the dominant cell type. Type III collagen predominates over type I.
  - Cytokines have also been implicated (TGF beta, epidermal growth factor, PDGF, connective tissue growth factor).
- **Associated Diseases:** alcoholism, diabetes mellitus, epilepsy, HIV infection
- *Dupuytren Diathesis: presents aggressively, with early onset and early recurrence; may require more extensive treatment. Characterized by three classic findings
  - Knuckle pads (Garrod pads)
  - Foot involvement (Ledderhose disease)
  - Penis involvement (Peyronie disease)

ANATOMY

- Bands are normal digital and palmar subcutaneous fibrous connective tissue
  - Spiral band
  - Lateral digital sheet
  - Natatory ligament
  - Pretendinous band
  - Grayson ligament: palmar to neurovascular (NV) bundle
  - Cleland ligament: dorsal to NV bundle and does not become diseased
- *Normal fascial bands become pathologic cords (Fig. 46-4)
  - Palmar
    - **Pretendinous cord:** diseased pretendinous band causes metacarpophalangeal joint contracture
  - Palmodigital transition
    - **Spiral cord:** components → pretendinous band, spiral band, lateral digital sheet, and Grayson ligament (mnemonic: Plastic Surgeons Look Good)
      - **Most important cord**
      - Cause of PIP Contracture
      - *This is the most dangerous surgically because it travels under the NV bundle and displaces it centrally and superficially
        - Best predictors of displacement are PIPJ flexion contracture and interdigital soft tissue mass
    - **Natatory cord:** from diseased natatory ligament; causes webspace contracture

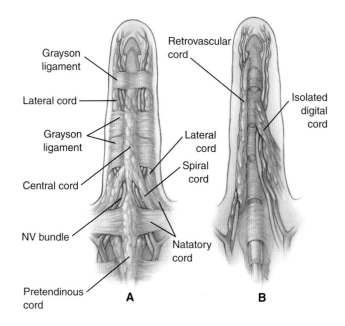

Figure 46-4 Pathological anatomy of the distal palmar and digital anatomy. **A.** The more superficial diseased elements. **B.** The deeper diseased elements.

- ○ Digital
  - ▪ **Central Cord:** from disease involving the pretendinous band. Inserts into the flexor sheath at the level of the PIPJ and causes MCP contracture
  - ▪ **Retrovascular cord:** originates from proximal phalanx and inserts onto the distal phalanx. Causes DIPJ contracture
  - ▪ Lateral cord
  - ▪ Digital cord
- ○ NOT involved in Dupuytren's → Cleland ligament and transverse ligament of the palmar aponeurosis

INDICATIONS FOR TREATMENT

- **MCP joint contracture is usually correctible;** operative release is indicated when
  - ○ Contractures interfere significantly with daily activities (ask the patient).
  - ○ Arbitrary contracture angles are less important, but usually an operation is done if MCP contracture is >30°-45°.
- **Any PIPJ contracture is difficult to fully correct,** so early intervention is warranted. Typically correct if contracture >15°.
- Contracture causing maceration or hygiene difficulties
- **"Table Top Test":** patient unable to have digit and palm simultaneously on the surface of a table top is a sign of significant contracture

NONOPERATIVE TREATMENT

- ROM Exercises
- Collagenase Injections (Xiaflex) With Manipulation

- o Thought to cause lysis and rupture of cords
- o Indications for its use are still evolving, but often patient preference
- o FDA approved to be used in Dupuytren disease with a palpable cord
- o Complications: skin tear, tendon rupture, swelling

OPERATIVE TREATMENT

- **Primary Operations**
  - o **Percutaneous needle aponeurotomy:** cords transected in clinic with sweep of a needle. Indicated in mild disease or medical comorbidities that preclude surgery
    - ▪ Outcomes
      - □ More successful for MCP contracture than PIP
      - □ Less improvement and higher recurrence rate than open surgery
  - o **Fasciectomy**
    - ▪ Indications: MCP flexion contracture >30°, PIP flexion contracture
    - ▪ Technique: limited fasciectomy (segment of cord tissue removed, most common), regional fasciectomy (all visibly diseased tissue removed), radical (both normal and abnormal fascia removed)
    - ▪ Outcomes
      - □ Partial palmar fasciectomy—most commonly used and preserves overlying skin. Recurrence rate roughly 30% at 1-2 years
      - □ Open palm technique (McCash)—reduced hematoma formation and reduced risk for stiffness. However, longer healing and greater recurrence than if the palmar defect were covered
      - □ Total/radical palmar fasciectomy—high complication rate and little effect on recurrence rate (also high)
  - o **Salvage**
    - ▪ Indicated for recurrent or advanced disease
    - ▪ Dermofasciectomy (excise skin + fascia), arthrodesis, amputation
- **Incision Design**
  - o Many skin incisions have been advocated
    - ▪ Palmar: transverse incision in proximal palmar crease is preferred.
    - ▪ Finger: longitudinal incision, broken up by Z-plasties over crease is preferred.
  - o Open palm technique heals well and prevents hematoma
- **Postoperative Considerations**
  - o Early active mobilization and nighttime splinting in extension, may need dynamic splinting.
  - o Dressing changes if open palm technique was used.
  - o Skin graft causes delay in early mobilization.
- **Complications**
  - o Hematoma (most common surgical complication → can lead to flap necrosis).
  - o Recurrence → 30% at 1-2 years.
  - o Nerve injury: remember that spiral cord pulls NV bundle proximally and abnormally centrally on the digit.
  - o Vascular injury.
  - o Stiffness (ie, failure to correct contracture, especially PIPJ).
  - o Complex regional pain syndrome (CRPS).

PEARLS

1. DMARDs ("disease-modifying agents") have made surgery in rheumatoid disease much less necessary, though the hand surgeon continues to play a crucial role in maintaining function.
2. Goals of surgery in a rheumatoid patient are to alleviate pain, improve function, and halt progression of disease. Surgery should not be performed for cosmesis alone, as many patients are functional even with significant deformity.

3. The surgeon should differentiate reducible joint deformities from fixed ones, as the treatment options are very different.
4. Nonoperative treatment should be maximized prior to offering surgical treatment in OA.
5. Spiral cord pushes the NV bundle volar, proximal, and midline. The NV bundle is often in a nonanatomic position, so be careful.

QUESTIONS YOU WILL BE ASKED

1. What is the mechanism of a swan-neck deformity?
   a. Synovitis at DIPJ → leads to rupture of distal extensor tendon → mallet deformity → extensor imbalance and volar plate laxity → PIPJ hyperextension.
   b. Synovitis at PIPJ → volar plate laxity → PIPJ hyperextension → extensor imbalance → DIPJ flexion.
   c. Intrinsic tightness → MP joint subluxations → extensor imbalance → PIPJ hyperextension and DIPJ flexion.
2. What is the mechanism of a boutonnière deformity?
   a. Synovitis at PIP joint → attenuation of central slip → flexion at PIPJ → volar subluxation of lateral bands.
   b. Shortened oblique retinacular ligaments → DIPJ hyperextension.
   c. Compensatory MPJ hyperextension.
3. What digital fascial structure is NOT involved in Dupuytren disease?
   Cleland ligament.

Recommended Readings
1. Adams JE. Surgical management of osteoarthritis of the hand and wrist. *J Hand Ther.* 2022;35(3):418-427.
2. Boe C, Blazar P, Iannuzzi N. Dupuytren contractures: an update of recent literature. *J Hand Surg Am.* 2021;46(10):896-906.
3. Chung KC, Pushman AG. Current concepts in the management of the rheumatoid hand. *J Hand Surg Am.* 2011;36(4):736-747; quiz 747.

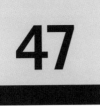

47

Breast Augmentation, Mastopexy, and Augmentation Mastopexy

Sarah Hart Kennedy

PREOPERATIVE WORKUP FOR ANY BREAST SURGERY

MEDICAL HISTORY

- Personal or family history of breast cancer
- Results of recent breast imaging
- Previous breast surgeries
- Pregnancies, breast-feeding, future childbearing plans
- Smoking history
- History of any bleeding disorders or diabetes
- History of deep vein thrombosis/pulmonary embolism or hypercoagulability (eg factor V Leiden, protein C or S deficiency, and use of birth control pills/HRT)

PHYSICAL EXAMINATION

- **Detailed breast examination** for masses and axillary examination for lymphadenopathy.
- **Assess breast size and shape** (eg, tuberous, wide, and loss of superior pole fullness).
- **Assess location of breast footprint on chest wall** (eg, high, middle, low).
- *Evaluate the degree of ptosis
  - Normal: nipple lies above the IMF.
  - Grade 1 (mild ptosis): nipple lies at the inframammary fold (IMF).
  - Grade 2 (moderate ptosis): nipple lies below the IMF but above the lowest contour of the breast.
  - Grade 3 (severe ptosis): the nipple is below the IMF and at the lowest contour of the breast.
  - Pseudoptosis: nipple is above IMF but lower pole breast tissue hangs below the fold.
- **Evaluate skin quality** (eg, tone, striae, elasticity).
- **Assess Symmetry**
  - Chest wall, sternum, ribcage, spine (pectus excavatum/carinatum, scoliosis, Poland syndrome)
  - Breast volume
  - Difference in direction and height of nipple-areolar complex (NAC)
  - Difference in IMF height
- **Key Measurements With Patient Sitting Upright**
  - Sternal notch to nipple
  - Nipple to IMF
  - Nipple to nipple distance
  - Base width

PREOPERATIVE MAMMOGRAM

If the patient is >35 years old or has positive family history

---

*Denotes common in-service examination topics.

BREAST AUGMENTATION

PREOPERATIVE CONSULTATION

- **History**
  - Motives for breast augmentation, current family situation, any recent life events influencing decision
  - Patient goals and expectations
  - Complete breast and medical history, as above
  - Obtain preoperative photographs
- **Physical**
  - Complete breast examination, as above.
  - Bring asymmetries to patient's attention prior to surgery. Asymmetries (eg, nipple position) may be amplified after augmentation.
  - Measure breast base width that will ultimately determine maximum size of the implant.
- **Patient Education**
  - Implants are not permanent and may need to be removed or replaced in the future.
  - Implants may impact cancer monitoring (see section "Breast Cancer Detection in Augmented Women")
  - Implants should be followed radiographically for rupture (see "Silicone Implant" section for FDA screening recommendations)
  - **Risk of BIA-ALCL** (breast implant associated—anaplastic large cell lymphoma), which is associated with textured implants.
  - **Breast implant illness (BII)**
    - FDA box warning that patients with implants have reported systemic symptoms (joint pain, muscle aches, confusions, chronic fatigue, autoimmune diseases, etc.).
    - Currently, no data to support an association but further research is ongoing

SURGICAL APPROACHES

- **Incision**
  - **Inframammary**
    - Most common.
    - Incision placed at final IMF crease location, start at medial nipple edge and extend lateral about 3-5 cm depending on implant type and size.
    - Allows excellent exposure and good control of implant position; places scar on breast surface.
    - Best for women with well-defined IMF, no hypertrophic scarring and mild ptosis.
    - Mark out limits of implant pocket
      - Second rib.
      - Laterally to mid-axillary line or anticipated lateral extent of breast.
      - Medially to most medial extent of pectoralis major but not to midline.
      - Center of implant should not be above the nipple level or it will be too high.
    - When dissecting laterally, dissect bluntly to avoid disrupting the lateral sensory intercostal nerve branches.
  - **Periareolar**
    - Incision placed along inferior half of areola from 3 o'clock to 9 o'clock position.
    - Dissection performed directly through gland, which may result in fat necrosis/ nodularity postop.
    - May get hypertrophic scar or hypopigmentation if within areola.

- ○ Transaxillary
  - ▪ Incision in uppermost axillary fold
  - ▪ Scar hidden within axilla; somewhat blind dissection unless endoscopy is used; less control of implant position, particularly with regard to IMF
  - ▪ Risk of injury to intercostobrachial nerve leading to axillary and posteromedial numbness of upper arm
- • Implant Type
  - ○ Saline
    - ▪ Advantages
      - □ Can use smaller incision since implant is inserted deflated.
      - □ May adjust fill volume to some degree.
      - □ Implant leakage easily detectable and safe since saline absorbed.
      - □ Lower rate of capsular contracture.
    - ▪ Disadvantages
      - □ Visible rippling of implant, especially in thin women
      - □ Less natural feel
    - ▪ **Air should be removed** prior to filling to prevent "sloshing." This is a time-limited effect, though, as the air will escape the implant over time.
    - ▪ **Overfilling** leads to less wrinkling but also makes implant more firm.
    - ▪ **Underfilling** leads to increased rupture rate.
  - ○ Silicone gel
    - ▪ Advantages
      - □ Look and feel more natural, similar to breast tissue
      - □ Less visible rippling
    - ▪ Disadvantages
      - □ Leaks can go undetected for long periods of time
      - □ Slightly higher risk of capsular contracture
    - ▪ *"Linguine sign" on MRI and "snowstorm" appearance of free silicone in the breast tissue on ultrasound are indicative of implant rupture.
    - ▪ *Food and Drug Administration (FDA) recommends MRI or ultrasound 5-6 years following implantation and then every 2-3 years to screen for silent rupture.
    - ▪ *Minimum age for silicone implants is 22.
- • Implant Shell Type
  - ○ Textured
    - ▪ Designed to reduce the incidence of capsular contraction, though only demonstrated with gel implants
    - ▪ Creates cohesion between the implant and the surrounding tissue, decreasing implant mobility
    - ▪ Associated with developing BIA-ALCL
      - □ Incidence: 33 per 1 million persons with textured breast implants
        - ▪ Overall risk is 1:30 000
        - ▪ Risk largely depends on textured implant type
          - • Allergan Biocell—1: 2 200 (implant was recalled in 2019)
          - • Mentor Siltex—1:53 000
      - □ Etiology
        - ▪ Distinct T-cell lymphoma that arises around textured breast implants
        - ▪ *Associated with biofilm from *Ralstonia* spp. bacteria
      - □ Presentation: patient with textured breast implant with late (>10 years) seroma, capsular contracture, or mass.
      - □ *Diagnosis: aspirate fluid and send for CD30 and cytology. BIA-ALCL is CD30+, whereas systemic ALCL is CD30−.
      - □ Treatment: explantation of implant, complete capsulectomy, medical oncology referral for staging, and assessment for radiation/chemotherapy.

- ○ **Smooth**
  - ▪ Higher rate of capsular contracture than textured gel implants but not textured saline
  - ▪ Moves freely within the breast pocket
  - ▪ No known association with BIA-ALCL at this time
- **Implant Shape**
  - ○ **Anatomic:** includes teardrop, contoured, or shaped implants. Intended to mimic the slope of a natural breast with decreased upper pole projection. Surface is textured to prevent the implant from moving.
  - ○ **Round:** assume a natural teardrop shape when the patient stands. Smooth or textured surface.
    - ▪ Low profile
    - ▪ Moderate profile
    - ▪ Moderate plus profile
    - ▪ High profile
      - □ Greater projection for a given base width
      - □ Greater projection with less volume
      - □ Advantageous if lower pole constriction or narrow breast base width
- **Pocket Position**
  - ○ **Subpectoral** (complete submuscular)
    - ▪ Superior implant under pectoralis major, inferolateral implant under serratus fascia.
    - ▪ Best for mammographic visualization of breast tissue
    - ▪ Lower risk of capsular contracture and visible rippling
    - ▪ Animation deformity: flexing of pectoralis can contract implant into unnatural position
    - ▪ Less risk of decreased nipple sensation
  - ○ **Dual plane** (partial submuscular)
    - ▪ Superior part of implant under pectoralis major, inferior part of implant under breast tissue only
    - ▪ Pectoralis major can be detached from inferior attachments, IMF and overlying gland (**Fig. 47-1**)
    - ▪ Risk of animation deformity if pectoralis released too much
    - ▪ Expands lower pole and decreases the risk of double-bubble appearance
    - ▪ Allows the implant to sit along IMF

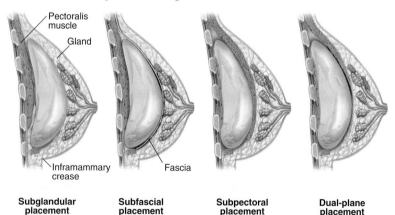

Figure 47-1 Options for planes of placement of the breast implant include subglandular, subfascial, subpectoral, and dual plane. (From Chung KC. *Grabb and Smith's Plastic Surgery*. 8th ed. Wolters Kluwer; 2020. Figure 55.3.)

- ○ **Subglandular**
  - Implant placed under breast tissue only, above pectoralis major
  - Less painful
  - Mammograms more difficult
  - Highest risk of visible or palpable wrinkling
  - Higher rate of capsular contracture

COMPLICATIONS

- **Early: hematoma, seroma, infection**—*Staphylococcus aureus* and *Staphylococcus epidermidis* most common, **loss of nipple sensation**
- **Late**
  - ○ **Capsular contracture:** firm fibrous scar forms periprosthetic shell around implant
    - *Baker classification describes the degree of capsular contracture
      - □ **I: Normal**—soft, no visible or palpable firmness
      - □ **II: Palpable**—minimal contracture with palpable but not visible firmness
      - □ **III: Visible**—moderate contracture with palpable and visible firmness
      - □ **IV: Painful**—severe contracture with palpable and visible firmness plus pain
    - Grade III and IV contractures can only be treated with open capsulotomy (release of scar tissue) or capsulectomy (removal of scar tissue)
      - □ Capsulectomy in subglandular plane—must be cautious anteriorly to avoid damage to overlying breast soft tissue and skin
      - □ Capsulectomy in submuscular plan—must be cautious posteriorly to avoid damage to pleura and pneumothorax
      - □ Capsulotomy done with radial scoring
    - Closed capsular release—not recommended due to high recurrence and complications
    - Rates close to 30% for subglandular and 10% for subpectoral
    - Higher rates in reconstruction (25%-30%) than in augmentation (10%)
  - ○ **Implant rippling:** more common with saline implants and in subglandular plane
  - ○ **Implant leak or rupture**
    - **Causes**
      - □ Underfilling
      - □ Fold flaw
      - □ Technical errors
    - **Diagnosis**
      - □ Physical examination
      - □ MRI or ultrasound for silicone implants (**see FDA recommendations in Silicone Implant section**)
  - ○ **Implant malposition or unsatisfactory shape**
    - **Double bubble:**
      - □ Type A: implant **above** the breast mound
        - Contour of implant visible above breast tissue secondary to excessively high implant placement and parenchyma descent inferior to implant
      - □ Type B: implant **below** the breast mound
        - With disruption of IMF, implant descends inferior to breast parenchyma and creates a second IMF inferior to the native IMF and breast mound
        - Native IMF is constriction band over the implant giving double buddle appearance
    - **Snoopy nose/waterfall deformity:** breast tissue hangs off inferior aspect of implant secondary to glandular ptosis
  - ○ **Upper arm numbness** secondary to injury to intercostobrachial nerve (transaxillary approach).
  - ○ **Nipple sensation is altered** in 15% of patients.

BREAST CANCER DETECTION IN AUGMENTED WOMEN

- Physical examination and mammography more difficult due to implants.
- American College of Radiology recommendations
  - Screening schedule should be same as for women without implants.
  - Imaging should be done at centers with experience reading augmented mammograms.
  - *Implant displacement views (*Eklund views*) should be performed to enable more breast tissue to be visualized.

SILICONE IMPLANT CONTROVERSY

- FDA mandated a moratorium on silicone implants in 1992 to investigate association between silicone implants and connective tissue diseases.
- Multiple large, population-based retrospective studies show no association.
- Silicone implants reapproved for cosmetic and reconstructive use in 2006.

MASTOPEXY AND AUGMENTATION MASTOPEXY

PATHOPHYSIOLOGY OF PTOSIS

- **Normal Breast Anatomy**
  - Gland spans from second to sixth rib.
  - NAC sits superior to IMF and centrally over breast mound.
  - Average sternal notch to nipple distance is 21-24 cm.
  - Average nipple to IMF distance is 6-7 cm.
  - Parenchymal blood supply
    - Perforators from internal mammary artery (main source)
    - Lateral thoracic artery
    - Thoracodorsal artery
    - Intercostal artery perforators
    - Thoracoacromial artery
  - Innervation
    - Branches of intercostal nerves T3-T5
    - NAC receives sensation from T4
  - Cooper ligaments connect parenchymal to dermis and are responsible for the degree of ptosis.
- **Anatomic Changes in Ptotic Breasts**
  - Nipple moves inferiorly, increasing sternal notch to nipple distance.
  - Parenchyma of breast gland hangs below IMF.
  - Connective tissue (Cooper ligaments) stretches due to loss of elasticity.
  - Etiologies include breast parenchyma involution after pregnancy, excess residual skin after weight loss, loss of skin elasticity secondary to aging, and gravitational forces.
- **Surgical Options for Breast Ptosis**
  - Breast augmentation only
  - Mastopexy only
  - Mastopexy with staged augmentation
  - Augmentation with staged mastopexy
  - Simultaneous augmentation mastopexy

PREOPERATIVE CONSULTATION

- **History** (Also, See Above "Breast Augmentation, Preoperative Consultation, History")
  - Complete medical history.
  - Mammographic studies.
  - History of previous/active weight loss. Confirm weight stable for 6 months.

- **Physical Exam** (Also, See "Breast Augmentation, Preoperative Consultation, Physical")
  - Degree of ptosis
  - Evaluate the amount and quality of excess skin
  - Note the patient's weight and body habitus
  - Volume of parenchyma
  - Breast and NAC asymmetry
  - Breast and axillary masses
- **Indications**
  - Ptosis of breast parenchyma
  - Ptosis of NAC
  - Patient willingness to accept potential scars
- **Patient Education**
  - Ptosis can recur with aging, weight gain or loss, pregnancy.
  - Scarring may be significant, depending on planned procedure.
  - Preoperative asymmetries may be more apparent postoperatively.

SURGICAL APPROACHES

- **The degree of ptosis** is the most important factor in determining which procedure to perform (**Table 47-1**).
- **Augmentation Only.** Patients with grade I ptosis may only require augmentation for correction of ptosis.
- **Mastopexy Only**
  - Key components
    - Correct NAC malposition
    - Improve glandular descent
    - Tailor skin excess
    - Modifying the skin envelope alone will not be a long-lasting correction
  - Periareolar mastopexy
    - Best for patients with grade I ptosis and good to fair skin quality
    - Periareolar incision with purse-string suture around NAC.
    - Minimal scarring
    - Limited NAC elevation (2-3 cm maximum)
    - NAC often widens over time and excessive skin resection deforms the areola
    - Does not correct parenchymal ptosis
    - "Donut" mastopexy flattens the breast and decreases projection
  - Liposuction-only mastopexy
    - Very limited role in correcting breast ptosis
    - Only fat removed, not gland
    - Nipple not repositioned
    - Least amount of scarring
    - Final result dependent on skin quality and extent of retraction
  - Vertical mastopexy
    - Best for patients with grade II ptosis
    - Final scar is periareolar plus vertical component from NAC to IMF
    - Corrects parenchymal malposition
    - Narrows the breast footprint and adds breast projection
    - Can add short horizontal component ("inverted-T") to increase skin resection
    - May takes several months for breasts to obtain final shape
    - Technique
      - Markings
        - Chest midline, breast meridian.
        - Mark 3 cm above IMF and transpose on breast meridian as new NAC.
        - Mark upper breast border and mark NAC position 8-10 cm down.
        - Compare two NAC markings as "check and balance."
        - Draw areola, ideal circumference of marking is 14-16 cm to leave 4-5 cm diameter areola.

TABLE 47-1 Augmentation Mastopexy Options

Degree of ptosis	Skin quality	Nipple elevation	Breast resection	Intervention	Notes
Minor glandular ptosis	Fair to good	0-1 cm	None	Augmentation only	
Glandular ptosis	Elastic	0-1 cm	None	Periareolar mastopexy with augmentation	Large areola
Minor ptosis	Fair	2-4 cm	None	Circumareolar mastopexy with periareolar purse-string closure	With augmentation of inadequate upper quadrant volume
Moderate ptosis	Fair	3-5 cm	0-100 g	Vertical scar mastopexy with augmentation	
Moderately severe ptosis	Fair to poor	5-7 cm	0-200 g	Vertical scar mastopexy with short horizontal incision and augmentation	
Severe ptosis	Poor	>7 cm	0-300 g	Wise pattern mastopexy	

- Displace breast medially and laterally to draw vertical lines and always stop 2-4 cm above IMF (ensure incision does not extend below new IMF).
- Limbs longer than with Wise pattern markings given increased projection. Vertical limbs may be 10-12 cm.
  □ Operation
    - Skin of pedicle is de-epithelialized, and areola is left *in situ*.
    - Excision of lower breast tissue or auto-augmentation (see Ribeiro flap below).
    - Closure of medial and lateral parenchyma pillars.
    - NAC transposition with inset into new position.
    - Placement of subcuticular stitch to close vertical and periareolar scar.
  □ Ribeiro inferior flap
    - "Autoaugmentation" during vertical mastopexy.
    - Repositioning of the lower parenchyma behind the NAC and suturing to chest wall behind a superior or superomedial flap
    - Medial and lateral pillars closed together, inferiorly caudal to the flap
  ○ **Inverted T or wise pattern mastopexy**
    - Best for patients with grade III ptosis.
    - Significant scarring including periareolar, vertical, and IMF scars.
    - Long horizontal component allows large skin resection in significantly ptotic breasts.
    - Predictable and straightforward, as the final shape of the breast is achieved in the operating room.
    - Does not modify the horizontal base diameter. Can look "boxy."

- Technique
  - Markings are similar to wise pattern breast reduction (see **Chapter 48 Section "Breast Reduction"**).
  - A superior, superomedial, medial, or inferior pedicle technique may be used.
  - The top of the new NAC is 1-2 cm above the IMF.
  - Limbs of the equilateral triangle are 7-8 cm.
- **Augmentation Mastopexy**
  - Patients with deficient breast tissue, lack of superior pole fullness, and ptosis may benefit from a combination of augmentation and mastopexy.
  - May be performed as a one-stage or two-stage procedure.
    - One-stage procedure is challenging and has high risk of wound healing complications and high reoperation rate (8%-23%) but may be performed successfully and with high satisfaction rate in the correct patient.
    - Two-stage procedure separates mastopexy and augmentation by 3-6 months to allow delay of skin flaps and preserve blood supply.
  - Any mastopexy that involves wide undermining of skin flaps should NOT be combined with augmentation due to the risk of flap necrosis.

COMPLICATIONS

- Overall complication rate is low: 2.4%-10.4%
  - Hematoma
  - Seroma
  - Unacceptable scarring—most common complaint
  - Nipple complications—distortion, asymmetry, reduction in sensation
  - Nipple loss and flap necrosis
  - Recurrent ptosis or pseudoptosis

PEARLS

1. Always point out asymmetries to patients prior to surgery.
2. Breast implants are not "permanent." Most women will need one or both replaced in their lifetime.
3. For patients receiving silicone implants, the Food and Drug Administration (FDA) recommends MRI or ultrasound 5-6 years following implantation and then every 2-3 years to screen for silent rupture.

QUESTIONS YOU WILL BE ASKED

1. How is breast ptosis categorized?
   Based on the nipple position relative to the IMF.
2. What classification scheme is used to describe the degrees of capsular contracture?
   Baker classification.
3. What are the advantages and disadvantages of saline and silicone gel implants?
   See "Breast Augmentation."

Recommended Readings
1. Nava MB, Adams WP, Botti G, Campanale A, et al. MBN 2016 aesthetic breast meeting BIA-ALCL consensus conference report. *Plast Reconstr Surg.* 2018;141(1):40-48.
2. Pferdehirt R, Nahabedian M. Finesse in mastopexy and augmentation mastopexy. *Plast Reconstr Surg.* 2021;148(3):451e-461e.
3. Tebbetts JB, Adams WP. Five critical decisions in breast augmentation using five measurements in 5 minutes: the high five decision support process. *Plast Reconstr Surg.* 2006;118(7S):35S-45S.

Section IV: Breast and Body Reconstruction

48

Reduction Mammoplasty, Top Surgery, and Gynecomastia

Sherry Tang

BREAST REDUCTION (REDUCTION MAMMOPLASTY)

PREOPERATIVE CONSULTATION

- **History** (see **Chapter 47: Breast Augmentation, Mastopexy, and Augmentation Mastopexy,** section "Preoperative Workup for Any Breast Surgery")
  - Patient's current and "desired" cup size—the patient should be counseled regarding relative anticipated cup size based on surgeon's estimate with regard to preop nipple to IMF length (longer = larger the smallest they can be reduced to) and width. Smaller outcomes are not often realistic, in terms of blood supply nor shape.
  - Previous/active weight gain/loss; ideally patient should have stable weight for 6 months.
- **Physical Exam** (See **Chapter 47: Breast Augmentation, Mastopexy, and Augmentation Mastopexy,** section "Preoperative Workup for Any Breast Surgery")
  - Degree of ptosis
  - Weight and BMI
  - Volume of parenchyma (cup size to surgeon, not just bra size)
  - Shape, size and NAC asymmetries
  - Breast masses
  - Measurements (Sternal notch to nipple, nipple to IMF and nipple to nipple)
  - Schnur sliding scale
    - Body surface area (BSA) is used to calculate the grams of tissue per breast needed to be removed to qualify the procedure to coverage by many insurance policies.
  - Schnur is not a valid clinical determinant "medical necessity" and should not be used for clinical targets. Studies have validated that many patients receive significant improvements in symptoms with less tissue removal.
- **Indications for Surgery**
  - Physical
    - Upper back, neck, and shoulder pain
    - Shoulder grooving
    - Recurrent intertrigo and maceration of inframammary skin
    - Exercise restriction
    - Inability to find clothes that fit
  - Psychological
    - Embarrassment
    - Feelings of physical unattractiveness
    - Uncomfortable in clothes, difficulty with clothing/bra fit
- **Patient Education:** important discussion points preop
  - **Breast reduction involves significant scarring.** Patient is trading larger breasts for smaller breasts with permanent scars.
  - **Everybody is asymmetric:** point out specific asymmetries in nipple position, size, and shape preop. Some asymmetries will persist postop.

---

*Denotes common in-service examination topics

○ **Approximately 30% of patients cannot breast-feed postoperatively** (the same percentage of patients with macromastia who cannot successfully breast-feed).
○ **Nipple sensation:** 5% of patients will have permanent nipple numbness.
○ **Partial or complete nipple loss:** approximately 2% risk.
○ **Smoking increases the risk of nipple or flap loss** and delayed healing. For most surgeons, this is an absolute contraindication.
○ **Weight gain or future pregnancies** can cause recurrent enlargement.
○ **All symptoms may not improve postoperatively.**
○ **New baseline mammogram** needed ∼6 months following surgery.
○ **Breast reduction patients** are generally one of the most satisfied groups of patients.

SURGICAL APPROACHES

• **Goals**
  ○ Reduction and reshaping of the gland
  ○ Creation of an NAC pedicle to preserve vascularity and sensibility while allowing for superior repositioning
  ○ Skin reduction and redraping
  ○ Remember, it is not what is removed but rather what is left behind that matters
• **Selecting the Appropriate Surgical Approach**
  ○ Skin removal: necessary to primarily adjust the skin envelope to the reduced breast volume and to reposition the nipple
  ○ Areas of breast resection
  ○ Amount of breast reduction
  ○ Incision length and placement
  ○ Lateral and abdominal fullness
  ○ Preservation of breast and nipple sensation
  ○ Size and position of the NAC
• **Wise Pattern Reduction**
  ○ **"Wise pattern" describes skin incisions (Fig. 48-1)**
    ▪ "W"-shaped incision allows significant skin resection, good for large volume or very ptotic breasts. Allows large movement of NAC.
    ▪ "Pedicle" describes the tissue bridge that keeps the NAC attached for blood/nerve supply. Wise pattern reduction can be used with any pedicle.
    ▪ **Choice of pedicle: there is no "best"; the choice is often dependent on surgeon preference and patient size and ptosis**
      ▫ Superior pedicle
        ▪ Blood supply: descending branch of the internal mammary artery (IMA) from the second intercostal space
        ▪ Indications: smaller reductions of <1000 g per breast
        ▪ Increased risk of pedicle folding and exaggerated projection in the immediate postoperative period but will eventually settle out with excellent final shape in the long term
      ▫ Medial pedicle
        ▪ Blood supply: branch of IMA from the third intercostal space
        ▪ Indications: small to moderate reductions
        ▪ Reduced risk of pedicle folding, allows for significant glandular resection laterally
      ▫ Superomedial pedicle
        ▪ Blood supply: branches of IMA from the second and third intercostal spaces
        ▪ Indications: small to moderate reductions
      ▫ Lateral pedicle
        ▪ Blood supply: superficial branch of the lateral thoracic artery
        ▪ Indications: can be use in larger reductions compared to superior pedicle
        ▪ Risk of persistent lateral fullness due to insufficient resection of the pedicle

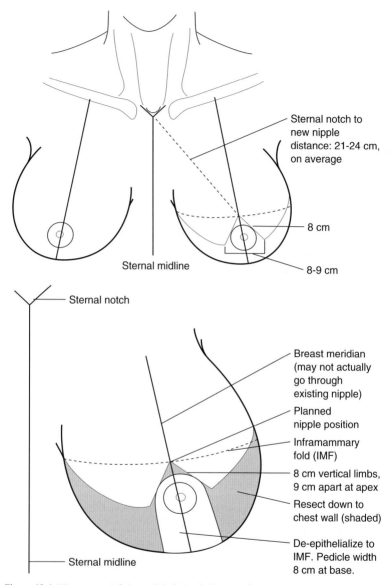

Figure 48-1 Wise pattern, inferior pedicle design for breast reduction.

□ Inferior pedicle
  ▪ Blood supply: branches of IMA from the fifth and sixth intercostal spaces
  ▪ Indications: larger reductions with high degree of ptosis
  ▪ Higher risk of bottoming out (sagging along the inferior pole of the breast)

- ○ **Advantages**
  - ▪ Reproducible, straightforward, and easily taught. To a large extent, skin incisions correspond to glandular incisions of breast parenchyma.
  - ▪ Applicable to large variety of breast shapes and sizes, especially when using inferior pedicle technique.
  - ▪ Breast-feeding is potentially more likely since a large amount of breast tissue is left beneath the nipple.
  - ▪ Higher rate of nipple sensory preservation.
- ○ **Disadvantages**
  - ▪ Produces more extensive scars than other techniques: "Anchor"-shaped scar starts around NAC, vertically down to IMF, and along entire IMF.
  - ▪ Breasts may "bottom out" over time.
- ○ **Markings (Fig. 48-1)**
  - ▪ Registration marks: sternal notch, midline, IMFs.
  - ▪ Breast meridian: from midpoint of clavicle to midpoint of the breast; this will not always transect the NAC.
    - □ Can drape a tape measure around patient's neck down to the nipple and trace a line along it to find breast meridian.
    - □ Line should be relocated medially if it is more than 10-12 cm from the midline.
  - ▪ New nipple position can be determined by several methods
    - □ Place hand under breast at level of IMF, transpose that point onto front of the breast along meridian.
    - □ Find Pitanguy point: 1-2 cm below mid-humeral point on breast meridian.
    - □ 21-24 cm from the sternal notch along breast meridian.
  - ▪ Vertical limbs are drawn obliquely from the intended nipple position. These will create an isosceles triangle—8 cm on each side and approximately 9 cm across the base (these numbers are variable based on patients' habitus and breast size).
  - ▪ Draw curvilinear lines from the base of triangle to medial and lateral endpoint of breast, connecting to IMF line.
  - ▪ If doing inferior pedicle, mark out the base of pedicle when the patient is supine on operating room table with a base width of 8-10 cm.
  - ▪ Mark out 42-mm areola when patient on table.
  - ▪ Can either dissect out pedicle first and then breast flaps or breast flaps first.
  - ▪ Important not to undermine pedicle.
  - ▪ Can be helpful to place medial tacking suture on pedicle to prevent it from migrating laterally.
  - ▪ Tailor tack after resection is done, sit the patient up, and place 38 nipple sizer.
- • **LeJour Vertical Reduction (Fig. 48-2)**
  - ○ **Markings**
    - ▪ IMF and chest midline and vertical axis of the breast are marked.
    - ▪ Future nipple position placed at the forward projection of the center point of the IMF:
      - □ 18-22 cm to sternal notch
      - □ 10-14 cm from midline
    - ▪ Lateral markings are determined by pushing the breast medially and laterally.
    - ▪ The lower margin is drawn 2-4 cm above the IMF connecting the medial to the lateral lines.
    - ▪ The periareolar markings are drawn in "mosque shape" and are typically 14-16 cm in length.
  - ○ **Gland reduction:** inferior central pole of breast, remaining medial and lateral pillars reapproximated to reshape the gland
  - ○ **Nipple pedicle:** superior
  - ○ **Redraping:** skin adapts to the breast shape

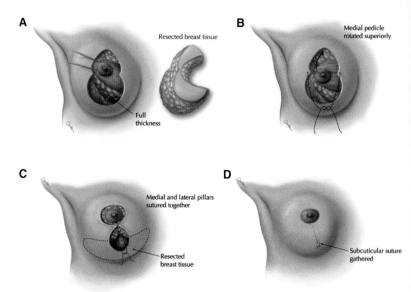

Figure 48-2 Vertical reduction technique (LeJour). A. Full-thickness breast tissue with overlying skin is resected following the markings. Most of the resection comes from the inferior pole of the breast. The skin resection leaves the nipple attached to the underlying dermis. The blood supply comes from the superomedial dermal pedicle. The gland is sutured to the superior pectoralis fascia to position it more superiorly. **B.** After securing the gland to the pectoralis fascia, the skin is sutured to form the lower closure of the areola. **C.** The medial and lateral pillars are sutured together. **D:** The skin is closed, leaving "gathers" that will smooth with time. The patient must be informed that the shape of the breast will improve over time. (From Thorne CH, ed. *Grabb and Smith's Plastic Surgery.* 7th ed. Lippincott Williams & Wilkins; 2014.)

- ○ Technique
  - ▪ Periareolar area is de-epithelialized to 3-4 cm inferior to the areola.
  - ▪ Liposuction is performed if desired.
  - ▪ Lateral vertical markings are incised, creating 1-cm-thick flaps going obliquely downward and terminating at the IMF.
  - ▪ From the IMF, the gland is undermined superiorly and a 6- to 8-cm-wide tunnel is created up to the third rib.
  - ▪ The lateral pillars and the superior gland are left intact.
  - ▪ The gland is sutured superiorly to the pectoralis fascia to elevate the areola, which is sutured to its new site.
  - ▪ The lateral pillars are brought together and sutured to shape the glandular cone.
  - ▪ Skin is closed with deep 3-0 and running subcuticular sutures around the areola and the vertical scar gathering the vertical component.
- ○ Advantages
  - ▪ Eliminates incision in IMF
  - ▪ Less "bottoming out" than with inferior pedicle technique
- ○ Disadvantages
  - ▪ Steep learning curve
  - ▪ On-table result not consistent with the final result. Will be significant puckering of the skin around nipple/vertical scar and flattening of lower pole which resolve within 4-6 weeks

- **Periareolar Reduction**
  - **Gland reduction:** central wedge
  - **Nipple pedicle:** superior
  - **Redraping:** skin redraped in purse-string manner around areola
  - **Advantages:** minimal scarring
  - **Disadvantages**
    - Tends to flatten breast in anteroposterior dimension
    - Areola may widen with time
    - Limited to small reductions
- **SPAIR Technique** (Short scar, PeriAreolar, Inferior pedicle Reduction)
  - **Gland reduction:** mostly periareolar
  - **Nipple pedicle:** inferior
  - **Redraping:** skin redraped around areola
  - **Advantages**
    - Maintains shape over time with less "bottoming out"
    - Minimizes scarring by eliminating IMF incision
    - Achieves attractive breast shape
  - **Disadvantages**
    - Steep learning curve and significant intraoperative decision making
    - Extensive glandular suturing required to obtain desired shape
- **Free Nipple Graft Technique**
  - **Indications**
    - Gigantomastia (>2500 g breast tissue)
    - Thresholds vary but strongly considered by some surgeons when nipple to IMF distance is >20-25 cm.
    - Comorbidities necessitating decreased operative time and blood loss.
  - **Technique**
    - Breast amputation combined with the removal of NAC with replacement as a full-thickness skin graft
    - Helps to keep an inferior mound that is de-epithelialized to maintain projection
  - **Advantages**
    - Decreased operative time
    - Straightforward, easy to perform
  - **Disadvantages**
    - Permanent nipple numbness
    - Eliminates the ability to lactate and nurse, so not ideal in younger patients
    - Risk of nipple graft loss
    - Risk of depigmentation of areola
- **Liposuction**
  - **May be performed alone or as an adjunct** to excisional reduction
  - **Indication:** useful in women with elastic skin, predominantly fatty breasts, and nipples in a nonptotic position
  - **Advantages**
    - Minimal external scarring
    - Symmetry easily achieved
  - **Disadvantages**
    - Specimen cannot be sent for pathologic evaluation
    - Does not address nipple ptosis or skin laxity
    - May be difficult in patients with dense breast tissue
    - Few patients are candidates: limited to small reductions in nonptotic breasts

COMPLICATIONS

- Wound healing delays, especially at T-junction in wise pattern reduction: 10%-15%
- Asymmetry: 8%-18%
- Changes in nipple sensitivity: 25%-60%

- Unacceptable scar: 18%
- Hematoma: 1%-2%
- Seroma: 2%
- Infection: 7%
- Fat necrosis: 8%
- Nipple loss: 1%
- Hypertrophic scarring
- Inability to breast-feed

GENDER-AFFIRMING CHEST RECONSTRUCTION

CRITERIA FOR SURGERY

- Patient must have formal diagnosis of Gender Identity Disorder (DSM-5 criteria) by a mental health professional.
- Operative plastic surgeon is not competent to decide who is ready for surgery.
- **Patient must meet WPATH (World Professional Association of Transgender Health) criteria prior to surgery.** The criteria for top surgery and bottom surgery are different.
- *WPATH criteria for top surgery. (See Chapter 54: Gender Affirming Pelvic Surgery for criteria for bottom surgery.)
  - Persistent, well-documented gender dysphoria.
  - Hormone therapy
    - Female to male patients: not a prerequisite unless patient is younger than 18
    - Male to female patients: not a prerequisite but recommended for minimum of 12 months to maximize breast growth to obtain better surgical results
  - One referral from qualified mental health professionals.
  - Capacity to make fully informed decision and able to give consent.
  - Stable medical and mental disease.
  - Patients younger than 18 may be candidates if the patient, their legal guardians and/or patients, their therapist, and their car team believe that delaying surgery would result in patient harm.

PREOPERATIVE CONSULTATION

- **History**
  - Patient's desired aesthetic outcome, including desired shape and size of chest/breast, nipple size and position, type of scars.
    - Most transmale patients desire to be flat.
    - Some patients may not want to keep their nipples.
  - Complete breast and medical history.
  - Use of hormonal therapy. Depending on surgeon preference, patient may be asked to stop hormones for several weeks prior to surgery.
  - Use of breast binding (decreases elasticity of the skin and results in higher degree of ptosis).
- **Physical Exam**
  - Complete breast examination.
  - Degree of ptosis.
  - Note nipple position.
  - Bring asymmetries to patient's attention prior to surgery.

FEMALE TO MALE CHEST RECONSTRUCTION

- **Goals**
  - Remove breast tissue and skin excess. This is not a cancer operation and thus excision of all breast tissue is not required, rather the breast tissue should be contoured to give a more masculine appearance.
  - Reduce and properly position of the NAC.
  - Eliminate the inframammary fold.
  - Minimize chest wall scars.

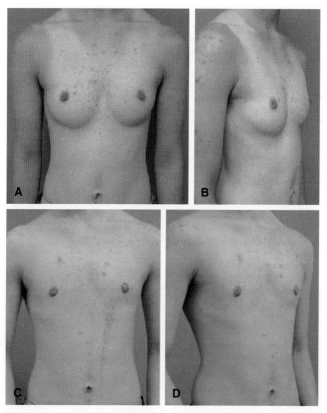

Figure 48-3 Female to male chest reconstruction using periareolar incision technique. A, B. Preoperative. **C, D.** Postoperative. (From Chung KC. *Grabb and Smith's Plastic Surgery*. 8th ed. Wolters Kluwer; 2020. Figure 100-5.)

- **Semicircular Circumareolar Approach or "Keyhole Mastectomy" (Fig. 48-3)**
  - Indications
    - Minimal excess breast tissue and skin
    - Good tissue elasticity
  - Technique
    - Make a semicircular incision along the inferior aspect of the NAC.
    - Resect excess breast tissue.
    - Can be combined with liposuction to eliminate the IMF and achieve the desired contour.
  - Advantages
    - Small and well-hidden scar
  - Disadvantages
    - Inability to reposition the NAC
    - Highest risk of surgical site complications requiring reoperation, including hematoma, seroma, infection, and nipple necrosis
- **Mastectomy With Periareolar Skin Excision**
  - Indications
    - Moderate excess breast tissue and skin

- Good tissue elasticity
  - ○ Technique
    - First mark out the size of the new NAC using a nipple sizer because the male nipple is usually smaller than the female nipple.
    - Then mark out the periareolar skin that needs to be excised. This should at least include the remaining areola.
    - Incise the areola circumferentially. Resect excess breast tissue and periareolar skin.
    - Close the incision in layers. Purse-string sutures around the NAC needed to prevent scar widening.
    - Can be combined with liposuction to eliminate the IMF and achieve the desired contour.
  - ○ Advantages
    - Able to remove excess skin and reposition the NAC
  - ○ Disadvantages
    - Circumareolar scar is unfavorable due to high risk of hypertrophy and widening.
    - High rate of revisions including scar revisions, correction of chest contour, and nipple-areolar correction.
    - Unable to reposition the NAC.
- **Double Incision Mastectomy With Free Nipple Grafting (Fig. 48-4)**
  - ○ Indications
    - Most commonly used technique

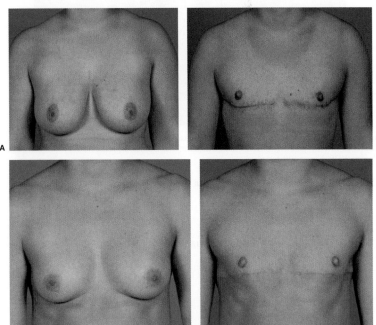

Figure 48-4 Female to male chest reconstruction using double incision mastectomy with free nipple grafts. A, C. Preoperative. **B, D.** Postoperative. In (B), the incisions are carried up laterally along the border of the pectoralis muscle to emphasize its shape. (From Gabriel A, Nahabedian MY, Maxwell GP, Storm T. *Spear's Surgery of the Breast.* 4th ed. Wolters Kluwer; 2021. Figure 117-6.)

- Large amounts of excess breast tissue and skin with high degree of ptosis
  ○ **Markings**
    - Mark sternal notch and midline.
    - Mark the superior incision: place hand under breast at level of IMF, transpose that line onto front of the breast.
    - Mark the inferior incision along the IMF.
  ○ **Technique**
    - **Preparation of the NAC**
      □ Mark the NAC using a 25-mm sizer and remove as a full-thickness graft.
      □ Defat the nipple graft.
    - **Mastectomy**
      □ Make the superior incision and elevate flaps.
      □ Then make the inferior incision and remove the excess breast tissue and skin superficial to the pectoralis fascia.
      □ Undermine inferiorly to eliminate the IMF.
      □ The skin is then closed in layers and drains are placed.
      □ If there is excess amount of tissue and skin along the midline causing contour irregularities or standing cutaneous deformities, it may be necessary to connect the two incisions at the midline.
    - **Placement of the free nipple graft**
      □ The female NAC is usually larger, lower, and more medial than the male NAC.
      □ Average male nipple is between 2 and 3 cm with a nipple height of 2.6 mm.
      □ The male nipple is usually located over the fifth intercostal space at the inferolateral borer of the pectoralis major muscle.
      □ Useful to sit the patient up and place paper templates onto the chest to judge the final size and position of the new NAC.
      □ Once the optimal location is determined, the area is de-epithelialized and the nipple graft is secured using sutures and a tie-on bolster.
  ○ **Advantages**
    - Provides excellent exposure during the operation
    - Able to resize and change the position of the NAC
    - Low revision rate
  ○ **Disadvantages**
    - Longer and more obvious scar
- **Postoperative care**
  ○ Important to wear circumferential compression garment for 6 weeks to maintain contour of chest and reduce risk of hematoma and seroma.
  ○ If free nipple grafting is performed, the bolster is removed after 5-7 days.
  ○ Avoid strenuous physical activity for 4-6 weeks.
  ○ Silicone sheeting, scar cream, and scar massage can be benefiting in preventing and treating hypertrophic scarring.
  ○ Patients need to continue routine breast cancer screening with primary care provider due to remnant breast tissue mostly along the upper pole.
- **Complications**
  ○ Hematoma: 6%-8%
  ○ Infection: 2%-3%
  ○ Delayed wound healing: 2%-3%
  ○ Hypertrophic scarring
  ○ Partial or total nipple necrosis: 4%-5%
  ○ Changes in nipple sensation: 45%-50%
  ○ Seroma
  ○ Inadequate amount of resection

MALE TO FEMALE CHEST RECONSTRUCTION

- Goals
  - Must understand patient's goals and preferences because aesthetic preferences in female breast size and shape vary widely.
- Hormonal therapy
  - Recommended as estrogen and antiandrogen therapies will produce modest breast development.
  - For some patients, hormonal therapy alone may be sufficient.
- Augmentation mammoplasty
  - The principles of breast augmentation in transfemales are adopted from those of aesthetic breast augmentation (see **Chapter 47: Breast Augmentation, Mastopexy, and Augmentation Mastopexy**, section "Breast Augmentation").
  - Can be submuscular or subglandular depending on the amount of overlying breast tissue.
- Challenges
  - **Insufficient skin envelope** may limit implant size
    - Can place tissue expanders first.
    - Can increase pocket size by releasing more pectoralis major muscle medially and undermine laterally. However, these may lead to suboptimal position of the implants, lateral migration, and symmastia.
  - NAC size and position
    - Male NAC are usually smaller, more oval in shape, and positioned more laterally.
    - Need to balance between centering the NAC on the breast mount and maximizing cleavage.
  - **Vertical constriction** caused by short nipple to IMF distance
    - Can perform radial scoring of the pectoralis major and overlying breast tissue.
    - Can lower the IMF, but this leads to an unpredictable result.
  - Shape of chest and shoulders
    - Wide sternum may lead to implants that are more lateral on the chest and lack of cleavage.
    - Tall stature and broad shoulder may need larger implants to achieve the best results, but this is limited by the size of the skin envelope.

GYNECOMASTIA

EPIDEMIOLOGY AND ETIOLOGY

- **Epidemiology:** peaks in incidence in infancy, puberty, and men ages 50-80
  - Overall incidence over 30%
  - Up to 65% of adolescent boys
- Etiology
  - Benign proliferation of glandular tissue of male breast
  - Infancy: transient gynecomastia secondary to high levels of maternal estrogen
    - Resolves 2-3 weeks after delivery
    - Most common hyperplastic childhood breast anomaly
  - Puberty: onset between 10 and 12 years, spontaneously resolves within 6 months to 2 years of onset in most cases.
  - **Medications and drugs**
    - Spironolactone, digoxin, cimetidine, alcohol, ketoconazole, finasteride, and tricyclic antidepressants
    - HAART (highly active antiretroviral therapy) for human immunodeficiency virus/AIDS (acquired immunodeficiency syndrome) treatment
    - Anabolic steroids
    - Alcohol, marijuana, heroin

- ○ Cirrhosis
- ○ Male hypogonadism: results in estrogen/androgen imbalance
  - ▪ Primary hypogonadism due to congenital abnormality such as Klinefelter syndrome.
  - ▪ Secondary hypogonadism due to a hypothalamic or pituitary abnormality.
  - ▪ Hyperprolactinemia: prolactin reduces the secretion of gonadotropins.
- ○ *Testicular neoplasm: germ cell, Leydig cell, or Sertoli cell tumors. All males presenting for the evaluation of gynecomastia must have a testicular examination.
- ○ Hyperthyroidism: due to Graves disease
- ○ Pseudogynecomastia: often seen in obese males, refers to fat deposition without glandular proliferation.
- ○ **Pneumonic: SACKED**
  - ▪ S = spironolactone
  - ▪ A = alcohol, age, alopecia medications, antidepressants
  - ▪ C = cimetidine, cirrhosis
  - ▪ K = ketoconazole, Klinefelter syndrome
  - ▪ E = excessive estrogen
  - ▪ D = digoxin, drugs

PREOPERATIVE CONSULTATION

- • **Presentation**
  - ○ Unilateral or bilateral
  - ○ Begins with subareolar enlargement
- • **Physical examination**
  - ○ **Breast**
    - ▪ Assess the amount and distribution of adipose tissue vs glandular tissue
      - □ Minimal adiposity gynecomastia: common in patients with low BMI and body builders. Glandular tissue is obliquely oriented, easily isolated, firm, and located more lateral than medial.
      - □ Adipose-laden gynecomastia: glandular tissue more spherical and has ill-defined borders.
      - □ Pseudogynecomastia: common in patient who are obese, older, or with prior massive weight loss. Glandular tissue sparsely interspersed in adipose tissue.
    - ▪ Ptosis
    - ▪ Skin excess
    - ▪ Masses
  - ○ **Testicular examination**
  - ○ **Feminizing characteristics**
  - ○ **Mass of thyroid, liver, or abdomen**
- • **Staging**
  - ○ **Grade I:** minimal hypertrophy (<250 g) and no ptosis
  - ○ **Grade II:** moderate hypertrophy (250-500 g) and no ptosis
  - ○ **Grade III:** severe hypertrophy (>500 g) with grade I ptosis
  - ○ **Grade IV:** severe hypertrophy with grade II or III ptosis
- • **Diagnosis (Fig. 48-5)**
  - ○ **Must rule out male breast cancer** if asymmetric. If concerning, order a mammogram.
  - ○ **If persistent, painful,** and/or no clear physiologic etiology, check labs: liver function tests, TSH, luteinizing hormone, follicle stimulating hormone, human chorionic gonadotrophin, prolactin, estradiol, testosterone, and androstenedione

SURGICAL APPROACHES

- • **Goals**
  - ○ Remove excess glandular tissue and skin.

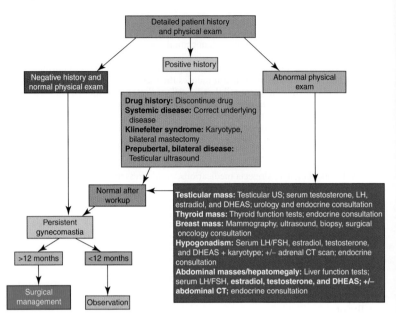

Figure 48-5 Gynecomastia workup algorithm. DHEAS, dehydroepiandrosterone-sulfate; LH/FSH, luteinizing hormone/follicle-stimulating hormone; US, ultrasound; CT, computed tomography. (From Thorne CH, ed. *Grabb and Smith's Plastic Surgery*. 7th ed. Lippincott Williams & Wilkins; 2014. Figure 57-1 and Rohrich RJ, Ha RY, Kenkel JM, Adams WP. Classification and management of gynecomastia: defining the role of ultrasound-assisted liposuction. *Plast Reconstr Surg*. 2003;111:909.)

- ○ Achieve smooth contour with surrounding tissue.
- ○ Maintain appropriate NAC position. Reduce NAC size if enlarged.
- **Surgical treatment** depends on the severity of disease
  - ○ Excess fat with minimal excess skin/gland: liposuction only
  - ○ Subareolar glandular tissue with minimal excess skin: liposuction + periareolar gland excision
  - ○ Excess skin, fat, and gland: inframammary incision with free nipple graft

PEARLS

1. Check a urinary cotinine test preoperatively in "former" smokers before performing a breast reduction. Exposure to secondhand smoke can also make this test positive.
2. Important to discuss with patients undergoing female to male top surgery that they still need routine breast cancer screening after surgery as some breast tissue remains.
3. A complete workup for gynecomastia always includes a testicular examination and review of medications.

QUESTIONS YOU WILL BE ASKED

1. How do the size and position of the female NAC differ from the male NAC? The female NAC is typically larger, lower, and more medial than the male NAC.
2. What is the most common complication after breast reduction?

Delayed wound healing. This is most often located at the T junction of wise-pattern breast reduction.
3. Describe the WPATH criteria for gender-affirming top surgery.
   Persistent and well-documented gender dysphoria, one referral from a mental health provider, ability to make informed decisions and consent, well-controlled medical and mental disease. Being on hormone therapy is not a prerequisite.

Recommended Readings

1. Hall-Findlay EJ, Shestak KC. Breast reduction. *Plast Reconstr Surg*. 2015;136:531e-5443e.
2. Hurwitz DJ, Davila AA. Contemporary management of gynecomastia. *Clin Plast Surg*. 2022;49(2):193-305.
3. Morrison SD, Wilson SC, Mosser SW. Breast and body contouring for transgender and gender nonconforming individuals. *Clin Plast Surg*. 2018;45(3):333-342.

49

Breast Disease

Emily Barrett

ANATOMY AND DEVELOPMENT OF THE BREAST

GLAND

- **Boundaries**
  - Superior: second rib or clavicle
  - Inferior: sixth rib
  - Medial: sternal edge
  - Lateral: midaxillary line—beware of lateral sensory intercostal nerves if dissecting this far, which can cause chronic neuropathic pain—often unnecessary to go this far posteriorly
  - Superolaterally: extends into axilla as the tail of Spence
  - Posterior: fascia of pectoralis major superomedially, fascia of serratus anterior inferolaterally
- **Composition:** skin, fat, and glandular tissue
  - 10%-15% epithelial; remainder is stromal
    - Large proportion of epithelial tissue found in upper outer quadrant, the most common site for both benign and malignant disease.
    - 15-20 radially arranged glandular lobes, supported by fibrous connective tissue with varying amounts of adipose tissue in between the lobes.
    - Lobes are subdivided into lobules and then into tubuloalveolar glands.
    - Each lobe concludes as a lactiferous duct.
    - Lactiferous ducts dilate into lactiferous sinuses beneath the nipple and then open through small orifices onto the nipple.
    - Cooper ligaments (suspensory ligaments) that divide the breast into segments can dimple the skin if involved with cancer "peau d'orange."
- **Nipple-Areolar Complex (NAC)**
  - Located at the fourth intercostal space in nonptotic breasts.
  - Composed of sebaceous glands and apocrine sweat glands.
  - Montgomery glands: at the areolar periphery, capable of secreting milk.
  - Tubercles of Morgagni: elevations formed by the openings of Montgomery glands.
  - Radial smooth muscle fibers beneath the nipple contribute to nipple erection.

BLOOD SUPPLY (FIG. 49-1)

- *Internal mammary artery: perforating branches supply the medial and central portions of the breast; dominant blood supply of the breast and NAC.
- Lateral thoracic artery: upper outer quadrant.
- Anterolateral and anteromedial intercostal perforators.
- Venous drainage: follows arterial supply.
- Batson plexus: valveless venous plexus that allows direct hematogenous metastasis of breast cancer to the spine.

---

*Denotes common in-service examination topics.

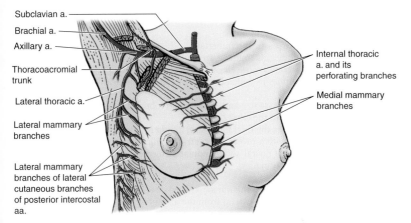

Subclavian a.

Brachial a.

Axillary a.

Thoracoacromial trunk

Lateral thoracic a.

Lateral mammary branches

Lateral mammary branches of lateral cutaneous branches of posterior intercostal aa.

Internal thoracic a. and its perforating branches

Medial mammary branches

Figure 49-1 Blood supply to the breast. (From Dalley AF II, Agur AMR, eds. *Moore's Clinically Oriented Anatomy.* 9th ed. Wolters Kluwer; 2023. Figure 4.24.)

INNERVATION
- Medial: second through fifth anteromedial intercostal nerves
- Lateral: third through sixth anterolateral intercostal nerves
- *NAC: lateral cutaneous branch of the fourth intercostal nerve

LYMPHATIC DRAINAGE
- **Skin, Nipple, and Areola:** superficial subareolar lymphatic plexus.
- **Breast:** deep lymphatic plexus, which is connected to the superficial plexus. About 97% of the breast drains directly into the axillary nodes, while the rest drains into the internal mammary nodes.
- **Axillary Space**
  - **Borders**
    - Apex: first rib, scapula, clavicle
    - Medial: serratus anterior, intercostal muscles of ribs 1-4
    - Lateral: intertubercular groove of the humerus
    - Anterior: pectoralis major, pectoralis minor
    - Posterior: subscapularis, latissimus dorsi, teres major
  - **Neural structures of clinical importance within the axilla**
    - Long thoracic nerve: innervates serratus anterior; injury results in winged scapula.
    - Thoracodorsal nerve: innervates and supplies latissimus dorsi; injury results in weak arm pull ups and adduction.
    - *Intercostobrachial nerve: provides sensation to upper medial arm. Most commonly injured nerve with modified radical mastectomy (MRM) or axillary lymph node dissection (ALND).
  - **Axillary lymph nodes: classified by relationship to pectoralis minor**
    - Level I: lateral to the pectoralis minor muscle
    - Level II: beneath the pectoralis minor muscle
    - Level III: medial to the pectoralis minor muscle
    - Rotter nodes: between the pectoralis major and pectoralis minor muscles
- **Supraclavicular Nodes:** contiguous with axillary apex
- **Internal Mammary Nodes:** in first six intercostal spaces with highest concentration of nodes in first three spaces, within 3 cm of sternal edge

DEVELOPMENT

- **Tanner Stages of Breast Development**
  - **Stage I:** no glandular tissue; prepubertal.
  - **Stage II:** breast bud begins to form; areola begins to widen.
  - **Stage III:** breast becomes more elevated and extends beyond borders of the areola, which continues to widen but remains in contour with the surrounding breast.
  - **Stage IV:** increased breast size and elevation; areola and papilla form a secondary mound projecting from the chest contour.
  - **Stage V:** breast reaches the final adult size; areola returns to contour of the surrounding breast with a projecting central papilla.
- **Menopause:** involution of ductal and glandular elements; breast becomes predominantly fat and stroma.
- **Embryology**
  - A pair of ectodermal ridges (mammary ridges) develop on the ventral surface of the embryo and initially extend from the axilla to groin, but later disappear everywhere except the fourth intercostal space on the chest wall.
  - The mesoderm creates the smooth muscle fibers of the nipple.
  - The surrounding ectoderm forms the areola.

CLINICAL EVALUATION OF BREAST MASSES

HISTORY

- Onset and duration of mass
- Pain, change in breast size or shape, nipple discharge, skin changes, weight loss, and/or fatigue
- Family history of breast cancer, including relationship, age of onset, and presence of bilateral disease
- Change in size with menstrual cycle or estrogen exposure
- Estrogen exposure: timing of menarche, pregnancy and menopause, and history of oral contraceptives or hormone replacement therapy (HRT)
- History of previous breast biopsy or other breast surgery
- History of any previous breast imaging

PHYSICAL EXAMINATION

- Chaperone: offer to have a chaperone for sensitive examinations.
- Patient supine, raise the arm above the head to examine the breast.
- Patient seated upright, support the arm to relax the pectoralis and examine the axilla.
- Masses and nodes are characterized by their location, number, size, firmness, and mobility.

BENIGN BREAST DISEASE

BENIGN BREAST DISEASE TYPES (TABLE 49-1)

NONPROLIFERATIVE BENIGN BREAST DISEASE

No increased risk of breast cancer.
- **Cysts**
  - **Epidemiology:** perimenopausal, ages 40-50 years
  - **Etiology:** lobular involution; acini within the lobule distend to form microcysts, which develop into macrocysts
  - **Presentation**
    - Well demarcated from the surrounding tissue, mobile, and firm

TABLE 49-1 Types of Benign Breast Disease

Classification	Risk of invasive disease	Examples
Nonproliferative	No increased relative risk	Cysts, macro or micro Ductal ectasia Fat necrosis/lipoma Simple fibroadenoma Fibrocystic change Mastitis Fibrosis Metaplasia, squamous or apocrine Mild hyperplasia
Proliferative	Relative risk of 1.5-2.0	Complex fibroadenoma Papilloma Phyllodes tumor Sclerosing adenosis Hyperplasia, moderate or severe
Proliferative with atypia	Relative risk of 4.5-5.0 (9.0 if there is a first-degree relative with breast cancer)	Atypical ductal hyperplasia Atypical lobular hyperplasia

- May fluctuate with patient's menstrual cycle (solid lesions do not)
- Uncommon in postmenopausal women who are not on HRT
  - ○ **Diagnosis/management**
    - Ultrasound differentiates simple cysts vs complex cysts.
    - Simple cyst: if asymptomatic, may be followed. If symptomatic, should be aspirated. If nonpalpable, no aspiration needed.
    - Complex cyst: biopsy.
    - Aspiration: may replace ultrasound as the initial step.
      - □ If aspirate is nonbloody and mass resolves, no further treatment needed. If fluid is bloody, mass does not resolve completely, or if it recurs multiple times, should be biopsied.
      - □ Cytologic analysis of fluid is of little value as malignant cells are seen in <1% of cases and atypical cells are often present even in benign disease.
    - Surgical biopsy
      - □ Indications: recurrent, bloody, persistent, or complex cysts.
      - □ Cyst wall tissue is required to determine the presence of malignancy.
- **Ductal Ectasia**
  - ○ **Epidemiology:** perimenopausal, ages 40-50 years.
  - ○ **Etiology:** chronic intraductal and periductal inflammation causes dilation of mammary ducts and thickening of secretions, leading to a blockage of the ducts.
  - ○ **Presentation**
    - Palpable subareolar mass
    - Nipple tenderness, irritation, or retraction
    - Thick black, gray, or greenish nipple discharge
  - ○ **Diagnosis/management**
    - Imaging: ultrasound or mammography.
    - Biopsy for definitive diagnosis.
    - Once diagnosed, no further treatment is needed as condition usually resolves on its own. However, if symptoms recur, excision of the affected duct may be indicated.
    - If duct becomes infected, treat with antibiotics.
- **Fat Necrosis**
  - ○ **Epidemiology:** most common in women with pendulous breasts or who are overweight.

- ○ **Etiology:** secondary to trauma, breast surgery, infection, or radiation therapy; 50% are idiopathic.
- ○ **Presentation**
  - Poorly defined, painless, firm mass
  - Usually occurs in superficial breast tissue
  - May be accompanied by skin thickening, dimpling, or retraction
- ○ **Diagnosis/management**
  - Diagnostic mammogram; however, diagnosis can only be made radiographically if an oil cyst (circumscribed mass of mixed soft tissue density and fat with a calcified rim) is seen.
  - Biopsy required to exclude malignancy in the absence of this finding or a clear history of trauma.
- • Fibroadenoma
  - ○ **Epidemiology**
    - Ages 15-5 years
    - *Accounts for 75% of breast biopsies in women younger than age 20
  - ○ **Etiology**
    - Aberrant lobular development; proliferation of epithelial and fibrous tissues.
    - Hormonal factors play a role in growth—fibroadenomas significantly increase in size during pregnancy and involute after menopause.
  - ○ **Presentation**
    - Well-defined, palpable mass that averages 2-3 cm diameter
    - Rubbery texture, mobile
    - Painless, slow growing
    - Solitary in 85%-90% of cases
  - ○ **Diagnosis/management**
    - Ultrasound: round or oval, well-circumscribed, solid, homogenous mass.
    - Biopsy, excision. pathology typically will be "simple" or "complex"— influences the risk of breast cancer.
  - ○ **Types**
    - **Simple fibroadenoma:** classified as nonproliferative breast disease, no proliferative histologic features
    - **Complex fibroadenoma**
      - □ Classified as proliferative breast disease and is associated with an increased risk of breast cancer
      - □ Contains cysts >3 mm in diameter and/or other proliferative changes, such as sclerosing adenosis, epithelial calcifications, and papillary apocrine changes
    - ***Giant fibroadenoma**
      - □ **Most common breast neoplasm in an adolescent patient**
      - □ Solitary, firm, and nontender
      - □ Presents near puberty as rapid, asymmetric breast enlargement with prominent veins over tumor and occasional skin ulceration due to pressure
      - □ Size >5.0 cm
      - □ Excise by enucleation, no adjuvant treatment indicated
- • Fibrocystic Changes or Disease
  - ○ **Epidemiology:** most common benign breast condition, affecting women during reproductive years or if taking hormone replacements after menopause.
  - ○ **Etiology:** related to fluctuations in hormone levels.
  - ○ **Presentation:** cyclic, bilateral breast pain and tenderness associated with nodularity that occurs most commonly in upper outer breast quadrant, symptoms peak just prior to menstruation.
  - ○ **Diagnosis/management**

- Observation for symmetrical tender nodularity.
- If asymmetric nodularity persists for one to two menstrual cycles, order mammogram and biopsy for definitive diagnosis.
- Lifestyle changes are beneficial to some patients, including restricting caffeine and methylxanthines and adhering to a low-salt diet.
- Bilateral mastectomy may be indicated in patients with intractable pain.
- **Mastitis in Lactating Women**
  - **Epidemiology:** most common during the first 4-6 weeks postpartum or during weaning
  - **Etiology:** proliferation of bacteria, most commonly *Staphylococcus aureus*, in poorly drained breast segments
  - **Presentation:** cellulitis with fever, pain, redness, swelling, and malaise
  - **Diagnosis/management**
    - Antibiotics: penicillinase-resistant cephalosporin.
    - Continue breastfeeding to help drain the engorged breast.
    - Consider abscess drainage if infection persists.
    - Consider biopsy if refractory to treatment to exclude malignancy.
- **Mastitis in Nonlactating Women**
  - **Epidemiology:** most common in premenopausal women
  - **Etiology**
    - Squamous epithelium extends abnormally into duct orifices trapping keratin, causing dilation and eventual rupture of ducts.
    - Recurrent infections associated with smoking secondary to promotion of squamous metaplasia of duct lining.
  - **Presentation:** periareolar inflammation, may have purulent nipple discharge
  - **Diagnosis/management**
    - Antibiotics: aerobic and anaerobic coverage
    - Aspiration if abscess present
    - Terminal duct excision for recurrent infections
    - Consider open drainage with biopsy if refractory to treatment

PROLIFERATIVE BENIGN BREAST DISEASE

Small increase in relative risk (1.5-2.0) for developing invasive breast cancer
- **Papilloma**
  - *****Epidemiology: most common cause of bloody nipple discharge in women 20-40 years old**
  - **Etiology:** intraductal epithelial tumor
  - **Presentation:** spontaneous bloody, serous, or cloudy nipple discharge; typically not palpable
    - Nipple discharge considered to be pathologic if it is spontaneous, arises from a single duct, is persistent, and contains blood.
    - Discharge is physiologic if it occurs only in response to nipple compression, originates from multiple ducts, and often bilateral.
  - **Diagnosis/management**
    - Increased malignant potential after age 60 or with atypia.
    - Mammography and ultrasound may reveal nonpalpable masses, calcifications, or dilated ducts.
    - Galactogram: mammography performed after the offending lactiferous duct has been cannulated and filled with a contrast agent; localizes peripheral lesions.
    - If biopsy reveals pathologic discharge, treat with terminal duct excision.
- **Phyllodes Tumor**
  - **Epidemiology:** average age 45 years
  - **Etiology**
    - Rapid growth of a fibroepithelial periductal tumor.
    - Malignant degeneration to sarcoma is reported in 6% of cases.

- **Presentation:** very large, firm mass that is mobile and painless and may be difficult to distinguish from a fibroadenoma
  - Metastatic involvement of lymph nodes is rare, although patients may have palpable axillary lymphadenopathy.
  - Metastases most frequently involve the lungs.
- **Diagnosis/management**
  - Core needle biopsy preferred method for diagnosis.
  - Treat with wide local excision with >1-cm margins.
  - If margins positive, patient should undergo reexcision to decrease the risk of local recurrence.
  - No axillary node dissection is required.
  - Postoperative radiation and chemotherapy is controversial but may be indicated for histologically malignant tumors or metastatic disease.

PROLIFERATIVE BENIGN BREAST DISEASE WITH ATYPIA

Higher relative risk (4.0-5.0) of developing into invasive breast cancer.
That relative risk increases to 9.0 with a first-degree relative with breast cancer.

- **Atypical Ductal Hyperplasia**
  - Resembles low-grade ductal carcinoma *in situ* (DCIS)
  - Characterized by proliferation of uniform, evenly spaced epithelial cells with low-grade nuclei involving a limited extent of a duct
- **Atypical Lobular Hyperplasia**
  - Resembles lobular carcinoma *in situ* (LCIS) and is characterized by monomorphic, evenly spaced cells with a thin rim of clear cytoplasm
  - Often containing clear vacuoles that involve <50% of the acini within a lobule
- **Risk Reduction Strategies for High-Risk Women**
  - Excision of abnormal cells vs prophylactic mastectomy
  - Annual surveillance mammograms
  - Discontinuation of oral contraceptives or HRT
  - Tamoxifen

PREMALIGNANT (NONINVASIVE) BREAST DISEASE

LOBULAR CARCINOMA *IN SITU*

- **Epidemiology:** premenopausal, ages 40-50 years.
- **Etiology:** >50% of acini are filled and distended with characteristic cells.
- **Presentation**
  - Usually incidental finding in women undergoing biopsy
  - Does not form a palpable mass
  - No specific mammographic finding
- **Prognosis:** regarded as a marker of increased risk rather than a true precursor
  - Relative risk of breast cancer is 2% per year.
  - When invasive cancer does develop, it is more commonly ductal than lobular.
  - Risk affects both breasts and persists indefinitely after diagnosis made.
- **Diagnosis/Management**
  - Controversial but includes lifelong surveillance with the goal of detecting subsequent malignancy at an early stage
  - Possible chemoprevention
  - Prophylactic bilateral mastectomy

DUCTAL CARCINOMA *IN SITU* OR INTRADUCTAL CARCINOMA

- **Epidemiology:** majority of *in situ* breast disease; risk increases with age.
- **Etiology:** abnormal proliferation of epithelial cells confined within basement membrane.
- **Presentation**
  - Usually first noted on mammography as clustered microcalcifications.
  - Less commonly may present as a palpable mass, pathologic nipple discharge, or Paget disease of the nipple.
- **Prognosis**
  - Classified based on nuclear grade (low, intermediate, and high) and necrosis.
  - About 50% of local recurrences after excision contain invasive carcinoma.
  - Younger women are at higher risk for recurrence.
- **Diagnosis/Management**
  - Mammography to evaluate the extent of calcifications
  - Diagnosis via image-guided core biopsy
  - Treated with breast conservation therapy (BCT, lumpectomy + radiation) or mastectomy
  - Adjuvant treatment with radiation therapy or endocrine therapy

PAGET DISEASE OF THE NIPPLE

- **Epidemiology:** rare, peak incidence ages 50-60 years
- **Etiology:** form of DCIS that spreads from ductal system into the epidermis of the nipple
- **Presentation**
  - Scaly, ulcerated nipple associated with erythema, pain, and/or pruritus
  - Palpable breast mass in 50% of cases
- **Diagnosis/Management:** diagnosed via full-thickness punch biopsy of the nipple
  - Hallmark is the presence of malignant, intraepithelial adenocarcinoma cells (Paget cells) within the epidermis of the nipple.
  - Treated with breast conservation therapy (BCT, lumpectomy + whole breast radiation) or mastectomy.

MALIGNANT (INVASIVE) BREAST DISEASE

EPIDEMIOLOGY

- The *most common cancer* in American women: incidence, one in eight women.
- Second most common cause of death in American women (heart disease is first).
- **Risk Factors**
  - **Age and ethnicity**
    - Greatest risk after age 65 years
    - Before age 40, African American women at higher risk; after age 40, Caucasian women at higher risk
  - **Family history**
    - About 20%-30% of women with breast cancer have a positive family history, but only 5%-10% have an inherited mutation in a breast cancer susceptibility gene.
    - *BRCA1 or BRCA2 mutations cause majority of hereditary breast cancer.
      - Lifetime risk of breast cancer of up to 85%
      - Increased risk of contralateral breast cancer and ovarian cancer (higher with *BRCA1*)
      - *BRCA2* increased the risk of male breast cancer, prostate cancer, and pancreatic cancer
      - Suspect hereditary breast cancer if 2+ first-degree relatives or 2+ generations with early-onset breast/ovarian cancer

○ **Hormonal factors:** risk increased with estrogen exposure
  ▪ Menarche <12 years old
  ▪ First pregnancy after age 35
  ▪ Nulliparity
  ▪ Increased age at menopause
  ▪ Obesity
  ▪ Estrogen replacement therapy >5 years
○ **Environment and diet**
  ▪ Ionizing radiation (medical or nuclear) >90 rads
  ▪ Increased alcohol intake
○ **Other risk factors include a history of other neoplasms** (contralateral breast, uterine or ovarian cancer, and major salivary gland carcinoma), atypical hyperplasia, and DCIS or LCIS.

EVALUATION AND DIAGNOSIS

- **Diagnostic Mammogram:** performed if abnormality detected on clinical examination or screening mammogram.
- **Ultrasound:** adjunct imaging study for women <40 years old and/or with palpable breast mass.
- **MRI:** indicated in some high-risk women and to evaluate for a primary breast tumor in patients presenting with axillary adenopathy.
- **Fine Needle Aspiration:** minimally invasive way to obtain cells for diagnosis.
- **Image-Guided Core Biopsy:** core of tissue obtained for histologic examination.
- **Excisional Biopsy:** complete removal of breast mass, serves as definitive therapy for benign breast mass, and may be therapeutic lumpectomy if margins are negative.
- **Incisional Biopsy:** reserved for masses too large to be completely excised.
- **Wire-Localization Biopsy or Lumpectomy:** lesion identified radiographically and marked with a wire prior to excision. After excision, specimen can be imaged to ensure removal of calcifications.

TYPES OF INVASIVE BREAST CANCER

- **Invasive cancer** refers to cases in which tumor cells have crossed the basement membrane and have the ability to metastasize.
- **Infiltrating Ductal Carcinoma**
  ○ Most common invasive breast cancer (65%-80%)
  ○ Presents as firm, fixed, irregular mass
- **Infiltrating Lobular Carcinoma**
  ○ Grows as single file of malignant cells circumferentially arranged around ducts and lobules and therefore does not usually produce distinct mass
  ○ Accounts for 10% of breast cancer
- **Histologic Subtypes**
  ○ Tubular: well differentiated, form normal-appearing tubules, no myoepithelial cells; nodal metastases rare; excellent prognosis.
  ○ Mucinous/colloid: large amount of extracellular mucus, relatively acellular; excellent prognosis.
  ○ Medullary: large, pleomorphic nuclei; high mitotic rate; grossly tumors are well circumscribed; nodal metastases unlikely; favorable prognosis.
  ○ Cribriform: well-differentiated gaps between cancer cells give a Swiss cheese appearance.
  ○ Adenoid cystic: rare subtype, cells resemble glandular and cystic cells.
  ○ Juvenile secretory: rare subtype, cells with clear vacuolated cytoplasm, most common type of breast cancer in children.

GRADING

Based on the degree of differentiation.
- **Nuclear:** well differentiated, intermediate, or poorly differentiated
- **Histologic:** differentiation, growth pattern, extent of tubule formation, nuclear hyperchromasia, and mitotic index

PROGNOSTIC MARKERS

- **Estrogen and progesterone receptors (ER/PR)**
  - Nuclear hormone receptors that function as transcription factors when bound to their appropriate ligand.
  - Approximately 70% of breast cancers are ER/PR positive, and ~60% of those respond to endocrine therapy.
  - ER/PR-positive tumors are candidates for hormonal therapy.
- **Human Epidermal Growth Factor Receptor 2 (HER2)**
  - Oncogene.
  - Overexpressed in 15%-30% of invasive breast cancers.
  - Associated with worse prognosis.
  - HER2-positive tumors are candidates for anti-HER2 therapy, including trastuzumab.

STAGING

- **Refers to the grouping of patients according to the extent of their disease.**
- **Staging is critical for**
  - Determining choice of treatment for a patient
  - Estimating prognosis
  - Comparing results of different treatment programs
- **Pathologic staging** is the most precise estimator of prognosis and end result and can only be performed if tumor has negative surgical margins at the time of excision.
- **Determined by the American Joint Committee on Cancer (AJCC)** using a system based on the TNM (tumor, node, metastasis) system.

TREATMENT OF MALIGNANT BREAST DISEASE

- **Local Therapy**
  - **BCT (breast conservation therapy):** removal of primary tumor with adequate (usually 1 cm) margins of normal tissue and subsequent radiation therapy (XRT)
    - Indicated when it is possible to reduce the tumor burden to a microscopic level that can be controlled by radiation; radiation can be delivered safely; and local recurrence can be promptly detected.
    - Absolute contraindications
      - Two or more tumors in different quadrants.
      - Persistent positive margins after surgery.
      - First and second trimester of pregnancy. In third trimester, BCT can be performed, and then, XRT can be given after delivery.
      - History of prior radiation to the breast.
      - Diffuse microcalcifications with malignant characteristics.
    - Neoadjuvant chemotherapy has not been shown to improve survival in BCT compared with postoperative therapy.
  - **MRM**
    - Traditionally, MRM includes excision of the NAC.
    - Nipple-sparing mastectomy can be controversial.

- □ *Indications: select patients with clinically negative axillae, tumor >2 cm from NAC, tumor size <3 cm, and no skin involvement.
        - □ Contraindications: locally advanced breast cancer, inflammatory breast cancer.
        - □ Must perform intraoperative biopsy of retroareolar ducts and send for frozen section. If positive, must excise NAC.
    - Biopsy scar(s) should be included in skin excision.
    - Skin flaps raised in the plane between the subcutaneous tissue and the underlying breast tissue.
    - Dissection should extend superiorly to clavicle, medially to sternum, inferiorly to rectus sheath, and laterally to latissimus dorsi to ensure removal of all breast tissue.
    - Fascia overlying pectoralis major is considered the deep margin of resection but can be preserved to facilitate reconstruction.
    - Breast flap viability should be assessed prior to placement of expander or implant. Adjunct perfusion scans (eg, fluorescence indocyanine green imaging) can be used to assess vascular perfusion to flaps.
  - Multiple prospective, randomized trials with long-term follow-up have compared mastectomy with BCT: None demonstrated 10-year survival differences, but local recurrence rate is slightly higher in the BCT group.
- Axillary Node Management
  - Sentinel lymph node (SLN) biopsy
    - The SLN is the first lymph node that receives drainage from a primary tumor.
        - □ Inject primary tumor with radioactive isotope–labeled colloid (ie, technetium), lymphazurin blue dye, or both.
        - □ SLN is detected via "hot" counts with a Geiger counter (radioactivity) or blue dye in node (lymphazurin).
        - □ Remove all SLNs with counts >10% of the most radioactive node.
    - SLN can be identified in 90% of patients and predicts the status of the remaining axillary nodes in >90% of those patients.
    - Contraindications to SLN biopsy
        - □ Clinically suspicious axillary lymphadenopathy
        - □ Inflammatory or other locally advanced cancer (T4 tumors)
        - □ Pregnant or lactating woman
        - □ Prior axillary surgery
  - ALND
    - Levels I and II: standard practice; identifies metastases in 98% of patients
    - Level III: performed only in patients with gross nodal metastases
    - Indications:
        - □ Patients with inflammatory breast cancer
        - □ Patients with three or more axillary sentinel nodes that are positive for cancer
        - □ Persistently positive lymph nodes after neoadjuvant therapy
        - □ Axillary lymph node recurrence after prior breast cancer treatment
        - □ Axillas with failed radiotracer and/or methylene blue during SLN biopsy
  - Complications of ALND
    - Injury to axillary vein or motor nerves traveling within the axilla
    - *Lymphedema: 15%-30% risk of development persists throughout a patient's lifetime and increases as the time from surgery increases
        - □ Highest risk following level III axillary dissections and axillary radiation
    - Intercostobrachial nerve paresthesia (numbness on medial arm): 70%-80% patients
    - Upper extremity pain and weakness: 20%-30% after 1 year

- **Radiotherapy (XRT)**
  - Indicated for BCT or 4+ positive lymph nodes, primary tumor size 5 cm or more, T4 disease, and positive surgical margin
  - Reduces the risk of local recurrence
  - Improves survival by eradicating residual local disease that may be resistant to systemic chemotherapy
- **Adjuvant Systemic Therapy**
  - Indicated to eliminate clinically occult micrometastases following local treatment of breast cancer to reduce recurrence and improve survival
  - Cytotoxic chemotherapeutic agents: doxorubicin, cytoxan, methotrexate, 5-fluorouracil, and paclitaxel
  - Endocrine agents
    - *Selective estrogen receptor modulators, that is, tamoxifen: has both estrogen antagonist and estrogen agonist properties
      □ Estrogen antagonist: competitive blockade of estrogen receptors in the breast.
      □ Estrogen agonist: preserves bone density, lowers cholesterol levels, and increases the risk of endometrial carcinoma.
      □ Indicated for ER/PR-positive tumors.
      □ Side effects include hot flashes, vaginal discharge, and increased risk of endometrial carcinoma and **venous thromboembolism.**
    - Aromatase inhibitor therapy: anastrozole
      □ Lowers estrogen levels by inhibiting the peripheral conversion of androgens to estrogen
      □ Indicated for postmenopausal women
      □ Side effect profile better than tamoxifen with fewer hot flashes, no endometrial effects, and fewer thromboembolic events
      □ Higher risk of osteoporosis, fractures, and severe joint pain

SPECIAL CONSIDERATIONS

MALE BREAST CANCER

- **Risk Factors**
  - Positive family history, *BRCA2* mutation, and radiation exposure
  - Hormonal imbalance leading to high ratio of estrogen to androgen, secondary to conditions such as cirrhosis and Klinefelter syndrome
  - No clear association with gynecomastia except with Klinefelter syndrome
- **Epidemiology**
  - Mean age of 65-70 years
  - 1% of all breast cancer cases
- **Presentation**
  - Mass beneath the NAC associated with retraction or ulceration of the nipple.
  - Differential diagnosis for a breast mass in a male includes gynecomastia, abscess, or metastases to the breast from remote primary tumor (ie, sarcoma).
- **Diagnosis/Management**
  - **Same diagnostic algorithm as female breast cancer.**
  - **Mastectomy** is the most common treatment.
    - Simple mastectomy if limited pectoral muscle involvement
    - Radical mastectomy if extensive pectoral muscle invasion present
  - **Hormonal therapy:** most beneficial if the tumor is hormone receptor positive.
    - Approximately 80% of male breast cancers are hormone receptor positive.
    - Tamoxifen: improves survival rates but may not be well tolerated in men and may cause weight gain and decreased libido.

- Orchiectomy: reserved for patients with metastatic disease refractory to other medical treatments.
- **Prognosis:** when matched by stage, survival is similar to women with breast cancer. Axillary nodal status is the major predictor of outcome.

PEARLS

1. The intercostobrachial nerve is a cutaneous nerve that transversely crosses the axilla to supply the skin of the medial aspect of the upper arm. Injury to this nerve during an ALND causes numbness of this region, and can lead to chronic neuropathic pain.
2. Depending on surgeon preference, patients may need to discontinue hormonal therapy prior to major operations.

QUESTIONS YOU WILL BE ASKED

1. What is the differential diagnosis for a breast mass?
   Cyst, fibroadenoma, fibrocystic changes, fat necrosis, and cancer.
2. What is the most common cause of bloody nipple discharge in women 20-40 years old?
   Papilloma.
3. What are the anatomic boundaries of the breast?
   Clavicle to the sixth rib, sternal edge to the midaxillary line, and posteriorly the fascia of pectoralis major and serratus anterior.
4. What is the dominant blood supply to the breast?
   Internal mammary artery.
5. What is the innervation of the NAC?
   Fourth intercostal nerve.

Recommended Readings
1. Kennedy RD, Boughey JC. Management of pediatric and adolescent breast masses. *Semin Plast Surg.* 2013;27(1):19-22.
2. National Comprehensive Cancer Network. *Breast Cancer (Version 2.2022).* Accessed April 18, 2022. https://www.nccn.org/professionals/physician_gls/pdf/breast.pdf
3. Sabel M. Overview of benign breast diseases. In: Chagpar AB, Chen W, eds, *UptoDate.* Available from https://www.uptodate.com/contents/overview-of-benign-breast-diseases#H4128255581

50 Breast Reconstruction

Sherry Tang

PREOPERATIVE EVALUATION

GOALS

- **Oncologic treatment comes first,** breast reconstruction comes second.
- **Meet the patient's needs:** breast reconstruction is elective, patient's goals for reconstruction should play a large role in decision-making.

HISTORY
(See Chapter 47: Breast Augmentation, Mastopexy, and Augmentation Mastopexy, section "Preoperative Workup for Any Breast Surgery—Medical History")

- **Complete Cancer History**
  - Diagnosis and cancer stage
  - Size and location of tumor
  - Previous treatment with dates (lumpectomy, mastectomy, chemo, and radiation)
  - Planned treatment by surgical oncologist (sentinel lymph node biopsy, lumpectomy/mastectomy, chemo, and radiation)
- **Breast History**
  - Previous breast diagnoses (cysts, masses, and cancer)
  - Previous breast surgeries (biopsies, reduction/augmentation, and lumpectomies)
  - Current breast size, desired breast size
- **Family History of Breast Cancer**
  - First-degree relative
  - BRCA status
- **Past Medical History, Medications, Past Surgical History, and Social History**
  - Medical conditions that could affect patient's ability to withstand long operation or wound healing (coronary artery disease, diabetes, autoimmune disease, and bleeding diatheses)
  - Medications that impact bleeding/wound healing (coumadin, steroids, etc.)
  - Surgeries that affect the use of certain donor sites: scars on abdomen, back, buttock, and thighs
  - Smoking status
  - Amount of social support

PHYSICAL EXAM
(See Chapter 47: Breast Augmentation, Mastopexy, and Augmentation Mastopexy, section "Preoperative Workup for Any Breast Surgery—Physical Examination")

- Height, weight, and BMI
- Current breast size/shape and inframammary fold (IMF) position. Note any asymmetries
- Degree of breast ptosis
- Note any scars on the breast and on potential donor site if considering autologous reconstruction (eg, abdomen, back, thighs)
- Palpable breast or axillary masses
- Nipple retraction, ulceration, and discharge

---

*Denotes common in-service examination topics.

BREAST RECONSTRUCTION DECISION ALGORITHM (FIG. 50-1)

TIMING OF RECONSTRUCTION

- **Immediate Reconstruction:** done at the same time as mastectomy
  - Early-stage disease
  - Low risk of needing radiation (based on cancer stage or negative sentinel lymph node biopsy)
- **Delayed Reconstruction:** done after cancer treatment complete
  - Advanced stage disease
  - Known need for radiation
  - Patient preference

TYPE OF MASTECTOMY INCISION

- **Nipple Sparing**
  - Oncologic indication: clinically negative axillae, tumor >2 cm from nipple-areolar complex (NAC), tumor size <3 cm, and no skin involve
  - Reconstructive indication: if the nipple will end up in an appropriate anatomic position postoperatively (ie, grade 1 ptosis)
  - Subareolar frozen biopsies are sent to confirm no cancer involvement of the NAC
  - Incision types: periareolar, IMF, radial, vertical
- **Skin Sparing**
  - For patients who are not candidates for nipple-sparing mastectomy, either from an oncologic or plastic surgery standpoint
  - For patients who wish to not have nipples
- **Wise Pattern**
  - Skin marking and incision similar to that of wise pattern breast reduction or mastopexy (**See Chapter 48: Reduction Mammoplasty, Top Surgery, and Gynecomastia, section "Wise Pattern Reduction"**).
  - Indications: grade II or III ptosis. Desired postoperative size significantly smaller than preoperative breast size.
  - Allows for good control of the skin envelope.
  - Inferior skin is typically deepithelialized to provide additional support to implant.

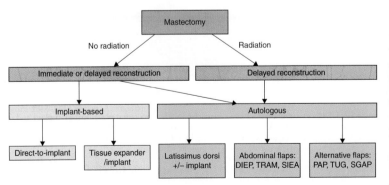

Figure 50-1 General breast reconstruction decision algorithm.

RECONSTRUCTIVE OPTIONS

IMPLANT-BASED RECONSTRUCTION

- Reconstruction following mastectomy is optional and based on patient preference. In patients who do not desire reconstruction or wish to delay reconstruction, breast prostheses can be fitted under a bra or bathing suit.
- **Direct to Implant (DTI):** placement of implant at the time of mastectomy (**Fig. 50-2**).
  - Ideal candidates
    - Preoperatively
      - Desire to stay the same size or smaller
      - Symmetric and relatively smaller breasts
      - Most common in nipple-sparing mastectomy

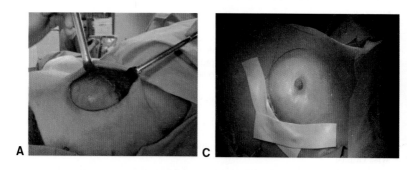

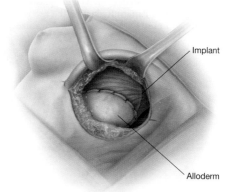

Figure 50-2 Direct to implant breast reconstruction with subpectoral placement of implant and use of acellular dermal matrix. A. Acellular dermal matrix is sutured to the chest wall and pectoralis muscle. **B, C.** After the implant is placed into the breast pocket, the acellular dermal matrix sutured to the inferior border of the pectoralis major muscle. (**A, C** from Colwell AS, Wright EJ. Direct-to-implant breast reconstruction. In: Chung KC, Disa JJ, Gosain A, et al. eds. *Operative Techniques in Plastic Surgery.* Wolters Kluwer; 2020:1398-1403. Tech Figure 4.17.2BCD; **B** from Colwell AS. Direct-to-implant breast reconstruction. In: Mulholland MW, ed. *Operative Techniques in Surgery.* Vol 2. Wolters Kluwer; 2015:1471-1475. Tech Figure 5.14.5.)

- Intraoperatively
  - Good quality and well-perfused mastectomy skin flap (most important): assess by physical exam and/or intraoperative indocyanine green angiography (eg, SPY system)
  - Can utilize weight of mastectomy specimen and base width to help determine implant size volume
- Benefits
  - Theoretically one stage although most patients will undergo some additional surgery
  - Less thinning of skin envelope
  - Most control of nipple position
- Limitations
  - Often need to use of acellular dermal matrix to provide additional support
  - Limited in the size of implant that can be placed
- **Tissue Expander (TE)/Implant:** placement of TE at time of mastectomy, exchange to implant once patient is expanded to desired volume (**Fig. 50-3**)
  - Most common type of reconstruction
  - Good candidates
    - Desire to make significant size changes
    - Asymmetry
    - Vascularity and quality of mastectomy skin is insufficient to tolerated DTI
  - Benefits
    - Safer choice than DTI
    - Patient has more input in final size of reconstruction
    - Better able to control size, symmetry, and implant position at time of exchange
  - Limitations
    - Two stages
    - Longer reconstructive timeline overall

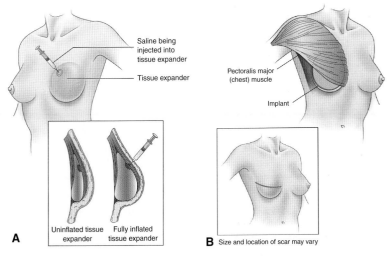

Figure 50-3 Tissue expander-implant–based breast reconstruction. A. Process of tissue expansion. **B.** Placement of permanent implant after tissue expansion has completed. Note: Can use serratus muscle or acellular dermal matrix to cover the inferolateral aspect of the tissue expander/implant (*not shown*). (From Mulholland MW, ed. *Greenfield's Surgery.* 5th ed. Lippincott Williams & Wilkins; 2011. Figure 113.3.)

○ Procedure
- First stage operation
  □ TE placement at time of mastectomy
  □ May start filling TE intraoperatively if skin quality is good. Important to not overfill to avoid tension-induced ischemia of the mastectomy flap
- Expansion
  □ Can start expansion 1 week after drain removal, usually 2-3 weeks post-op.
  □ Expansions occur weekly, typically 60-120 cc saline injected each time, depending on patient's tolerance of expansion.
  □ Expansion stops when patient's desires size is achieved. Usually overexpand by 10% or more past goal size to account for recoil at the time of expander removal.
  □ Must wait for several months following expansion to allow the expanded skin to settle into new position.
- Second stage operation
  □ TE is exchanged for permanent silicone or saline implant.
  □ Revisions to pocket made at this time: capsulotomies, IMF adjustments (resuspension or lowering as needed), and skin tailoring.
  □ For unilateral reconstruction, symmetrizing procedures (mastopexy, reduction, augmentation) can be done for the contralateral breast.
- **Use of Support Matrix for Coverage of Implant and/or TE**
  ○ Ideal material: have good flexibility and is soft. Able to thicken soft tissue envelope. Long-lasting and durable. Ability to be biointegrated to reduce risk of matrix exposure and infection
  ○ Acellular dermal matrix (ADM)
    - Most commonly used.
    - Made from human skin (eg, FlexHD, AlloMax, AlloDerm) or animal skin (SurgiMend) where cells are removed, and support structure is left in place.
  ○ Synthetic mesh: short-term absorbable mesh or titanium mesh
    - Less expensive but inconsistent outcomes
  ○ Dermal graft
    - Used with wise-pattern mastectomy.
    - Inferior mastectomy flap is deepithelialized and sutured to the chest wall to act as a sling over the TE or implant.
- **Plane of Implant/TE Placement**
  ○ Subpectoral plane (total muscle coverage)
    - Pectoralis major covers superior implant. Serratus anterior muscle or fascia to cover the inferolateral implant.
    - No longer used much due to lack of inferior pole projection and painful expansions.
  ○ Dual-plane (partial muscle coverage): most common
    - Pectoralis major covers superior implant and ADM covers inferior implant.
    - Provides good inferior pole projection.
  ○ Prepectoral plane (no muscle coverage): increasing in popularity
    - Implant placed superficial to the pectoralis major muscle.
    - ADM can be used to cover the anterior surface of the implant, with or without posterior coverage.
- **Complications**
  ○ Early: hematoma (3.5%), seroma (2.9%), infection (10%), mastectomy flap necrosis (6.6%), wound dehiscence (1.6%).
  ○ Late: implant rupture or deflation (1.1%), implant malposition (0.5%), capsular contracture (0.8%).
  ○ **See Chapter 47: Breast Augmentation, Mastopexy, and Augmentation Mastopexy, section "Breast Augmentation"** for more details on implant-related complications.

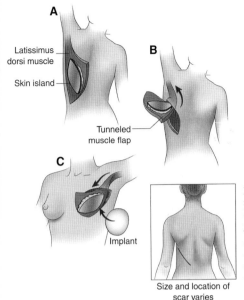

Figure 50-4 Latissimus dorsi flap reconstruction. **A.** A skin island overlying the latissimus dorsi muscle is designed, and the flap is elevated. **B.** The flap is tunneled through the axilla to the chest. **C.** The flap is inset on the chest, and an implant or tissue expander is placed. (From Mulholland MW, ed. *Greenfield's Surgery.* 5th ed. Lippincott Williams & Wilkins; 2011. Figure 113.4.)

AUTOLOGOUS RECONSTRUCTION

- Pedicled Flaps
  - Latissimus dorsi ± tissue expander/implant (Fig. 50-4)
    - *Mathes-Nahai type V flap: blood supply from (1) thoracodorsal artery (off subscapular) and (2) intercostal perforators. Thoracodorsal is primary blood supply for use in breast reconstruction.
      - Thoracodorsal artery enters latissimus muscle 8.7 cm distal to origin of subscapular artery and 2.6 cm medial to the lateral border of muscle.
      - Upon entry into latissimus, artery splits into lateral and medial branches.
      - If thoracodorsal vessels are damaged, latissimus can also survive on retrograde flow from serratus branch.
    - Harvested with elliptical skin paddle (up to 10 cm wide will close primarily).
    - Can be used in the setting of radiation or as a salvage procedure to bring in healthy tissue to support implant-based reconstruction.
    - Benefits: "workhorse flap." Very reliable, easy to harvest, relatively short operative time, excellent option for patients who need autologous tissue but are not good candidates for larger operations.
    - Limitations: small flap volume, almost always requires TE/implant under flap to provide adequate breast size.
    - **Complications: seroma (up to 50%), hematoma, capsular contracture, and partial flap loss.**
  - Latissimus dorsi and immediate fat transfer procedure
    - Combines a pedicled latissimus dorsi flap with fat grafting
    - Uses
      - Patients who desire autologous reconstruction but are not candidates for abdominally based free flaps
      - Salvage previous failed reconstruction using free flaps or implant-based reconstruction

- Benefits: avoids risks associated with TEs/implants, ability to use patient's own tissue without a free flap
- Limitations: final size of the reconstructed breast is limited by the amount of available fat
  - Pedicled transverse rectus abdominis myocutaneous (TRAM) flap
    - *Mathes-Nahai type III flap: dual blood supply from superior epigastric artery (off internal mammary artery) and deep inferior epigastric artery (DIEA) (off external iliac).
    - This procedure has lost its favor due to reduced donor site morbidity of deep inferior epigastric perforator (DIEP) flap.
    - Technique
      - Blood supply: superior epigastric artery.
      - Rectus muscle attached superiorly, DIEA, and rectus detached inferiorly.
      - Muscle and skin flap are turned and passed through a subcutaneous tunnel at the IMF up to mastectomy defect.
      - Delay 1-2 weeks prior to operation by ligating the DIEA might improve outcomes by increasing size and flow through superior epigastric vessels.
- Free Flaps
  - Recipient vessels
    - Internal mammary vessels (preferred): allows for medial position of flap, maximizes superior and medial pole fullness
    - Thoracodorsal vessels: disrupts ability to use latissimus dorsi muscle for salvage reconstruction
  - Abdominal-based flaps
    - Free TRAM
      - Rectus muscle with transverse abdominal skin island.
      - Bloody supply: deep inferior epigastric vessels.
      - Advantage: allows for greater manipulation of flap position on chest wall compared to pedicled TRAM.
      - Disadvantage: risks associated with free flap. Increased risk of hernia and abdominal wall bulges compared to free muscle-sparing TRAM or DIEP and due to this is not frequently performed.
    - Free muscle-sparing TRAM
      - Transverse abdominal skin with a strip of rectus muscle overlying blood supply, leaving behind most of rectus
      - MS-1: preserves lateral segment of rectus; MS-2: preserves medial and lateral segments of rectus
      - Blood supply: deep inferior epigastric vessels
      - Advantage: lower risk of hernia and bulges
    - DIEP flap (Fig. 50-5)
      - Free transverse island of abdominal skin and subcutaneous tissue with no muscle
      - Gold standard for abdominal based breast reconstruction
      - Blood supply: perforators from deep inferior epigastric vessels
        - DIEA runs from lateral to medial deep to the rectus abdominis muscle.
        - It sends perforators through the rectus muscle and pierce the rectus fascia to supply the overlying skin and fat.
        - There are medial row and lateral row perforators.
        - Obtain preoperative CT angiogram of abdomen to assess the branching pattern, location, and caliber of perforator vessels.
      - Technique
        - Lower incision placed transversely above the pubic bone and extends laterally. Upper incision placed above umbilicus and curves laterally to meet the lower incision.
        - Flap is elevated lateral to medial and perforator and identified and protected.

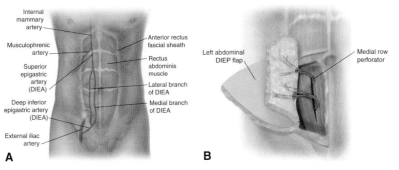

Figure 50-5 DIEP flap reconstruction. A. DIEP flap anatomy showing the right hemiabdomen with the medial and lateral branches of the deep inferior epigastric artery, giving off branches to become the medial and lateral row perforators. **B.** The right hemiabdomen DIEP flap is reflected laterally with the medial row perforators penetrating through the rectus abdominis muscle to supply the overlying skin and soft tissue. (From Chevray PM. DIEP flap breast reconstruction. In: Chung KC, Disa JJ, Gosain A, et al., eds. *Operative Techniques in Plastic Surgery.* Wolters Kluwer; 2020:1429-1437. Tech Figure 4.22.1.)

- Once large perforators are identified, small perforators can be ligated.
- Perforator dissection is done by incising the rectus fascia longitudinally around the perforator and tracing the perforator through the muscle.
- Dissection continues once the origin of the DIEA vessel are reached and the vessels and divided to be ready for anastomosis.
- The rectus muscle and rectus sheath are repaired.
- The remaining abdominal wall is then undermined to the costal margin and closed over drains.
  - □ Advantage: preserves entire rectus muscle
  - □ Disadvantage: tedious dissection
- **Superficial inferior epigastric artery flap (SIEA)**
  - □ Free transverse island of abdominal skin and fat only without violation of fascia or muscle.
  - □ Blood supply: superficial inferior epigastric artery off of the femoral artery.
  - □ Advantage: complete preservation of rectus muscle and fascia.
  - □ Disadvantage: few patients are candidates (<30% have SIEA large enough), higher risk of fat necrosis/flap complications.
  - □ Superficial dominance phenomenon: in some patients, the primary venous drainage of the abdominal wall is via the SIEV. In cases where the SIEA is not selected as the primary pedicle, it is still important to preserve these vessels so they can serve as lifeboat if free TRAM or DIEP has venous congestion.
  - o Gluteal-based flaps
    - **Superior gluteal artery perforator (SGAP) flap**
      - □ Free elliptical flap from upper lateral buttock includes skin, subcutaneous tissue, but preserves gluteus maximus muscle.
      - □ *Blood supply: perforators from superior gluteal artery (SGA) (off of internal iliac). SGA emerges one-third of the way from posterior superior iliac spine to greater trochanter of the femur.
      - □ Advantages: scar can be concealed in clothing.
      - □ Disadvantages: buttock fat and tissue are less malleable/harder to contour, difficult dissection requires experience, contour deformity of donor site possible leading to asymmetry. Much higher rate of flap loss compared to abdominal flaps.
    - **Inferior gluteal artery (IGA) perforator flap**
      - □ Free flap from lower buttock includes skin, subcutaneous tissue, and small segment of gluteus maximus muscle overlying perforators.

- Must less commonly used than SGAP flap.
- Blood supply: descending branch of inferior gluteal artery (IGA) (off of internal iliac). IGA emerges between the posterior superior iliac spine and the ischial tuberosity, at the junction between the middle and distal third.
- Advantages: scar concealed in infragluteal crease.
- Disadvantages: similar to SGAP.
○ **Thigh-based flaps**
  ▪ **Transverse upper gracilis flap**
    - Free gracilis muscle with overlying skin
    - Blood supply: medial circumflex femoral artery (off of profunda femoris) and venae comitantes
    - Short pedicle 6-8 cm
    - Advantages: hidden donor site, alternative for patients without adequate abdominal tissue
    - Disadvantages: small flap volume, donor site complications (scarring, medial thigh sensory changes)
  ▪ **Profunda artery perforator flap**
    - Free flap from medial thigh comprised of skin and subcutaneous tissue
    - Blood supply: perforator from the profunda femoris artery
    - Pedicle usually 10-12 cm with artery measuring 2 mm in diameter
    - Can be oriented longitudinally or transversely
      ▪ Transverse orientation: requires presence of an adequate proximal perforator. More favorable scar that is hidden in the infragluteal crease
    - Advantages: well-concealed scar
    - Disadvantages: small flap volume, risk of lymphedema if the dissection proceeds too medially
  ▪ **Anterolateral thigh flap**
    - Free elliptical flap from lateral thigh soft tissue
    - Blood supply: perforator from lateral circumflex femoral artery
    - Rarely used due to small size and conspicuous donor site scar
○ **Neurotization of free flaps**
  ▪ Goal: create a sensate flap by coaptation of a nerve supplying the flap to most commonly the third intercostal nerve.
  ▪ Can be done with direct nerve coaptation or via a nerve graft or conduit.
  ▪ Has not gained wide acceptance due to conflicting outcomes.
○ **Complications**
  ▪ **Breast complications:** total flap loss (1.4%-2.1%), acute partial flap necrosis (2.5%-5.2%), mastectomy flap necrosis (6.2%-7.7%), hematoma (4.1%-6.0%), infection (2.8%-.1%), wound dehiscence (1%-3.6%), fat necrosis (5.2%-9%)
  ▪ **Donor site complications:** wound dehiscence (3.1%-8.5%), wound infection (2.1%-3.3%), hematoma (0%-2.7%), seroma (2.1%-5.2%), fat necrosis (0%-1.9%)
- **Goldilocks Procedure**
  ○ Goal: use residual mastectomy flap to create an autologous tissue breast mound.
  ○ Ideal candidates
    ▪ Patients who are poor candidates for traditional reconstruction
    ▪ Macromastia or significant breast ptosis (usually have large amount of excess skin and fat left following mastectomy)
  ○ Technique
    ▪ Incision options: IMF, circumareolar, inverted T, wise pattern.
    ▪ The superior mastectomy flap is maintained and elevated superiorly.
    ▪ The inferior, medial, and lateral mastectomy flaps are deepithelialized.
    ▪ The medial and lateral deepithelized flap are folded beneath the inferior flap to provide extra projection.
    ▪ The inferior deepithelized flap is advanced superiorly and sutured to the chest wall.
  ○ Advantages: single-stage procedure. Does not need to use implants or additional flap donor site.

- Disadvantages: resulting size and projection of breast mound is limited by the amount of tissue present following mastectomy and the incision use. Not a complete substitute for formal breast reconstruction.

AUGOLOGOUS FAT GRAFTING IN BREAST RECONSTRUCTION

- Uses
  - Breast reconstruction with fat grafting only
    - Best suited for small- or medium-sized breasts and patients with sufficient donor site fat
    - Typically require 3-4 sessions for nonirradiated breasts and 4-6 sessions for radiated breasts
  - Latissimus dorsi and immediate fat transfer procedure (see above section on autologous breast reconstruction)
  - Secondary revision procedures following implant-based or autologous breast reconstruction
  - Enhance skin quality and mastectomy flap thickness prior to planned autologous or implant-based reconstruction
  - Correction of asymmetry and volume deficiency following lumpectomy
- Technique
  - Fat harvest via liposuction from abdomen, flanks, and thighs
  - Process of fat via filtration, centrifugation, decanting, or closed-system devices
  - Injection of fat into breasts
- Drawbacks
  - Fat graft resorption: volume retention of fat is approximately 50% necessitating need for multiple rounds for fat grafting to achieve the desired volume and shape.
  - Impact of fat grafting on breast cancer screening and detection:
    - On mammography, fat grafts may appear as fat necrosis, calcifications, and scar tissue.
    - High rates of biopsy of suspicious imaging finding following fat grafting.
- **See Chapter 6: Fat Grafting for more details on fat grafting**

NIPPLE-AREOLAR RECONSTRUCTION

- Can be done as early as 2-3 months after final breast mound reconstruction is complete
- **Papule reconstruction**
  - Nipple sharing: graft from contralateral nipple.
  - Composite graft (ear and hallux).
  - Prosthetic material (AlloDerm and polyurethane).
  - Local flap (most popular): uses local breast skin/fat to build papule. Choice of technique is surgeon dependent. Examples include skate flap (**Fig. 50-6**), CV flap, star flap, bell flap, S-flap, H-flap, double-opposing tab flap.
  - Biggest problem with all techniques is loss of papule projection, 50% or more, after 1 year. Many surgeons will overcompensate initially to account for loss over time.
- **Areola Reconstruction**
  - Tattoo: pigment applied to simulate areola
  - Skin graft: doughnut-shaped full-thickness skin graft applied around papule gives color and texture contrast
  - *In situ* skin graft: lifting the skin surrounding papule and then sewing back down
- **3D Nipple Areola Tattooing:** nonsurgical way to apply pigment and given the illusion of papule projection

RECONSTRUCTION OF LUMPECTOMY DEFECTS (ONCOPLASTIC BREAST SURGERY)

- **Definition:** oncoplastic breast surgery combines breast conserving therapy (lumpectomy) with plastic surgery techniques.

A Skate Flap Design

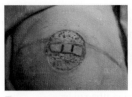

B De-epithelialization

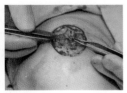

C Raised and rotated flaps

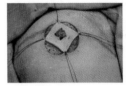

D Skin graft placement

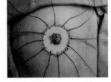

E Completed

Figure 50-6 Nipple-areolar reconstruction with skate flap (A-E).

- **Goals:** ensure a complete oncologic resection with negative margins, while obtaining a satisfying aesthetic result.
- **Preoperative Evaluation**
  - Oncologic perspective: tumor size compared to total breast volume, tumor location, microcalcification, multifocal breast cancer, need for chemotherapy or radiation
  - Reconstructive perspective: breast volume, degree of ptosis, breast shape, nipple asymmetries
- **Techniques**
  - **Simple glandular reshaping**
    - Indications: tumor volume less than 20% of total breast volume
    - Technique
      - Incisions: periareolar with or without radial extension, IMF.
      - Glandular tissue is mobilized and repositioned to achieve address asymmetry between both breasts created by the lumpectomy defect.
  - **Oncoplastic breast reduction**
    - Indications: large breasts, high degree of ptosis.
    - Benefits: larger tumor volume can be resected. Reducing glandular tissue can decrease amount of tissue being irradiated and reduce risk of ipsilateral recurrence.
    - Technique
      - Incisions: wise pattern incision most commonly used.
      - Pedicle choice is dependent on tumor location. Choose a pedicle that does not include the tumor in it.
      - In most cases, the tumor is located within the tissue resected as part of the reduction. However, if the tumor is located outside of this area, the tissue defect created can be filled in using the remaining breast tissue.
  - **Mastopexy**
    - Indications: small and slightly ptotic breasts, tumor size is more than 20% of the total breast volume.
    - Technique
      - Incisions: wise pattern, batwing, periareolar, etc.
      - Various approaches but common to all is that skin envelope is reduced and redistributed following lumpectomy, and NAC is repositioned to an ideal position.
      - No additional glandular tissue is resected.

○ Pedicled flaps
  ▪ Indications: small breast volume but insufficient to replace volume loss following lumpectomy
  ▪ Flap options: latissimus dorsi, intercostal artery perforator flap, laterothoracic artery perforator flap, thoracodorsal artery perforator flap
○ Fat grafting (see section "Autologous Fat Grafting in Breast Reconstruction")
  ▪ Indications: small lumpectomy defects and sufficient donor fat
  ▪ May require multiple rounds of fat grafting

PEARLS

1. All patients undergoing mastectomy should be offered breast reconstruction, but reconstruction is optional and is a personal choice. It always comes second to oncologic treatment.
2. The type and timing of breast reconstruction is dependent on multiple factors: patient preference, surgeon experience/preference, need for radiation, viability of mastectomy flap, and patient specifics (BMI, age, past medical/surgical/social history).
3. Do not hesitate to delay immediate reconstruction if there is questionable viability of the mastectomy flaps. Flap necrosis over a reconstruction can be devastating.
4. For patients undergoing autologous reconstruction, abdominal-based flaps such as a DIEP flap or muscle-sparing TRAM flap is the first choice. Medial thigh-based flaps such as the profunda artery perforator flap are the next choice.

QUESTIONS YOU WILL BE ASKED

1. What are the different types of breast reconstruction available to a patient?
   No reconstruction/prosthesis, implant-based reconstruction (DTI vs TE), autologous reconstruction.
2. What is the blood supply to the DIEP flap?
   Deep inferior epigastric perforators.
3. What is the blood supply to the latissimus dorsi flap?
   Thoracodorsal artery.
4. In direct to implant reconstruction, what is the most important factor to assess following mastectomy?
   Must assess viability and perfusion of the mastectomy skin flap.

THINGS TO DRAW

Markings for a nipple reconstruction flap (**see Fig. 50-6**).

Recommended Readings

1. Chang EI. Latest advancements in autologous breast reconstruction. *Plast Reconstr Surg.* 2021;146:111e-122e.
2. Colwell AS, Taylor EM. Recent advances in implant-based breast reconstruction. *Plast Reconstr Surg.* 2020;145:421e-432e.
3. Dancey A, Blondeel PN. Technical tips for safe perforator vessel dissection applicable to all perforator flaps. *Clin Plast Surg.* 2010;37(4):593-606. xi-vi.
4. Gougoutas AJ, Said HK, Um G, Chapin A, Mathes DW. Nipple-areola complex reconstruction. *Plast Reconstr Surg.* 2018;141(3):404e-416e.
5. Honart J, Reguesse A, Struk S, et al. Indications and controversies in partial mastectomy defect reconstruction. *Clin Plast Surg.* 2018;45:33-45.

Section IV: Breast and Body Reconstruction

51 Thoracic Reconstruction

Megan Lane and Paige L. Myers

OVERVIEW

ANATOMY

- Skeleton
    - Posterior—12 thoracic vertebrae, bilateral scapulae
    - Anterior: sternum, manubrium, xiphoid, and bilateral clavicles
    - Ribs
        - 10 pairs with costal cartilage, 2 pairs without
        - Superior 7 articulate directly with the sternum ("true ribs")
        - 8th, 9th, and 10th ribs ("false ribs") have indirect articulation
        - 11th and 12th ribs have articulation only posteriorly with vertebral bodies
- Vascular Anatomy (**Fig. 51-1**)
    - Internal Mammary Vessels
        - Arises from subclavian artery near its origin, travels down on ~1 cm from the costosternal junction
        - Runs deep to internal intercostal muscles
        - Divides into superior epigastric around the 6th intercostal
        - Critical to assess patency if using rectus abdominis flap in chest wall reconstruction as it is frequently utilized in prior coronary artery bypass
        - Useful recipient sites for microvascular reconstruction. Most suitable and consistent for microsurgery at the third intercostal space.
    - Intercostal Vessels—run alongside the intercostal nerve between the inner and innermost intercostal muscles inferior to the rib
- Innervation
    - 11th intercostal nerves arise from the corresponding spinal cord level; the nerve arising from T12 is the subcostal nerve. All intercostals are inferior to the rib.
    - Each intercostal is connected to the sympathetic chain via rami communicantes, which splits into two rami. The posterior rami gives off a posterior cutaneous branch, and anterior rami gives off an anterior cutaneous branch.
    - Each branch enters the intercostal space between the internal and innermost intercostal muscles.
    - Lateral cutaneous branches arise at approximately the midaxillary line, and anterior cutaneous branches arise at the sternum.
- Musculature
    - Muscles of the chest wall aid in respiration and posture stabilization.
    - Primary Muscles of Inspiration
        - Diaphragm
            - Insert on T6-T12 ribs laterally, the xiphoid anteriorly, and L1-L3 intervertebral discs posteriorly.
            - C3, C4, and C5 *keep the diaphragm alive.*
- Intercostals—three layers (external, internal, and innermost). External and internal used within respiration.

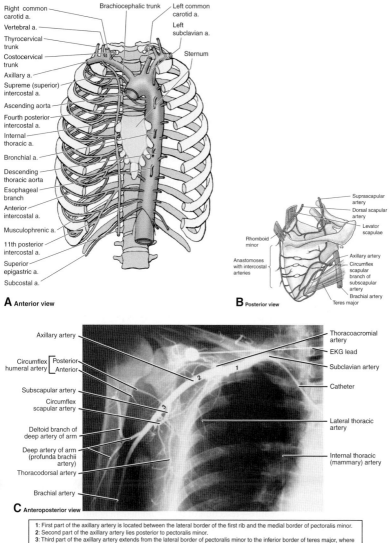

Figure 51-1 Vascular anatomy of the A) Chest wall, B) Posterior shoulder, C) Upper arm (angiogram) (From Dalley AF II, Agur AMR. *Moore's Clinically Oriented Anatomy.* 9th ed. Wolters Kluwer; 2023. Figure 4.19.)

- Secondary Muscles of Inspiration—pectoralis major and minor, scalene, sternocleidomastoid, rectus abdominis, and internal and external oblique
- Posture and Upper Extremity Stabilization—erector spinae, quadratus lumborum, trapezius, latissimus, levator scapulae, supraspinatus, infraspinatus, rhomboid major and minor, and subscapularis

- Physiology
  - ○ Inspiration is an active process with generation of negative intrathoracic pressure → lung inflation.
  - ○ Expiration is passive with creation of positive intrathoracic pressure → lung deflation.
  - ○ Pulmonary function testing (PFTs) can be useful in evaluating chronic pulmonary disease as well as determining physiologic impact of pectus excavatum and carinatum.

EVALUATION AND INITIAL MANAGEMENT

HISTORY

- Past medical history, surgical history, and smoking status is essential to determining the best reconstructive options. Also, ask about cardiac status, history of cardiac surgery, and history of intra-abdominal operations.
- High mortality with defects in the setting of infection, thus adequate understanding of entire clinical picture for patient (history, current medications, labs) is essential.
  - ○ Untreated empyema has a mortality rate of 15%-20%.
  - ○ Bronchopleural fistula has a mortality rate of 18%-67%.
  - ○ Mediastinitis has a mortality rate of 14%-42%.

IMAGING AND STUDIES

- Previous CT imaging should be reviewed to assess patency of internal mammary arteries (IMAs). Consider CT chest to assess for fluid collections, mediastinal widening in setting of possible infection.
- Pulmonary function testing (PFTs) can be useful to assess physiologic impact of structural deformities in pectus excavatum and carinatum.
- There should be a low threshold for consultation to cardiac or thoracic surgery if they are not involved in the care of a patient.
- For infective etiologies, adequate bony resection and source control must be achieved prior to reconstruction.

ETIOLOGY OF CHEST WALL DEFECTS

INFECTION

- **Empyema and Bronchopleural Fistula**
  - ○ Chronic empyema surgical treatments include the following:
    - ■ Clagett procedure—historical three-stage procedure, which included removing the posterolateral ribs, creating a window into the pleural space to drain and irrigate the empyema cavity, and finally closure of the thoracotomy wound.
      - □ Eloesser procedure—resection of the rib immediately inferior to empyema cavity with skin and subcutaneous flap sewn to the pleura. This drains the empyema acts as a one-way valve and allows the lung to expand into the dead space created by the empyema.
      - □ Thoracoplasty—removal of ribs in order to close the dead space.
  - ○ Flaps used to fill intrathoracic dead space and reinforce/bolster fistula repair
- **Deep Sternal Wounds and Mediastinitis**
  - ○ Defined as having one of the following:
    - ■ Positive culture from mediastinal fluid or tissue
    - ■ Evidence of mediastinal widening on imaging
    - ■ Fever, sternal instability, or chest pain with purulent drainage from the chest, mediastinal widening on imaging, or positive blood cultures
  - ○ Average presentation is 14 days post-op, but there are reports of delayed presentations.

- Risk factors for deep sternal wound infection: obesity, IMA harvest, COPD, diabetes, tobacco use
- Adequate bony débridement and removal of infected foreign material such as sternal wires are essential for reconstructive success.
- Once source control is achieved, flap coverage is dependent on the size of the defect.
  - Wounds in the upper sternum are frequently closed with pectoralis flaps.
  - Wounds in the lower sternum and larger wounds are frequently closed with rectus abdominis or omental flaps.
- Risk factors for reconstructive failure: female sex, history of coronary artery bypass graft procedure, IMA harvest, and obesity.

NEOPLASM

- Most common indication for chest wall resection and reconstruction followed by desmoid tumors and bronchopleural fistula.
- Primary chest wall tumors are rare: most commonly breast CA and sarcoma.
- Most common primary tumors are soft tissue.
- Ninety-six percent of sternal primary bone tumors are malignant.
- Desmoid Tumors
  - Benign tumors originating in muscle/fascia (40% in the shoulder or chest wall areas)
  - Aggressive local invasion with high recurrence rate if resected with positive or close margins

IATROGENIC (ie, OSTEORADIONECROSIS)

- *Should have high suspicion for malignancy in chronic radiation wounds; rule out with biopsy
- Common after chest wall radiation in the setting of breast cancer treatment or lymphoma

CONGENITAL

- *Poland syndrome (sequence)
  - Pathophysiology
    - Defective development of a unilateral proximal subclavian artery
    - Right side more common than left 2:1; no difference in prevalence between male and female
  - Clinical characteristics
    - Congenital absence of the sternal head of the pectoralis major muscle that may present with other ipsilateral anomalies such as:
      - *Brachysyndactyly or hypoplasia of ipsilateral extremity
      - Absence of costal cartilages
      - Hypoplasia of breast and subcutaneous tissue that might affect nipple-areolar complex
      - Axillary hair deficiency
  - Related conditions
    - Mobius syndrome (underdeveloped cranial nerves VI and VII)
    - Klippel-Feil syndrome (fusion of cervical vertebrae)
  - Treatment for females
    - General goals: breast symmetry, recreate anterior axillary fold, and provide adequate infraclavicular fullness.
    - Implant vs autogenous tissue-based reconstruction often with latissimus dorsi or combination of latissimus and implant.
    - If implant-based reconstruction used, tissue expander placed until patient's growth has stopped.

- ○ Treatment for males
  - General goals: provide a symmetric chest wall contour
  - Can use latissimus flap or custom-designed tissue expander and implant placed through open or endoscopic techniques
- **Pectus excavatum and carinatum**
  - ○ Excavatum ("funnel chest")
    - Chest wall concavity due to retrodisplaced sternum. Typically in lower one-half to one-third of the sternum.
    - Most common congenital chest wall deformity.
    - Male to female incidence is 4:1.
    - Indications for repair: cosmetic or cardiopulmonary impairment.
    - Surgical options
      - □ Ravitch (classic approach): cartilage resection/detachment and bar placement.
      - □ *Nuss: "turnover" bar is placed providing retrosternal deformation pressure. Optimal age at repair is 10-13 years.
      - □ Fat grafting, implant-based repair to fill defect without changing intrathoracic mechanics.
      - □ Other/nonsurgical: vacuum, magnetic, orthotics.
- **Carinatum ("bird chest")**
  - ○ Chest wall convexity
  - ○ Incidence only 20% of all pectus deformities
  - ○ Associated with scoliosis, familial pectus deformity (any), mitral valve prolapse, and osteogenic syndromes
  - ○ Surgical options: Ravitch; reverse Nuss procedure; orthotics/bracing

TECHNICAL ASPECTS OF RECONSTRUCTION AND MATERIALS

SKELETAL DEFECTS

- *Indications for Skeletal Repair
  - ○ Skeletal injury/resection >5 cm in diameter.
  - ○ Greater than 4-5 ribs with potential flail chest.
  - ○ Goal: avoid flail chest, restore protective structure, maintain physiologic function.
  - ○ Defects <5 cm diameter usually recover well without rigid reconstruction.
  - ○ Radiated chest wall is stiff secondary to fibrosis and many times does not need rigid reconstruction.
- **Autologous Reconstructive Options** (Bone Grafting)
  - ○ Potential donor sites: split rib, iliac crest, and fibula
  - ○ Useful in possibly contaminated cases but cannot cover large defects
  - ○ Drawbacks: flaccidity, prone to infection, poor protective barrier, donor site morbidity
- **Prosthetic Materials**
  - ○ Methyl methacrylate (poly-MMA): exothermic polymer. Inexpensive and customizable with multiple potential complications possible including embolization, burns, difficulty fixing to bone, infection, or erosion.
  - ○ Gore-Tex, Marlex, Vicryl, Prolene, and other available synthetic mesh materials. Prone to infection and can loosen over time.
  - ○ SurgiMend, AlloDerm, and other available biologic mesh materials. More expensive but have less likelihood of becoming infected.

SOFT TISSUE COVERAGE

- **Skin Grafting**—rarely used in isolation but can be performed in conjunction with other flap reconstruction

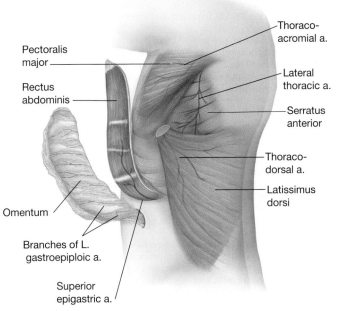

Figure 51-2 Common pedicled flaps for thoracic or abdominal wall reconstruction and their arterial anatomy. (From Thorne CH, ed. *Grabb and Smith's Plastic Surgery*. 7th ed. Lippincott Williams & Wilkins; 2014. Figure 92.7D.)

- ○ Considerations: must have tissue with viable blood supply at base, which will accept graft and cannot be used for exposed bone; will not fill dead space or cavities, poor candidate in irradiated areas
- **Local Reconstructive Options (Fig. 51-2)**
  - ○ The goal for thoracic reconstruction is complete débridement followed by closure and dead space obliteration with well-vascularized tissue (typically muscle flaps).
  - ○ *Pectoralis major flap (Mathes-Nahai type V) is the workhorse for midline upper sternal wound defects.
    - ▪ Dominant blood supply: thoracoacromial vessels (regional artery: subclavian).
    - ▪ Minor blood supply: internal mammary perforators.
    - ▪ Considerations: IMAs must be present to divide thoracoacromial (commonly used in cardiac procedures).
    - ▪ Can be used as an advancement or turnover flap.
  - ○ **Latissimus dorsi flap (Mathes-Nahai type V)**—useful in reconstruction of anterior and posterior defects
    - ▪ Dominant blood supply: thoracodorsal vessels (regional artery: subscapular)
    - ▪ Minor blood supply: posterior intercostal perforators, retrograde flow from the artery serratus (terminal branch of thoracodorsal artery)
  - ○ **Rectus abdominis flap (Mathes-Nahai type III)**—useful in anterior reconstructions as pedicled flap or used as a free flap
    - ▪ Both pedicled and free flap options possible
    - ▪ Common variations: deep inferior epigastric artery perforator flap, superficial inferior epigastric artery flap, transverse rectus abdominis musculocutaneous (TRAM) flap, free TRAM flap, vertical rectus abdominis musculocutaneous flap

- Major blood supply: superior epigastric from the internal mammary and inferior epigastric off of the external iliac
- Considerations
  - For pedicled TRAM flaps, internal mammary artery generally needs to be patent.
  - Can still harvest as a pedicled flap if the IMA on that side has been used for coronary artery bypass graft, by basing blood supply on the highest intercostal to the rectus muscle, though this can be unreliable.
  - Should know any history of major abdominal surgery that could compromise blood supply.
  - High donor site morbidity and complications.
- **Trapezius flap (Mathes-Nahai type II)**
  - Muscle or musculocutaneous can reconstruct superior aspect of the chest wall with pivot at posterior base of the neck.
  - Dominant blood supply: transverse cervical vessels (off thyrocervical trunk [80%]) or subclavian artery (20%)
  - Minor blood supply: posterior intercostal perforators and occipital vessels
- **Parascapular flap (fasciocutaneous flap, Mathes-Nahai type B)**
  - Useful in reconstruction of the shoulder, axilla, and lateral chest
  - Dominant blood supply: circumflex scapular a. (with venae comitantes)
  - Pivot point at vascular pedicle in the triangular space
  - Can be incorporated into chimeric flap with latissimus
- **Serratus anterior flap (Mathes-Nahai type III)**
  - Dominant blood supplies: lateral thoracic a. and thoracodorsal a.
  - Can be used as muscle, musculocutaneous, or fascial flap
  - Cannot take entire muscle or winged scapula will result
  - Useful in filling intrathoracic cavities
- **External oblique flap (Mathes-Nahai type IV)**
  - Dominant blood supply: posterior intercostal vessels
  - Useful in lower one-third chest wall defects in which the latissimus/rectus may be compromised by previous radiation or surgery
- **Omental flap (Mathes-Nahai type III)**
  - Salvage option that can provide coverage for large defects
  - Dominant blood supplies: right and left gastroepiploic vessels
  - Can be harvested laproscopically or with a laparotomy
  - Tunnel necessary through costal margin or diaphragm usually
  - Need to ensure no history of significant abdominal surgery or use of omental flap in previous cardiothoracic procedures
  - Pivot on right: first portion of the duodenum
  - Pivot on left: splenocolic ligament
- Free Flap Considerations
  - Aids in decision-making tree when vascular supply may be compromised and increased freedom in flap positioning
  - Can include rectus abdominis, ALT, latissimus, chimeric flaps

PEARLS

1. Bony reconstruction is recommended for chest wall resection >5 cm in diameter or >4-5 ribs, in a nonradiated field (radiation stiffens chest wall and lessens need for bony reconstruction).
2. Soft tissue reconstruction should not only provide coverage but also fill dead space.
3. An understanding of a patient's surgical history, specifically previous cardiac and abdominal surgery, is critical to determining available reconstructive options.
4. Poland's syndrome can be associated with multiple additional congenital anomalies, most commonly ipsilateral upper extremity anomalies (brachysyndactyly).

Recommended Readings

1. Althubaiti G, Butler CE. Abdominal wall and chest wall reconstruction. *Plast Reconst Surg.* 2014;133(5):688e-701e.
2. Isaac KV, Elzinga K, Buchel EW. The best of chest wall reconstruction: principles and clinical application for complex oncologic and sternal defects. *Plast Reconst Surg.* 2022;149(3): 547e-562e.
3. Jones G, Jurkiewicz MJ, Bostwick J, et al. Management of the infected median sternotomy wound with muscle flaps. 4. 4. The Emory 20-year experience. *Ann Surg.* 1997;225(6):766-776; discussion 776-778. doi:10.1097/00000658-199706000-00014

52 Abdominal Reconstruction

Brigit Baglien

OVERVIEW

ANATOMY AND PHYSIOLOGY

- The Anterior Abdominal Wall
  - Layers lateral to the linea semilunaris
    - Skin
    - Subcutaneous tissue/Camper fascia
    - Scarpa fascia
    - External oblique muscle: fibers course superolateral to inferomedial
    - Internal oblique muscle: fibers course inferolateral to superomedial
    - Transversus abdominis muscle: fibers course horizontally
    - Transversalis fascia
    - Peritoneum
  - Central abdomen
    - Paired rectus muscles
    - Linea alba: midline fusion of anterior and posterior rectus sheaths
    - Linea semilunaris: convergence of deep fascia lateral to rectus muscles bilaterally
  - **The rectus sheath and the arcuate line of Douglas**
    - Rectus sheath above the arcuate line
      - Anterior: external oblique and the anterior leaf of the internal oblique aponeuroses
      - Posterior: posterior leaf of the internal oblique aponeurosis, transversus abdominis, and transversalis fascia
    - Rectus sheath below the arcuate line
      - Anterior: external and internal oblique aponeuroses and transversus abdominis muscle
      - Posterior: transversalis fascia
- Arterial Supply of the Abdominal Wall (**Fig. 52-1;** also **see Chapter 64: Liposuction, Panniculectomy and Abdominoplasty** for cutaneous blood supply categorized by Huger zones)
- Innervation of the Abdominal Wall
  - Via ventral rami of T7-T12 running between internal oblique and transversus abdominis

FORM AND FUNCTION

- Protection: vital organs of the abdomen.
- Forces: the abdomen is under cylindrical forces with the inward abdominal wall and diaphragm pressures equilibrating with outward intraperitoneal pressures.
- Physiology: abdominal strength derived from tendinous connections and soft tissue.
  - Valsalva: used to brace body and increase intraperitoneal pressure
  - Herniation: results in pressure outlet and inability to effectively control abdominal pressure with Valsalva forces

---

*Denotes common in-service examination topics.

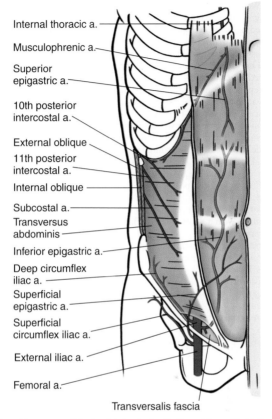

Internal thoracic a.

Musculophrenic a.

Superior epigastric a.

10th posterior intercostal a.

External oblique

11th posterior intercostal a.

Internal oblique

Subcostal a.

Transversus abdominis

Inferior epigastric a.

Deep circumflex iliac a.

Superficial epigastric a.

Superficial circumflex iliac a.

External iliac a.

Femoral a.

Transversalis fascia

Figure 52-1 Arterial anatomy of the hemiabdominal wall. (From Moore KL, Dalley AF, Agur AM. *Clinically Oriented Anatomy*. 6th ed. Lippincott Williams & Wilkins; 2010. Figure 5.4A.)

- **Goals of Reconstruction**
  - Protection for the abdominal viscera
  - Prevention of fluid losses
  - Fascial support
  - Aesthetics
  - Restore normal abdominal counterpressure forces and cylinder continuity; thus restoring proper muscle function and trunk mechanics
  - Minimize risk of hernia recurrence

ETIOLOGY OF ABDOMINAL WALL DEFECTS

- **Congenital**
  - **Gastroschisis**
    - Midline full-thickness umbilical defect with eviscerated bowel
    - Failure of midline mesoderm embryologically
  - **Omphalocele**
    - Periumbilical partial-thickness defect with sac of amnion and peritoneum enveloping abdominal viscera
    - Associated with chromosomal abnormalities including trisomies 18, 13, and 21; Turner syndrome; and triploidy

- Beckwith-Weidman syndrome
  - Sporadic syndrome related to mutations on chromosome 11, characterized by increased tissue growth (large features—tongue, gigantism, hemihypertrophy), ear pits, nevus flammeus, increased cancer risk, and midline abdominal defects.
  - Diastasis recti, umbilical hernia, or omphalocele may occur.
- Congenital umbilical/inguinal hernias
  - Most pediatric surgeons recommend repair of inguinal hernia.
  - Delay repair of congenital umbilical hernias until 4 to 5 years of age with conservative observation, as many resolve spontaneously.
- **Surgical Dehiscence/Incisional Hernia**
  - **A separation of the layers of a wound following previous abdominal surgery.** May be partial, superficial, or complete with separation of all layers and full interruption. Complete dehiscence of an abdominal wound may lead to evisceration (see section "Technical Aspects of Soft Tissue Reconstruction and Materials").
  - Risk factors: Increased age, obesity, genetic predisposition, smoking, diabetes, infection, fluid collection, postoperative trauma, or technical error.
- **Diastasis Recti**
  - **Spreading of the linea alba** resulting in widening of parallel rectus muscles.
  - Do not confuse with a ventral hernia. There is no palpable fascial edge with rectus diastasis.
  - May be amenable to physical therapy, fascial plication but typically does not require surgical intervention.
- **Full-Thickness Tissue Loss**
  - Tumor resection
  - Necrotizing soft tissue infection
  - Trauma
  - May require serial débridement prior to definitive reconstruction

SURGICAL MANAGEMENT OF ABDOMINAL WALL DEFECTS

- **Planning for Abdominal Reconstruction**
  - Optimize nutrition status.
  - Ensure that comorbid conditions are under control.
  - Treat inflammation/infection.
  - Examine exposed viscera (is exposed bowel "frozen" or free).
  - Assess defect size.
  - Ask about prior reconstruction including presence of mesh.
- **Evisceration**
  - Principles
    - Pristine wounds may be closed primarily (rare).
    - Delay definitive closure until wound is decontaminated.
    - Avoid wet-to-dry or other debriding dressings on bowel.
    - Vacuum assist devices effective for swelling (not used in grossly contaminated, infected, or malignant wounds).
  - Large wound with exposed viscera may need to be closed with skin grafting directly on bowel if long delays to closure occur; can be performed after granulation tissue present on bowel.
  - Fistula management: tube drainage, grafting, closure after 3-6 months.

MIDLINE ABDOMINAL HERNIATION

- **Direct repair:** reserved for defects <3 cm or with easily opposable edges
- **Repair with mesh:** hernias >3 cm may be amenable to laparoscopic vs open repair with mesh. Allow additional 3 cm of overlap of mesh and posterior rectus sheath
  - *Mesh placement: lower recurrence rates found with retro-rectus and underlay placement

- **Onlay:** mesh secured superficial to abdominal wall repair.
- **Inlay:** mesh sewn to margins of defect without fascial reapproximation, inferior in terms of recurrence rates.
- **Retro-rectus:** mesh is placed posterior to the rectus muscles and anterior to posterior rectus sheath.
- **Underlay:** mesh is placed anterior to the peritoneum and posterior to the rectus sheath.
  - **Synthetic mesh:** generally used for clean cases; lower cost, increased risk of bowel adhesion
    - **Polypropylene** (Prolene, Marlex): highly porous, good incorporation; common. May be paired with polytetrafluoroethylene (PTFE), with Gore-Tex layer on bowel contact surface
    - **PTFE** (Gore-Tex, polytetrafluoroethylene): smooth, nonporous; lower foreign body reaction, low bowel adherence, and low fistula rates. Low adhesion/incorporation to body wall
    - **Polyester** (Mersilene, Dacron): persistent chronic inflammation at prosthetic interface
    - **Polygalactin** (Vicryl): satisfactory in contaminated wounds, but only as a temporary solution, since it is biodegradable
  - **Biologic mesh:** increased resistance to infection, used in contaminated fields, increased cost, reabsorbs and remodels over time
    - **Human dermis** (AlloDerm, AlloMax, FlexHD): differences in sterilization techniques; very few indications to use in abdominal ventral hernia repair due to high recurrence and infection rates; may be placed intraperitoneally or as adjunct to alloplastic repair or separation of parts
    - **Porcine dermis** (Permacol, Strattice, Collamend, XenMatrix): may be a good alternative in contaminated fields, with low overall recurrence rates (0%-15%), variable cross-linkage (ie, Permacol has chemically cross-linked diisocyanate bonds)
- **Separation of Parts (SOP;** also referred to as "component release" or "component separation": midline advancement of innervated rectus muscle to achieve complete fascial closure; **Fig. 52-2)**
  - **Anterior components separation**
    - Division of external oblique aponeurosis from costal margin to near inguinal ligament from semilunar line.
    - Blunt separation of external oblique from internal oblique to allow for movement medially.
    - Cut posterior rectus sheath unilaterally vs bilaterally if additional length is needed.
    - *Bilateral SOP can allow movement of:
      - *Superior abdomen: 10 cm
      - *Umbilicus: 20 cm
      - *Inferior abdomen: 6 cm
    - If open approach, preservation of periumbilical perforators decreases skin loss.
    - Can use of endoscopic techniques improve visualization and decrease dissection.
    - Can be augmented with the use of mesh underlay.
  - **Posterior components separation, transversus abdominis release**
    - Release transversus abdominis muscle medial to linea semilunaris
    - Plane developed between transversus abdominis and transversalis fascia laterally to allow anterior and posterior rectus sheath reapproximation at midline
    - Sublay mesh placed between rectus muscle and posterior sheath
    - Increased mobility while preserving innervation to the rectus muscle

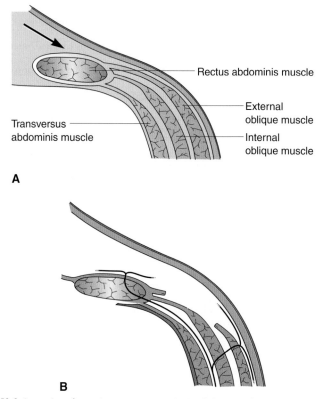

Figure 52-2 Separation of parts (component separation) technique. A. The anterior rectus sheath is often accessed through a vertical midline abdominal incision. **B.** The external oblique fascia is divided at the semilunar line. Note that the nerve supply to the abdominal wall musculature is preserved. (From Dimick JB. *Mulholland & Greenfield's Surgery.* 7th ed. Wolters Kluwer; 2022. Figure 72.37.)

RECONSTRUCTION WITH AUTOGENOUS TISSUE

- Skin and subcutaneous defects 5-15 cm: local advancement or split-thickness skin graft (STSG)
- Defects >15 cm: local random flaps, axial skin flaps, regional pedicled flaps
  - ○ Tissue expansion may be considered as an adjunct after STSG.
  - ○ Regional pedicled flap options (**see Table 52-1**).
- Musculofascial or complete defect: free flap
  - ○ Nonfunctional free flap reconstruction
    - ▪ When both rectus abdominis muscles are intact and functional
    - ▪ Options: ALT, tensor fasciae latae, latissimus dorsi, gracilis
  - ○ Functional free flap reconstruction
    - ▪ When motor function of the anterior abdominal wall is severely impaired, such as when both rectus abdominis are missing, or when one oblique muscle and the ipsilateral rectus muscle are missing
    - ▪ Options: innervated chimeric ALT, rectus femoris, tensor fasciae latae

TABLE 52-1 Common Pedicled Flaps Used in Abdominal Wall Reconstruction

Flap	Flap type	Type	Pedicle	Size (cm)
Tensor fascia lata	Musculocutaneous	Upper, middle, lower 1/3	Ascending branch of lateral circumflex femoral artery	15 × 5
Latissimus dorsi	Musculocutaneous	Upper 1/3	Thoracodorsal artery	25 × 35
Rectus femoris	Musculocutaneous	Middle, lower 1/3	Descending branch of lateral femoral circumflex artery	20 × 8
ALT	Fasciocutaneous	Middle and lower 1/3	Descending branch of lateral circumflex femoral artery	18 × 25
Vastus lateralis	Musculocutaneous	Lower 1/3	Lateral femoral circumflex artery	10 × 26
Gracilis	Musculocutaneous	Lower 1/3	Medial femoral circumflex artery	6 × 24

ABDOMINAL WALL TRANSPLANT

- Rigorous patient selection process including exhaustion of all other options and concurrent other organ transplantation given requirment of lifelong immunosuppression
- Full-thickness abdominal wall composite allotransplantation based on iliac or inferior epigastric vessels
- Remains a cutting-edge reconstructive technique requiring advanced care and multidisciplinary teams

COMPLICATIONS

- Intra-abdominal hypertension and abdominal compartment syndrome
  - Tense abdomen, increasing pain, decrease venous return, decreased cardiac output, increase ventilatory pressures
  - Bladder pressure > 20 mm Hg
  - Treatment: emergent decompressive laparotomy
- Hematoma
- Seroma
- Infection

PEARLS

1. Delay definitive closure in cases of excessive contamination. May require temporizing measures such as vacuum-assist devices.
2. Anterior component separation can gain 10, 20, and 6 cm of advancement in the superior, middle, and inferior thirds of the abdominal wall, respectively.
3. Understand healing aspects and applications of biologic and synthetic mesh.
4. Understand the difference between ventral hernia and diastasis recti.
5. Hernia recurrence rates are lowest when primary fascial closure of the abdominal wall is reinforced with underlay mesh placement.

QUESTIONS YOU WILL BE ASKED

1. What muscles of the abdomen are divided in a posterior SOP technique?
   The transversus abdominis medial to linea semilunaris allowing medialization of the posterior rectus sheath-transversalis fascia complex.
2. What layers of the abdomen are separated in a ventral hernia repair using anterior SOP technique?
   The external and internal oblique laterally allowing medialization of the rectus abdominis.
3. What is blood supply to the abdomen?
   Midabdomen: deep epigastric arcade *(zone I)*; lower abdomen: external iliac artery *(zone II)*; and the lateral abdomen: intercostal, subcostal, and lumbar arteries *(zone III)*.
4. What muscles do the nerves innervating the rectus abdominis travel between?
   Internal oblique and transversus abdominis.
5. How large of a hernia defect can be closed with an anterior component separation closure?
   Unilateral: 5 cm in the epigastric region, 10 cm at the umbilicus, and 3 cm in the suprapubic region.

Recommended Readings
1. Lak KL, Goldblatt MI. Mesh selection in abdominal wall reconstruction. *Plast Reconstr Surg.* 2018;142(3S):99-106.
2. Novistsky YW, Elliott HL, Orenstein SB, Rosen MJ. Transversus abdominis muscle release: a novel approach to posterior component separation during complex abdominal wall reconstruction. *Am J Surg.* 2012;204(5):709-716.
3. Patel NG, Ratanshi I, Buchel EW. The best of abdominal wall reconstruction. *Plast Reconstr Surg.* 2018;141(1):113e-136e.
4. Ramirez OM, Ruas E, Dellon AL. "Components separation" method for closure of abdominal-wall defects: an anatomic and clinical study. *Plast Reconstr Surg.* 1990;86(3):519-526.

53 Perineal, Penile, and Vaginal Reconstruction

Kyle R. Latack and Widya Adidharma

OVERVIEW

DEVELOPMENT

- Structures are derived from
  - Mesoderm (wolffian/müllerian ducts)
  - Endoderm (cloaca, membrane)
  - Ectoderm (external genitalia)
- Wolffian Ducts: epididymis, vas deferens, and seminal vesicles
- Müllerian Ducts: fallopian tubes, uterus, and upper two-third of vagina
- Gonads begin as ridges, differentiate after 6 weeks
- Male Differentiation
  - H-Y antigen on Y chromosome initiates gonadal differentiation into testes.
  - Testes contain Sertoli cells and Leydig cells.
  - Müllerian inhibiting substance (MIS) secreted from Sertoli cells in testes causes regression of müllerian ducts.
  - Leydig cells produce testosterone analog → development of wolffian ducts.
  - Dihydrotestosterone → virilization of external genitalia.
- Female Differentiation
  - Female differentiation is the default.
  - No H-Y antigen → gonads become ovaries, no MIS and müllerian ducts develop.

ANATOMY

- Male
  - **Penis:** superficial to deep (**Fig. 53-1**)
    - Skin
    - Dartos (superficial) fascia
    - Buck (deep) fascia
    - Neurovascular bundle: deep dorsal vein, paired dorsal artery, and dorsal penile nerves
    - Tunica albuginea (surrounds each corpora individually)
    - Erectile tissue: paired corpora cavernosa, corpora spongiosum surrounds urethra
  - **Arterial supply:** internal pudendal artery branches into
    - Perineal artery to perineum and scrotum.
    - Common penile artery branches to bulbourethral artery, dorsal artery, and deep cavernosal artery.
  - **Nerve supply:** sensory via the dorsal nerves.
    - These nerves travel with the dorsal arteries.
    - Originate from sacral nerves and travel via pudendal nerve.
    - Cavernous nerve supplies sympathetic and parasympathetic innervation, which arises from the pelvic plexus.
  - **Urethral divisions**
    - Posterior: proximal to the bulb (prostatic and membranous portions)

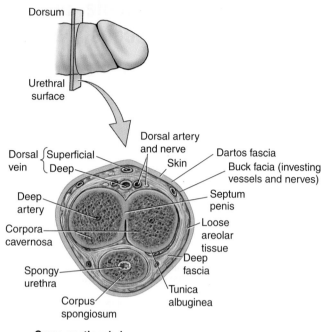

Cross-sectional view

Figure 53-1 Cross-sectional anatomy of the penis. (From Agur AMR, Dalley AF, eds. *Grant's Atlas of Anatomy*. 15th ed. Wolters Kluwer; 2021. Figure 5.56C.)

- Anterior: distal to bulb; contained within corpus spongiosum (bulbar and penile/pendulous portions, fossa navicularis)
- **Female (Fig. 53-2)**
  - **Vulva**
    - Female external genitalia found on the anterior perineal triangle.
    - Vulva contains numerus apocrine sweat glands, which can become chronically infected in hidradenitis suppurativa.
    - Mons: hair-bearing skin over a cushion of adipose on the pubic bone.
    - Labia majora
      - Extend posteriorly from mons
      - Composed of similar hair-bearing skin and adipose tissue
    - Labia minora
      - Hairless skin folds
      - Each splits anteriorly to run over and under glans of clitoris
      - No underlying adipose but rather connective tissue
      - In dermatologic diseases such as lichen sclerosis, can significantly atrophy or disappear
    - Innervation: pudendal nerve
      - Terminal branches: dorsal nerve of the clitoris, perineal nerve, and inferior anal nerve.
      - Inferior hypogastric plexus also provides cavernous nerve fibers that are critical to sexual function as well as voiding.

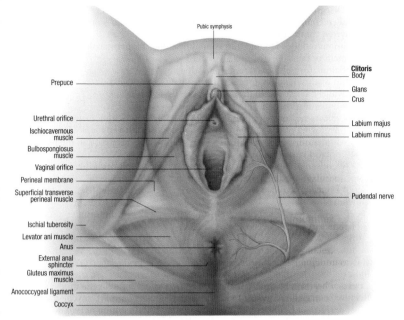

Figure 53-2 Female anatomy. (Asset provided by Anatomical Chart Co.)

- ○ **Pelvic viscera**
  - ▪ Vagina
    - □ Three layers: nonkeratinized squamous epithelium that lines the lumen, then muscular layer, and an outer adventitial layer
  - ▪ Seven potential or avascular spaces in the pelvis: retropubic, vesicovaginal, paravesical (bilateral), rectovaginal, and pararectal space bilaterally.
  - ▪ Blood supply: descending branch of uterine artery and the vaginal artery, which is a branch from the internal iliac artery. There is also flow from the middle rectal artery (posteriorly) and the pudendal artery distally.

PENILE AND SCROTAL RECONSTRUCTION

PENILE RECONSTRUCTION

- **Goals of Reconstruction**
  - ○ Sufficient length and adequate skin for unrestricted erections
  - ○ Protective sensation to prevent chronic skin breakdown
  - ○ Ability to spontaneously void standing up
  - ○ Erectile function
- **Defects of Penile Surface**
  - ○ Can occur due to SCC of shaft, glans, or traumatic injury
  - ○ Split-thickness skin graft (STSG) or full-thickness skin graft (FTSG) is viable option.
  - ○ Urethral exposure requires more durable coverage with local flap.

- **Peyronie Disease:** 1% males age 40-60 years
  - **Painful erections, chordee curvature, firm nodules or plaques** on shaft, 10% have Dupuytren contracture
  - **Evaluation:** requires Doppler ultrasound of induced (pharmacologic) erection
  - **Treatment options**
    - Inflammatory phase: vitamin E may help
    - Mild disease/sexually functional: treatment discouraged
    - Advanced disease/sexually disabled
      - Implant prosthesis if impotent.
      - Plication procedure (mild curve, 30°-45°): circumcising incision with degloving of shaft. Tunica albuginea opposite area of maximal curvature is identified and an ellipse excised. This will slightly shorten the penis but correct curvature.
      - Excision/dermal graft (curves >45°): excise plaques and use defatted dermal graft for patch.
      - Erections avoided for 6 weeks; full recovery takes months.
  - **Outcomes**
    - 10%-15% rate of impotence postop: venous leak phenomenon vs psychogenic
    - 85% successful (straight penis, spontaneous erections, and successful intercourse)
- **Penis Replantation**
  - Indicated for sharp, nonavulsive injuries.
  - **Contraindications:** gross contamination, extended warm ischemia time >8 hours.
  - **Relative contraindication:** self-mutilating injury and uncontrolled psychiatric disease.
  - Must perform debridement of nonviable tissue, and dissection of two dorsal arteries, two dorsal veins, and two dorsal nerves for anastomosis.
  - Spatulated urethral repair over Foley catheter.
  - Direct repair of tunica albuginea or corporal bodies.
  - **End to end anastomoses of dorsal arteries and veins**
  - Close Buck fascia and skin
  - Dressings must be supportive, Foley × 2-3 weeks to prevent urethral stricture.
- Reconstructive options
  - **Radial forearm flap:** most common method for reconstruction. Fasciocutaneous flap vascularized by the radial artery and contains forearm fascia and skin. Harvested from nondominant forearm. Ensure adequate blood supply via Allen test.
    - Disadvantages of this type of flap include forearm donor site deformity (can be reconstructed), development of cold intolerance of donor side hand, and forearm grows hair. Recipient vessels include deep inferior epigastric vessels.
  - **Anterolateral thigh:** common alternative site especially in gender affirming phalloplasty. Blood supplied by lateral femoral circumflex vessels and innervation from lateral femoral cutaneous nerve.

SCROTAL RECONSTRUCTION

- **Fournier Gangrene:** necrotizing fasciitis of the perineum
  - Higher incidence in immunosuppressed and those with diabetes.
  - Mixed aerobic/anaerobic bacteria.
  - Fournier gangrene is a surgical emergency. Surgical debridement is necessary to control infection.
  - Testes are often spared of direct infection secondary to independent blood supply and lymphatic drainage.
  - Initial management can be wet to dry dressings between serial debridement, which are typically required until infection is under control.
  - Scrotal defect—STSG over testes, which are sutured together in midline, meshed graft. Medial thigh pockets are a temporary option as higher temperature will alter sperm production.

MALE PERINEAL DEFECTS

- Most commonly encountered secondary to cancer resection.
- Patients s/p XRT have high risk of delayed wound healing and fistulas.
- **Flap Options**
  - **Vertical rectus abdominis musculocutaneous flap** (VRAM): obliquely oriented skin paddle may give more length to traverse the very long and narrow male pelvis. Be cautious with patients requiring lifelong ostomies (s/p abdominopelvic resection for rectal cancer).
  - **Pedicled anterolateral thigh flap** (ALT): flaps based on descending branch of lateral circumflex femoral artery: tunnel under sartorius and rectus femoris.
  - **Bilateral gracilis:** myocutaneous or muscle only flaps with primary closure over the flap or STSG.
  - **Bilateral posterior thigh flaps.**
  - **Singapore flap.**

VAGINAL RECONSTRUCTION

- **Goals**
  - **Sufficient depth** of vaginal wall.
  - **Adequate transverse dimension** of introitus and pouch for intercourse.
  - **Consider pelvic floor physical therapy** for all reconstruction patients.

CONGENITAL ABSENCE

- **MRKH (Mayer-Rokitanski-Kuster-Hauser syndrome)**
  - 1/4000-1/80 000 live births
  - Maldevelopment of müllerian duct system (upper vagina, uterus, fallopian tubes).
  - Patients are 46XX with normal ovaries, rudimentary uterus, and female external genitalia. Typical female hormone profile. However, patients may often have active endometrium in uterine remnants (ie, uterine horns).
  - Often present with primary amenorrhea.
  - Vaginal atresia and absent cervix noted on examination.
  - Associated with rib and vertebral anomalies, 25%-50% with renal duplications, agenesis, and ectopy.
  - Need intravenous pyelogram and renal ultrasound prior to surgical intervention.
  - Child bearing is possible with surrogate and *in vitro* fertilization.
  - Timing of procedure—14-20 years old, start with dilation.
  - **Treatment options**
    - **Serial dilation:** can be very successful in motivated patients, requires daily dilation either with manual dilators or with manufactured seats. Requires continued therapy (usually 2-3×/daily) after successful vaginal creation
      - **Complications:** recurrent urinary tract infections and stress urinary incontinence
    - **Abbe-McIndoe technique**
      - Blind pouch dissected in areolar space between urethra and rectum, STSG harvested, and placed over obturator.
      - Obturator removed at 7 days and dilation started at 14 days.
      - Majority of patients report satisfactory sexual relationships postop.
      - PAP smears recommended in future to monitor for graft conversion to SCC.
      - Complications: around 14% and include injury to nearby structures (bladder or rectum), vaginal stenosis (9.3%), lack of lubricant, vaginal hair growth, and rejection of graft (9.3%).
    - **Vecchietti procedure**
      - Placement of "olive" at perineum and advanced through vaginal space and into abdominal cavity
      - Requires several day hospitalization with analgesia

- ▫ Complications: perforation of nearby organs, stress incontinence, vaginal prolapse
  - **Sadove and Horton:** FTSG into dissected blind pouch, advantage over STSG is that it may grow with patient if she is still young.
  - **Fasciocutaneous flaps** (ie, Singapore flaps)
    - ▫ Based on terminal branches of internal pudendal a. (posterior labial a.)
    - ▫ Hairless skin just lateral to labia is used, 15 cm × 6 cm may be harvested.
    - ▫ Sensate flap: posterior labial branches of pudendal nerve and perineal branches of posterior cutaneous nerve of thigh.
    - ▫ Not typically performed as it alters external anatomy in young patients.
  - **Colonic/small bowel interpositions:** salvage procedure, associated with persistent foul-smelling secretions, requires laparotomy, friable mucosa bleeds with intercourse.
    - ▫ Complications: 16%-26% overall. Organ prolapse (3%-8%), stenosis (14%).
  - **Davydov (sliding peritoneal flap):**
    - ▫ Initial approach similar to McIndoe until vaginal peritoneum is encountered. Pulled through into abdomen laparoscopically. Avoid in those with suspected endometriosis or adhesions.
    - ▫ Complications: bladder/bowel injury (7%), fistula (3.6%), vaginal stenosis (14.3%).
- Other causes of congenital absence of the vagina
- Transverse vaginal septum, androgen insensitivity syndrome, and 17α-hydroxylase deficiency.

ACQUIRED DEFECTS

ACQUIRED ABSENCE OF THE VULVA

- Most commonly secondary to resection of SCC or melanoma.
- Reconstructive options.
  - ○ **Rhomboid flaps** and laterally based advancement flaps excellent options.
  - ○ **Skin grafts for large defects** (FTSG from lower abdomen, closed primarily) require a bolster for 7 days. Postop Foley and constipating medications improve graft take.
  - ○ **Superficial external pudendal artery (SEPA) flap**
    - More reliable anatomy than superficial inferior epigastric artery (SIEA) flap.
    - Small skin territory is OK for unilateral vulva reconstruction.
  - ○ **Gracilis myocutaneous V-Y advancement flap**

ACQUIRED ABSENCE OF THE VULVA

- Most commonly result of resection of urologic, gynecologic, and GI malignancies.
- Prior radiation therapy is indication for flap at the time of resection though increases risk of complications.
- Be cautious using abdominal-based flaps when patient has diverting ostomy.
- Try to avoid circumferential incision at introitus—will stricture with time.
- **Flap options**
  - ○ **VRAM (Fig. 53-3)**
    - Skin paddle can provide epidermis for perineum and posterior vaginal wall.
    - Rolled VRAM can reconstruct circumferential vaginal defect and is the treatment of choice for total absence of the vagina.
    - Based on deep inferior epigastric artery and vein.
    - Thought to have better outcomes and less complications than other types of flaps.
  - ○ **Pedicled ALT**
    - Excellent option with favorable donor site, best in thin patients
    - Based on descending branch of lateral femoral circumflex

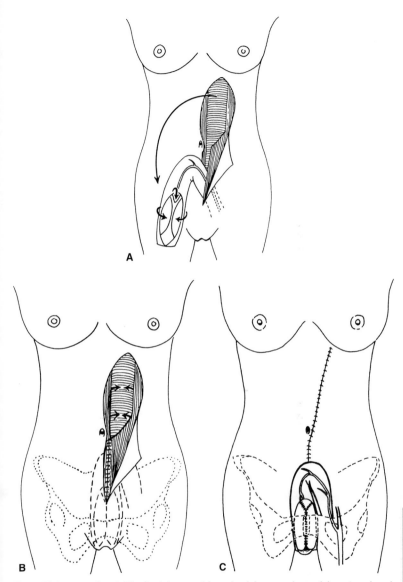

Figure 53-3 VRAM flap. A. The flap is harvested from the abdomen and turned down into the pelvis on its pedicle. **B.** The abdominal fascia is repaired. **C.** The flap is inset at the recipient site. (From Tobin GR, Persell SH, Day TG. Refinements in vaginal reconstruction using rectus abdominis flaps. *Clin Plast Surg.* 1990;17(4):705-712.)

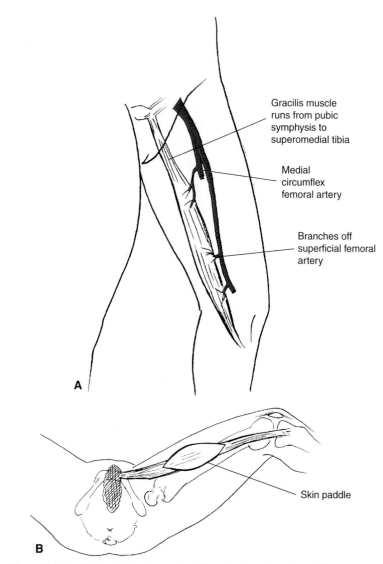

Gracilis muscle runs from pubic symphysis to superomedial tibia

Medial circumflex femoral artery

Branches off superficial femoral artery

A

Skin paddle

B

Figure 53-4 Gracilis flap. A. Vascular supply. **B.** Example of overlying skin paddle design. Innervation is from obturator nerve. (From Friedman J, Dinh T, Potochny J. Reconstruction of the perineum. *Semin Surg Oncol.* 2000;19:282. Figure 4, with permission.)

- **Bilateral gracilis flaps**
  - □ Minimal donor site morbidity but with temperamental skin paddle, may require STSG
  - □ Based on medial circumflex femoral (**Fig. 53-4**)
- **Posterior thigh flaps** (**Fig. 53-5**): may have difficulty reaching vaginal defect
- **Singapore (pudendal thigh) flaps** (**Fig. 53-6**): May be difficult to contour if patient is previously radiated

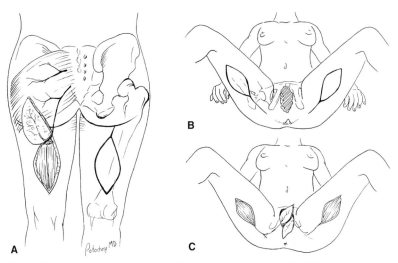

Figure 53-5 Posterior thigh flaps (steps A-C shown). (From Friedman J, Dinh T, Potochny J. Reconstruction of the perineum. *Semin Surg Oncol.* 2000;19:282. Figure 5, with permission.)

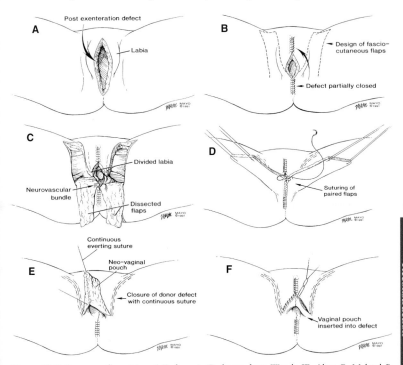

Figure 53-6 Singapore flaps (steps A-F shown). (Redrawn from Woods JE, Alter G, Meland B, et al. Experience with vaginal reconstruction utilizing the modified Singapore flap. *Plast Reconstr Surg.* 1992;90:280 and Strauch B, Vasconez LO, Hall-Findlay E. *Grabb's Encyclopedia of Flaps.* JB Lippincott; 1998:1477.)

○ Simplified algorithm
  ▪ Partial defect: involving vaginal walls but not circumferential
    □ Anterior or lateral wall: Singapore flap
    □ Posterior: rectus flap
  ▪ Circumferential defect
    □ Upper two-thirds: rolled rectus flap

Total circumferential: bilateral gracilis flaps

LABIAPLASTY

- **Surgical reduction of labia minora** for functional and/or aesthetic reasons. Often in cases where labia minora extend past labia majora and cause dyspareunia, pain, or discomfort wearing clothing.
- Causes of Labial Hypertrophy
  ○ Most are congenital
  ○ Acquired causes: exogenous androgenic hormones in infancy, sensitivity to topical estrogen, stretching of the labia, vulvar lymphedema, myelodysplastic diseases
- Franco Classification System for Labial Hypertrophy
  ○ Stage I: <2 cm
  ○ Stage II: 2-4 cm
  ○ Stage III: 4-6 cm
  ○ Stage IV: >6 cm
- Surgical techniques
  ○ **De-epithelialization:** preserves the natural border of the labia minora but may not be suited for patients with a wider labia.
  ○ **Direct distal trimming:** simple technique but removes the natural contour, texture, and color of the free edge of the labia minora.
  ○ **Wedge resection:** preserves the natural shape and color of the free edge of the labia minora, but there may be an abrupt transition in color at the scar.
  ○ **Composite reduction:** reduces labia minora and addresses clitoral hooding.
- Complications: hypoesthesia and paresthesia due to innervation. Some thought that there is increased innervation in distal labia compared to proximal. Must take care to avoid dorsal nerve of the clitoris.

PEARLS

1. In patients who require an ostomy, be cautious about using VRAM flaps. Abdominal wall integrity is important to prevent parastomal hernias.
2. Beware of local tissue rearrangement or Singapore flaps to close a previously irradiated perineum. These tissues will have also been irradiated. The tissues may be difficult to move into defect and will have a high rate of delayed wound healing and breakdown.

QUESTIONS YOU WILL BE ASKED

1. What is the path of the pedicled ALT in perineum reconstruction?
   The flap must be tunneled under the rectus femoris and sartorius muscles.
2. Where are your ALT flap perforators of the descending branch of lateral femoral circumflex artery?
   Located within 3 cm of midpoint on axis from anterior superior iliac spine to lateral aspect of patella.

3. What is unique about the blood supply to the penis?

   The glans and the shaft have separate blood supplies. The skin of the shaft is supplied by a dermal plexus while the dorsal artery supplies the glans. This allows these structures to remain viable after they are divided to create vaginal lining and neoclitoris in gender reassignment surgery.

4. Describe the layers of the penis.

   See **Figure 53-1**.

Recommended Readings

1. Cordeiro PG, Pusic AL, Disa JJ. A classification system and reconstructive algorithm for acquired vaginal defects. *Plast Reconstr Surg*. 2002;110(4):1058-1065.
2. Hoffman BL, Schorge JO, Halvorson LM, Hamid CA, Corton MM, Schaffer JI, eds. *Williams Gynecology*. 4th ed. McGraw Hill; 2020.
3. Hollenbeck ST, Toranto JD, Taylor BJ, et al. Perineal and lower extremity reconstruction. *Plast Reconstr Surg*. 2011;128(5):551e-563e.
4. Monstrey S, Hoebeke P, Selvaggi G, et al. Penile reconstruction: is the radial forearm flap really the standard technique? *Plast Reconstr Surg*. 2009;124(2):510-518.
5. Wong S, Garvey P, Skibber J, Yu P. Reconstruction of pelvic exenteration defects with anterolateral thigh-vastus lateralis muscle flaps. *Plast Reconstr Surg*. 2009;124(4):1177-1185.

54

Gender-Affirming Pelvic Surgery

Caleb Haley

OVERVIEW

DEFINITIONS

- Gender Identity: personal sense of one's gender
- Transgender: a person whose gender identity differs from their sex assigned at birth
- Gender Dysphoria: distress due to discrepancy between a person's gender identity and sex
- Transmale: a person who was assigned female at birth but whose gender identity is male
- Transfemale: a person who was assigned male at birth but whose gender identity is female
- Gender-Affirmation Surgery: surgery to align anatomy with gender identity
- WPATH: World Professional Association of Transgender Health

GENERAL CONCEPTS OF GENDER-AFFIRMING SURGERY

- Per WPATH Standards, gender affirmation surgery is effective and medically necessary for many transgender and nonbinary individuals to alleviate gender dysphoria.
- Gender is biologically derived, not a learned condition.
- Patients must have formal diagnosis of Gender Dysphoria (DSM-5 criteria) and undergo assessment by a qualified mental health professional. The operative plastic surgeon is not able to decide who is ready for surgery.
- A multidisciplinary approach is recommended.
- Very high incidence of depression, anxiety, addiction, suicidality, alienation from social support systems, homelessness, poverty, and poor health care access in this patient population.
- Three major subsets of gender-affirmation plastic surgery: facial, chest/breast, and pelvic gender-affirmation surgery.
- Patients must meet WPATH criteria prior to operative intervention.

CRITERIA FOR SURGERY

- WPATH criteria for pelvic gender-affirming surgery have been updated as of September 2022 and have become congruent among all gender affirming surgery. There are now individual criteria for adults and adolescents (See **Chapter 48: Reduction Mammoplasty, Top Surgery, and Gynecomastia,** section "Criteria for Surgery").

TRANSMALE PELVIC GENDER-AFFIRMING SURGERY

- Surgical options include hysterectomy, salpingo-oophorectomy, metoidioplasty, phalloplasty, urethroplasty, scrotoplasty, and erectile/testicular prosthesis implantation.
- Goals
  - Creation of a perineum that is aesthetically similar to a cis-male perineum
  - Tactile and erogenous sensation
  - Standing micturition (+/− with metoidioplasty)
  - Ability for erectile function and penetrative intercourse (with erectile prosthesis)

---

*Denotes common in-service examination topics.

METOIDIOPLASTY

- Goals: clitoral enlargement and urethral transfer to create a neophallus.
- Preoperatively: hormone therapy provides modest clitoral enlargement.
- **Technique**
  - Suprapubic catheter (SPC) placement.
  - Release clitoris from both dorsal and ventral attachments to maximally expose the clitoris as the neophallus.
    - Dorsal: superficial and deep clitoral suspensory ligaments are divided.
    - Ventral: clitoris partially released from ventral chordae.
  - Urethra lengthened to the end of the clitoris by harvesting buccal mucosal grafts and securing proximally to the urethral plate and distally to the clitoral glans.
  - The inner mucosal edge of the bilateral labia minora is de-epithelialized. One de-epithelialized labia minora is used to reconstruct the ventral aspect of the urethra. The contralateral de-epithelialized labia minora is wrapped around the ventral aspect of the neophallus to cover the urethral reconstruction.
  - Confirm urethral patency by passing a Foley catheter.
- **Postoperative care:** SPC for 4-6 weeks until passes voiding urethrogram
- **Complications**
  - Urethral fistula (16.9%) and stricture (9.1%)
- **Advantages:** erogenous sensation maintained, shorter operation with less morbid donor site, no risk of flap failure
- **Disadvantages:** suboptimal appearance and variable ability to urinate in standing position

PHALLOPLASTY

- Multiple components, often done in staged fashion, which varies across institutions: (1) vaginectomy and removal of reproductive organs, (2) phalloplasty, (3) urethral lengthening, (4) scrotoplasty, (5) glansplasty, and (6) testicular and erectile implants
- Autologous tissue creation of a neophallus
  - Pedicled flap options: ALT, extended groin flap, tensor fascia lata flap, SIEA skin flap, rectus flap
  - Free flap options: radial forearm flap, ulnar forearm flap, lateral upper arm flap, scapular flap, dorsalis pedis flap, fibula flap with pre-op tissue expansion
- **Radial forearm free flap (gold standard)**
  - Preoperative
    - Laser hair removal of the donor site
    - Demonstrate a normal Allen test of nondominant upper extremity
  - Technique
    - Flap design and donor site dissection
      - Rectangular radial forearm flap on the nondominant upper extremity with an ulnar-based urethra and a radial-based shaft
      - Flap incorporates the radial vascular system, cephalic vein, median antebrachial cutaneous nerve, lateral antebrachial cutaneous nerve, and a venous branch that becomes the urethral vein
      - Construct based on a tube within a tube flap:
        - Ulnar aspect of flap de-epithelialized and wrapped around a Foley catheter to create the neourethra.
        - Radial aspect of the flap then wrapped in the opposite direction around the neourethra to create the penile shaft.
        - The neourethral meatus is then inset into the distal tip of the shaft.
    - Recipient site preparation
      - The clitoral shaft is degloved along dartos fascia. The skin of the clitoral glans is removed, taking care not to damage the dorsal neurovascular bundle.
      - Recipient vessels from the femoral system and saphenous venous system.

- □ Recipient nerves: ilioinguinal and dorsal clitoral nerves.
  - ▪ Microsurgical anastomoses
    - □ Lateral antebrachial cutaneous nerve to clitoral nerve
    - □ Medial antebrachial cutaneous nerve to ilioinguinal nerve
    - □ Radial artery to branch of femoral artery
    - □ Cephalic vein to saphenous vein
    - □ Side branch of cephalic vein to urethral vein
  - ▪ The proximal neourethra is inset to the native urethral plate.
  - ▪ A split-thickness skin graft is secured onto the donor site.
  - ○ **Complications**
    - ▪ Urethral fistulae (26.60%) and strictures (12.28%)
    - ▪ Wound healing problems (7.38%)
    - ▪ Risk of anastomotic revisions (7.82%) and total and partial flap failure (1.69% and 5.43%, respectively) as with other microsurgical operations
    - ▪ Donor site regrafting (1.42%)
- **Anterior lateral thigh (ALT) pedicle flap phalloplasty**
  - ○ **Technique**
    - ▪ Design ALT flap from the ASIS to the lateral border of the patella.
    - ▪ Identify perforators via Doppler.
    - ▪ Incise the medial border of the flap and dissect down to the deep muscular fascia over the rectus femoris.
    - ▪ Elevate the flap laterally until perforators and the septum between the rectus femoris and vastus lateralis are identified.
    - ▪ Incise the proximal and distal aspect of the flap until nerve branches of the lateral femoral cutaneous nerve are identified. These will be clipped for future coaptation.
    - ▪ Open the septum between the rectus femoris and vastus to identify the descending branch of the lateral circumflex femoral neurovascular system.
    - ▪ Incise the lateral aspect of the flap and dissect medially toward the perforators.
    - ▪ After determining the perforators of choice, trace these vessels back to the origin vessels of the descending branch of the lateral femoral circumflex neurovascular system.
    - ▪ Make an omega incision over the pubic symphysis just above the vulva.
    - ▪ Locate the ilioinguinal nerve by opening the external inguinal ring and round ligament.
    - ▪ Dissect the clitoris to locate the clitoral nerve.
    - ▪ Pass the flap under rectus femoris and sartorius to get the ALT flap to its site of inset in the perineum and secure the dorsal aspect of the flap.
    - ▪ Coapt one branch of the lateral femoral cutaneous nerve to the ilioinguinal nerve and one branch of the lateral femoral cutaneous nerve to the clitoral nerve.
    - ▪ Tubularize the flap.
    - ▪ Place a purse-string suture at the distal aspect of the phallus to create the penile meatus. Secure the base of the phallus.
    - ▪ Close the ALT donor site in the usual fashion, using a Split-thickness skin graft from the contralateral thigh if needed.
    - ▪ Urethroplasty is generally done as a second stage with assistance from urology.
  - ○ **Complications**
    - ▪ Urethral fistulas (22.2%) and stricture (6.7%)
    - ▪ Partial flap loss (2.2%)
- **Subsequent stages**
  - ○ Glansplasty: Norfolk technique of coronal ridge and sulcus construction to produce circumcised appearance—triangle flaps at the distal end of neophallus create conical glans and sagittal slitted urethral meatus.

○ Erectile prosthesis for erectile function is possible, but high risk of wound breakdown and extrusion.
• Advantages: urinate standing up, aesthetic result similar to cis-male phallus

SCROTOPLASTY

• **Technique**
  ○ Bilateral superiorly based labia majora flaps are raised, rotated medially, and reapproximated at midline at the base of the neophallus.
  ○ Perineal defect is closed primarily in layers.
  ○ Testicular implants can be placed at later date.

TRANSFEMALE PELVIC GENDER-AFFIRMING SURGERY

• Surgical options include but are not limited to orchiectomy, penile inversion vaginoplasty, sigmoid vaginoplasty, and zero-depth vaginoplasty.
• Goals
  ○ Creation of a perineum that is aesthetically similar to a cis-female perineum
  ○ Creation of a neovagina that is hairless and of similar length to a cis-female vagina (average 9.6 cm, range 6.5-12.5 cm); not applicable in zero-depth vaginoplasty
  ○ Ability to urinate in a sitting position without obstruction
  ○ Ability to achieve orgasm

PENILE INVERSION VAGINOPLASTY

○ **Structures**
  ▪ Neoclitoris created from glans penis
  ▪ Labia majora created from scrotal skin
  ▪ Neovagina created from penile shaft and scrotal skin
  ▪ Urethra created from native urethra (shortened)
○ **Preoperative considerations**
  ▪ Laser hair removal of the entire pubic region
  ▪ Hold estrogen therapy for 3 weeks to reduce the risk of VTE
  ▪ Bowel preparation to decompress the bowel
○ **Technique**
  ▪ Design perineal triangular flap with base above the rectum and the apex on posterior scrotum to create the posterior vaginal vault lining.
  ▪ Design and harvest rectangular full-thickness skin graft (FTSG) from scrotum and tubularize. This later becomes the neovaginal lining.
  ▪ Perform bilateral orchiectomy.
  ▪ Create the neovagina by blunt dissection of perineal canal between prostate and rectum (*separated by Denonvilliers fascia), about 15 cm in length. Assess for rectal perforation, repair if present.
  ▪ Deglove penile shaft leaving dartos fascia up and Buck fascia down, careful not to injure the dorsal neurovascular pedicle.
  ▪ Deliver degloved penis through the flap and undermine the mons into the infra-abdominal region.
  ▪ Open the corpus spongiosum and urethra circumferentially 5 cm from the meatus.
  ▪ To create the neoclitoris, raise the glans penis W-plasty pedicled flap based on dorsal neurovascular bundle to the base of the penis. Secure to the pubic tubercle at the level of the **adductor longus tendons**.
  ▪ Dissect the corpus cavernosa from the corpus spongiosum bilaterally. Next, dissect the corpus spongiosum away from the urethra.
  ▪ Shorten the urethra and secure the dorsal aspect to the base of the neoclitoris.

- Suture the scrotal FTSG to the distal penile skin tube to create the neovagina.
- Invert the neovagina and place into the neovaginal canal (the space created between the prostate and rectum).
- Secure the perineal flap to the posterior neovaginal canal and the perineal body.
- Pass the neoclitoris and urethra through this opening and suture in place.
- The scrotal skin is contoured to create the labia majora and secured to the base of the perineal triangular flap bilaterally.
- Place packing in the neovagina and bolster over the neoclitoris.
  ○ Postoperative care
- 1 week post-op: remove Foley, remove vaginal packing, and start vaginal rinses.
- 3-4 weeks post-op: start vaginal dilation (lifelong to prevent vaginal stricture).
- Life long prostate cancer screening as prostate is not removed during surgery.
  ○ Complications
- Vaginal and urethral stricturing (11%)
- Rectovaginal fistula (1%)
- Delayed wound healing
- Inadequate vaginal depth
- High incidence of revisional surgeries
  ○ Advantages
- Excellent aesthetic result
- One stage operation

SIGMOID VAGINOPLASTY

○ Technique
- An alternative to penile inversion vaginoplasty where the neovaginal canal is created from a pedicled segment of sigmoid colon with assistance from a colorectal surgeon.
- Blood supply is from the sigmoid arteries.
- The proximal end of the sigmoid colon is closed. The distal end is left open.
- The plastic surgeon follows steps above for PIV including creation of a perineal canal between the prostate and rectum (**separated by Denonvilliers fascia**).
- The colorectal surgeon connects the abdomen and perineal canal.
- The pedicled sigmoid colon is passed through this opening with the open end of the sigmoid colon passed through first so that this can be sutured to the inverted penile skin and become the neovaginal canal.
○ **Advantages:** good for patients with limited penile-scrotal skin quantity or failed prior PIV, self-lubrication, texture, and appearance similar to cis-female vagina
○ **Disadvantages:** discharge and malodor, need for neovaginal colon cancer screening
○ Complications
- Fistula (2%)
- Vaginal stenosis (14%)
- Vaginal prolapse (6%)
- Discharge and malodor
- Abdominal surgery risks such colitis, peritonitis, intestinal obstruction, ileus, etc.
○ **Zero-Depth Vaginoplasty/Vulvaplasty**
○ Similar to penile inversion vaginoplasty without creation of a neovaginal canal
○ For patients who do not want the more morbid PIV procedure nor vaginal intercourse

PEARLS

1. Patients must meet WPATH criteria prior to undergoing gender-affirming surgery.
2. Patients who undergo gender-affirming surgery are best cared for by multidisciplinary teams to provide comprehensive care.
3. Many surgical options are available for pelvic gender-affirming surgery. For transmale phalloplasty, the radial forearm free flap is most common. For transfemale vaginoplasty, penile inversion vaginoplasty is most common.

QUESTIONS YOU WILL BE ASKED

1. What separates the prostate and bladder from the rectum where the neovaginal canal will be created?
   Denonvilliers (rectoprostatic) fascia.
2. What structure must be preserved when raising the glans penis to create the neoclitoris in penile inversion vaginoplasty?
   Dorsal neurovascular bundle.
3. Describe the outer layers of the penis, superficial to deep.
   Skin > dartos (superficial) fascia > alveolar tissue > Buck (deep) fascia > tunica albuginea.

Recommended Readings
1. Chen ML, Reyblat P, Poh MM, et al. Overview of surgical techniques in gender-affirming genital surgery. *Trans Androl Urol.* 2019;8(3):191-208.
2. Salim A, Poh M. Gender-affirming penile inversion vaginoplasty. *Clin Plast Surg.* 2018;45(3):343-350.
3. Schechter LS, Safa B. Introduction to phalloplasty. *Clin Plast Surg.* 2018;45(3):387-389.

55

Pressure-Induced Skin and Soft Tissue Injuries

Humza N. Mirza and Geoffrey E. Hespe

PRESSURE INJURY DIAGNOSIS AND MANAGEMENT

- **Definition:** localized tissue injury caused by compression of underlying tissue
- **Etiology/Mechanism of Injury**
  - *Tissue ischemia from external pressures exceeding the closing pressure of nutrient capillaries (32 mm Hg) for a prolonged duration.
  - *Pressures exceeding 70 mm Hg for 2 hours result in irreversible ischemia.
  - Shear forces can induce tissue ischemia: vessel stretch leading to thrombosis.
  - Ischemia-reperfusion cycle has been implicated.
  - Friction may cause epidermal injury (eg, during transfers).
  - Excess moisture especially from incontinence: skin maceration and increased pressure sore risk.
  - Decreased autonomic control leading to spasm, loss of bladder and bowel control, and excessive sweating seen in paraplegics.
  - Advanced age: decreased skin tensile strength.
  - Malnutrition: important to supplement calories and vitamins.
  - Sensory loss: inability to experience discomfort or tissue ischemia.
  - Impaired lymphatic drainage: impaired fluid transport and direct damage.
- **Epidemiology/Biology/Natural History**
  - Prevalence
    - 15% in general acute care, long-term, and home care setting
  - Incidence
    - 0.5%-38% in general care settings
    - 2%-24% in long-term care settings
    - 0%-17% in home care settings
  - 15% of elderly patients develop pressure sores in the first week of hospitalization; patients >70 years old make up over 60% of patients with pressure sores
  - Other risk factors
    - Cerebrovascular disease
    - History of pressure sore
    - Immobility (debility or paralysis)
    - Undernourishment, low BMI
    - End-stage renal disease
    - Small vessel occlusive disease: diabetes mellitus and smoking
    - Neurological dysfunction: sensory loss, decreased level of consciousness
  - **Chronic polymicrobial colonization** (count $>1 \times 10^5$)
    - *Staphylococcus aureus* and *Streptococcus* are most common bacteria
    - Decreased growth factor level
    - Increased matrix protease activity
  - **Chronic wound:** increased risk of malignant degeneration (**Marjolin ulcer**)
- **Surface Anatomy (Fig. 55-1)**
  - **Dependent on patient positioning,** and underlying condition
    - Supine: sacral (17%) and heel sores (9%) most common
    - Seated: ischial sores most common overall (28%)

---

*Denotes common in-service examination topics.

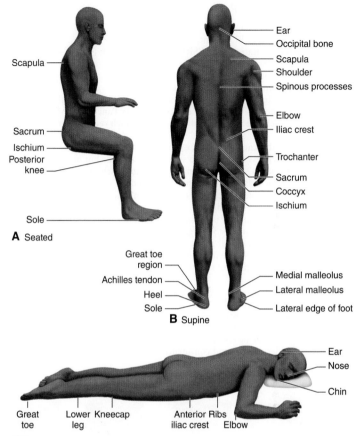

Figure 55-1 Common sites of pressure on the human body when seated, prone, and supine.

PREVENTION

- **Decrease moisture:** bladder/bowel hygiene, avoiding soilage → consider colonic diversion
- **Control of spasticity**
  - Baclofen or diazepam treatment
  - Physical rehabilitative medicine consult
- **Proper pressure distribution**
  - Air fluidized, low air loss, and alternating air cell mattresses (head of bed <45°)
  - Proper wheelchair Roho cushions when sitting, dispersion cushions
- **Pressure relief protocols**
  - Reposition patients every 2 hours for at least 5 minutes.
  - Patients in wheelchairs should be lifted for >10 seconds every 10 minutes.

DIAGNOSIS/WORK-UP

- **Laboratory studies and imaging**
  - ○ Complete blood cell (CBC) count with differential
  - ○ **Erythrocyte sedimentation rate (ESR)/C-reactive protein (CRP) → important to set baseline markers**
  - ○ Glucose/hemoglobin A1c
  - ○ Albumin/prealbumin (nutritional status)
  - ○ MRI → evaluate for underlying abscess or osteomyelitis if clinically indicated
- ***Stages defined by the National Pressure Ulcer Advisory Panel (NPUAP) (Fig. 55-2)**
  - ○ Stage I: nonblanchable erythema of intact skin, which remains for >1 hour after pressure relief
  - ○ Stage II: partial-thickness skin loss, exposed dermis
  - ○ Stage III: full-thickness skin loss into subcutaneous tissue but not through fascia
  - ○ Stage IV: full-thickness skin loss through fascia into muscle, bone, tendon, or joint
  - ○ Unstageable: when eschar or slough present, cannot be staged until fully débrided
- **Muscle is more susceptible to ischemia than skin:** muscle necrosis may have occurred with skin erythema as the only sign.
- **Nutritional status:** malnutrition is a risk factor for poor wound healing.
  - ○ In the past, serum albumin <3.5 mg/dL was used as a proxy for malnutrition.
  - ○ Recent studies show these labs may complement a nutrition-focused physical examination (NFPE) but are not reliable by themselves.
- **Osteomyelitis (OM):** infection of the bone must be determined. Initial studies include the following:
  - ○ ESR, CRB, and CBC.
  - ○ *MRI can identify OM and extent of disease. However, bone biopsy remains the gold standard for diagnosis.
- **Identify contractures and spasticity** in paraplegic and quadriplegic patients: patient may need physical medicine consult.
- **Assess bowel/bladder routine and continence.**

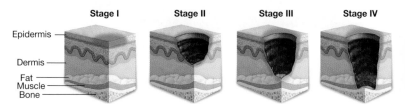

Figure 55-2 The International National Pressure Ulcer Advisory Panel Pressure Ulcer Stages/Categories. Stage I: Nonblanchable erythema. Intact skin with nonblanchable redness of a localized area usually over a bony prominence. Darkly pigmented skin may not have visible blanching; its color may differ from the surrounding area. The area may be painful, firm, soft, warmer, or cooler as compared to adjacent tissue. **Stage II:** Partial thickness. Partial-thickness loss of dermis presenting as a shallow open ulcer with a red pink wound bed, without slough. May also present as an intact or open/ruptured serum-filled or serosanguinous-filled blister. Presents as a shiny or dry shallow ulcer without slough or bruising. **Stage III:** Full-thickness skin loss. Subcutaneous fat may be visible but bone, tendon, or muscle is not exposed. Slough may be present but does not obscure the depth of tissue loss. May include undermining and tunneling. The depth of a stage III pressure ulcer varies by anatomical location. The bridge of the nose, ear, occiput, and malleolus do not have (adipose) subcutaneous tissue, and stage III ulcers can be shallow. In contrast, areas of significant adiposity can develop extremely deep stage III pressure ulcers. **Stage IV:** Full-thickness tissue loss. Full-thickness tissue loss with exposed bone, tendon, or muscle. Slough or eschar may be present. Often includes undermining and tunneling. The depth of a stage IV pressure ulcer varies by anatomical location. The bridge of the nose, ear, occiput, and malleolus do not have (adipose) subcutaneous tissue, and these ulcers can be shallow. Stage IV ulcers can extend into muscle and/or supporting structures (eg, fascia, tendon, or joint capsule) making osteomyelitis or osteitis likely to occur.

- **Assess motivation and social support structure.**
  - Adherence to pressure relief protocols
  - Adherence to wound care routines
  - Maintenance of adequate nutrition (20 kcal/kg)
  - Participation in risk factor modification (eg, smoking cessation)

MANAGEMENT OF PRESSURE INJURIES

TREATMENT OVERVIEW

- **Goals**
  - Avoid new and prevent worsening of current pressure sores.
  - Prevent soft tissue infection and osteomyelitis.
  - Eventual wound closure. Surgical closure is not attainable in all patients (eg, poor surgical candidates, nonoptimal social circumstances, etc.).
- **Management Strategies**
  - Débride devitalized tissues
  - Wound care
  - Antibiotic therapy
  - Surgical closure when appropriate
- **Stage I and II wounds: nonsurgical**
  - **Stage I:** wound dressing to prevent desiccation and protect tissue
  - **Stages I and II**
    - Pressure relief with patient repositioning every 2 hours
    - Appropriate pressure dispersion (eg, low-air loss mattress bed)
  - **Stage II**
    - Silver sulfadiazine ointment (Silvadene) to prevent bacterial invasion.
    - Impregnated gauze (Xeroform and petrolatum gauze) are useful alternatives for sulfa-allergic patients.
- **Stage III and IV wounds: surgical**
  - **History and physical**
    - Identify etiology, risk factors, type of bed/wheelchair cushion.
    - Current wound care regimen for chronic wounds.
    - Social circumstances, level of activity and mobility.
    - Prior surgical and nonsurgical treatments.
    - Assess wound characteristics (stage, three-dimensional size, palpable bone, type of tissue present in wound bed [eg, granulation, fibrinous, necrotic]), nature and volume of exudate, integrity of tissue surrounding wound.
    - Rule of associated soft tissue infection.
    - Assess history of wound and progression with current dressing regimen.
  - **Modify risk factors**
    - Treat spasticity when present.
    - Eliminate excess moisture with bladder/bowel regimen or diversion (eg, Foley catheter/diverting ostomy).
    - Eliminate pressure (specialty mattresses, cushions, and pressure relief protocols).
    - Optimize nutritional status.
  - **Assess for OM → high suspicion in chronic wounds with exposed bone**
    - CBC, CRP, and ESR (ESR >100 is diagnostic for OM).
    - MRI (may confirm OM when ESR is 50-100, shows extent of disease for surgical and overall treatment planning) → should only order in clinically indicated.
    - ***Bone biopsy for culture and pathology is diagnostic standard.**
  - **Surgical débridement → key for management of pressure injuries**
    - Excise devitalized skin, soft tissue, muscle, and bone.
    - Resected bone should be sent to microbiology and pathology only after proper débridement of outer bone.
    - Wound care regimen initiated (discussed later in this chapter).

- Postdébridement IV antibiotic course for osteomyelitis: initially broad-spectrum and then tailored when bone culture results available typically lasting 6 weeks.
- Depending on patients condition, this can be done at bedside vs in the operating room.
  - ○ **Preparing for wound closure**
    - Appropriate wound care regimen
    - Assessments of the wound to ensure healing is taking place (eg, there is healthy granulation and wound shrinkage)
  - ○ **Definitive closure**
    - Use well-vascularized tissue
    - May allow wound to heal secondarily if reasonably small, healing well and aligns with patient preference
- **Unstageable injuries**
  - ○ **Definition**
    - A full-thickness tissue loss where the depth of injury is unable to be determined.
    - Classically eschar or slough will obscure the depth of the pressure ulcer.
  - ○ **Assessment and treatment**
    - Stability and location dictates management → stable eschar can be treated conservatively with silver sulfadiazine while planning definitive management.
    - Débride to remove necrotic tissue and determine injury depth.
    - Débridement could reveal a stage 3 or 4 pressure injury.
    - Stable eschar (dry, nonfluctuant, adherent) on the heel or ischemic limb should not be softened or removed.
    - Upon staging, treat accordingly (see above).
- **Suspected deep tissue injuries**
  - ○ **Definition**
    - Internal injury where the skin remains intact, and soft tissue deformation progresses outward
    - Originates in muscular tissue over bony prominences
  - ○ **Pathophysiology**
    - Ischemic/hypoxic/reperfusion damage, structural damage, and lymphatic/interstitial fluid drainage lead to deformation of plasma membranes and loss of cell homeostasis.
  - ○ **Assessment**
    - Injury progresses outward until appears on skin surface as intact, discolored purple/maroon skin leading to blood blisters.
    - May be harder to detect in patients with darker skin tones; studies have shown that patients identifying as Black are twice as likely to get pressure-related injuries.
    - Often precedes stage III and IV ulcers.

WOUND DRESSINGS (STAGE III/IV SORES)

- **Goals**
  - ○ **Achieve warm, moist, and clean environment for wound healing**
    - Desiccated wound needs hydration.
    - Wound with excess drainage needs absorbent.
    - Wound with necrosis needs débridement.
    - Infected wound needs antimicrobial treatment.
- **Wet to Dry Dressing**
  - ○ **With normal saline or Dakin solution and mesh gauze**
  - ○ **In clean wounds:** prevents desiccation for optimal fibroblast and keratinocyte development and epithelial migration
  - ○ **In dirty wounds:** When dressing dries and is removed it will result in mechanical debridement of the wound
- **Debriding Dressing**
  - ○ **Chemical:** enzymatic agents such as collagenase

- ▪ Liquefy devitalized tissue; works well for management of overlying eschar
  - ○ **Autolytic:** hydrocolloids inner gel forming absorbent layer keeps wound moist
    - ▪ Moisture softens devitalized slough
- **Antiseptic Dressings**
  - ○ **Used in heavily contaminated wounds to decrease bacterial counts.**
    - ▪ Acetic acid thought to be effective in controlling *Pseudomonas*.
    - ▪ Other options include silver sulfadiazine (can cause neutropenia) or Dakin solution (sodium hypochlorite and boric acid).
  - ○ **Several of these agents have detrimental effects on wound healing** (eg, impair fibroblast proliferation). Switch to other dressings when wound is clean typically after 3 days.
- **Absorbent Dressings (eg Alginates)**
  - ○ Hydrophilic gels with ability to absorb up to 20 times their weight
  - ○ Have antimicrobial properties
  - ○ Used in excessively exudative wounds
- **Negative Pressure Wound Therapy**
  - ○ Increase granulation tissue, shrinking size of larger wounds prior to closure
  - ○ Appropriate for stage III and IV wounds
  - ○ Contraindicated with OM, necrotic tissue, infection, malignancy, and fistulas

SOFT TISSUE INFECTIONS (STAGE III/IV SORES)

- **Local Infections**
  - ○ Presents as cellulitis, a malodorous wound and purulent drainage
  - ○ Can lead to systemic infections with leukocytosis, fever, and sepsis → typically associated with underlying abscess/fluid collection
- **Obtain deep tissue specimens after débridement with clean instruments for quantitative bacterial counts, culture, and sensitivity.**
  - ○ *Staphylococcus aureus, Pseudomonas aeruginosa, Enterococcus faecalis*, and *Proteus mirabilis* are the most common culprits.
  - ○ Mixed aerobic/anaerobic infections not uncommon.
  - ○ There is little clinical value in swabbing an open pressure wound as this will be polymicrobial.
- **Treat promptly with drainage, irrigation, débridement, antibiotics guided by appropriate cultures.**

BONE INFECTIONS (OM)

- **Diagnosis**
  - ○ **Exposed/palpable bone** on initial evaluation: OM until proven otherwise
  - ○ **Bone biopsy:** gold standard for diagnosis
  - ○ Obtain bone biopsy during initial evaluation with a rongeur if patient is insensate
    - ▪ Make sure to débride overlying bone exposed to environment and take deep clean bone biopsy with a clean rongeur.
  - ○ **Bone scans:** not specific for diagnosing OM but can rule out OM if negative
  - ○ **MRI**
    - ▪ 80%-100% sensitivity and 70%-100% specificity in diagnosis of OM
    - ▪ Can also use to determine extent of disease
    - ▪ Enhancement of bone and marrow in T2 signal
- **Treatment**
  - ○ **Débridement** of devitalized and infected bone typically in the OR with pre- and postdébridement cultures.
  - ○ **A 6-week IV antibiotic course** tailored to causative organism typically guided by infectious disease.
  - ○ **Some patients' OM may be unresectable due to extent of disease** (extension to acetabulum and pubic rami).
    - ▪ Flap closure is contraindicated in these instances due to high rate of failure.
    - ▪ Management: chronic suppressive antibiotics and wound dressings indefinitely.

SURGICAL MANAGEMENT

PREOPERATIVE AND INTRA OPERATIVE CONSIDERATIONS FOR WOUND CLOSURE

- Minimize Risks of Recurrence
  - Recognize that not all patients are candidates for closure.
    - Patients who have not optimized conservative measures such as bowel and bladder regimens and contractures
    - Patients with significant medical comorbidities
    - Patients with unresectable osteomyelitis
  - Optimize nutritional status: evaluate with nutrition focused physical examination ± albumin.
  - Optimize spasticity management, for example, diazepam, baclofen, dantrolene.
  - Optimize comorbidities management, that is, glycemic control in diabetics.
  - No smoking or nicotine use.
  - Optimize bladder/bowel regimen (prevent moisture/soilage): consider urinary and fecal diversion if bladder/bowel regimen is not effective.
  - Establish history of adherence to wound care regimen, pressure relief protocols.
  - Motivated patient
    - Mood disorders (not uncommon in pressure sore patients) are detrimental to motivation.
  - Social support for the postoperative convalescence when restrictive regimens are in place to protect flap.
  - Wound must demonstrate capacity to heal after débridement and treatment with systemic antibiotics. If signs of no wound shrinkage after débridement/antibiotics, or infection (increased drainage, malodor, soft tissue infection), then halt plans for closure and reevaluate: CBC, ESR, CRP, bone biopsy, and MRI.
  - Postdébridement monitoring should include the following:
    - Weekly ESR, CRP, and CBC during antibiotic treatment.
    - Evaluate the trend of these test results before embarking on closure to ensure ESR is not elevated or trending up.
  - Patient should be off antibiotics for at least 7 days before closure to get an accurate microbiological assessment of intra-op bone cultures.
  - Intra-op
    - Excise entire ulcer and bursa, scar tissue, and soft tissue calcifications.
      - Can paint entire ulcer with methylene blue to ensure complete resection, that is, make sure no blue is left at end of debridement
    - Send tissue for quantitative counts, culture, and sensitivities.
    - Resect devitalized bone until firm, bleeding bone is encountered.
    - Send bone to microbiology and pathology.
    - Exercise caution with partial ischiectomy: overly radical ischiectomy increases risk of recurrence and perineal pressure sores.
- Other Considerations for Wound Closure
  - Need bulk to fill dead space and pad underlying bone with muscle, musculocutaneous flaps, or fasciocutaneous flaps.
  - *Preserve lower extremity function in ambulatory patients by using perforator flaps rather than myocutaneous flaps.
  - Design large flap to prevent tension after closure and place suture line away from direct pressure.
  - Do not violate adjacent flap territories to preserve options for recurrence or development of new pressure sores.
  - Rotation and V-Y advancement flaps can be re-advanced if recurrence occurs.
  - If possible, bring sensate tissue into the wound for protective sensation.
  - In OR, pad all pressure points appropriately to avoid new pressure sores.

FLAPS AND OTHER PROCEDURES

- **Sacral Pressure Sores (Fig. 55-3)**
  - Gluteal flaps (**gluteus maximus**): muscle, musculocutaneous flaps, and fasciocutaneous flaps
    - **Mathes/Nahai type III muscle supplied by superior and gluteal artery branching off of internal iliac**
    - Musculocutaneous and fasciocutaneous flaps can be designed as rotation, V-Y advancement flaps (unilateral or bilateral) or island flaps
    - **In ambulatory patients, preserve origin and insertion of gluteus maximus**
    - Unilateral rotational gluteal musculocutaneous flap
      - Landmarks: greater trochanter, lateral edge of sacrum, and posterior superior iliac spine (PSIS)
      - Incision: arc from sacral wound edge through PSIS through trochanter to ipsilateral ischial tuberosity
      - Elevate in plane between gluteus maximus and medius detaching muscle from sacral insertion
      - Preserve inferior/superior gluteal arteries
      - Rotate flap into defect (eliminate dead space)
      - Superior gluteal artery perforator flap as an alternative when only skin is required
      - Lumbosacral flaps
- **Ischial Pressure Sores (Fig. 55-4)**
  - Gluteal flaps (**gluteus maximus**): include rotational musculocutaneous and island musculocutaneous flaps
    - **Inferior gluteal artery-based rotational musculocutaneous flap.**
    - Landmarks are PSIS and trochanter.
    - Incision: arc just superior to the PSIS through trochanter to the ischial wound.
    - Divide only insertion of gluteus maximus laterally and inferiorly.
    - Elevate at fascial level until mobile enough to rotate into the defect.
    - Preserve inferior gluteal artery and sciatic nerve.

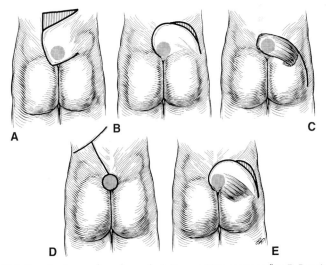

Figure 55-3 Flaps for closure of sacral wounds. A. Transposition cutaneous flap. **B.** Rotation cutaneous flap. **C.** Gluteus maximus muscle flap. **D.** Double cutaneous rotation flap. **E.** Rotation musculocutaneous flap. (From Thorne CH, ed. *Grabb and Smith's Plastic Surgery.* 7th ed. Lippincott Williams & Wilkins; 2014. Figure 98.7.)

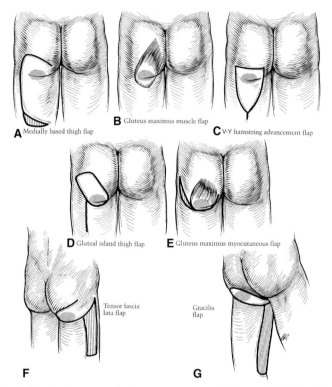

Figure 55-4 Flaps for closure of ischial pressure sores. A. Medially based thigh flap. **B.** Gluteus maximus muscle flap. **C.** V-Y hamstring advancement flap. **D.** Gluteal island thigh flap. **E.** Gluteus maximus musculocutaneous flap. **F.** Tensor fascia lata musculocutaneous flap. **G.** Gracilis musculocutaneous flap. (From Thorne CH, ed. *Grabb and Smith's Plastic Surgery.* 7th ed. Lippincott Williams & Wilkins; 2014. Figure 98.6.)

- Eliminate dead space.
- *Not appropriate for ambulatory patients.
  - ○ Posterior/gluteal thigh flap
    - Fasciocutaneous flap based on descending branch of inferior gluteal artery
    - May be designed as laterally based rotation flap or V-Y advancement flap
    - Rotational posterior gluteal thigh flap
      - □ Landmarks are ischial tuberosity and greater trochanter.
      - □ Distal limit is 10 cm above popliteal fossa and width should be approximately 10 cm.
      - □ Incision: extends from medial aspect of ischial defect inferior to distal limit and then back cut up toward greater trochanter (should not extend more proximal than 10 cm to ischial tuberosity).
      - □ Elevate superficial to hamstrings.
      - □ Preserve posterior femoral cutaneous nerve and profunda femoris perforators.
      - □ Rotate flap into the defect.
      - □ *May be used in ambulatory patients.
- **Trochanteric Pressure Sores**
  - ○ **Tensor fascial ata (TFL) flap:** muscle and musculocutaneous flaps

- Mathes/Nahai type I flap supplied by descending branch of lateral femoral circumflex artery (enters muscle 10 cm inferior to anterior superior iliac spine [ASIS]).
- Musculocutaneous flap can be designed as rotation (transposition) or V-Y advancement flaps.
- Muscle only flap will require split-thickness skin graft (STSG).
- May need STSG to cover donor defect.
- Transposition TFL flap.
  - Pedicle landmarks: a line connecting ASIS to lateral knee.
  - Anterior margin of the flap is 3 cm anterior to pedicle landmark line.
  - Distal extent of flap is junction of proximal two-third and distal one-third of thigh.
  - Incision: anterior margin of flap through distal limit and back up to trochanteric sore (width should be approximately 10 cm at widest point).
  - Elevate deep to TFL.
  - Transpose into the defect.
  - Inferiorly based V-Y flap, rotation advancement flap.
- Girdlestone procedure
  - Indication: communication of trochanteric pressure sore with the hip joint.
    - Communication may cause pyarthrosis and is commonly missed.
    - Pyarthrosis: purulent drainage, fever, and signs of sepsis on presentation. Need a high index of suspicion to diagnose.
  - Trochanteric pressure sores tend to have small openings with extensive bursas.
    - Thoroughly examine patients to ensure no communication with the joint.
  - Magnified "coned down" radiographic views of the joint may show OM.
  - Arthrogram: may demonstrate communication of pressure sore with the hip joint.
  - Treatment: incision and drainage as indicated, proximal femur resection with antibiotics course followed by flap coverage (to fill the joint space).
  - Operative technique
    - Resect proximal femur.
    - Distally, débride until healthy bone encountered.
    - Proximally, strip all cartilage from acetabulum until cancellous bleeding surface is encountered.
    - Postoperatively: antispasmodics and abduction pillow to prevent pistoning of femur into the defect.
- Vastus lateralis is the flap most used for coverage after Girdlestone procedure
  - Pedicle is a descending branch of lateral circumflex femoral artery (10 cm distal to greater trochanter).
  - Divide muscle 8 cm proximal to patella.
  - Posterior dissection should not cross lateral intermuscular septum.
  - Elevate up to vascular pedicle and transpose.
  - May require skin grafting.

NONOPERATIVE TREATMENT (STAGE III/IV)

- Goals
  - Prevent invasive infection, the wound from enlarging and new wounds from developing
- Patients With Resectable OM Who Are Not Surgical Candidates
  - Débridement with bone cultures and specimens
  - IV antibiotics and monitoring of CBC, ESR, and CRP
  - Appropriate wound care regimen
  - Pressure off-loading every 2 hours for at least 5 minutes and pressure dispersion
  - Proper bladder/bowel regimen or diversion as appropriate
  - Treatment of spasticity

- ○ Nutritional optimization
- ○ Management of comorbid conditions and long-term follow-up with wound care team
- **Patients With Unresectable OM** (Extension to Acetabulum and Pubic Rami)
  - ○ Require the same treatments as resectable OM (above)
  - ○ Also require chronic suppressive antibiotics monitored by infectious specialists and appropriate wound care regimen

POSTOPERATIVE CARE (STAGE III/IV WOUND CLOSURES)

- **General Considerations**
  - ○ Pressure relief protocols
  - ○ Pressure dispersion: air-fluidized mattress, alternating air overlay, dispersion cushions
  - ○ Protection of flap from pressure, shear, and friction
  - ○ No pressure on the flap/wound bed for 6 weeks
  - ○ Optimize nutrition
  - ○ Control spasticity/spasms
  - ○ Bladder and bowel regimen
  - ○ Surgical drains essential
  - ○ Antibiotic treatment if indicated by intraoperative cultures
- **Sitting Protocol**
  - ○ For closed ischial pressure sores.
  - ○ **No sitting for 3-6 weeks**.
  - ○ Advance sitting duration over 1-2 weeks: start with 30 minutes twice a day with at least 1 hour in between.
  - ○ Advance by 15 minutes a day until 2 hours achieved.
  - ○ Evaluate flap after each sitting session for signs of dehiscence or compromise (erythema).
  - ○ Sitting is not resumed until erythema is resolved. Sitting time not increased if erythema persists 30 minutes after a sitting session.
  - ○ During each sitting session, the patient must be lifted for >10 seconds every 10 minutes.

POSSIBLE COMPLICATIONS (FLAP PROCEDURES) AND OUTCOMES

- **Hematoma (~20%)**
  - ○ May compromise flap viability or be a nidus of infection.
  - ○ Evacuate the hematoma.
- **Seroma**
  - ○ Prevent by filling dead space.
  - ○ Place drains or drain percutaneously.
- **Infection (~6%-25%)**
  - ○ Reduce risk with perioperative antibiotics.
  - ○ If superficial, treat with antibiotics, otherwise débridement is required.
- **Wound Dehiscence (~10%-30%)**
  - ○ Avoid tension with closure.
  - ○ Leave sutures in place for 3 weeks.
  - ○ If dehiscence is small, manage with wound care otherwise débridement and flap re-advancement.
- **Partial Flap Loss (~13%)**
  - ○ Prevent with proper flap design.
  - ○ If small area of flap loss, manage with wound care otherwise débride.
- **Recurrence (5%-90%)**
  - ○ Very high in stage III/IV pressure sores.
  - ○ Proper patient selection and proper postoperative management reduce this risk.

PEARLS

1. Many healed or surgically closed pressure ulcers recur. Recurrence usually occurs within 1 year.
2. Recurrence of pressure sores is mostly due to inadequate débridement and patient nonadherence to pressure-relief protocols.
3. Outpatient support, patient motivation, and modification of risk factors also significantly influence success in maintaining a closed wound.
4. Operative closure is not appropriate for every patient. Surgical candidates need both social and clinical factors optimized for sustained wound closure.
5. Important considerations when making clinical decisions
   a. Is there devitalized tissue?
   b. Is the amount of devitalized tissue more than could likely be débrided with dressing changes alone?
   c. Has the patient had recent improvement in the wound with current dressing regimen?
   d. Is the patient stable for the operating room? Has anticoagulation been held?
   e. Have comorbidities been optimized? Is the patient nourished?
   f. Have all social issues been optimized? Will this sore reoccur when discharged?

QUESTIONS YOU WILL BE ASKED

1. What are the three stages of wound healing?
   Inflammatory, proliferative, and remodeling.
2. Besides pressure and noncompliance, what else should you consider in the differential diagnosis for nonhealing wounds?
   Residual infection of soft tissue, untreated OM, and Marjolin ulcer.
3. What are several flap options for ischial ulcer closure?
   Gluteus rotation advancement flap, V-Y hamstring flap, and inferior gluteal artery-based fasciocutaneous flap from posterior thigh.
4. Which flap is ideal for ischial pressure ulcer in an ambulatory patient and what is the blood supply?
   Posterior thigh flap and descending branch of inferior gluteal artery.
5. What is gold standard to diagnose OM?
   Bone biopsy.
6. How may pressure sores be avoided?
   Relief of pressure for at least 5 minutes every 2 hours, use specialty beds and wheelchair with proper cushioning, control moisture, and spasticity.

Recommended Readings
1. Brown DL, Kasten SJ, Smith Jr DJ. Surgical management of pressure sores. In: Krasner DL, Rodeheaver GT, Sibbald RG, eds. *Chronic Wound Care: A Clinical Source Book for Healthcare Professionals*. 4th ed. HMP Communications; 2007:653-660.
2. Levi B, Rees R. Diagnosis and management of pressure ulcers. *Clin Plast Surg.* 2007;34(4):735-748.
3. Ricci JA, Bayer LR, Orgill DP. Evidence-based medicine: the evaluation and treatment of pressure injuries. *Plast Reconstr Surg.* 2017;139(1):275-286.
4. Tchanque-Fossuo CN, Kuzon Jr WM. An evidence-based approach to pressure sores. *Plast Reconstr Surg.* 2011;127(2):932-939.

56 Lower Extremity Reconstruction

Connor Mullen

OVERVIEW

GOALS

- **Form:** major component of body image.
- **Function:** weight-bearing stability, sensate organ, pain-free mobility. An intact leg without function is a hindrance to rehabilitation and recovery.
- **Vitality:** débride devitalized tissue and obtain healthy wounds.
- **Amputation may result in:**
  - Quicker recovery course
  - Improved mobility
  - Improved wound healing
  - Improved level of activity

ANATOMY AND PHYSIOLOGY

- **Skeleton**
  - Femur
  - Patella
  - Tibia: bears 85% of weight, no anteromedial muscular coverage
  - Fibula: primarily serves as anchor for muscular attachments
  - Tarsals: calcaneus, cuboid, navicular, and cuneiforms (medial, intermediate, and lateral)
  - Metatarsals (5)
  - Phalanges (14)
- **Musculature and Soft Tissue**
  - Thigh (**Fig. 56-1** and **Table 56-1**).
  - Lower leg (**Fig. 56-2** and **Table 56-2**).
  - Four compartments: anterior, lateral, superficial posterior, deep posterior.
  - Plantar foot (**Table 56-3**).
  - Sensory innervation and nerve anatomy (**Fig. 56-3**).
  - Muscular loss is not a contraindication to limb salvage since even a fused ankle can be ambulatory.
- **Vascular**
  - **Thigh and knee (Fig. 56-4)**
    - Common femoral artery: gives rise to superficial circumflex iliac artery and superficial inferior epigastric artery.
    - Common femoral artery bifurcates 5 cm distal to inguinal ligament into the deep (profunda femoris) and superficial femoral artery.
    - Lateral circumflex iliac artery from deep femoral artery divides into ascending, transverse, and descending branches.
    - Popliteal artery: continuation of superficial femoral artery.
  - **Leg and foot**
    - Popliteal trifurcation: anterior tibial, posterior tibial, peroneal arteries.
    - Posterior tibial divides into medial and lateral plantar arteries.
    - Anterior tibial continues as dorsalis pedis.

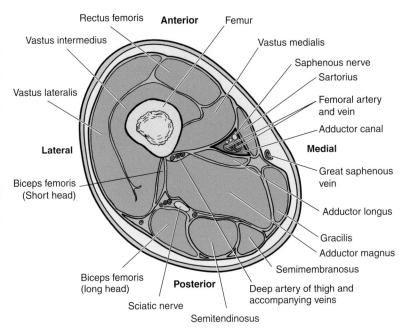

Inferior view

Figure 56-1 Anatomy of the midthigh in cross section. (From Dalley AF II, Agur AMR. *Moore's Clinically Oriented Anatomy.* 9th ed. Wolters Kluwer; 2023. Figure 7.44B.)

TABLE 56-1 Thigh Anatomy

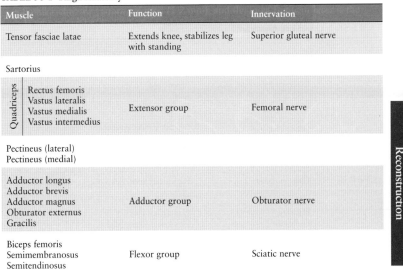

Muscle		Function	Innervation
Tensor fasciae latae		Extends knee, stabilizes leg with standing	Superior gluteal nerve
Sartorius			
Quadriceps	Rectus femoris Vastus lateralis Vastus medialis Vastus intermedius	Extensor group	Femoral nerve
Pectineus (lateral) Pectineus (medial)			
Adductor longus Adductor brevis Adductor magnus Obturator externus Gracilis		Adductor group	Obturator nerve
Biceps femoris Semimembranosus Semitendinosus		Flexor group	Sciatic nerve

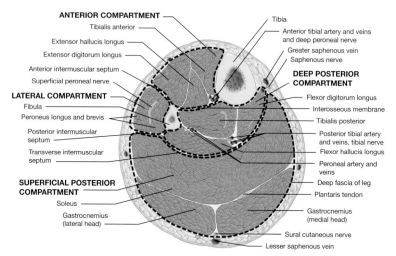

Figure 56-2 Lower leg in cross section.

- Innervation
  - Thigh
    - Compartments: anterior—femoral nerve (L2-L4), posterior—sciatic nerve (L4-S3), medial—obturator nerve (L2-L4)
    - Femoral nerve
      - Superior to inguinal ligament branches to psoas and iliacus muscle
      - Inferior to inguinal ligament
        - Sensory: anterior cutaneous branch—ant. thigh and knee, saphenous nerve—medial leg and foot

TABLE 56-2 Lower Leg Anatomy

Compartment	Muscle	Function	Innervation
Anterior	Tibialis anterior	Dorsiflex foot, invert foot	Deep peroneal nerve
	Extensor digitorum longus	Extend toes II-V, dorsiflex foot	
	Extensor hallucis longus	Extend great toe, dorsiflex foot	
	Peroneus tertius	Dorsiflex foot, evert foot	
Lateral	Peroneus longus	Plantarflex foot, evert foot	Superficial peroneal nerve
	Peroneus brevis	Plantarflex foot, evert foot	
Superficial posterior	Gastrocnemius	Plantarflex foot, flex knee	Tibial nerve
	Soleus	Plantarflex foot	
	Plantaris	Plantarflex foot	
	Popliteus	Flex knee, rotate tibia	
Deep posterior	Flexor hallucis longus	Flex great toe, flex foot	Tibial nerve
	Flexor digitorum longus	Flex toes II-V, flex foot	
	Tibialis posterior	Plantarflex foot, invert foot	

TABLE 56-3 Plantar Foot Anatomy

Layer	Muscles	Innervation
1 (Superficial)	Flexor digitorum brevis Abductor hallucis Abductor digiti minimi	Medial plantar N. Lateral plantar N.
2	(FHL tendon) (FDL tendon) Lumbricals Flexor digitorum accessories (also known as quadratus plantae)	 1 = Medial plantar 2-5 = Lateral plantar N. Lateral plantar N.
3	Flexor hallucis brevis Flexor digiti minimi brevis Adductor hallucis	Medial plantar N. Lateral plantar N.
4 (Deep)	(Tibialis posterior tendon) (Peroneus longus tendon) Interossei	Lateral plantar N.

- Obturator nerve—branches into anterior and posterior division after exiting obturator canal
  - Anterior branch: motor—adductor longus, gracilis, adductor brevis; sensory—medial thigh
  - Posterior branch: motor—obturator externus and adductor magnus; sensory—none
- Sciatic nerve—travels superficial to adductor magnus and deep to long head biceps femoris, lateral to semitendinosus and semimembranosus muscle
  - Motor to all posterior compartment muscles—biceps femoris, semimembranosus, semitendinosus, ischial portion of adductor magnus
  - Sensory to leg and foot, except medial leg, which is innervated by saphenous nerve
  - Divides dividing into the tibial and common fibular nerves at the popliteal fossa
  - Leg and foot
    - Tibial nerve (L4-S3): supplies posterior compartment of the leg
      - Motor branches to gastrocnemius, soleus, plantaris, popliteus, flexor hallucis longus, flexor digitorum longus, tibialis posterior
      - Divides into medial and lateral plantar nerves
    - Common peroneal nerve (L4-S2): supplies anterior and lateral compartments of the leg
      - Anterior compartment, motor to tibialis anterior, extensor hallucis longus, extensor digitorum longus, and peroneus tertius.
      - Lateral compartment, motor to fibularis longus and brevis.
      - Common peroneal nerve divides into superficial and deep peroneal nerves.
        - Superficial peroneal nerve sensory to lateral leg and dorsal foot
        - Deep peroneal nerve sensory to space between first and second toe
    - Sural nerve (S1-S2)
      - Purely sensory to lateral foot, heel, and ankle
      - Formed by medial sural cutaneous nerve from tibial nerve and lateral sural cutaneous nerve from the common peroneal nerve
        - Travels posterolateral between two heads of gastrocnemius, aside the short saphenous vein, becoming superficial midcalf
        - Passes 2.5 cm posteriorly to lateral malleolus

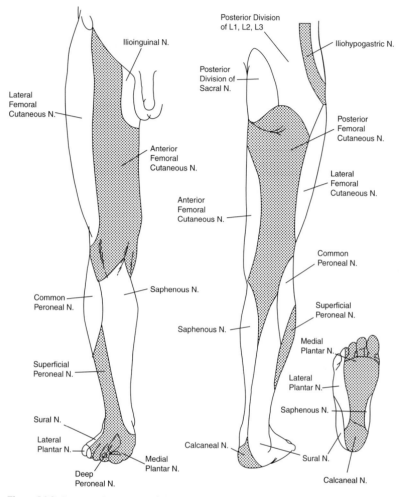

Figure 56-3 Cutaneous innervation of the lower extremity.

ETIOLOGY OF LOWER EXTREMITY WOUNDS AND INJURIES

- Trauma: falls, MVAs, military etiologies have high likelihood of penetrating component.
- Vasculopathies: diabetic lower extremity wounds, peripheral vascular disease
- Infection: chronic osteomyelitis, iatrogenic, postoperative wounds.
- Neoplasm.
- Irradiated tissue.
- Iatrogenic/postoperative wounds.
- Compartment syndrome is a risk in any lower extremity injury/reconstruction.

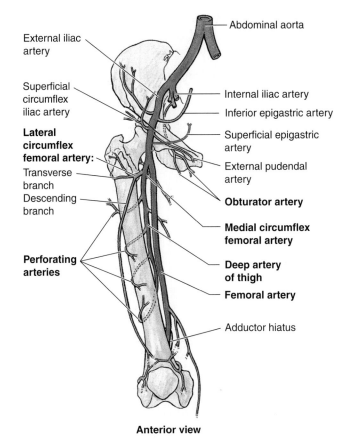

Anterior view

Figure 56-4 Arterial anatomy of the lower extremity. (From Moore KL, Dalley AF, Agur AM, eds. *Clinically Oriented Anatomy.* 6th ed. Lippincott Williams & Wilkins; 2010.)

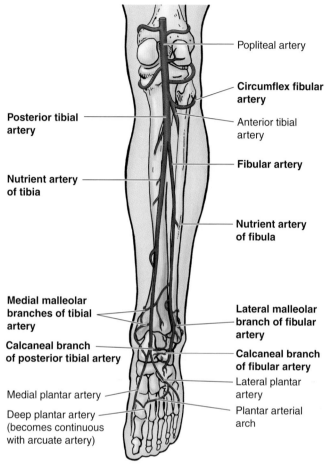

Popliteal artery

Circumflex fibular artery

Anterior tibial artery

Fibular artery

Nutrient artery of fibula

Posterior tibial artery

Nutrient artery of tibia

Medial malleolar branches of tibial artery

Lateral malleolar branch of fibula artery

Calcaneal branch of posterior tibial artery

Calcaneal branch of fibular artery

Lateral plantar artery

Medial plantar artery

Deep plantar artery (becomes continuous with arcuate artery)

Plantar arterial arch

Posterior view with foot plantar flexed

Figure 56-4 *(Continued)*

LOWER EXTREMITY RECONSTRUCTION

EVALUATION

- **Principles of management of trauma patients:** treat the whole patient; amputation can be lifesaving.
- **Pertinent history**
  - When/where did injury occur; potential contaminants; duration of devascularized tissues?
  - Mechanism of injury
  - Past medical, surgical, and social history (smoking status, home support, expectations)

- **Physical examination**
  - Neurovascular status: absence of plantar sensation maybe due to neuropraxia or reversible ischemia.
  - Skeletal and joint stability: joint above and below injury
  - "Fracture + laceration": assume open fracture until proven otherwise
- **Wound assessment**
  - Extent of injury: depth, tissues involved or devitalized
  - Exposure of vital structures: nerve, vessels, bone, joint, and hardware
  - Contamination: soil, chemical, marine, machinery, etc.
    - Length of time/chronicity
    - Prior cultures (type/reliability of cultures)
    - Prior débridements/dressings
- *Gustilo classification (Table 56-4) and Tscherne classification: severity of soft tissue injury predicts clinical course and healing probability.
- **Multidisciplinary considerations.**
- Lower extremity reconstruction is a labor, resource, and time intensive for patient and care team including preoperative optimization, inpatient stay, but most importantly, postoperative follow-up and maintenance.
- A multidisciplinary approach includes plastic, vascular, podiatric, and orthopedic surgeons, in addition to hospitalists, endocrinology, infectious disease specialists, and occupational and physical therapy, social workers, durable medical equipment vendors, community transportation programs, outreach and education teams, among others.

CONSIDERATIONS IN LOWER EXTREMITY RECONSTRUCTION

- **Acute Treatment of an Open Fracture**
  - Life over limb, ATLS.
  - Assess limb viability: ankle-brachial indices (ABIs), if <0.9, get angiogram and consult vascular surgery.

TABLE 56-4 Gustilo Classification of Open Tibial Fractures and Tscherne Classification for Open Fractures and Soft Tissue Injury

Gustilo classification		Tscherne classification	
Type	Criteria	Type	Criteria
I	Open fracture with wound <1 cm	I	• Open fracture without skin contusion • Minimal contamination • Low-energy fracture pattern
II	Open fracture with wound >1 cm without extensive soft tissue damage	II	• Open fracture with small skin and soft tissue contusion • Moderate contamination • Variable fracture pattern
III	Open fracture with extensive soft tissue damage A) With adequate soft tissue coverage B) With soft tissue loss with periosteal stripping and bone exposure C) With arterial injury requiring repair	III	• Open fracture with extensive soft tissue damage • Often, arterial and neural injuries • Severe contamination • High-energy fracture pattern
		IV	• High-energy open fracture with incomplete or complete amputation

Section IV: Breast and Body Reconstruction

- Evaluate for compartment syndrome: if present, emergent four-compartment fasciotomy.
- Imaging: x-ray including joint above and below. CT for periarticular/arthrotomy injuries.
- *IV antibiotics (within 3 hours of injury) tetanus prophylaxis, extremity stabilization and dressing.
- I&D within 24 hours (disproven dogma argue 6 hours), temporary fracture stabilization, local antibiotic administration, soft tissue coverage of vital structure.
- Delayed definitive closure vs serial débridements.
- Patients may benefit from early flap coverage.
- **Decision Point: Limb Salvage vs Primary Amputation**
  - Decisions must be made on individualized, patient-oriented basis.
  - Helpful to include physical medicine and rehabilitation into discussion to educate patient on amputation.
  - **Indications for primary amputation**
    - Devitalized or unsalvageable limb: consider both short- and long-term
    - Risk to life: intractable bleeding, overwhelming infection, etc.
  - **Relative indications for primary amputation**
    - *High tibial nerve transection (insensate plantar foot is not an indication)
    - Major soft tissue injury/fractures with significant devascularized tissue
    - Combined diaphyseal and major joint fractures
    - Open long-bone fracture with significant burns
    - Consider the patient: elderly, obtunded and/or neurologic injury, morbid obesity, severity of fractures (not necessarily location)
  - **Cost-utility analyses** indicate that when technically possible, reconstruction is always preferable over amputation. Reconstruction results in less long-term costs and increased utility when compared to amputation.
- **Complicating Factors**
  - **Vascular injury**
    - Fracture reduction may improve spasm or compression of vessels.
    - Consider temporary vascular shunts if stabilization process prolonged and limb is ischemic.
    - **Single vessel is usually adequate to perfuse distal lower extremity.**
    - If revascularization is performed, consider early fasciotomies.
    - Saphenous vein is common vein graft source.
  - **Soft tissue avulsion**
    - Injury often more significant than can initially be appreciated.
    - Requires resection of avulsed tissue with skin harvesting for skin grafting.
  - **Nerve injury**
    - Nerve grafting has not shown to be effective historically, better in pediatric patients.
    - Loss of posterior tibial nerve is not a contraindication to salvage.
    - Sural nerve grafts
      - Minimal donor site morbidity (lateral foot numbness)
      - Limited to use in clean and closed wounds
    - Prognosis of primary repair, if attempted, is guarded: most patients require lifetime splinting or tendon transfers.
  - **Osteomyelitis**
    - **Diagnostic testing/studies**
      - Erythrocyte sedimentation rate (ESR): better for ruling out osteomyelitis initially.
      - C-reactive protein (CRP): distinguishes osteomyelitis from soft tissue infection in diabetic patients hospitalized for foot infections.
      - *Bone culture and biopsy: gold standard for diagnosis; identification of the organism and diagnosis confirmation via histology not microbiology.
      - X-ray: findings lag behind the progression of the disease (not accurate).
      - Tc99: false positives if blood flow is poor.

□ Gallium: false positives with soft tissue inflammation.
□ MRI: T1-weighted images demonstrate decreased signal in infected bone; significant interference from hardware.
□ **Standards: ESR, CRP, MRI, and bone culture/biopsy.**
- Treatment
  □ Débridement
  □ IV antibiotics (often 6 weeks)
  □ Reconstruction as needed for coverage of vitalized/healthy tissue
○ Bone gaps
- **Cancellous bone grafting**
  □ Needs well-vascularized bed and delayed 6-12 weeks from trauma
  □ >90% effective in gaps of a few centimeters
- **Distraction osteogenesis (Ilizarov technique)**
  □ Bone lengthening with distraction osteogenesis
  □ Best in gaps 4-8 cm
  □ Requires external pins, risk of pin track infections
- **Vascularized fibular grafts**
  □ Indicated for bony defects >6 cm
  □ Must preserve the proximal and distal 6 cm of donor fibula to maintain knee/ankle function; up to 25 cm theoretically harvestable
  □ 87.5% reported success rate; non–weight bearing until evidence of radiographic union, single fibula ~15 months vs "twin-barreled" fibula ~6 months.
  □ Vascular supply: peroneal artery (via nutrient artery) and periosteal
○ Compartment syndrome
- **Compartments of lower leg (Fig. 56-2):** anterior, lateral, deep posterior, superficial posterior
- **Pathophysiology**
  □ Life- and/or limb-threatening condition.
  □ Compartments function as closed containers. Pressure can build without adequate release.
  □ High compartment pressures decrease venous outflow relative to arterial inflow perfusion pressures, leading to myoneural necrosis.
  □ Can cascade: hematoma increases pressure, causes inflammation increasing pressure, etc.
  □ Do not be fooled: an open fracture does not protect against compartment syndrome; patient still requires full fasciotomies.
  □ Systemic damage from necrotic debris, rhabdomyolysis, or even reperfusion injury following correction. Consider alkalizing urine (HCO_3 in IV fluids) with goal urine pH >8.
- **Signs and symptoms ("cardinal signs")**
  □ Pain (out of proportion and with passive movement)
  □ Pallor
  □ Poikilothermia
  □ Pulselessness (LATE)
  □ Paresthesia (LATE)
  □ Paralysis
- **Diagnosis**
  □ Clinical diagnosis
  □ Can check compartment pressure
    - Stryker pressure needle is the gold standard but can use standard needle or even arterial line kit.
    - Threshold pressures for diagnosis are controversial.
      • Compartment pressure >30 mm Hg
      • Delta pressure <30 mm Hg. Delta pressure = diastolic pressure – measured compartment pressure
- **Treatment:** four-compartment fasciotomy

TECHNICAL ASPECTS OF RECONSTRUCTION

- **Amputation**
  - **Preserve length**
    - Practice limb salvage through amputation.
    - *Ideal below-knee amputation (BKA) length is 10 cm below the tibial tuberosity.
      - The transverse incision is made 10 cm distal to the tibial tuberosity.
      - Its length is equal to two-thirds of the circumference of the leg at that level.
      - The length of the posterior flap is equal to 2 times the distance from midtibia to lateral extent of incision (gastrocnemius/soleus complex).
      - Transect the tibia just proximal to the transverse skin incision angled distally so anterior part of the tibia does not bear excess weight.
      - Fibula is transected with a bone cutter at least 1 cm cephalad to the tibia.
    - Person with a BKA has an increased energy demand.
    - Benefits of BKA vs above-knee amputation (AKA)
      - BKAs require less work for ambulation than AKAs.
        - 25% vs 68% increase in energy expenditure than with no amputation
        - 40% increase in energy expenditure for patients with bilateral BKA
      - BKAs report better quality of life than AKAs.
      - Midfoot amputations show no added benefit over BKAs.
  - **Keep "spare" parts**
    - Fillet flaps (commonly fasciocutaneous flaps) may be used in tissue transfer.
    - Skin grafts (full or split thickness) can be obtained from the amputated part.
  - **Contaminated wounds:** delayed closure/reconstruction; guillotine amputation
- **Primary Reconstruction**
  - **Timing**
    - Immediate coverage indicated for clean wounds with exposed vital structures.
    - Early coverage has been advocated to limit complications (**Table 56-5**).
    - Goal prior to reconstruction: débride nonviable tissue until there is a well-vascularized wound bed with no exposed vital structures.
    - Note: platelets increase fourfold as acute phase reactant and may contribute to subsequent complications.
  - **Delaying reconstruction with negative pressure wound therapy (NPWT)**
    - In conjunction with excisional débridement, NPWT has demonstrated its utility of expediting wound bed preparation for closure or coverage.
    - NPWT allows for temporary coverage of the wound in a sterile environment while applying negative pressure at the wound bed.
      - NPWT is hypothesized to improve angiogenesis, local vascular flow, and lymphatic drainage; to contract wound edges; and to reduce lateral stress.
      - Effect is decreased bacterial contamination and surgical site infections, promote stronger scar formation, and shorten healing time.
  - **Skeletal stabilization**
    - First goal of operative management to provide stable fixation
    - Skeletal blood supply

TABLE 56-5 The Godina Timing Considerations for Open Fracture Coverage and Outcomes

Timing to close	Failure rate	Infection rate	Bone healing time	Hospital time
<72 h	1%	2%	68 mo	27 d
72 h-3 wk	12%	18%	123 mo	130 d
>3 wk	10%	6%	29 mo	256 d

- □ Periosteal and nutrient arteries
  - Periosteal supplies outer third of the cortex and runs long axis of bone.
  - Nutrient via endosteal circulation supplies inner two-thirds of the cortex.
- □ Periosteal stripping should be minimized.
- Techniques
  - □ **Traction:** if patient unstable, temporary measure
  - □ **Cast immobilization:** adequate for closed fractures or open fractures with a stable/clean wound
  - □ **Intramedullary nailing**
    - Useful with minimal comminution and no significant bone loss
    - Reamed nails: early mobility, but tight fixation results in endosteal vascular obliteration
    - Nonreamed nails: risk in Gustilo grade IIIB/C for intramedullary infection; can be very effective
    - Early, stable coverage necessary
  - □ **Plate/screw fixation**
    - May require significant soft tissue and periosteal stripping
    - Early, stable coverage necessary
  - □ **External fixation**
    - Gold standard with significant trauma to soft tissue
    - Minimizes additional soft tissue/vascular trauma
    - May obstruct subsequent reconstruction efforts
    - Pin tract infection risk
    - May be combined with procedures for bone gaps
- ○ Débridement
  - Thorough débridement of devitalized tissue is the most important factor for the management of open, lower extremity fractures.
  - May require multiple trips to the operating room to achieve.
- ○ Soft tissue reconstructive ladder vs elevator
  - **Observation/dressing changes**
    - □ Unavailable if exposed vital structures
    - □ Must keep tendon moist to avoid desiccation
    - □ **NPWT** devices shown to be useful
      - Removes interstitial fluid, decreases pressure below capillary filling pressure, increases wound bed blood flow, promotes granulation tissue formation.
      - Microstrain on cell activates VEGF and angiogenesis.
      - *Reduces wound metalloproteinases.
      - Often temporizing for final reconstruction
  - **Primary closure:** requires low tension, healthy, and clean wounds
  - **Skin grafting**
    - □ Poor coverage on weight-bearing areas (ie, heel and plantar midfoot)
    - □ Inappropriate over hardware, bone, vital structures, or bare tendon
  - **Tissue expansion:** poor results, high complication rates (>75%)
  - **Local flaps (see Table 56-6 and Table 56-7)**
  - **Regional flaps**
    - □ Cross-leg flaps are of historic significance only
      - Local flap necrosis ~40%. Infection ~28%
      - Can base on axial blood supply of posterior descending subfascial cutaneous branch of popliteal artery
  - **Free flaps**
    - □ Valuable in complicated wounds or wound with significant local soft tissue loss.
    - □ Contouring of muscle flaps improves over time (secondary to atrophy from denervation and disuse).

◻ No difference in peri-op complications for anastomosis performed proximal, distal, inside, or out to zone of injury.
◻ Two-vein anastomoses demonstrate up to a fourfold reduction in complications.
◻ Vein size mismatch >1 mm can increase risk of total flap failure.
◻ End-to-side anastomosis beneficial: single vessel runoff not a contraindication, must go end-to-side, does not sacrifice distal circulation.
◻ Preoperative imaging (CTA, ultrasound, or angiography) allows for improved preoperative planning.
◻ Reconstruction by anatomic location.

RECONSTRUCTIVE CHOICES BY LOCATION

• **Thigh reconstruction** (Table 56-6)
  ○ Ample muscle/soft tissue surrounding femur is an advantage.
  ○ Rarely requires distal free flap reconstruction.
  ○ Common options: tensor fascia lata, gracilis, rectus femoris, vastus lateralis.
• **Knee reconstruction**
  ○ **Skin graft** satisfactory if joint capsule intact (may be unstable or result in limiting joint contracture)
  ○ **Gastrocnemius muscle flap** (medial or lateral head)

TABLE 56-6 Thigh Flaps

Flap type	Flap	Class	Pedicle and comments
Fasciocutaneous	Posterior thigh	B	Descending inferior gluteal a. [good for perineal wounds; can be raised as sensate flap with posterior femoral cutaneous n.]
	Anterior lateral thigh	B&C	Branches (septocutaneous and musculocutaneous) of descending branch of lateral circumflex femoral a.
Muscle and musculocutaneous	Rectus abdominis	III	Superior and inferior epigastric aa. [reliable, large skin paddle; good free flap]
	Vastus lateralis	II	Lateral femoral circumflex a. [good for infected hip wounds; good for middle and lower thigh; skin paddle rarely used]
	Vastus medialis	II	Profunda femoris branch [good for middle and lower thigh; skin paddle rarely used]
	Rectus femoris	I	Medial femoral circumflex and distal segmentals [must reconstruct quadriceps/patellar tendon after harvest]
	Gracilis	II	Medial femoral circumflex a. and SFA segmentals [reliable skin paddle; good for perineal wounds; good free flap]
	Sartorius	IV	8-10 segmental pedicles from superficial femoral vessels [flap of choice for small anterior defects, exposed groin vessels]
	Tensor fasciae latae	I	Terminal branch of lateral femoral circumflex a. [flap of choice for posterior defects; reliable skin paddle to 10 cm above knee; can be raised as a sensate flap with lateral femoral cutaneous n.]

- ▪ *Medial gastrocnemius provides wider arc of rotation (4 cm more) and broader belly.
- ▪ Lateral gastrocnemius requires identification of common peroneal nerve to avoid injury.
- ▪ Dominant blood supply: medial and lateral sural arteries off the popliteal, respectively.
- ▪ Muscle fascia can be scored to provide additional coverage area.
  - ○ **Alternatives**
    - ▪ Distally based gracilis, sartorius, vastus lateralis muscle flaps.
    - ▪ Random flaps can be designed off of anastomosis of superior geniculate vessels and the descending branches of the lateral circumflex femoral artery.
    - ▪ Consider distally based anterior lateral thigh fasciocutaneous flap.
  - ○ May require patellar tendon reconstruction: consider tensor fascia lata flap
- • **Lower leg reconstruction: "Rule of Thirds" (Fig. 56-5; Table 56-7)**

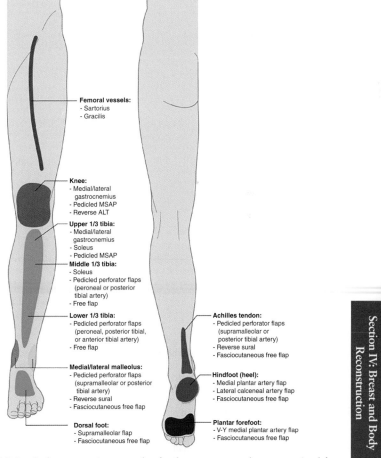

Figure 56-5 Standard reconstructive approaches for the most common lower extremity defects. (Reprinted with permission from Fang F, Lin CH. Lower extremity reconstruction In: Wei FC, Mardini S, eds. *Flaps and Reconstructive Surgery.* 2nd ed. Elsevier; 2017:259. Figure 22.5.)

TABLE 56-7 Lower Leg Flaps

Flap type	Flap	Class	Pedicle [comments]
Fasciocutaneous	Medial calf flap	A	Perforators from saphenous a., medial geniculate a., and posterior tibial a. [unsightly donor site; requires skin graft]
	Retrograde peroneal flap	C	Retrograde peroneal a. [depends on distal communication between peroneal and anterior and/or posterior tibial aa.]
	Reverse superficial sural artery flap	B	Superficial sural a. [can cover nearly any ankle or proximal foot defect]
Muscle and musculocutaneous	Gastrocnemius: medial (larger) and lateral heads	I	Paired (medial/lateral) sural branches of the popliteal a.: [pedicle enters just below knee joint; skin paddle can extend to 5 cm above medial malleolus; ugly donor defect when skin taken]
	Soleus: medial and lateral heads	II	Medial portion: posterior tibial & popliteal aa.; lateral portion: peroneal a. [delicate muscle; harder to elevate than gastrocnemius; distal end unreliable]
	Tibialis anterior	IV	Anterior tibial a. [not expendable; raise as bipedicled flap or "book flap" for middle or distal one-third]
	Extensor digitorum longus	IV	Anterior tibial a. [not expendable; must preserve function]
	Flexor digitorum longus	IV	Posterior tibial a. [used with soleus for small tibial defects]
	Peroneus longus	II	Peroneal a. [can be used for small middle one-third defects]
	Extensor hallucis longus	IV	Anterior and posterior tibial aa. [for small defects in distal one-third]
	Peroneus brevis	II	Peroneal a. [for small defects in distal one-third]
Any	Cross-leg flap	N/A	Varies [rarely used; can be fasciocutaneous, musculocutaneous, or muscle alone]

- ○ **Proximal third**
  - ▪ First choice: medial head of the gastrocnemius
    - □ Larger than lateral head. Proximal single pedicle. No functional deficit.
    - □ Scoring fascia can increase muscle belly surface area.
  - ▪ Alternatives: lateral head of the gastrocnemius
  - ▪ Smaller: no functional deficit
    - □ Soleus, proximally based
  - ▪ Can dissect to 5 cm above its tendinous insertion. No functional deficit
- ○ **Middle third**
  - ▪ First choice: Soleus, proximally based
  - ▪ Alternatives: medial head of the gastrocnemius
    - □ Lateral head of the gastrocnemius
    - □ Flexor digitorum longus

- Less common, used for small wounds of lower middle third defects. Pedicle enters at junction of middle and proximal third.
  - ○ Distal third
    - First choice: typically free flap
      - ▫ Consider regional flaps, if free flap is contraindicated; options include soleus, peroneus brevis, extensor digitorum longus, extensor hallucis longus, tibialis anterior, lateral supramalleolar flaps
      - ▫ Random, multiply delayed flaps
      - ▫ Dorsalis pedis flap
    - Reverse superficial sural artery flap
      - ▫ Pedicle is distal peroneal artery perforators located 4-7 cm proximal to malleolus. Small saphenous vein is always included.
      - ▫ "Neuro-skin" flap—sural nerve runs with median superficial sural artery.
      - ▫ Also uses vascular plexus of sural nerve and lesser saphenous vein.
      - ▫ Increased complications with (1) age >40 years and (2) comorbidity (peripheral vascular disease, venous insufficiency, and diabetes).
      - ▫ 21% reported local flap necrosis.
      - ▫ Can delay at time of initial wound débridement.
  - ○ Sural artery flap
    - Most reliable perforators near midline raphe in the distal half of the medial gastrocnemius
    - Venous drainage can be unreliable
  - ○ Propeller flap
    - Unequal length **island fasciocutaneous** flap based on **single perforator**
    - Prevent occlusion by maintaining **pedicle length >2 cm**
    - Venous congestion ~8%, partial flap loss ~11%
- **Foot reconstruction** (Table 56-8)
  - ○ **Dorsum of the foot:** reconstruct with thin flap with high surface area (ie, fasciocutaneous flaps)
  - ○ **Plantar foot**
    - Thickest skin on the body (up to 3.5 mm thick).
    - First choice: medial plantar artery (Instep) flap vs fasciocutaneous flap.
    - Alternatives: skin graft (unstable).
    - Attempts should be made to preserve sensation.
- Tissue expansion.
  - ○ Primary use is resurfacing. Results better in buttocks, thigh.
  - ○ High complication rate when placed below the knee: ~10%-30%.
  - ○ One of the most common causes for implant exposure is inadequate pocket dissection.

CHRONIC ULCERS AND THE DIABETIC FOOT

GENERAL CONSIDERATIONS

- Why does an acute wound become chronic? (see **Chapter 1: Complex Wound Care**)
- **Useful Labs and Studies**
  - ○ Amputation independent risk factors
    - Diabetic population: end-stage renal disease (30-fold increase risk), hindfoot wounds (4.5-fold), elevated HbA1c > 7.5-8.4 (variable increase risk), and positive post-debridement wound cultures (6-fold)
    - Trauma population: diabetes mellitus, any arterial injury and, notably, posterior tibial artery injury, one-vessel runoff, osteomyelitis
  - ○ **Hemoglobin A1c > 7.5-8.4** independent risk factor for amputation
    - No evidence intensive glycemic control in type 2 diabetes mellitus, delays onset or progression of microvascular complication (retinopathy,

TABLE 56-8 Foot Flaps

Flap type	Flap	Pedicle [Comments]
Skin/subcutaneous	Reversed dermis flap	Dermal/subdermal plexus [turn-over flap of dermis to cover adjacent wound; may be useful for Achilles coverage]
	Fillet of toe flap	Digital a. [sensate flap via deep peroneal n. or digital nerves]
	Lateral calcaneal artery skin flap	Lateral calcaneal a. (branch of peroneal a.) [can cover Achilles tendon and posterior heel]
	Suprafascial rotational flap	Proximal subcutaneous vascular plexus via dorsalis pedis and medial calcaneal aa. [sensate flap via medial calcaneal n.]
	Cross-foot flap (also cross-thigh and cross-groin flaps)	Multiple musculocutaneous perforators [seldom used; can transfer plantar skin to opposite foot in theory]
	Medial plantar flap	Cutaneous branch of medial plantar a. [versatile; can elevate abductor hallucis brevis m. with flap]
Fasciocutaneous	Flexor digiti minimi brevis	Lateral plantar a. [can reach proximal 5th metacarpal]
Muscle	Abductor digiti minimi	Lateral plantar a. enters near origin [can reach lateral heel and beneath lateral malleolus]
	Flexor digitorum longus	Perforators from posterior tibial a. [may reach distal one-third anteromedial ankle wounds]
	Flexor hallucis brevis	Medial plantar a. and first plantar metatarsal a. [can reach around to dorsum of foot; often used in combination flaps]
	Extensor digitorum brevis	Dorsalis pedis a. via lateral tarsal a. [thin; ok for local defects of dorsum]
	Abductor hallucis brevis flap (w/skin = medial plantar flap)	Medial plantar a. enters on lateral side [can reach to posterior heel; sensate flap if medial plantar n. preserved]
Muscle or musculocutaneous	Flexor digitorum brevis (w/skin = plantar artery-skin-fascia flap)	Dominant = lateral plantar a.: enters undersurface of the proximal 1/3 muscle; minor = reverse flow via plantar arch [can reach to heel and Achilles if dominant pedicle divided (risky); harvest results in loss of arch support]

nephropathy, neuropathy) or macrovascular (peripheral arterial disease [PAD]). Only shown in type 1 diabetes mellitus.

- ○ **Osteomyelitis workup** (see section on *Lower Extremity Reconstruction— Osteomyelitis*)
- ○ **Cultures and biopsies** (do not forget possibility of malignancy—Marjolin ulcer, etc.)
- ○ **Rule out vascular cause of ulcer: ABI testing**
  - ▪ Involve vascular surgery if abnormalities exist
  - ▪ History of claudication and/or rest pain

- Physical examination: cool extremity with dry, shiny, and hairless skin
- Other studies per vascular consult: arteriogram, CTA, MRA, etc.
- ABI: >1.30 noncompressible abnormal calcifications, 1.00-1.29 normal, 0.91-0.99 borderline, 0.41-0.90 mild to moderate PAD, <0.40 severe PAD necessitates vascular surgery consultation
- ABI = highest pressure in (R or L) lower limb (DP or PT) divided by highest pressure of both arms
  - *Quantitative cultures: generally >1 × 10^5 of most species will impair wound healing and prevent skin grafts from taking. This may be lower for Streptococcus pyogenes species (1 × 10^3 may impair healing).
  - Venous stasis ulcers and lymphedema (see Chapter 8: Lymphedema and Vascular Anomalies): mainstay treatment is compression.
  - Consider labs for rheumatologic/vasculitic disease if appropriate.
  - Meggitt-Wagner system: most commonly diabetic foot ulcer classification system.
- **Six Essentials of American Diabetes Association (ADA) Treatment Guidelines**
  - Off-loading
    - Most important aspect of neuropathic diabetic foot wound healing.
    - Goal is to off-load and keep patient ambulating.
    - Gold-standard off-loading modality: total contact casts.
  - Débridement early and often
  - Moist wound healing
  - Treatment of infection
  - Correction of ischemia (below-knee disease)
  - Prevent amputation
- **Other Considerations**
  - Foot baths macerate skin and are contraindicated.
  - Topical antibiotics are not recommended for noninfected ulcers.
  - Data do not support silver-based dressing in infected wounds.

ETIOLOGY

- **Neuropathy**
  - **Most important risk factor** for development of diabetic foot ulcers and amputations
    - Strict glucose control is only way to preserve sensory function.
  - Pathophysiology
    - Alerted neuronal metabolism due to prolonged hyperglycemia
    - Buildup of sorbitol in perifascicular connective tissue leading to intraneural compression
    - Decreased rate of anterograde axoplasmic flow (decreased nerve healing)
  - Sensory neuropathy: leads to inability to detect, sense, or protect injuries/wounds
    - Diagnosis: 10 g of pressure using a 5.07 Semmes-Weinstein filament
  - Autonomic neuropathy: decreased sweat and oil gland function and arteriovenous shunting lead to dry and cracked skin.
  - Motor neuropathy: alerted mechanics and function, leading to joint/toe deformity like claw toes, dislocated metatarsophalangeal joints
- **Ischemia**
  - Arterial insufficiency is from atherosclerosis of large vessels, but micro- and macrovascular disease are contributory.
  - "Trashed trifurcation" disease: destruction and arteriosclerosis of the infrapopliteal branches; foot branches may be spared.
  - ABIs: falsely elevated due to calcification (incompressible vessels). TBIs may be a better indicator of blood supply.
- **Immune Dysfunction and Immunosuppression**
  - Involves both cellular and humeral immune systems

- Superficial infections usually Gram-positive cocci
- Deep infections usually polymicrobial, including anaerobes
- **Mechanical/Traumatic**
    - Charcot foot: collapse of midfoot bones (rate: 1 in 800 diabetics)
        - Radiologic findings may mimic osteomyelitis
    - Shortening of the Achilles tendon: due to loss of collagen elasticity
- Most common location for a diabetic foot ulcer is **under the hallux.**

TREATMENT AND RECONSTRUCTION

- Conservative Medical Management
    - Six essentials of ADA guidelines, see above
    - Off-load—keeps patient ambulatory without pressure on ulcer
    - Wet to dry dressing changes: mechanical débridement
    - Autolytic and enzymatic débridement: break down necrotic tissue
    - Maggot (larval) débridement
        - Larvae of green blowfly (*Phaenicia sericata*) only eat necrotic tissue.
        - Dressing stays in place for 3 days.
        - Poor tolerance, need frequent clinic visits to get new batch of maggots, may be painful.
        - Maggots can eat methicillin-resistant *Staphylococcus aureus*–infected and vancomycin-resistant *Enterococcus*–infected tissue.
    - For moderate-severe cellulitis, attempt to obtain deep culture (abscess, postdébridement or surgery).
    - Can start empiric antibiotic while awaiting cultures, and the most common diabetic foot infection pathogens are aerobic Gram-positive cocci, especially *Staphylococcus aureus*.
    - Risk factors for Gram negative: recent hospitalization or antibiotic, gangrene, moderate-severe cellulitis.
        - Antibiotic treatment of 10-14 days is sufficient for most soft tissue infections, and treatment for 4-6 weeks is adequate for bone infection.
- Key predictive factors of healing, amputation, and final amputation level: wound depth, infection, PAD
- **Superficial injury (with or without infection):** pressure relief and topical antibiotics as necessary
- **Cellulitis**
    - Gold standard: trust only deep tissue cultures (swabs are notoriously misleading).
    - Antibiotics: typically polymicrobial; consider coverage for β-hemolytic *Streptococcus* and methicillin-resistant *Staphylococcus aureus*.
    - Consider fungal infections, for example, tinea pedis, in persistent cellulitic infections.
- **Deep Ulcers**
    - **Assessment**
        - Exposed bone: obtain bone biopsy, begin osteomyelitis workup.
        - Sequestrum: devitalized and infected bone and soft tissue that must be débrided thoroughly.
        - Consider infectious disease involvement, will likely need 6 weeks of IV antibiotics if osteomyelitis is suspected or confirmed.
        - Severe osteomyelitis generally necessitates some level of amputation, especially in patients who are poor candidates for subsequent reconstruction.
        - Depending on clinical scenario, toe amputation, ray amputation, midfoot amputation, or BKA may be appropriate.
    - **Postoperative care** includes pressure off-loading, optimization of nutrition, diabetic or wedge shoes in ambulatory patients, and regular foot examinations.

PEARLS

1. Débridement of all devitalized tissue is key to successful staged reconstruction.
2. Understand different options for soft tissue coverage of the lower leg including the following workhorse flaps: gastrocnemius for the upper third, soleus for the middle third, and free tissue transfer for the distal third.
3. Limb salvage should be the default operation, but understand the relative indications for amputation.
4. Understand the concept of perforator flaps and the vascular anatomy of the lower extremity.
5. Chronic wounds can be properly managed with off-loading, nutrition, edema control, and bacterial management.

QUESTIONS YOU WILL BE ASKED

1. Mathes-Nahai flap classification of flap types (know dominant and minor vessels) **See Tables 56-6 and 56-7.**
2. A patient undergoes open reduction and internal fixation of an open tibial fracture and develops purulent drainage. An extensive débridement is performed with subsequent flap coverage. IV antibiotics are continued for 8 weeks. The patient does well initially, but at a post-op appointment 3 months later, a recurrence of the infection is present. Why?
   If hardware is left in place, bacteria may survive on a biofilm. If hardware was removed, inadequate bone débridement with retained sequestrum is likely the cause.
3. What is the most appropriate reconstruction for an open distal third tibia fracture?
   The classic answer is that free flap reconstruction is necessary for these types of injury. However, recent literature has shown that peroneal or posterior tibial-artery-based propeller flaps can be useful as well.
4. What nerve is most at risk in dissection of lateral gastrocnemius flap?
   Common peroneal nerve.

THINGS TO DRAW

1. Draw the lower extremity vascular anatomy in detail, including the thigh, knee, lower leg, and foot (**Fig. 56-4**).
2. Draw the lower extremity dermatomes (**Fig. 56-3**).
3. Draw a cross section of the leg at different levels within the thigh and lower leg (**Figs. 56-1 and 56-2**).

Recommended Readings

1. Azoury SC, Stranix JT, Othman S, et al. Outcomes following soft-tissue reconstruction for traumatic lower extremity defects at an orthoplastic limb salvage center: the need for Lower Extremity Guidelines for Salvage (L.E.G.S.). *Orthop Surg.* 2021;3:1-7.
2. Godina M. Early microsurgical reconstruction of complex trauma of the extremities. *Plast Reconstr Surg.* 1986;78(3):285-292.
3. Gustilo RB, Anderson JT. Prevention of infection in the treatment of one thousand and twenty-five open fractures of long bones: retrospective and prospective analyses. *J Bone Joint Surg Am.* 1976;58(4):453-458.
4. Soltanian H, Garcia RM, Hollenbeck ST. Current concepts in lower extremity reconstruction. *Plast Reconstr Surg.* 2015;136(6):815e-829e.

57 Evaluation of Facial Aging

Jaclyn T. Mauch

OVERVIEW

COMPONENTS OF FACIAL AGING (FIG. 57-1)

- **Skin Changes**
  - Chronologic aging
    - Decrease in dermal and epidermal thickness (especially reticular dermis), loss of elasticity, and reduction in dermal appendages cause **fine rhytides.**
    - Repetitive muscle contractions lead to superficial and deep rhytides in the orbicularis oculi and oris, risorius, frontalis, and corrugator orientations (**Fig. 57-2**).
    - Total collagen decreases, while the proportion of collagen type III increases.
    - Larger sebaceous glands.
    - Deep rhytides result from fat compartment descent.
  - Actinic damage from chronic sun exposure (photoaging)
    - Hyperpigmentation, dyschromia, increased rhytides, skin laxity
    - Solar keratoses
    - Increased intracellular reactive oxidative intermediates lead to
      - Epidermal thinning
      - Solar elastosis: histologic appearance of the photoaged dermal extracellular matrix, which shows accumulation of abnormal elastin surrounding decreased and disorganized collagen fibrils
      - Increased collagenases and matrix metalloproteinases
  - Other chronic damage from acne or dermatologic conditions
  - Environmental factors such as **smoking** can result in similar damage to sun exposure
  - Skin classifications:
    - Fitzpatrick skin type classification (**Table 57-1**) prognosticates degree of photoaging.
    - The Glogau Scale categorizes patients based on cumulative sun exposure (**Table 57-2**).
    - Facial wrinkling can be categorized using Fitzpatrick Classification of Facial Wrinkling (**Table 57-3**).
- **Soft Tissue Changes (Figs. 57-3 and 57-4)**
  - Overall loss of volume, most pronounced in middle and upper facial thirds.
  - Progressive laxity of the retaining ligaments of the face
    - Attenuation of the zygomatic-cutaneous, masseteric, orbitomalar, and mandibular retaining ligaments creates a hammock for the atrophied fat compartments causing tear trough deformity, malar bags, and jowling.
  - Muscle atrophy.
  - Deflation and descent of fat compartments leading to skin laxity, nasolabial folds, periorbital folds, and jowling
    - The fat of the face is divided into distinct superficial and deep compartments, which age at different times and affect facial aging in various ways.
  - Irregularities and facial creases occur from a juxtaposition of lax tissues with fixed retaining ligaments (eg, nasojugal groove, jowls, etc.).

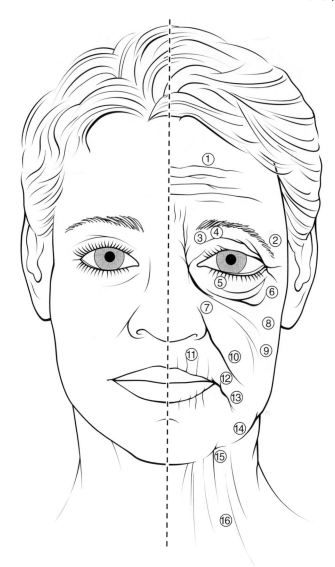

Figure 57-1 Aging changes in the face. 1. Forehead and glabella creases. 2. Ptosis of the lateral brow. 3. Redundant upper eyelid skin. 4. Hollowing of the upper orbit. 5. Lower eyelid laxity and wrinkles. 6. Lower eyelid bags. 7. Deepening of the nasojugal groove. 8. Ptosis of the malar tissues. 9. Generalized skin laxity. 10. Deepening of the nasolabial folds. 11. Perioral wrinkles. 12. Downturn of oral commissures. 13. Deepening of labiomental crease. 14. Jowls. 15. Loss of neck definition and excess fat in neck. 16. Platysmal bands.

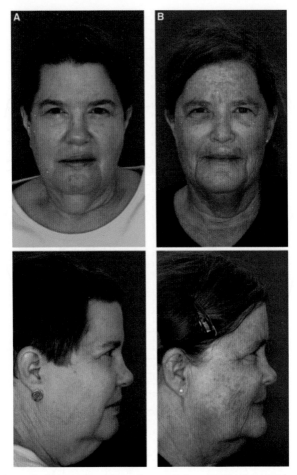

Figure 57-2 Muscle-rhytid correlates. (From Guyuron B, Rowe DJ, Weinfeld AB, Eshraghi, Y, Fathi A, Iamphongsai S. Factors contributing to the facial aging of identical twins. *Plast Reconstr Surg.* 2009;123(4):1321-1331. Figure 6.)

- Facial Skeletal Changes
  - Bone mass resorption with age in superomedial and inferolateral aspects of the orbital rim (larger orbital aperture), anterior maxilla (leading to posterior displacement of the maxilla), pyriform region of the nose, and prejowl area of the mandible contributes to decreased mid and lower facial height.
  - Loss of dentition decreases alveolar bone and causes loss of lower facial height.
  - Increased prominence of the chin, supraorbital rim, and zygomatic arch.

FACIAL ANATOMICAL CHANGES WITH AGING

- Upper Face: Temples, Eyebrows, Superior Orbital Area
  - **Temporal narrowing** causes decreased brow support/brow ptosis and pseudodermatochalasis of the upper lid
    - Dermatochalasis: excess and laxity of eyelid skin

TABLE 57-1 Fitzpatrick Skin Type Classification

Skin type	Sun exposure history/skin color
Type I	Always burns, never tans, extremely fair complexion
Type II	Always burns, sometimes tans, fair complexion
Type III	Sometimes burns, always tans, medium complexion
Type IV	Rarely burns, always tans, olive complexion
Type V	Never burns, always tans, medium brown complexion
Type VI	Never burns, always tans, markedly dark brown/black complexion

Derived from Ward WH, Lambreton F, Goel N, et al. Clinical presentation and staging of melanoma. In: Ward WH, Farma JM, ed. *Cutaneous Melanoma: Etiology and Therapy*. Codon Publications; 2017. TABLE 1, Fitzpatrick Classification of Skin Types I through VI. Available from: https://www.ncbi.nlm.nih.gov/books/NBK481857/table/chapter6.t1/. doi: 10.15586/codon.cutaneousmelanoma.2017.ch6

- ○ **Periorbital hollowing/bone resorption** superomedially and inferolaterally causes a vertically lengthened orbital aperture and lower lid hollowing with contour deformities (**Fig. 57-5**).
- ○ **Soft tissue atrophy**
  - ■ Temple: atrophy of the deep temporal fat pad and the temporal extension of the buccal fat pad
  - ■ Forehead and lateral brow: thinning of the subcutaneous plane
    - □ Glabellar creases and central forehead furrows from procerus and corrugator activation
    - □ Frontalis activation leads to transverse forehead rhytides
    - □ Stronger depressor muscles overpower brow elevators and weak attachments of skin to periosteum cause brow laxity and lengthening
    - □ Lateral temporal fat pad descent results in lateral brow ptosis
  - ■ Upper lids: retro-orbicularis oculi fat pad and medial and middle orbital fat pad volume loss; ptosis of the eyelid due to attenuation of the levator aponeurosis
    - □ Ptosis of the lacrimal glands
- ○ **Hairline recession and hair thinning**
  - ■ Androgenic alopecia:
    - □ Male pattern baldness
      - ▪ Genetically driven by the presence of androgen; X-linked dominant
      - ▪ Characterized a receding frontal hairline and thinning on the crown

TABLE 57-2 Glogau Scale

Severity	Findings	
Mild	No wrinkles	No keratosis; wears little to no makeup
Moderate	Wrinkles in motion	Early keratosis, sallow complexion; usually needs makeup
Advanced	Wrinkles at rest	Many actinic keratosis, telangiectasias; always wears makeup
Severe	All wrinkles	Severe keratosis, severe photoaging; wears makeup with poor coverage

Derived from Glogau RG. Aesthetic and anatomic analysis of the aging skin. *Semin Cutan Med Surg.* 1996;15(3):134-138. doi: 10.1016/s1085-5629(96)80003-4

TABLE 57-3 Fitzpatrick Classification of Facial Wrinkling

Class	Score	Wrinkling	Degree of elastosis
I	1-3	Fine wrinkles	Mild (fine textural changes with subtly accentuated skin line)
II	4-6	Fine to moderate	Moderate (distinct papular elastosis, individual papules with yellow translucency under direct lighting, dyschromia); intermediate number of lines
III	7-9	Moderate to deep	Severe (multipapular and confluent elastosis, thickened yellow and pallid wrinkles, cutis rhomboidalis); numerous lines with or without redundant skin

Derived from Shoshani D, Markovitz E, Monstrey SJ, Narins DJ. The modified Fitzpatrick Wrinkle Scale: a clinical validated measurement tool for nasolabial wrinkle severity assessment. *Dermatol Surg.* 2008;34 (Suppl 1):S85-S91; discussion S91.

- □ Female pattern hair loss is the term for androgenic alopecia in females, potential causes include polycystic ovarian syndrome
  - ▪ Frontoparietal pattern
- • **Midface Face: Inferior Periorbital Area, Malars, Maxilla, and Nasolabial Fold**
  - ○ **Loss of malar projection** and nasal support secondary to bony loss of orbit and maxilla; maxillary posterior rotation causing a decrease in the maxillary angle and widening of the pyriform aperture
  - ○ **Attenuation of lower eyelid contour**
    - ▪ Protrusion of the periorbital fat due to laxity of the orbital septum
    - ▪ Atrophy of inferior lid fat compartments/suborbicularis oculi fat
    - ▪ Laxity of the orbicularis oculi and orbitomalar ligament
    - ▪ Decrease in the lateral canthal angle, descent of the lateral canthal tendon, loss of lower eyelid tone/hollowing, and tear trough deformity

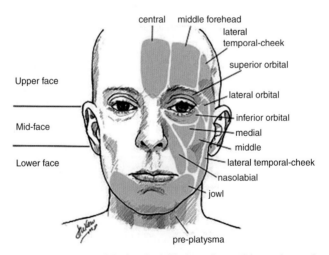

Figure 57-3 Fat compartments of the face divided by lower face, mid face, and upper face. Image of fat compartments by area of face (mid, upper, lower). (From Wilson AJ, Taglienti AJ, Chang CS, Low DW, Percec I. Current applications of facial volumization with fillers. *Plast Reconstr Surg.* 2016;137(5):872e-889e.)

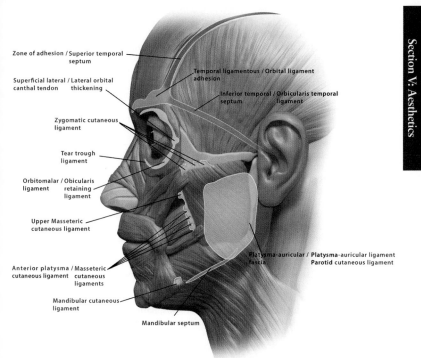

Zone of adhesion / Superior temporal septum

Superficial lateral / Lateral orbital canthal tendon thickening

Temporal ligamentous / Orbital ligament adhesion

Inferior temporal / Orbicularis temporal septum ligament

Zygomatic cutaneous ligament

Tear trough ligament

Orbitomalar / Obicularis ligament retaining ligament

Upper Masseteric cutaneous ligament

Platysma-auricular / **Platysma**-auricular ligament fascia **Parotid** cutaneous ligament

Anterior platysma / Masseteric cutaneous ligament cutaneous ligaments

Mandibular cutaneous ligament

Mandibular septum

Figure 57-4 Retaining ligaments of the face. (From Miotto GC, Nahai F. Facelift and Necklift. In: Chung KC, ed. *Grabb and Smith's Plastic Surgery*. 8th ed. Wolters Kluwer; 2020:510-518. Figure 51.1.)

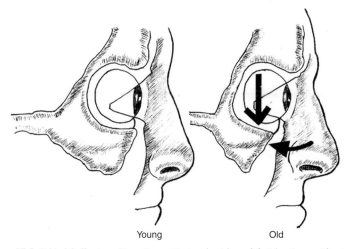

Young   Old

Figure 57-5 Orbital hollowing. (From Pessa JE. An algorithm of facial aging: verification of Lambros' theory by three-dimensional stereolithography, with reference to the pathogenesis of midfacial aging, scleral show, and the lateral suborbital trough deformity. *Plast Reconstr Surg.* 2000;106(2):479-488; discussion 489-90 and Farkas JP, Pessa JE, Hubbard B, Rohrich RJ. The science and theory behind facial aging. *Plast Reconstr Surg Glob Open.* 2013;1(1):e8-e15.)

- □ **Tear trough deformity:** develops within the boundary of the orbicularis oculi muscle. Medial periorbital hollow extending obliquely from medial canthus to mid-pupillary line.
  - Correlates to junction between preseptal and orbital portions of orbicularis oculi (location of the orbitomalar ligament).
  - This results in a sunken appearance of the lower lid and creates a shadow over the medial lower eyelid.
  - With age, soft tissue atrophy and orbital fat herniation accentuate deformity.
  - Not the same as nasojugal groove, which is inferomedial to the tear trough and bounded by the orbicularis oculi and the levator labii superioris alaeque nasi.
- □ Lid-cheek junction/palpebromalar groove: lateral lid-cheek junction at midpupillary line, below and along the infraorbital rim
- □ Factors associated with aging of the tear trough deformity and lid-cheek junction:
  - Herniation of the infraorbital fat.
  - Atrophy of the skin and the orbicularis oculi muscle.
  - Loosening and shifting of the malar fat pad.
  - Surface puckering caused by contractions of the orbicularis oculi muscle.
  - Malar retrusion.
  - Most of these anatomical changes result from the aging of the suborbital ligament-muscle system.
- Lateral brow laxity leads to orbital hooding and crow's feet
- ○ Exaggerated transitions between cheek fat pads, flattening of the malar prominence, increased nasolabial folds, lengthening of the cutaneous upper lip
- **Lower Face: Jawline, Perioral Region, Lips**
  - ○ **Widening of lower face** due to increased jowl volume, decreased jawline prominence and perioral/lip volume, and radial expansion
  - ○ **Jowling**
    - Unlike other fat compartments, jowl fat does not atrophy with age, so as surrounding facial fat atrophies, jowls become more apparent.
    - Descent of jowl fat compartments.
    - Masseteric ligaments attenuate, allowing jowl fat to descend into the neck and radially expand; jowl fat is separated from the submandibular fat by a septum adherent to the mandibular body.
    - Worsened by volume loss in the prejowl sulcus and volume loss posterior to the masseter in the posterior jawline and inferior preauricular region.
  - ○ **Perioral area**
    - Superficial and deep atrophy causing lengthening and flattening of the upper lip complex (1 mm loss of incisor with each decade of age)
    - Loss of vermillion and vermilion border volume with vertical perioral rhytides
    - Downturning of oral commissure
    - Flattening/ptosis of mentalis region
    - Mandibular atrophy associated with decreased vertical ramus height, widening of the mandibular angle, and loss of anterior mandibular (mental) projection
    - Deepening of the nasolabial folds and formation of marionette lines around the chin
  - ○ **Cervical changes**
    - Skin laxity and wrinkling.
    - Formation of vertical platysmal bands from diastasis of the platysma muscles.
    - With laxity and increase in submental fat, a more obtuse cervicomental angle develops.
    - Ptosis of the submandibular glands.

EXACERBATING FACTORS

- **Skin**
  - Sun damage (photoaging): atrophy, loss of skin tone, and pigmentation changes
    - DNA and urocanic acid: UV spectrum chromophores in the skin that absorb UVA/UVB radiation
      - UVA damages DNA but primarily causes damage through reactive oxygen species and free radicals
      - UVB mainly absorbed in the epidermis; thus, UVA alone causes dermal damage
    - Epidermis
      - Epidermal hyperplasia.
      - Increased fibroblast and Langerhans cells.
      - Slower keratinocyte turnover with proliferation, and decreased melanocyte counts, combined with regions of increased melanocyte concentration/melanin production and keratinocyte deposition causing solar lentigines.
      - Keratinocyte proliferation can form seborrheic and actinic keratoses.
      - UV radiation increases angiogenesis, creating telangiectasias.
    - Dermis
      - Solar elastosis
      - Decreased fibroblast and Langerhans cells
      - Matrix metalloproteinases degrade collagen
      - Shows chronic inflammation
      - Increased extracellular matrix components: glycoproteins and glycosaminoglycans (usually decreased with age and now found in the reticular dermis, not the usual papillary dermis)
  - Acne and other dermatologic conditions
  - Traumatic injuries/scarring
  - Smoking
    - Increased reactive oxidative species cause epidermal thinning and dermal collagen disorganization
- **Soft Tissue**
  - Significant weight gain or loss: increased facial fat deposits will confer a more youthful appearance.
  - Facial paralysis leads to muscle atrophy.
- **Skeletal:** facial trauma
- **Other Considerations:** radiation, surgery, chronic diseases

PEARLS

1. Facial aging can be analyzed through three components: skin changes, soft tissue atrophy, and skeletal resorption.
2. Overall loss of volume is most pronounced in middle and upper third of the face.
3. Rhytides are caused by a combination of thinning of the dermis and epidermis, fat pad descent, and muscle contractions.
4. Factors associated with aging of the tear trough deformity and lid-cheek junction include herniation of the infraorbital fat, atrophy of the skin and the orbicularis oculi muscle, loosening and shifting of the malar fat pad, surface puckering caused by contractions of the orbicularis oculi muscle, and malar retrusion.

QUESTIONS YOU WILL BE ASKED

1. Horizontal rhytides at the root of the nose and between the eyebrows are caused by the action of the procerus muscle.
2. For aesthetic analysis, the face can be divided into equal horizontal thirds and vertical fifths.
3. "Hollowness" of the cheeks is caused primarily by deflation of facial fat compartments and attenuation of facial retaining ligaments.

Recommended Readings
1. Farkas JP, Pessa JE, Hubbard B, Rohrich RJ. The science and theory behind facial aging. *Plast Reconstr Surg Glob Open*. 2013;1(1):e8-e15. doi:10.1097/GOX.0b013e31828ed1da
2. Mendelson B, Wong CH. Changes in the facial skeleton with aging: implications and clinical applications in facial rejuvenation. *Aesthetic Plast Surg*. 2020;44(4):1151-1158. doi:10.1007/s00266-020-01823-x
3. Wilson AJ, Taglienti AJ, Chang CS, Low DW, Percec I. Current applications of facial volumization with fillers. *Plast Reconstr Surg*. 2016;137(5):872e-889e. doi:10.1097/PRS.0000000000002238

58 Nonoperative Facial Rejuvenation

Galina G. Primeau

FACIAL AGING

FACTORS AFFECTING FACIAL AGING

- **Chronic Sun Exposure**
  - Ultraviolet (UV) radiation causes DNA damage and production of free radicals resulting in collagen and elastin damage, diminished dermal robustness, loss of skin elasticity, and increased risk for development of skin cancers.
  - Elastic fibers rearrange in abnormal distribution.
  - Overall decrease in collagen fibers.
  - Creates fine rhytids and skin laxity.
- **Chronologic Aging**
  - Diminished collagen and elastin deposition with increasingly disorganized structure.
  - Fewer fibroblasts and diminished supply of blood.
  - Fewer elastic fibers.
  - Thinning of the dermis due to these effects ultimately results in rhytid development.
  - Aging is related with time-dependent exposure to gravity, resulting in deep rhytids.
  - Sebaceous glands produce less oil resulting in decreased skin moisture.
  - The subcutaneous fat thins, resulting in a more hollowed appearance.
- **Other Exposures**
  - Cigarette smoke results in fine rhytids secondary to local irritants from smoke and systemic hypoxia; production of matrix metalloproteinases; inhibits procollagen synthesis.
  - Radiation therapy—DNA damage and free radical production similar to UV radiation.
  - Weight gain can result in dermal thinning, which is persistent despite weight loss.
- **Higher Fitzpatrick types (darker skin) have higher resistance to photoaging**.
  - Describes skin types in relation to color, sensitivity to UV light, and whether the skin type characteristically burns or tans with sun exposure.
  - Photoaging—changes associated with UV exposure

STIGMATA

- **Rhytids**
  - Fine rhytids caused by facial muscle forces and chronic changes in dermis.
  - Deep rhytids are caused by gravity fixed structures, such as retaining ligaments.
- **Dyschromia**—changes in the coloration of the skin. In older patients, the number of melanocytes decreases causing the skin to appear pale. The remaining melanocytes increase in size, resulting in patchy appearance and pigmented spots.

---

*Denotes common in-service examination topics.

NONOPERATIVE REJUVENATION OPTIONS

CHEMICAL PEELS

- Background
  - Chemically induced injury to epidermis and superficial dermis
  - Healing via epithelial advancement from skin appendages
    - Epidermal regeneration begins at 48 hours; complete by 7 days. Cell uniformity, columnar shape (vertical polarity), increased melanocytes, decreased melanin
    - Collagen deposition in the dermis begins 2 weeks after peel application; lasts up to 1 year. Homogenization of dermal collagen, dense parallel collagen bundles
- Pretreatment
  - Generally, indicated in patients undergoing medium (trichloroacetic acid [TCA]) or deep (phenol) peels
  - Use is variable—tretinoin and/or hydroquinone (4%) 2 weeks to 3 months prior
    - **Tretinoin**
      - □ Stimulates papillary dermal collagen synthesis and angiogenesis
      - □ Enhances basement membrane structure—increased deposition of glycosaminoglycans
      - □ Increases depth of penetration of actual peel by exfoliating the stratum corneum
    - **Hydroquinone**—tyrosinase inhibitor
      - □ Blocks tyrosinase (enzyme that produces melanin)
      - □ Helps prevent postpeel hyperpigmentation
  - Keratinolytics such as Jessner solution, salicylic acid, lactic acid, and resorcinol
- Factors to Change Depth of Penetration
  - Peeling agent characteristics—concentration, type of formula, storage and age of acid
  - Skin preparation—degreasing, skin cleansing, abrasion
  - Method of application—number of coats, occlusion
- Superficial Peels (Fig. 58-1)
  - Affects superficial epidermis; use for mild dyschromia
  - Alpha hydroxy acid (AHA)
    - Primarily used as exfoliant
    - May include acids such as lactic acid, glycolic acid, tartaric acid, or malic acid
  - Jessner solution
    - Similar to alpha hydroxy acid in depth of effect
    - Can be used as pretreatment for TCA peel
  - Salicylic acid
- Medium Depth Peels
  - TCA
    - Derivative of acetic acid
    - Medium or deep depending on the concentration used
- Deep Peels
  - Phenol
    - **Baker-Gordon peel**—3 mL phenol, 2 mL tap water, 8 drops liquid soap, 3 drops croton oil—vesicant that enhances keratolytic and penetrating action. It is believed that the croton oil is the active ingredient, not the phenol.
      - □ Number of coats does not affect depth of penetration as in TCA peels.
    - **Patient selection**
      - □ Good for type I-III skin (less risk of hypopigmentation)
      - □ Not suitable for acne, telangiectasia, and skin grafts
      - □ Contraindicated in patients with cardiac disease
    - **Metabolism**
      - □ Absorbed through skin, metabolized by liver, renally excreted.

□ High risk for cardiac dysrhythmia if >50% of face resurfaced in <30 minutes. For large areas, take 15-minute breaks between subunits or apply slowly over 1 hour.
- **Complications**
  - ○ Infection
    - ▪ Viral: herpes prophylaxis for peels in individuals with a history of herpes
    - ▪ Bacterial: rare, prompt diagnosis and treatment to limit scarring
  - ○ **Scarring**
    - ▪ Do not resurface people with keloid scar history due to risk of abnormal scarring.
    - ▪ Constant moisturizing fosters reepithelization and decreases healing time.
  - ○ **Pigmentary changes** hyperpigmentation (usually transient) vs hypopigmentation (may be permanent)
  - ○ **Milia,** keratin-filled epidermal inclusion cysts

LASERS IN AESTHETIC SURGERY (TABLE 58-1)
- **Background (see Chapter 9: Lasers in Plastic Surgery)**
- **Ablative Lasers**
  - ○ Vaporizes the superficial epidermal tissue and coagulates deeper tissues
  - ○ Proliferation of progenitor cells in adnexal structures results in reepithelization
  - ○ Increased collagen synthesis
    - ▪ Type I collagen deposition in subepidermal layer of papillary dermis (Zone of Grenz)
    - ▪ Heat-induced collagen contraction
    - ▪ Reorientation of disorganized collagen fibers
  - ○ Reorganization of elastic fibers to become parallel and more bundled
  - ○ **Contraindications**
    - ▪ Active infection (viral, bacterial, or fungal)
    - ▪ *Isotretinoin use in previous 12 months
  - ○ CO_2 laser (10 600 nm)
    - ▪ *Water is the chromophore
    - ▪ Depth of ablation—number of passes and cooling time
    - ▪ Greatest effect in papillary dermis: disorganized collagen replaced by compact collagen bundles, parallel to the skin
    - ▪ Side effects
      - □ Hypopigmentation—most pronounced in Fitzpatrick I/II (opposite chemical peels)
      - □ Erythema for 2-4 months after use
      - □ Hyperpigmentation
      - □ Milia
      - □ Acne
      - □ Infection: bacterial, viral, or fungal
      - □ Hypertrophic scarring
      - □ Ectropion
  - ○ **Erbium:yttrium-aluminum-garnet (Er:YAG, 2940 nm)**
    - ▪ Rarely used compared to CO_2; not as effective at collagen remodeling
    - ▪ Shorter recovery time
    - ▪ *Water is the chromophore
    - ▪ Useful for thin skin (dorsum of hand, tip of nose)
    - ▪ Useful for superficial, fine wrinkles. Need more passes to get deeper effect
- **Nonablative**
  - ○ **ND:YAG (1064 nm)**
    - ▪ *Energy nonspecifically absorbed—targets: blood vessels, red blood cells, collagen, and melanin
    - ▪ Secondary target: water

TABLE 58-1 Facial Lasers

Ablative	Produces heat-induced injury to dermis and removes epidermis. Stimulates collagen synthesis and reorganization to improve skin texture and tone.			
	Fractionated CO_2	10 600 nm	Water	Resurfacing laser
	Er:YAG (erbium)	2940 nm	Water	Does not completely destroy epithelium; more superficial treatment with faster recovery. Less risk of hypopigmentation than CO_2
Nonablative	Produces heat-induced injury to dermis without epidermal ablation. Stimulates collagen synthesis and reorganization to improve skin texture and tone.			
	Nd:YAG (neodymium)	1046 nm	Multiple	Resurfacing, vascular lesions, hair removal. Targets melanin less efficiently, allowing for safer treatment of all skin types. May be used for hair removal on darker skin types
	Pulsed dye laser (PDL)	577-585 nm	Hgb	Cutaneous vascular lesions. Minimal discomfort and down time
	Q-switched	532 and 1064 nm	Melanin, pigment	Commonly used for tattoo removal; high-intensity pulse spares skin not containing pigment
	Alexandrite	755 nm	Melanin	Hair removal, pigmented lesions. Less commonly used in-office
	Broad band light (BBL)	Multiple	Multiple	Vascular lesions, pigmented lesions, acne, hair removal. Able to treat multiple conditions with interchangeable filters to select desired wavelength

- Greatest effect 1-2 mm below skin in dermis
- Epidermis not ablated
- Less blistering but less dramatic effect than ablative lasers
- **Postlaser Care**
  - Moist wound environment with lipid-based ointment
  - Valacyclovir or acyclovir for 1 week to prevent herpes simplex activation
  - Hydroquinone and sunscreen to prevent hyperpigmentation
- **Intense Pulsed Light**
  - Not a laser
  - Emits photons in the range of 500-1300 nm, with multiple targets
  - Indications—telangiectasias, rosacea, solar lentigines, melisma, or freckling
  - Contraindications—isotretinoin, pregnancy, Fitzpatrick VI, and photosensitizing medications
  - Series of four to seven treatments needed

DERMABRASION AND MICRODERMABRASION

- **Dermabrasion**
  - **Background**
    - Mechanical abrasion of the epidermis and superficial dermis.
    - Facial skin is excellent surface for dermabrasion due to increased healing potential from abundant vascular network and ample adnexal structures.
  - **Indications**
    - Most commonly used to improve scars from acne
    - Traumatic scars
    - Perioral and periorbital rhytids
    - Telangiectasia, actinic keratoses, pigmented nevi, and rhinophyma
    - Higher risk of dyspigmentation for skin types III and above
  - **Contraindications**
    - Recent or current history of isotretinoin
    - Current outbreak of herpes
    - History of herpes—acyclovir pre- and postprocedure 2 weeks
    - History of hypertrophic or keloid scarring
    - Patients with coagulation disorders or taking anticoagulants
  - **Preprocedure preparation**
    - Topical tretinoin for 1-2 months prior
    - Avoid direct sunlight for 2 months prior
  - **Postprocedure**
    - Antibiotic ointment and dressing.
    - Skin reepithelializes in 7-10 days.
    - Redness will persist for up to 2-3 weeks.
    - Collagen remodeling occurs over the next 3-6 months.
    - Avoid sun exposure to reduce risk of skin hyperpigmentation.
  - **Complications**
    - Uneven pressure or uneven skin tension may result in streaky or blotchy outcome.
    - Abrasion of subcutaneous fat may result in scarring due to dermal discontinuity. Dermis should be reapproximated with suture if subcutaneous fat is entered.
    - Milia formation may occur.
    - Hypopigmentation.
- **Microdermabrasion**
  - **Background**
    - Noninvasive method of mechanical rejuvenation, not requiring physician oversight.
    - Inert crystal particles (aluminum oxide or sodium chloride) cause superficial ablation of the epidermal stratum corneum.

- Indications
  - To improve the tone and texture of already healthy skin
  - To correct photodamage, superficial rhytids, actinic keratoses, stretch marks
- Complications
  - Extremely rare due to superficial nature of procedure
  - Prolonged erythema may occur

BOTULINUM TOXIN

- **Mechanism**
  - Protein naturally produced by bacteria *Clostridium botulinum.*
  - Toxin consists of two parts—heavy chain (binds to presynaptic terminals) and light chain (translocated across cell membrane, prevents release of acetylcholine at neuromuscular junction).
  - Function restored in 2-6 months after new axon terminals sprout and replace deactivated end plates.
- **Indications:** FDA approved for glabellar frown lines, crow's feet, forehead lines, hyperhidrosis, migraines, cervical dystonia, spasticity, and urinary incontinence
- **Serotypes**
  - **There are seven different serotypes** of the toxin, A-G
  - **Type A**—the most commonly used and most potent; FDA approved for glabellar frown lines, periorbital crow's feet, forehead lines, and hyperhidrosis
  - **Type B**—less potent; approved for cervical dystonia
- **Commercially Available Toxins**
  - **Botox** (onabotulinumtoxinA, type A)
    - Reconstitute in 2.5 4 mL to make 2.5-4 units/0.1 mL
    - Lethal dose 2700 units in 70-kg human
  - **Dysport** (abobotulinumtoxinA, type A)
  - **Xeomin** (incobotulinumtoxinA, type A)
  - **Myobloc** (rimabotulinumtoxinB, type B)
- **Dose Preparation**
  - Expressed in mouse units. 1 U is the amount that kills 50% of Swiss Webster mice
  - Relative units: 1 U Botox = 1 U Xeomin = 2-3 U Dysport = 50-100 U Myobloc
- **Effect**
  - 3- to 6-day latency period (Dysport may have slightly faster onset than Botox)
  - Paralysis lasts 2-6 months
- **Contraindications**
  - Disorders of neuromuscular transmission—myasthenia gravis, Lambert-Eaton syndrome, multiple sclerosis, amyotrophic lateral sclerosis.
  - Women who are pregnant or breast-feeding.
  - Patients with allergies to albumin, milk, or other ingredients in the formulation.
  - Use of aminoglycosides and calcium channel blockers can potentiate toxin effects.
  - Do not inject near sites of active infection.
- **Complications**
  - Bruising: discontinue anti-inflammatory agents 1 week before injection; avoid prominent veins when injecting; apply pressure and ice after injection.
  - Eyelid ptosis: avoid injecting too deep as the toxin may penetrate the orbital septum and paralyze the levator palpebrae muscle.
  - Diplopia: iatrogenic effect on the extraocular muscles—inject outside the orbital rim and avoid deep injection, which can lead to oblique or recti muscle paralysis.
  - Pain: greater pain associated with injection of type B.
- **Antibody Formation**
  - Occurs in 5%-15% of patients, leading to reduced toxin effectiveness
  - Risk increased with more than 200 units in a session or repeat injection within 1 month
- **Treatment Locations (Fig. 58-1)**

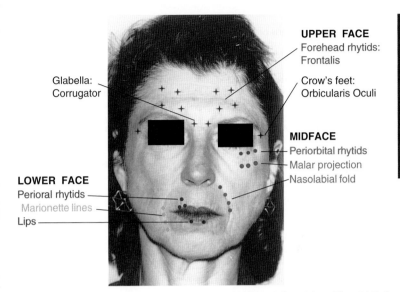

Figure 58-1 Common injection sites for Botox (crosses) and fillers (circles). (Adapted from Mulholland MW, ed. *Greenfield's Surgery*. 4th ed. Lippincott Williams & Wilkins; 2006.)

- ○ **Forehead:** horizontal lines
  - ▪ Target: frontalis; 4-6 injection points in the occipitofrontalis muscle in the middle of the forehead, 2-3 cm above the orbital rims.
  - ▪ **10-30 U total.**
  - ▪ Direct injections more medial in women to allow greater lateral eyebrow elevation.
  - ▪ Avoid low lateral brow injections to prevent ptosis.
- ○ **Glabella**
  - ▪ *Target: corrugator supercilii, procerus, and orbicularis oculi
  - ▪ 3-7 injection points, with a total of **20-40 U**
  - ▪ Placed outside of the orbital rim to avoid paralysis of the levator palpebrae superioris
- ○ **Crow's feet and lower eyelid**
  - ▪ Target: orbital, palpebral, and lacrimal portions of orbicularis oculi.
  - ▪ Typically 3-5 injection sites above zygomatic arch.
  - ▪ 4-12 U per side are placed approximately 1 cm lateral to the orbital rim.
  - ▪ The lower eyelid is treated with 1-2 injections using a total of 1-2 U per side.
  - ▪ Snap test—if sluggish, lower eyelid should be avoided (ectropion).
  - ▪ Avoid injecting the zygomaticus muscle—cheek ptosis and lip asymmetry.
- ○ **Bunny lines**—develop on the lateral or dorsal portion of the nose
  - ▪ Target: nasalis and procerus.
  - ▪ Typically, one injection is given on each side; total of 2-5 U.
  - ▪ Avoid deep injection which causes bruising.
  - ▪ Avoid levator labii superioris alaeque nasi and levator labii superioris, which will cause external nasal valve collapse.
- ○ **Nasolabial folds**
  - ▪ Primarily treated with dermal fillers.
  - ▪ Targets: levator labii superioris (primary target), levator labii superioris alaeque nasi, zygomaticus minor, zygomaticus major, and levator anguli oris.
  - ▪ A single injection of 1-3 U is given per side.

- ○ Perioral wrinkles
  - Target: orbicularis oris muscle.
  - Fine lines of the upper lip; total of 1-2.5 U per side.
  - Treatment should be limited and lateral injections avoided to prevent drooling.
  - Dermal fillers are often used in conjunction.
  - Avoid in singers, public speakers, and musicians who play wind instruments.
  - Stay within 5 mm of vermilion border.
- ○ Marionette lines
  - The depressor anguli oris muscle draws down the corner of the mouth.
  - Two injections are given per side.
    - □ One targeting the depressor anguli oris at least 1 cm away from the mouth
    - □ Second injection laterally to treat the platysmal bands, total up to 5 U per side
- ○ Cobblestone chin
  - Target: mentalis muscle
  - 1-3 injection points 0.5-1 cm above the chin; 2-8 U
- ○ Platysmal bands
  - Target: platysma
  - 4-8 injection points per band, approximately 1 cm apart; 2-2.5 U per injection

INJECTABLES

- Background
  - ○ Autologous materials include fat, platelet-rich plasma, collagen, fascia, and fibroblasts
  - ○ Biological materials include collagen and hyaluronic acid
  - ○ Synthetic materials include polylactic acid (PLLA), calcium hydroxylapatite, and polymethylmethacrylate
- Absorbable
  - ○ Platelet-rich plasma
    - Autologous blood plasma.
    - Platelets are activated by the addition of calcium and release a variety of growth factors, cytokines, and chemokines that stimulate collagen production.
    - Two to three treatments 1 month apart.
    - Effects have 6- to 12-month duration, retreatment often performed every 6 months.
  - ○ Collagen—FDA approved to treat fine to deep facial wrinkles and folds and acne
    - Bovine origin: Zyderm, Zyplast
    - Porcine origin: Evolence
    - Human origin: CosmoDerm, CosmoPlast
    - Injected into the superficial or mid dermis to treat fine to medium lines
    - Deep rhytids and nasolabial folds—injection into the middle to deep dermis
    - 2- to 6-month duration
    - *Allergy skin testing for hypersensitivity prior to use of bovine collagen
    - Lip augmentation technique—at the vermilion border or within the muscle
    - Nasolabial fold effacement technique
      - □ A "threading" technique is used in which multiple passes are used.
      - □ It is important to retain part of the nasolabial fold and not efface all of it.
    - Glabellar folds/scars/other hollow areas—linear threading technique is used
  - ○ Hyaluronic acid
    - Brands: Restylane, Perlane, Captique, Hylaform, and Juvéderm.
    - Hydrophilic glycosaminoglycan from by Streptococcus or from rooster comb.
    - Cross-linking improves duration of effect by resisting degradation.
    - FDA approved to treat moderate to severe facial wrinkles and folds.
    - Small particle sizes.

- □ Restylane Fine Lines, Juvederm 18, and Hylaform Fine Lines.
- □ Inject into the superficial dermis or dermal epidermal junction to treat fine lines.
  - Intermediate particle sizes
    - □ Restylane, Juvederm 24, and Hylaform.
    - □ Inject into middle dermis to treat moderate wrinkles.
  - Larger particle
    - □ Perlane, Juvederm 30, and Hylaform Plus.
    - □ Inject into the deep dermis to treat more pronounced wrinkles and folds.
  - Lip augmentation—within vermillion and not above to avoid shortening the lip.
  - Higher concentration gels absorb more water and swell more following injection.
  - 6- to 12-month duration.
  - For undesired outcome or concern for injection necrosis, hyaluronidase can be injected to break down the hyaluronic acid.
- ○ Poly-L-lactic acid (PLLA)
  - Brand: Sculptra.
  - Synthetic biodegradable lactic acid polymer microparticles suspended in cellulose.
  - FDA approved to treat nasolabial folds and deep facial wrinkles.
  - Volume enhancement effect occurs through fibroblast stimulation of collagen synthesis and replacement of degraded PLLA.
  - Results may not appear for at least 4 weeks, 2-5 treatments 4-6 weeks apart.
  - 2+ years duration and degrades and is replaced with collagen.
  - Immunologically inert, sensitivity testing is not required.
  - Delayed appearance of palpable but nonvisible subcutaneous nodules may occur.
  - *Approved for HIV lipoatrophy—inframalar hollow; concavities adjacent to zygomatic bone; zygomatic arch.
  - Must be injected deep (deep dermis or periosteum).
- ○ Calcium hydroxylapatite
  - Brand: Radiesse.
  - Main mineral component of bone, microparticles suspended in a polysaccharide gel that acts as a scaffold for collagen and tissue growth.
  - FDA approved for moderate to severe facial wrinkles and folds and lipoatrophy.
  - Injected just below the dermis to treat deep wrinkles, glabellar lines, midfacial atrophy, and nasolabial folds and for cheek and chin augmentation.
  - 6- to 18-month duration.
  - Sensitivity testing is not required.
  - Nodules may form if injected into the dermis.
- • Nonabsorbable—Polymethyl Methacrylate
  - ○ Brand: Artefill.
  - ○ Nonbiodegradable synthetic polymer microspheres suspended in bovine collagen.
  - ○ Induces fibroblast collagen synthesis, leading to tissue ingrowth and connective tissue encapsulation of the microspheres.
  - ○ FDA approved only for correction of nasolabial folds.
  - ○ Injected into the deep dermis or subcutaneous layer.
  - ○ Massage after injection to decrease lumps.
  - ○ May take 6-8 weeks for results to appear.
  - ○ Effects considered permanent, but additional may be required after 18 months.
  - ○ Skin testing performed prior to use due to bovine collagen component.
- • Kenalog—Triamcinolone Acetonide
  - ○ Inhibits fibroblast proliferation and promotes collagen degeneration

○ Used for hypertrophic and keloid scar management
○ Requires multiple injections; should be spaced out in time by 3+ months
○ Adverse effects—dermal atrophy, hypopigmentation, telangiectasia, and pain

PEARLS

1. Increasing Fitzpatrick skin type – increasingly dark skin with easier tanning and less burning.
2. Risks of facial peels: hyperpigmentation (usually transient), hypopigmentation (more likely to be permanent), and infection (herpes).
3. CO_2 and Er:YAG are ablative. Water as a chromophore. CO_2 has a deeper effect.
4. Dermabrasion allows for a more controlled depth of resurfacing compared to peels.
5. *Botox is FDA approved for glabellar frown lines, crow's feet, forehead lines, hyperhidrosis, migraines, cervical dystonia, spasticity, and urinary incontinence.

QUESTIONS YOU WILL BE ASKED

1. How does reepithelialization occur after a chemical peel?
   Through dermal appendages, which remain intact in the deep dermis and subcutaneous tissues.
2. Do fine wrinkles occur parallel or perpendicular to facial muscle fibers?
   Repetitive contraction results in fine wrinkles perpendicular to muscle fibers.
3. What can you do to diminish the risk of hyperpigmentation after a chemical peel?
   Hydroquinone prior to the procedure inhibits tyrosinase, an enzyme that is involved in melanin production. Patients should also use sunscreen after the peel.
4. What is the concern with performing chemical peels or laser resurfacing in patients at the time of operative facial procedures (eg, face-lift)?
   Operative procedures require significant undermining of tissue resulting in loss of some vascular supply. Chemical peels and laser resurfacing cause damage to the epithelial and superficial dermis – without a robust blood supply, they can be slow to heal and may scar.
5. How will injection of Botox into the lateral orbicularis oculi affect brow position?
   The lateral orbicularis is involved in lateral brow depression. Paralysis of the lateral orbicularis will result in some lateral elevation of the brow.
6. How many days after injection of Botox can you expect to see a significant change?
   Generally, it takes about 3-5 days for patients to notice the effects of Botox.

Recommended Readings
1. AlKhawam L, Alam M. Dermabrasion and microdermabrasion. *Facial Plast Surg.* 2009;25:301-310.
2. Beer K, Beer J. Overview of facial aging. *Facial Plast Surg.* 2009;25:281-284.
3. Nahai F, Lorenc ZP, Kenkel JM, et al. A review of onabotulinumtoxinA (Botox). *Aesthet Surg J.* 2013;33(1_Supplement):9S-12S.
4. Goldberg D. *Facial Rejuvenation.* Springer; 2007.
5. Nguyen AT, Ahmad J, Fagien S, Rohrich RJ. Cosmetic medicine: facial resurfacing and injectables. *Plast Reconstr Surg.* 2012;129:142e-153e.
6. Pathak A, Mohan R, Rohrich RJ. Chemical peels: role of chemical peels in facial rejuvenation today. *Plast Reconstr Surg.* 2020;145(1):58e-66e.
7. Roy D. Ablative facial resurfacing. *Dermatol Surg.* 2005;23:549-559.

59

Periocular Rejuvenation: Blepharoplasty, Eyelid Ptosis, and Brow Lift

Peter M. Kally and Jane S. Kim

See **Chapter 19: Facial Palsy** for complete anatomy of the eyelid and periocular structures (**eFigure 59-1**).

UPPER EYELID BLEPHAROPLASTY

- A surgical procedure to remove excess skin from the upper eyelid to restore a youthful contour and appearance, preserving underlying eyelid function.

PREOPERATIVE ASSESSMENT

- Goal: to rejuvenate and restore upper eyelid appearance and visual function
- Etiology: dermatochalasis (excess skin) weighing down the upper eyelids
- **History**
  - Is the heaviness of the upper lids interfering with ability to perform specific activities: driving, computer use, reading, ambulation, activities of daily living?
  - Headaches, dermatitis from redundant skin folds, skin-lash overhang
  - History of smoking, diabetes, myasthenia gravis, Graves disease, bleeding disorders, abnormal scarring, dry eyes, ocular allergies, glaucoma, cataracts, visual impairment, or contact lens use
- **Examination and documentation** (Table 59-1)
  - Dermatochalasis (upper lid skin) with or without skin-lash overhang
  - Measurement of upper lid height (MRD1), lagophthalmos, levator function, Bell phenomenon (upward rolling of the globe with the eye closed, which will protect the cornea in the event of lagophthalmos), vertical skin distance (from lash line to brow-eyelid skin junction), nasal fat pad prolapse, concomitant brow ptosis
  - Visual field testing with lids taped and untaped to document visual improvement
  - Photographic frontal and oblique (flash and unflash) documentation
- **Examination tips**
  - For the aesthetically minded patient, using a mirror or clinical photos is valuable to directly address their concerns both pre- and postoperatively.
  - A tuck of the redundant tissue with a cotton-tipped applicator or creaser device can reveal the tarsal platform, detail the amount of skin to be removed, and show the buried incision location in the supratarsal lid crease.
  - Additional components to discuss when indicated include lacrimal gland prolapse causing lateral fullness, medial orbital fat pad herniation, and the contribution of lateral brow ptosis to temporal hooding. These can be addressed concurrently with lacrimal gland pexy, herniated orbital fat excision or brow lift, respectively. (**See Chapter 57: Evaluation of Facial Aging** for further discussion of brow, upper, and lower lid aging.)
- Additional testing
  - Schirmer test for dry eye: strip placed into lower lid fornix for 5 minutes to document tear production (normal >15 mm)

---

*Denotes common in-service examination topics.

TABLE 59-1 Periocular Measurements

Measurement	Definition	Approximate normal value(s)
Palpebral fissure (PF)	Distance between upper and lower eyelid margins (vertical) or medial and lateral commissure (horizontal)	8-10 mm (v) 28-30 mm (h)
Margin-reflex distance 1 (MRD1)	Distance between corneal light reflex and upper eyelid margin in primary gaze with direct illumination	3.0-4.5 mm
Margin-reflex distance 2 (MRD2)	Distance between corneal light reflex and lower eyelid margin in primary gaze with direct illumination	4.0-5.0 mm
Levator function (LF)	Maximum upper lid excursion from full downgaze to upgaze (with brow fixated)	12.0-18.0 mm
Lagophthalmos (lag)	Measured PF with gentle eyelid closure	0-0.5 mm
Supratarsal lid crease	Height of lid crease measured from upper eyelid margin centered over pupillary axis	8-10 mm
Lateral canthus position	A positive vector superior to medial canthus	1-2 mm

- Relative Contraindications
  - Lagophthalmos, corneal exposure
  - Severe dry eye or compromised blink
  - History of skin cancers, as excess skin can be used in periocular reconstruction
  - *History of LASIK within previous 6 months

OPERATIVE APPROACHES AND VARIATIONS

- Markings are made prior to injection of local anesthetic with the patient awake. Can be done either sitting upright or once patient is lying on the operating table.
- The minimum vertical skin distance from upper eyelid margin to brow-lid skin junction is 20 mm to prevent postoperative lagophthalmos (**Fig. 59-1**).
- Markings are carried along the planned supratarsal lid crease from the medial upper puncta to the lateral canthus and then flaring at a 30°-45° angle ~1 cm laterally to encompass the lateral skin fold usually in a periorbital rhytids.
- Prevention of lagophthalmos and appropriate skin excision can be confirmed in addition to measuring and marking with the pinch technique.
  - "Pinch method": eyelid skin is plicated or pinched from the supratarsal lid crease mark to the superior proposed mark for maximal skin removal using nontoothed forceps. Lagophthalmos should not occur with the eyes gently closed to confirm appropriate skin removal. Should see a superior tilt of the upper eyelashes.
- Skin-only flap is removed; orbicularis oculi is maintained to preserve blink efficiency. Variably, a thin strip of orbicularis is removed by some surgeons.
- Nasal fat pad is sculpted by some, with careful dissection into the superonasal pocket and gentle depression of the globe to identify fat prolapse.
  - The nasal fat pad is whiter than the preaponeurotic fat pad, and the color difference is useful in identification and appropriate removal.
  - Complication of retrobulbar hemorrhage from deep vascular trauma in this area can occur with aggressive pulling during removal.
  - **Judicious fat removal is essential to avoid superior sulcus hollowing.**

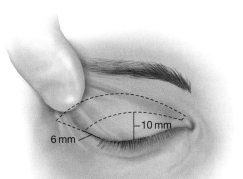

Figure 59-1 Upper lid blepharoplasty markings. (From Thorne CH, ed. *Grabb and Smith's Plastic Surgery*. 7th ed. Lippincott Williams & Wilkins; 2014.)

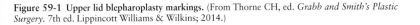

- Lateral hooding secondary to concomitant brow ptosis can be addressed at the time of blepharoplasty or later.
- Lateral fullness from lacrimal gland prolapse can be addressed with lacrimal gland repositioning.
- Closure is performed with dissolving or nondissolving sutures in running, interrupted, or subcuticular fashion as per surgeon preference.
- **The Asian Eyelid (Fig. 59-2)**

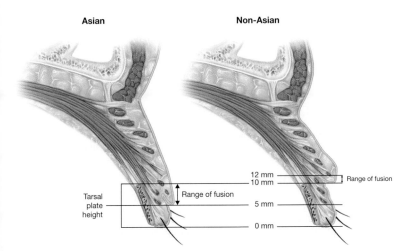

Figure 59-2 Asian vs non-Asian upper lid anatomy. (From Thorne CH, ed. *Grabb and Smith's Plastic Surgery*. 7th ed. Lippincott Williams & Wilkins; 2014.)

- Classically differentiated from the prototypical Caucasian eyelid by the insertion of the septum over the tarsus allowing fullness to the upper eyelid from the preaponeurotic fat pad.
- A low lid crease, narrower palpebral fissure, and epicanthal fold are common.
- Careful preoperative planning of lid crease position and discussion of the desired aesthetic outcome are critical.
- Lid crease formation sutures are used with variable techniques to anchor some levator aponeurosis fibers to the subcuticular tissue at the planned crease height.

POSTOPERATIVE CARE AND COMPLICATIONS

- **Postoperative Care**
  - Limit postoperative swelling and edema.
    - Use ice packs for 15-20 minutes every hour while awake for 72 hours.
    - Elevate head while sleeping on back for first week as able.
    - Avoid lifting weights >5 lb, bending over, straining, etc.
  - Apply topical ophthalmic ointment over sutures.
  - Lubricate eyes with artificial tears.
  - Patient should check vision with each eye covered independently every hour while awake during the first 24 hours.
- **Complications**
  - Orbital hemorrhage and blindness are rare (incidence 1:20 000). Requires emergency lateral canthotomy/cantholysis and management of bleed.
    - Significant unilateral pain, firm globe proptosis, and elevated intraocular pressure, with difficulty opening eyelids.
    - Permanent ischemic nerve and retina injury occurs within 1-2 hours.
  - Globe injury is incredibly rare but a devastating complication of inadvertent trauma.
  - Wound dehiscence can be repaired with interrupted sutures.
  - Lagophthalmos may be secondary to periorbital edema or excessive skin removal. Start with aggressive ocular lubrication and evaluate in 1-2 weeks. Can also consider taping or massage.
  - Medial canthal webbing due to medially overextended incision can be corrected with Z-plasty, W-plasty, or Y-V advancement flaps.
  - Scar hypertrophy can be treated with massage, topical or intralesional corticosteroid, and silicone gel/pads.
  - For suture granulomas (more common with absorbable sutures), remove the offending suture. May need topical or intralesional corticosteroid.
  - Ptosis may be secondary to edema or result from trauma to the levator complex inadvertently incurred with deep dissection.

LOWER EYELID BLEPHAROPLASTY

A surgical procedure to restore the natural contour of the lower lid by removing prolapsed orbital fat pads with or without conservative skin tightening and tightening of the lower lid.

PREOPERATIVE ASSESSMENT

- **Goal:** to rejuvenate and restore a youthful lower eyelid appearance by addressing lower lid orbital fat protrusion and dermatochalasis
- **History:** careful discussion of patient concerns and expectations in addition to all elements discussed above in the history for upper lid blepharoplasty
- **Examination and documentation**
  - Evaluate each clinical fat pad protrusion in upgaze and primary gaze.

- Degree of dermatochalasis, rhytidosis, tear trough deformity, and Fitzpatrick skin type.
- Evaluate for concomitant periorbital edema or festoons.
- Assess risk factors for lower lid postoperative lid malposition
  - Determine lower lid laxity (can be measured in millimeters of distraction from the globe or in subjective severity grading).
  - Preexisting lower lid retraction with an MRD2 > 5 mm, indicating a lower lid support failure.
  - Snapback testing, a measurement of lower lid elasticity by distracting and quickly releasing the lower lid to assess the speed and completeness of the lid's return to appropriate position without allowing blinking.
  - Midface descent: evaluate for drooping facial skin and a prominent nasolabial sulcus.
  - Assess for the presence of negative vector with globe prominence over inferior orbital rim.
  - Tear trough deformity, concavity at the border of the eyelid and cheek junction medially. This trough is created by the juxtaposition of protruding orbital fat above tight septal attachments at the arcus marginalis along the orbital rim.
- Examination tips
  - Cosmetically optimal results rely on an excellent examination and discussion of desired results.
  - Main features of aging will characteristically cause lower lid laxity, slower snapback (less elasticity), and a combination of orbital fat herniation and midface decent, which accentuates the tear-trough junction.
  - Determine the contribution of these factors during your examination and discuss the appropriate components and their corrective surgery: lower lid laxity—lateral tarsal strip, negative vector—canthopexy, midface decent—midface/SOOF lift, tear trough deformity—fat redraping and repositioning.
- Additional testing
  - If significant periorbital edema, evaluate kidney and thyroid function.
- **Relative Contraindications**
  - Use of anticoagulation
    - If medically able, stop anticoagulants prior to surgery.
  - Significant lower lid retraction, lagophthalmos, or severe dry eye

OPERATIVE APPROACHES AND VARIATIONS

- **Transconjunctival Approach**
  - Preferred method to eliminate anterior skin incision and minimize risk of cicatricial ectropion.
  - Preseptal and postseptal approaches based on location of incision in the palpebral conjunctiva.
  - Exposure maintained with Desmarres retractor and conjunctival traction sutures. Rarely an inferior cantholysis is required for additional exposure.
  - The inferior oblique muscle is visualized between the medial and central fat pads.
  - Fat pads are either sculpted with globe ballottement or pedicalized and redraped with percutaneous or absorbable sutures.
  - Can be paired with a skin pinch excision for excess skin. Additional methods of dealing with skin include TCA peel and CO_2 laser resurfacing.
- **Transcutaneous Approach (Fig. 59-3)**
  - An infraciliary incision is placed 1-2 mm below the lash line. A skin-muscle flap deep to orbicularis is dissected inferiorly to the infraorbital rim to expose the orbital fat pads.

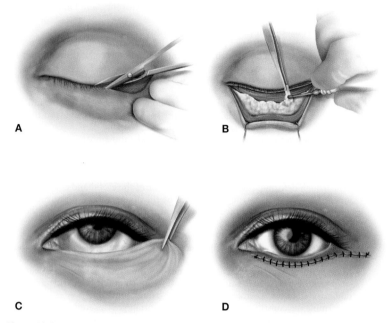

Figure 59-3 Transcutaneous lower lid blepharoplasty. A. Lower lid incision placed in the infraciliary groove. **B.** Excision of fat, after orbital septum and fat capsule have been incised. **C.** Determination of the amount of excess skin and muscle for excision by draping skin in a superior and lateral direction while the patient is looking up with the mouth open. **D.** Closure with running infraciliary 6-0 Prolene suture.

- - Orbitomalar ligament resuspension and lateral canthopexy can be concurrently performed to address midface descent and lid position.
- Variations in Approach
  - Dermatochalasis and rhytidosis can be addressed with a subciliary skin-pinch, laser skin resurfacing, or a chemical peel.
  - Infraorbital hollowing at tear trough may need fat redraping, fat grafting, or filler injections.
  - Lateral canthopexy or canthoplasty is often performed to reduce the risk of postoperative ectropion or retraction.
  - Preoperative presence of midface descent may require SOOF/midface lift, anchored to orbital rim periosteum.
  - Some perform fat grafting to blend the lid-cheek junction.

POSTOPERATIVE CARE AND COMPLICATIONS

- Postoperative care
  - Limit postoperative swelling and edema.
    - Use ice packs for 15-20 minutes every hour while awake for 72 hours.
    - Elevate head while sleeping on back for first week as able.
    - Avoid lifting weights >5 lb, bending over, straining, etc.
  - Use combination steroid-antibiotic eye drops for first week.

- Check vision before discharge and have patient check vision with each eye covered independently every hour while awake during the first 24 hours.
- **Complications**
  - Orbital hemorrhage causing blindness (0.05%). Intervention to relieve orbital compartment syndrome from retrobulbar hemorrhage requires rapid identification of the bleed, followed by emergent lateral canthotomy/cantholysis.
    - Significant unilateral pain, firm globe proptosis, and elevated intraocular pressure, with difficulty opening eyelids.
    - Permanent ischemic nerve and retina injury occurs within 1-2 hours.
  - Inferior oblique muscle injury causing diplopia.
    - Binocular diplopia worse in adduction and upgaze on affected side.
    - Direct injury or transection needs strabismus specialist evaluation.
    - Hematoma or bruising of muscle may take months to recover.
  - Lower eyelid retraction from scarring of the middle lamella.
  - Cicatricial ectropion from anterior lamellar shortage (secondary to aggressive skin excision).
  - Infection is rare. Orbital cellulitis requires IV antibiotics and prompt ophthalmology evaluation.

UPPER EYELID PTOSIS

PREOPERATIVE ASSESSMENT

- Goal: to determine cause of eyelid ptosis and improve visual function. (Not all lid ptosis is surgically treated.)
- Etiology: depends on type (acquired or congenital), see section II below.
- **History**
  - Onset, sudden or gradual; degree of ptosis, variable or progressively worsening; any changes during the day.
  - Associated headaches, recent trauma, neck surgery, or botulinum toxin use.
  - Record the presence or absence of dysphagia, dysphonia, diplopia, etc.
  - Is the drooping of the upper lids interfering with ability to perform specific activities: driving, computer use, reading, ambulation, activities of daily living?
- **Examination and documentation**
  - Corrected vision, extraocular motility, pupil evaluation for anisocoria and presence of afferent pupillary defect
  - Measurement of upper lid height (MRD1), levator function, lid crease height, lagophthalmos, Bell phenomenon
    - Significant ptosis = generally, MRD1 $\leq$ 2 mm
  - **If unilateral, lifting the affected lid removes Hering law of equal innervation to evaluate for compensated contralateral ptosis.**
  - Visual field testing with lids taped and untaped to document visual improvement.
  - Photographic frontal and oblique (flash and unflash) documentation.
- **Additional testing**
  - Schirmer test for dry eye: strip placed into lower lid fornix for 5 minutes to document tear production (normal >15 mm)
  - Phenylephrine testing for stimulation of Müller muscle to determine possibility of internal ptosis repair (Müller muscle-conjunctival resection, MMCR)
  - Ice pack test (apply ice pack to eyes for 2-3 minutes) or rest test (have patient lie down and close eyes for 30 minutes) in cases of variable ptosis to evaluate for myasthenia gravis
- Relative Contraindications
  - Lagophthalmos, corneal exposure.

- ○ Severe dry eye or compromised blink.
- ○ Significant lower lid retraction should be corrected prior to ptosis repair.

TYPES OF EYELID PTOSIS

- **Aponeurotic (Involutional/Senile)**
  - ○ **Most common type,** secondary to dehiscence of levator aponeurosis, typically involutional
  - ○ Presents with ptosis in an older patient with full levator function and high lid crease
- **Myogenic:** motor function abnormality with systemic disease
  - ○ **Myasthenia gravis:** variable ptosis, diplopia, positive ice-pack testing. Confirm with serology testing (eg, antiacetylcholinesterase, anti-MUSK) and single-fiber EMG testing.
  - ○ **Chronic progressive external ophthalmoplegia:** mitochondrial inheritance, decreased extraocular motility (ophthalmoplegia) and levator function, and myocardial conduction defects (need EKG). Typically do not subjectively experience diplopia.
  - ○ **Oculopharyngeal muscular dystrophy:** Autosomal dominant inheritance (OPMD gene), French-Canadian descent. Decreased extraocular motility and levator excursion, dysphagia, and dysphonia.
  - ○ **Myotonic dystrophy:** Autosomal dominant inheritance. Prolonged muscle contractions (locked grip on handshake), temporal wasting.
- **Neurogenic**
  - ○ **Third nerve palsy:** possible fatal finding! Worst etiology is due to posterior communicating artery aneurysm, often with dilated pupil from compression of parasympathetic fibers running with the oculomotor nerve, and severe ptosis with eye positioned in down and outward direction from loss of third nerve function.
    - ▪ Dilated pupil with anisocoria more pronounced in light
    - ▪ CT angiography of the brain and orbits urgently indicated
    - ▪ Ophthalmology evaluation to assess for other causes
  - ○ **Horner syndrome:** disruption of the sympathetic pathway including the cervical sympathetic chain affecting Müller muscle (typically 1-2 mm of ptosis). Worst etiology is carotid dissection or apical lung mass. Triad of mild ptosis, miosis, and anhidrosis. Note: All three signs are not always present.
    - ▪ Constricted pupil with anisocoria more pronounced in dark
    - ▪ CT angiography of the head and neck urgently indicated
    - ▪ Also recommend imaging of chest to evaluate for apical lung mass
    - ▪ Ophthalmology evaluation to assess for other causes
- **Traumatic**
  - ○ Direct injury to the levator muscle or neural pathway
- **Mechanical**
  - ○ Direct mass effect lowering lid height (eg, upper eyelid dermatochalasis, eyelid lesions, eyelid edema, orbital mass, orbital inflammation, etc.)
- **Congenital**
  - ○ Etiology from dysgenesis of the levator palpebrae superioris resulting in a thickened septum and thin fibrous or fatty-infiltrated levator muscle.
  - ○ Presents with poor levator function, poorly defined lid crease, and **lagophthalmos on downgaze** due to septal and levator fibrosis.
  - ○ Surgical correction is delayed until age 3-5 years unless visual obstruction risks amblyopia.
    - ▪ Unilateral ptosis has highest risk of amblyopia (poor visual development).
  - ○ Alternative congenital presentations include the following
    - ▪ **Horner syndrome or third nerve palsy at birth.**
      - □ Congenital Horner's is associated with neck birth trauma, neuroblastoma, and iris heterochromia (affected eye is lighter).

- **Blepharophimosis syndrome** presents with ptosis and triad of short palpebral fissures, epicanthus inversus, and telecanthus.
- A **Marcus-Gunn jaw wink** results from aberrant innervation of the levator palpebrae superioris muscle. A congenital aberrant connection between the muscles of mastication (motor branches of CN V) and the ipsilateral levator (superior division of CN III) causes eyelid elevation with chewing or jaw thrust.
  - *Surgical approaches depend on levator palpebrae superioris function
    - Poor function (<5 mm): frontalis suspension preferred (needs good frontalis function in order to be an effective approach)
    - Fair function (5-7 mm): large levator resection preferred
    - Good function (8-12 mm): levator advancement or resection
    - Excellent function (>13 mm): levator advancement or MMCR

OPERATIVE APPROACHES AND VARIATIONS

- **Levator Advancement**
  - Performed under minimal IV sedation with ability to sit up patient, who can then open their eyes to evaluate lid height, contour, and symmetry under natural conditions.
  - External approach: incision along supratarsal lid crease with dissection over tarsus.
  - Isolation of levator aponeurosis with separation of septal attachments.
  - Suture placed with a horizontal, ~5 mm, partial-thickness pass at superior 1/3 of tarsus. Length of pass, number of sutures used, type of suture, and height of placement are patient and surgeon specific.
  - Typically a double-armed pass through levator, with height of placement patient specific. **Can be affected by Hering phenomenon.**
  - Sutures can be adjusted as needed after determination of lid position and symmetry while patient is seated in upright position with eyes open.
  - Sutures are finalized, and skin closure is performed as with a blepharoplasty incision.
- **Levator Resection**
  - Predominantly performed in congenital ptosis repair
  - Similar approach to levator advancement but with large resection of levator aponeurosis, using resection nomogram based on degree of ptosis and lid excursion
- **Tarsoconjunctival Müllerectomy (Fasanella-Servat Procedure)**
  - Local anesthetic injected subconjunctivally in a posterior approach at superior border of tarsus with the lid everted.
  - Internal approach: amount of Müller muscle/conjunctiva and tarsus predetermined; this amount is patient and surgeon specific. Always resect <3 mm of tarsus to preserve eyelid stability. Generally, a 2:1 ratio of Müller's-to-tarsus resection.
  - Hemostat or Putterman clamp is placed along markings, and a double-armed gut suture is woven in a horizontal-mattress fashion under the clamp, plicating the tissues.
  - A #15 blade is slid in, with metal-on-metal fashion, angled away from the globe and suture line to remove the redundant tissue.
  - The sutures can be externalized though the lid at the lateral superior eyelid crease.
  - Bandage contact lenses can be variably used for the first week. Topical fluoroquinolone eye drops are recommended to decrease risk of corneal infection with postoperative contact lens use.
- **Müller Muscle Conjunctival Resection (Putterman Procedure)**
  - Patient must have adequate response to phenylephrine test.
  - Similar approach to Fasanella-Servat procedure with clamp placement at superior tarsal border but plicating only Müller muscle and conjunctiva.
  - Approximately 8 mm of total resection (markings placed at 4 mm for plication fold.
  - Variably, surgeons adjust this amount, tailoring to phenylephrine response.

- **Frontalis Suspension (Sling)**
  - Sling material is attached to tarsus ~2-3 mm superior to the lash line and tunneled in a postseptal plane to the arcus marginalis and anchored in the frontalis to allow lid elevation with frontalis activation.
  - Sling materials include silicone, autologous or banked fascia lata, permanent nonabsorbable suture.
  - Sling configurations: triangle, double triangle, rhomboid, and double rhomboid.
- **Frontalis Muscle Advancement Flap**
- **Nonsurgical Management**
  - Sympathomimetic ophthalmic drops
    - Oxymetazoline hydrochloride 0.1% ophthalmic solution or alpha-adrenergic agonists.
    - Stimulate Müller muscle for ~1-2 mm temporary correction in ptosis.
    - Phenylephrine testing can simulate effect in office, evaluate response.
    - Can be used for nonsurgical candidates, temporizing measures, mild degrees of ptosis, or temporary treatment of botulinum toxin ptosis.
  - Ptosis crutches: a physical-stenting attachment to glasses to lift the lid

POSTOPERATIVE CARE AND COMPLICATIONS

- **Postoperative Care**
  - Limit postoperative swelling and edema.
    - Use ice packs for 15-20 minutes every hour while awake for 72 hours.
    - Elevate head while sleeping on back for first week as able.
    - Avoid lifting weights >5 lb, bending over, straining, etc.
  - Apply topical ophthalmic ointment over sutures.
  - Lubricate eyes with artificial tears.
  - Patient should check vision with each eye covered independently every hour while awake during the first 24 hours.
- **Complications**
  - Lid asymmetry or under correction; reoperation ~5% in ptosis repair
  - Lagophthalmos secondary to ptosis overcorrection or tethering septum
  - Exposure keratopathy and corneal ulceration (secondary to lagophthalmos or exposed tarsal suture)
  - Scarring, symblepharon (scar or palpebral to bulbar conjunctiva)

BROW LIFT

ANATOMY (SEE TABLE 59-2)

- **Forehead Musculature**
  - **Frontalis Muscle**
    - Origin: occipitalis posteriorly, skin of eyebrow anteriorly
    - Insertion: galea aponeurotica
      - Galea aponeurotic is a dense fibrous aponeurosis from the occipitalis muscle posteriorly to the frontalis.
      - Temporal fusion line (conjoint tendon) = fusion of galea, temporalis, and periosteum at the temporal crest laterally.
    - Action: elevation of brow, **causing transverse rhytids**
    - Innervation: frontal branch of facial nerve
- **Corrugator supercilii muscle**
  - Origin: supraorbital ridge
  - Insertion: forehead skin near eyebrow
  - Action: central paired brow depressor causing **vertical glabellar frown lines**
  - Innervation: frontal and zygomatic branches of facial nerve

TABLE 59-2 Anatomic Layers of the Upper Face

	Scalp	Forehead	Brow	Temporal
	Skin	Skin	Skin	Skin
	Subcutaneous fat	Subcutaneous fat	Subcutaneous fat	Subcutaneous fat
	Galea aponeurotica	Superficial galea	Superficial galea	Superficial temporal fascia (AKA temporoparietal fascia)
Anterior		Frontalis muscle	Sub-brow fat (ROOF) + Corrugator	Deep temporal fascia (superficial layer)
↓				
Posterior	Loose connective tissue	Deep galea	Deep galea	Deep temporal fascia (deep layer)
				Temporalis muscle
	Pericranium	Pericranium	Pericranium	Pericranium
	Frontal bone	Frontal bone	Frontal bone	Temporal bone and greater wing of sphenoid bone

- **Procerus Muscle**
  - Origin: nasal bone and lateral nasal cartilage
  - Insertion: skin of glabella and fibers of frontal belly of frontalis
  - Action: brow depressor causing **horizontal glabellar rhytids**
  - Innervation: frontal branch of facial nerve

NERVES

- **Frontal (temporal) branch of the facial nerve (CN VII):** motor
  - Course follows Pitanguy line, running 0.5 cm below the tragus to 1.5 cm above the lateral eyebrow. Inserts onto underside of forehead muscles
  - Arises in deep fascia dividing the deep and superficial lobe of parotid and transitions to the underside of the superficial temporalis fascia (temporoparietal fascia) over the zygomatic arch
- **Supraorbital branch (V1) of trigeminal nerve (CN V):** Sensory
  - Forehead sensation exiting either from supraorbital foramen or notch generally 2.0-3.2 cm from midline. Can be generally located superior to the medial iris in primary gaze.
- **Supratrochlear nerve (V1) of trigeminal nerve (CN V):** Sensory
  - Forehead sensation exiting the orbit from frontal notch ~1.6-2.2 cm from midline. Medial to supraorbital nerve.
  - "Zone of safety" is generally set to 1.6-3.2 cm from midline to protect nerve branches during brow lift.

PREOPERATIVE ASSESSMENT

- Goal: to rejuvenate the upper aesthetic unit of the face by repairing brow ptosis and improving forehead rhytids. May also be performed for visually significant brow ptosis and facial nerve paralysis
  - Feminine eyebrow follows a "C" shape with the peak height at the lateral limbus and minimized frontal bossing; usually located above the orbital room.
  - Male eyebrow shape in a "T" pattern; usually located at the orbital rim.

- **History**
  - Cosmetic and functional concerns regarding appearance, visual function, heaviness, headaches/brow fatigue
  - History of dry eye or preexisting ocular comorbidities, facial paralysis
- **Examination and documentation**
  - Frontalis action, brow height (normal: 5-6 cm), brow shape/symmetry, hairline, and scars. Severity of glabellar/forehead/lateral canthi rhytids, lateral hooding, and upper eyelid superior sulcus hollowing or fullness.
  - Evaluate for lagophthalmos, Bell phenomenon.
  - Photograph frontal, oblique, and side view at rest, eyes open and closed.
- **Additional testing**
  - Visual field testing may be performed in functional cases.
- **Contraindications**
  - Lagophthalmos or severe dry eye
  - Psychological/psychiatric instability or unrealistic expectations

OPERATIVE APPROACHES AND VARIATIONS

- **Direct Brow Lift**
  - Advantages: best for visually significant brow ptosis with lateral hooding. Exact lift based directly on skin excised. Most appropriate for older males with thick eyebrows and deep rhytids, with male-pattern balding. Minimal sedation required.
  - Disadvantages: visible scar. Unable to address glabellar rhytids or significantly raise the medial brow.
  - Technique: manual lift of brow to desired height measured at three points. Lower line drawn just above brow cilia and ellipse created off medial and lateral tapering lines. Dissection of flap taken to frontalis muscle, except medially where the incision is more superficial to avoid damage to the neurovascular bundles. Wound closure is performed in layered fashion with excellent wound eversion. The authors prefer buried 5-0 absorbable suture and running cross-hatched or horizontal-mattress 5-0 nonabsorbable suture.
- **Internal Browpexy**
  - Advantages: able to be performed though concurrent blepharoplasty incision. Best for mild to moderate lateral brow ptosis.
  - Disadvantages: lift is predominantly lateral and does not address glabellar lines or forehead rhytidosis. Modest effect and duration.
  - Technique: amount of brow ptosis correction determined with patient in supine position at natural resting position. Dissection carried from blepharoplasty incision in suborbicularis plane to superior orbital rim. Preperiosteal dissection under the ROOF performed laterally. ROOF and surrounding connective tissue engaged in double-armed mattress fashion with nonabsorbable polypropylene or slowly absorbable 4-0 suture through the periosteum at the desired natural brow height. This is repeated for a total of two to three sutures.
    - Caution against excessive skin dimpling from superficial suture placement.
- **Endoscopic Forehead Lift**
  - Advantages: full elevation of temporal and medial brow ptosis. Minimally invasive approach with concealed incisions behind the hairline. No need to cut or shave hair. Excellent periosteal deep release with ability to adjust height and symmetry. Ideal for foreheads <6 cm.
  - Disadvantages: hairline elevation and surgical dissection not ideal for >7-cm foreheads. Increased cost to patients for equipment and fixation anchors. Does not address deep forehead rhytids.
  - Technique
    - Markings are placed behind hairline, with three vertical incisions (one central and two paracentral locations marked at the desired area of maximal brow elevation for fixation anchor placement). Next, a temporal incision behind

the hairline is marked perpendicular to an imaginary line running though the ipsilateral lateral canthus and nasal ala. Lastly, a safety zone with a 1.5-cm radius is placed around the palpated supraorbital notch or foramen.

- Temporal incisions are created, and dissection is carried out to the deep temporal fascia. A pocket is then endoscopically dissected to the lateral orbital rim no more than 1.5 cm lateral to the rim to minimize risk of facial nerve injury. The **zygomaticotemporal vein** (**sentinel vein**) is used as a landmark for the extent of lateral dissection, as it indicates the likely location of the facial nerve just temporally.
- Central incisions are made in the scalp through the periosteum. An endoscope and periosteal elevator are used to raise the periosteum down over the supraorbital rim where the periosteum is bluntly separated, and the supraorbital and supratrochlear neurovascular bundles are visualized and avoided.
- Full periosteal release of the temporal fusion line (conjoint tendon) connecting the temporal pockets to the central dissection is performed, and the brow is confirmed to freely elevate without attachments. Medial brow depressors are variably released as per surgeon preference.
- Anchoring fixation of the periosteum is placed at the planned paracentral incisions at the hairline. Variably, a bone tunnel with polypropylene suture or bioabsorbable fixation anchors can be used. The brow is elevated to anchors, and symmetry confirmed.
- A single suction drain is placed along the brow, typically removed on postoperative day 1.
- Closure is performed with deep buried interrupted 3-0 PDS through superficial temporalis fascia and anchored to deep temporalis fascia. Surgical skin staples are placed for wound eversion and removed at 1 week.
- After thorough hair cleaning, a pressure headwrap dressing is placed for 24 hours to limit hematoma formation.

- **Temporal Forehead Lift**
  - Performed as detailed above without central dissection or anchoring. Variably, a 1.5-cm ellipse is removed from the temporal incisions to assist in brow elevation.
- **Pretrichial Forehead Lift**
  - Advantages: directly addresses forehead rhytidosis and moderate to severe brow ptosis that decreases forehead height. Excellent exposure and release.
  - Disadvantages: long incision along hairline can leave visible scar if poorly performed. Patients with alopecia or frontal balding are poor candidates.
  - Technique
    - Markings: 3 mm behind the frontal hairline and then curved down into the temples from conjoint tendon toward the superior root of the helix.
    - Incision made in a sinusoidal or irregular pattern to minimize scarring appearance. Dissection carried in subgaleal plane along forehead and deep temporal fascia plane laterally.
    - Subgaleal dissection carried with a monopolar cautery inferiorly and joined to temporal pockets at the temporal line of fusion. At 1 cm before the brow ridge, the dissection is carried subperiosteal, releasing the periosteum from the arcus marginalis from lateral canthus to lateral canthus. Care to visualize and protect the neurovascular bundles.
      □ Corrugator release is generally performed to limit glabellar lines.
    - Fixation performed with deep buried galeal 2-0 or 3-0 PDS sutures at the frontal incision line and laterally after redraping to appropriate height and symmetry. Redundant tissue is excised.
    - Closure is performed with a tension-free closure using buried interrupted 2-0 or 3-0 PDS for fixation, buried interrupted 5-0 absorbable suture, and surgical skin staples or running nonabsorbable suture.
    - After thorough hair cleaning, a pressure headwrap dressing is placed for 24-48 hours to limit hematoma formation.

- **Coronal Approach**
  - Approach similar to pretrichial with incision made 4-6 cm behind the hairline.
- **Midforehead Approach**
  - Approach similar to pretrichial with incisions placed in two deep horizontal rhytids in the midforehead. Dissection of flap is taken to frontalis muscle similar to direct brow ptosis repair, with excision of redundant skin. Meticulous multilayer closure is performed with attention to good wound eversion.
- **Botulinum Toxin Injections** (nonsurgical): Utilizes principle of antagonistic muscle action to preferentially paralyze brow depressors, favoring brow elevators
  - Advantages: nonsurgical approach to attain mild brow elevation, predominantly laterally. Able to address glabellar lines concurrently
  - Disadvantages: temporary effect, does not address moderate to severe brow ptosis. Does not improve forehead rhytids. Risk of eyelid ptosis by proximity of injections to orbital rim and levator
  - Technique: injections placed in the corrugator supercilii and at the lateral aspects and tail of the brow cilia superior to the orbital rim superficially at the orbicularis oculi

POSTOPERATIVE CARE AND COMPLICATIONS

- **Postoperative Care**
  - Limit postoperative swelling and edema.
    - Use ice packs for 15-20 minutes every hour while awake for 72 hours.
    - Elevate head while sleeping on back for first week as able.
    - Avoid lifting weights >5 lb, bending over, straining, etc.
    - Head dressing is removed after first 24-48 hours as based on surgeon preference.
- **Complications**
  - Hematoma: one of the most common complications, over 1/3 due to nausea/vomiting postoperatively. Immediate percutaneous drainage or evacuation with redressing should be performed based on size and bleeding rate (arterial vs venous).
  - Nerve paralysis
    - Facial nerve: neuropraxia from blunt trauma generally has slow recovery of facial nerve function. Complete transection is a rare complication with full paralysis.
    - Trigeminal nerve: transection is rare but may result in loss of brow and periorbital sensation. Some cross-coverage of sensation is present from supratrochlear and supraorbital nerve bundles. Every patient will have decreased sensation to the scalp and hairline and will generally recover over 2-6 months.
  - Scarring/alopecia: widened scars can be excised and repaired after complete recovery. Common where excessive cautery or wound tension occurs.
  - Asymmetry/patient dissatisfaction: attention to patient-specific complaints.

PEARLS

1. For upper eyelid blepharoplasty, 20 mm of skin should always be maintained to prevent lagophthalmos.
2. In blepharoptosis repair, always assess the degree of levator function to aid in surgical planning and evaluation.
3. Unilateral ptosis always needs a pupil evaluation to look for any anisocoria in light and dark conditions as well as an assessment of extraocular movements.
4. Understanding eyelid and brow anatomy is critical to avoiding surgical complications. Always be prepared to draw upper and lower cross-sectional eyelid anatomy.

QUESTIONS YOU WILL BE ASKED

UPPER EYELID BLEPHAROPLASTY

1. What is the absolute minimum skin to preserve during upper eyelid blepharoplasty, as measured from the lash line to the brow-eyelid skin junction?
20 mm.
2. Carrying the upper eyelid incision medial to the upper eyelid punctum can cause what complication?
Medial canthal webbing.
3. Injection of lidocaine with epinephrine during upper eyelid blepharoplasty may cause mild lagophthalmos secondary to stimulation of what muscle(s)?
Müller muscle.
4. For patients having undergone corneal refractive surgery (LASIK), what is the recommended time to wait before proceeding with blepharoplasty or ptosis repair?
At least 6 months.

LOWER EYELID BLEPHAROPLASTY

1. Lower lid retraction after lower blepharoplasty is predominantly secondary to what preexisting examination finding?
Horizontal lid laxity.
2. What is the most common motility defect noted as a complication of lower eyelid blepharoplasty?
Limitation of ipsilateral extortion and elevation.
3. When performing fat transposition for lower eyelid blepharoplasty with herniated orbital fat, which structure is important to release?
Orbitomalar ligament.
4. What is the response to a postoperative lower lid blepharoplasty patient with sudden unilateral pain, eye proptosis, and tense lids.
Perform emergent lateral canthotomy and cantholysis.

UPPER EYELID PTOSIS

1. What is a defining characteristic of aponeurotic (involutional) blepharoptosis?
High lid crease, good levator function.
2. What is the function of the meibomian glands?
Secretes lipid to prevent evaporative dry eye.
3. The law of equal innervation to the bilateral levator muscles can cause what complication postoperatively?
Asymmetric ptosis.
4. A patient presents with pseudoptosis, with MRD1 of 6 mm on the left and 4 mm on the right, without change after correcting for Hering law. What is the most likely etiology for this finding?
Thyroid eye disease.

BROW LIFT

1. When would a pretrichial forehead lift be an appropriate surgical choice?
High hairline.
2. On medial dissection, what structure is at risk of injury?
Supraorbital neurovascular bundle.
3. Dissection or cauterization lateral to the sentinel vein in the temporal pocket can cause injury to what structure?
Frontal branch of facial nerve.
4. Postoperative hematoma can be limited by addressing what factors during and after surgery?
Antiemetics and a pressure dressing.

Recommended Readings

1. Carraway JH. Surgical anatomy of the eyelids. *Clin Plast Surg.* 1987;14(4):693-701.
2. Fasanella R, Servat J. Levator resection for minimal ptosis: another simplified operation. *Arch Ophthalmol.* 1961;65:493-496.
3. Henderson JL, Larrabee WF Jr. Analysis of the upper face and selection of rejuvenation techniques. *Facial Plast Surg Clin North Am.* 2006;14(3):153-158. doi:10.1016/j.fsc.2006.05.003
4. Jelks GW, Jelks EB. Preoperative evaluation of the blepharoplasty patient. Bypassing the pitfalls. *Clin Plast Surg.* 1993;20(2):213-223. Discussion 224.
5. May JW Jr, Fearon J, Zingarelli P. Retro-orbicularis oculus fat (ROOF) resection in aesthetic blepharoplasty: a 6-year study in 63 patients. *Plast Reconstr Surg.* 1990;86:682.
6. Weinberg DA, Baylis HI. Transconjunctival lower eyelid blepharoplasty. *Dermatol Surg.* 1995;21(5):407-410.

60 Rhinoplasty

Johnny Yanjun Xie and Rami D. Sherif

NASAL ANATOMY (FIG. 60-1)

- **Skin:** the thickness of nasal skin is a crucial consideration during preoperative analysis.
  - Thickness varies between ethnic populations.
  - Thin skin will readily reveal the underlying structural irregularities and is less forgiving to dissection while thick and sebaceous skin is prone to postoperative edema and scar formation.
  - The skin overlying the rhinion (the distal edge of the nasal bones) is the thinnest area. The skin of the lower third of the nose is almost twice the average thickness of the skin of the upper two-thirds. In addition, the lower skin is much less mobile and contains more sebaceous glands.
- **Muscle**
  - **There are four groups of paired nasal muscles** that are draped by the superficial musculoaponeurotic system (SMAS).
    - **Depressors** lengthen the nose and dilate the nostrils: the alar portion of the nasalis muscle (dilator naris posterior) and depressor septi (can be hyperactive causing decreased tip projection when smiling).
      - The depressor septi nasi is commonly divided during rhinoplasty to increase tip projection with smiling.
    - **Elevators** shorten the nose and dilate the nostrils: procerus, levator labii superioris alaeque nasi (opens external valve), and anomalous nasi.
    - **The minor dilator** is the dilator nasalis anterior.
    - **Compressors** lengthen the nose and narrow the nostrils: the transverse nasalis muscle and compressor narium minor.
  - **The blood vessels and nerves run on the undersurface** of the SMAS. Therefore, the proper plane of dissection is within a relatively avascular plane deep to the SMAS and just superficial to the periosteum and perichondrium.
- **Blood Supply:** a rich vascular network is comprised of branches of the ophthalmic, internal maxillary, and facial arteries. Venous drainage accompanies the arterial supply.
  - **The dorsal nasal artery** (branch of ophthalmic) perforates the orbital septum superior to the medial canthal ligament and courses inferiorly along the nasal sidewall.
  - **The facial artery** bifurcates into the **angular artery** and the **superior labial artery.** The latter supplies the nostril sill and the columella, via the columellar artery.
  - **The nasal tip** receives blood from the **columellar artery,** the external nasal branch of the anterior ethmoidal artery, and the **lateral nasal artery** (branch of angular).
    - *The traditional approach to open rhinoplasty involves a transcolumellar incision that divides the columellar artery; therefore, the primary blood supply to the nasal envelope in open rhinoplasty is the lateral nasal artery, which runs 2 mm superior to the alar groove. Therefore, alar base excision should be performed conservatively in these instances.
- **Innervation:** motor innervation is from the zygomatic and buccal branches of the facial nerve. Sensation to the external nose is through divisions of CN V.
  - The radix, the upper dorsum, and upper nasal side walls are supplied by supratrochlear and infratrochlear branches of the ophthalmic nerve.

---

*Denotes common in-service examination topics.

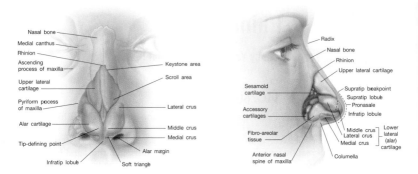

Figure 60-1 Frontal (*left*) and lateral (*right*) views of the anatomy of the external portions of the nose.

- ○ *The external nasal branch of the anterior ethmoid nerve (V1), which emerges between the nasal bones and the upper lateral cartilages (ULCs), supplies sensation to the distal dorsum and the nasal tip.
  - ○ Sensation to the lower half of the nasal sidewall, columella, and ala is supplied by the infraorbital branches of the maxillary nerve.
- **Osseocartilaginous Framework**
  - ○ **Upper vault (bony vault)**
    - Comprised of the paired nasal bones and the ascending frontal processes of the maxilla
    - Upper one-third to one-half of the nose
    - Average length of nasal bones ~2.5 cm
  - ○ **Middle vault**—comprised of **upper lateral cartilages (ULCs)**
    - The cartilaginous vault is comprised of the ULCs and the cartilaginous septum.
    - At the "keystone" area, the nasal bones overlap the cephalic aspect of the ULCs by about 8-10 mm.
    - **Internal nasal valve:** formed by the caudal edge of the ULC, the nasal septum, and the anterior head of the inferior turbinate (**Fig. 60-2**).
      - □ Narrowest portion of nasal airway and, therefore, site of greatest airway resistance
      - □ Should be between 10° and 15°
    - There is a contiguous perichondrial lining from the undersurface of the ULCs to the septum.
  - ○ **Lower vault**—comprised of **lower lateral cartilages (LLCs)**
    - Also known as the alar cartilages, the paired LLCs may be viewed as a tripod, which supports the nasal tip.
    - Each LLC is subdivided into the medial crus, middle crus, and the lateral crus. The cephalic edge of the domal segment of the middle crus creates the important "tip-defining point" or pronasale.
    - The junction between the lateral crus of the LLC and the caudal edge of the ULC is known as the **"scroll area."** At this location, the ULC edge is rolled deep to the more superficial LLC edge.
    - The lateral crus does not extend to the pyriform aperture. Instead, the patency of the posterior aspect of the ala depends on dense fibrofatty connective tissue and accessory cartilages. These structures contribute to the arch of the vestibule and provide support for the **external nasal valve** (made up of alar rim, nasal floor, the columella).
  - ○ **Septum**—the cartilaginous component is the quadrangular cartilage. This articulates with the posterior bony septum, consists of the perpendicular plate of

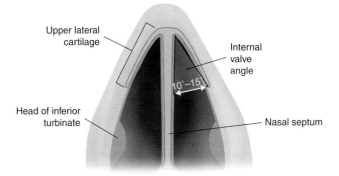

Figure 60-2 **The internal nasal valve.** (From Thorne CH, ed. *Grabb and Smith's Plastic Surgery.* 7th ed. Lippincott Williams & Wilkins; 2014. Figure 48.5.)

the ethmoid bone, the vomer, the nasal crest of the maxilla, and the nasal crest of the palatine bone.
○ **Turbinates**
  ▪ Paired structures that come off the lateral nasal wall that warm and humidify air. Turbinates swell and contract to regulate level of moisture in air.
  ▪ Three pairs—inferior (most clinically relevant), middle, and superior.
  ▪ Comprised of a bony component with overlying mucosa. Hypertrophic turbinates are a common cause of unilateral vs bilateral nasal obstruction.
  ▪ *Addressing inferior turbinates is an integral part of rhinoplasty when addressing airway issues; however, overresection can lead to empty nose syndrome—the sensation of nasal obstruction with an open nasal airway.

PREOPERATIVE CONSIDERATIONS

GOALS AND PATIENT SELECTION

• **Patients seek rhinoplasty for cosmetic and/or functional reasons.**
  ○ In addition to the patient's concerns about the nose, the surgeon should also respect nasofacial balance, gender-specific characteristics, and ethnic congruence.
  ○ In cosmetic patients without nasal obstruction, an important goal is to preserve the nasal airway.
• **Selection of appropriate patients is key to good outcomes.**
  ○ Ask the patient specifically what they dislike about their nose and commit to a set of aesthetic/functional goals. Then examine the patient to determine if those goals can be achieved.
  ○ Be wary of patients with uncorrectable problems, unrealistic expectations, or unhealthy motivating factors. Poor patient satisfaction after rhinoplasty is often due to emotion dissatisfaction and not technical failure.
  ○ **The acronym SIMON represents some red flags:** single, immature, male, overly expectant, and narcissistic.
  ○ **Body dysmorphic disorder** (BDD)
    ▪ Somatoform disorder marked by excessive preoccupation with a trivial or perceived defect in physical appearance, which causes significant psychological or social impairment.
    ▪ *Affects 7%-15% of all plastic surgery patients (general population 1%-2%).** Most common sites of patient concern: skin, hair, and nose.
    ▪ BDD is a contraindication for surgery. Refer the patient to the psychiatrist.

○ Surgeons now commonly use image manipulation software to give patients an idea of what their postoperative result can look like. This can be very helpful, but make sure to caution patients that you can never guarantee a surgical result.

PREOPERATIVE ASSESSMENT

• **History and Primary Complaints:** a patient's nasal history must be elicited in detail, as certain medical conditions, trauma, allergies, sinusitis, medications, or previous interventions may affect the final outcome.
   ○ Carefully illicit a patient's **primary functional and aesthetic complaints.** It can be helpful to have a patient list their top three concerns, as often patients struggle to narrow down specific issues.
   ○ Evaluate for **nasal obstruction:** alteration in normal aerodynamic flow from increased resistance due to medical or anatomic reasons. Diagnosis is made by history and rhinoscopic examination. It is important to elicit whether a patient has a structural nasal obstruction, mucosal disease (ie, rhinosinusitis), or both.
      ▪ *The Cottle maneuver: lateral cheek traction by the examiner using a small metal prong or skinny Q-tip opens a narrow internal valve and results in clinically noticeable improvement in airflow.
      ▪ **Inferior turbinate hypertrophy:** compensatory enlargement occurs on the side opposite of septal deviation. Combined with the internal valve, the anterior aspect of the inferior turbinate can account for up to two-thirds of upper airway resistance.
      ▪ **Anterior rhinoscopy:** examine whether the mucosal lining generally looks inflamed (mucous stranding, erythema, even purulence if infected).
      ▪ If your patient has mucosal disease, consider ENT referral.
      ▪ Consider if septoplasty alone can address the patient's complaints.
   ○ **Inquire about medications** (especially antihypertensives and blood thinners), smoking, drug abuse, previous nasal trauma, and sinus or nasal surgeries.
   ○ **Document allergic disorders and symptoms:** hay fever, asthma, vasomotor rhinitis, sinusitis, nasal stuffiness, dry raw pharynx, postnasal drip, and alterations in taste or smell.
   ○ **Previous operative notes** may be helpful if the patient has had prior rhinoplasty.
• Nasal Analysis
   ○ **Nasal analysis begins with complete facial analysis.**
      ▪ The ideal face is divided into equal vertical fifths and horizontal thirds.
      ▪ Preexisting asymmetries and the appearance of the patient's maxilla and mandible should be noted prior to surgery.
      ▪ Patients typically have a long facial half and a short facial half.
      ▪ Look for underlying craniofacial diagnoses such as vertical maxillary excess or malocclusion, which may necessitate intervention prior to rhinoplasty.
      ▪ Skin type and thickness is important to evaluate.
      ▪ It is more important for a nose to be in harmony with the rest of the patient's face than to achieve ideal relationships within the nose itself.
      ▪ In rhinoplasty surgery, "cephalic" means toward the root of the nose and "caudal" means toward the tip of the nose.
      ▪ Standard photographs are taken at Frankfort horizontal planes: frontal, profile (L and R), oblique (L and R), and base views.
   ○ The nose should be analyzed from a frontal, lateral, and basal view.
      ▪ Frontal
         □ Evaluate nasal deviation as well as dorsal aesthetic lines
            ▪ Dorsal aesthetic lines originate at the supraorbital ridges and curve down through the glabella terminating at the nasal tip. In males, these lines should be wider and straighter while in females the dorsum is narrower with a gentle curve to the aesthetic lines.
         □ Examine shape and width of bony vault and midvault.

- The bony width should typically be ~80% of alar width.
  □ Analyze nasal tip shape (see tip analysis below), alar base width.
    - Alar base width should be equal to intercanthal distance.
- Lateral
  □ Radix position and angle of the nasofrontal angle
    - **Radix:** the area where the nose meets the brow is called the radix.
    - *The nasion is at the deepest point of the radix and is the apex of the nasofrontal angle (ideal = 134° for women, 130° for men)
  □ Nasal dorsum
    - On lateral view, the dorsal line is drawn from the nasion to the tip-defining point. For women, the ideal line is slightly concave and for men, slightly convex.
    - **The nasofacial angle** (ideal = 34° for women, 36° for men) is created from a vertical line through the nasion and the dorsal line.
    - The distance between the anterior septal angle and the tip-defining point on lateral view determines the presence of a **supratip break**. This measurement should be 7 mm for thin-skinned patients and 10 mm for thick-skinned patients.
  □ Nasal length
  □ Tip projection and tip rotation
    - Projection—if a vertical line is drawn at the anterior most point of the upper lip, ~50-60% of the nose should lie anterior to this line.
    - Rotation—the nasolabial angle should be ~90° in men and between 95 and 110° in women.
  □ Chin position
    - In the frontal view, the lower third of the face should be equal in height to the middle and upper thirds.
    - On the lateral view, chin projection must be carefully evaluated. Riedel line describes a line connecting anterior-most points along upper and lower lip. The chin should touch this line. If significantly behind this line, consider implant vs osseous genioplasty in conjunction with planned rhinoplasty (**see Chapter 62: Genioplasty**).
- Basal
  □ Nostril shape and nostril:columella relationship
  □ Alar base and alar flare
○ **Six characteristics of the tip should be evaluated**—volume, width, definition, rotation, projection, and shape. Interventions to the delicate cartilages of the tip should be judicious because often a change in one characteristic will result in a change in another. Note the 3 major tip support mechanisms (attachment of the medial crura to the septum; quality, strength, and resiliency of the LLC, and the scroll) and minor tip support mechanisms (dorsal septum, interdomal ligaments, membranous septum, nasal spine, soft tissue envelope, minor accessory cartilages).
  - **Excision of excess cephalic lateral crura** (cephalic trim) will reduce tip volume and will also result in some increased tip projection.
  - One important landmark of a refined tip is the **tip-defining point,** which is created by the domal segment of the middle crus. The most aesthetic LLC configuration is a convex domal segment adjacent to concave lateral crura.
  - **Tip rotation is measured by the *nasolabial angle (ideal = 95-110° for women, 90-95° for men),** which is measured between a line perpendicular to the natural horizontal facial plane and a line drawn through the most anterior and posterior points of the nostril on lateral view. The nasolabial angle is not the same as the columellar-labial angle.
  - **The columellar-lobular angle** is produced by the junction between the columella and the infratip lobule (ideal = 30-45°). Fullness can be due to a prominent caudal septum; deficiency will usually require grafting.

- **Tip projection** is measured from a line tangent to the alar-cheek junction (ACJ) and a perpendicular line drawn to the tip-defining point. Tip projection is affected by maxillary projection, columellar length, and abnormalities of the LLCs.
- **The depressor septi nasi muscle** can cause downward tip rotation and decreased tip project on animation and may require transposition.
  - ○ **Ala:** the ala should demonstrate a slight outward flare in an inferolateral direction. Note that the width of the base will change with alterations in tip projection.
    - On frontal view, the width of the alar base should be about the same as the intercanthal distance.
    - The relationship between the alar rims and the columella should allow slight nostril show and give a gentle "seagull in flight" appearance.

A Byrd analysis can be very helpful with perioperative planning. This technique utilizes known aesthetic norms of nasal appearance to manipulate 1:1 photographs to elicit surgical goals. This can be then transposed to acetate tracing paper to provide the patient with an idea of potential surgical outcomes. See additional reading for resources to perform a Byrd analysis.

KEY PRINCIPLES OF RHINOPLASTY

- Detailed descriptions of rhinoplasty techniques can be found within the listed references, but major points are discussed here.
- **Anesthesia:** an oral RAE endotracheal tube should be used and taped to midline at the lower lip.
  - ○ **Topical:** nasal packing with pledgets soaked with either 1% lidocaine with 1:100 000 epinephrine, oxymetazoline (Afrin), or 4% cocaine.
  - ○ **Local:** 1% lidocaine with 1:100 000 epinephrine is infiltrated throughout the nose and around the nose, providing complete anesthesia and bloodless operative field. Sites injected can include infraorbital foramen (infraorbital artery), lateral nasofacial groove (lateral nasal artery), alar base (angular artery), columella (columellar artery), dorsum (anterior ethmoid artery), tip, and radix (infratrochlear artery). Next the incisions and septum are injected.

EXPOSURE

- **Approach:** the **open approach** allows for complete exposure, precise diagnosis of defects, and multiple surgical techniques to be performed, but results in a columellar scar, creates more tip edema, and requires suture stabilization of nasal structures. The **endonasal (closed) approach** offers no external scars, less edema, and rare need for suture fixation but involves working with restricted exposure, relies heavily on grafts, and is difficult to master.
- **Incisions (Fig. 60-3)**
  - ○ **Intercartilaginous:** the incision is placed at the junction of the ULC and the LLC. However, due to the scrolling relationship of these two structures, an incision is in reality a cut made into the cephalic lateral crura.
  - ○ **Intracartilaginous:** the incision is placed purposefully within the substance of the cephalic lateral crura and is determined by the amount of cephalic trim needed.
  - ○ **Infracartilaginous (aka marginal):** the incision is placed just caudal to the caudal edge of the LLC. In open rhinoplasty, this incision is connected with the transcolumellar incision.
  - ○ **Transcolumellar:** used for open rhinoplasty. Most use a chevron or stairstep incision at the narrowest aspect of the columella.
- **Transfixion:** an incision is made through-and-through the membranous septum, causing downward rotation of the nasal tip. When only one side of the incision is made, this is known as a **hemitransfixion** incision.
- **Septal Exposure**
  - ○ Bilateral mucoperichondrial flaps are elevated to fully expose and examine the septum.

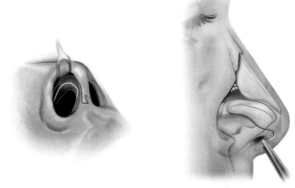

Figure 60-3 Incisions. The transcolumellar stairstep with intranasal marginal incisions (shown in red) is standard for open rhinoplasty. The cartilage-splitting incision (shown in yellow) is often used in closed rhinoplasty. The intercartilaginous incision (shown in green) is often used in combination with marginal incision to "deliver" cartilage in closed rhinoplasty. (From Chung KC. *Grabb and Smith's Plastic Surgery*. 8th ed. Wolters Kluwer; 2020. Figure 52.11.)

- This allows visualization of any septal deviations or deformities that need to be addressed to improve breathing. It also allows for harvesting of septal cartilage for grafting in the nose.

SPECIFIC COMPONENTS OF RHINOPLASTY

- **Dorsal Hump Reduction:** prominent dorsal hump is one of the primary reasons that patients seek rhinoplasty. The dorsum consists of both bony and cartilaginous components, and a dorsal hump can have one or both components.
  - Submucosal tunnels are created by gently elevating the mucoperichondrium off the septum using a Cottle elevator.
  - The ULCs are then separated from the septum, and component dorsal hump reduction is performed by trimming these structures incrementally.
  - *The dorsum should be reduced before septal harvest to ensure that at minimum, a 10-mm dorsal and a 10-mm caudal strut (together known as "L-strut") remain to provide support to the nose.
  - Overresection of the dorsal strut will predispose to **saddle-nose deformity**, which is when the nasal dorsum collapses due to weak dorsal support.
  - **An osteotome** or bone rasp is used to reduce the bony dorsum.
  - Reduction to the bony dorsum typically leaves an "**open roof deformity,**" which is when the bony dorsum is wide and there is a gap between the nasal bones. Osteotomies are required to close the roof.
  - It is important to resuspend the midvault to prevent an **inverted V deformity**— sharp transition between caudal border of the nasal bones and the cephalic border of the ULC.
- **Septal Work and Cartilage Harvest**
  - A portion of cartilaginous septum can be harvested to be used as a variety of cartilage grafts (see below).
  - As previously mentioned, it is critical to leave a 10-mm x 10-mm L strut of cartilage to support the dorsum and prevent inverted V deformity.
  - Other maneuvers can be performed to ensure correction of any previously noted septal deviation or warping.
- **Osteotomy**

- ○ Used to correct **nasal bone deviation, close an open roof deformity** after dorsal reduction, and to **narrow a wide bony base.**
  - ▪ **Medial osteotomies:** performed along the medial border of the nasal bone. Separate nasal bones from septum. These can be used to mobilize the entire nasal sidewall in conjunction with lateral osteotomies. Can also be used as part of an effort to widen the bony dorsum.
    - ▫ Either medial oblique or paramedian, depending on the trajectory of the osteotomy. Medial oblique refers to an osteotomy that is initiated medially and then curves to meet the lateral osteotomy as progress is made superiorly. This type of osteotomy decreases the likelihood of a rocker-bottom deformity when compared with a paramedian osteotomy that travels superiorly without lateral curvature.
  - ▪ **Lateral osteotomies:** performed along the ascending process of the maxilla (NOT through the nasal bones), used to narrow the bony dorsum, correct asymmetry, and close an open roof. Can be done in a "high-low-high," "low-low," or "high-high" (or other combinations) fashion. These terms are used to refer to the anatomic position of the osteotomy from the lateral view of the nose. "Low" would be postero/lateral while "high" refers to anteromedial. The exact definitions of these and the nuances between the techniques are beyond the scope of this text.
  - ○ The angular artery can be at risk with lateral osteotomies. **To avoid the angular artery,** sweep down the lateral nasal sidewall in subperiosteal plane. **Once osteotomies completed,** put pressure from the thumb and index finger only at the superior aspect (not lower or will close off internal valve) to perform greenstick fracture of nasal bones.
- • **Nasal Tip**—tip shaping is a critical part of rhinoplasty. Detailed analysis of the tip must be performed as there are a variety of maneuvers that can be used to address nasal tip deformities. Generally, nasal tip shaping has three components: (1) cartilage trimming/resection, (2) tip suturing, and (3) cartilage grafts.
  - ○ **Cartilage resection:**
    - ▪ *Excess tip volume is addressed by performing cephalic trim of the lateral crura. A minimum width of 6-8 mm of intact lateral crus should be left to ensure stability.
  - ○ **Tip suturing:** a **variety of suturing techniques** have been described to effectively increase tip definition, affect tip rotation, influence projection, and reduce tip width (**see Table 60-2** later in this chapter).
  - ○ Tip grafts: see section that follows for details on various cartilage grafts used in rhinoplasty.
    - ▪ Columellar strut graft
    - ▪ Tip grafts: infralobular or onlay
  - ○ Septal extension grafts
- • **Common Cartilage Grafts (Table 60-1)**
- • **Ala:** alar base resection (sometimes called Weir excision) can be used to decrease nostril flaring. Care must be taken to avoid injury to the lateral nasal artery. Alternatively, nostril sill excision can be performed.
- • **Inferior Turbinate:** hypertrophic inferior turbinates can be addressed by a variety of techniques including submucous resection, outfracture, cautery, or partial turbinectomy.
- • Care must be taken to **avoid overresection of the inferior turbinates,** as this can cause **empty nose syndrome,** which is the sensation of nasal obstruction despite clear/open nasal airways.
- • **Postoperative Care**
  - ○ Nasal taping is performed for several weeks to reduce swelling.
  - ○ An external nasal splint is worn for 1 week for protection.

TABLE 60-1 Common Cartilage Grafts

Graft	Goal of graft	Location and other information
Dorsum grafts		
Spreader grafts 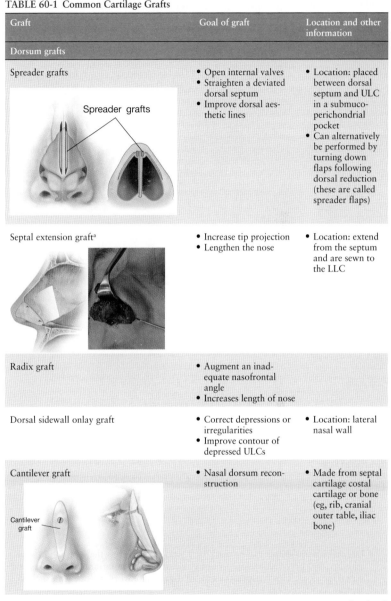 Spreader grafts	• Open internal valves • Straighten a deviated dorsal septum • Improve dorsal aesthetic lines	• Location: placed between dorsal septum and ULC in a submuco-perichondrial pocket • Can alternatively be performed by turning down flaps following dorsal reduction (these are called spreader flaps)
Septal extension graft[a]	• Increase tip projection • Lengthen the nose	• Location: extend from the septum and are sewn to the LLC
Radix graft	• Augment an inadequate nasofrontal angle • Increases length of nose	
Dorsal sidewall onlay graft	• Correct depressions or irregularities • Improve contour of depressed ULCs	• Location: lateral nasal wall
Cantilever graft Cantilever graft	• Nasal dorsum reconstruction	• Made from septal cartilage costal cartilage or bone (eg, rib, cranial outer table, iliac bone)

(continued)

Section V: Aesthetics

TABLE 60-1 Common Cartilage Grafts (*Continued*)

Graft	Goal of graft	Location and other information
Alar grafts		
Alar strut graft	• Used to support the external valve	• Location: Sutured to the lateral crura and extend over the pyriform aperture
Alar contour graft[b]	• Support the alar rims and prevent notching or retraction • Support external nasal valves	• Location: placed along the alar rims in a subcutaneous pocket
Nasal tip grafts		
Columellar strut graft	• Help to define columellar strut shape, strength within the central limb of the LLC tripod, and maintain or increase tip projection	• Location: placed between the medial crura
Tip grafts	• Provide definition to symmetry to the nasal tip, increase tip projection and improved deficiency infra tip lobular	

[a]Figure from Chung KC, Disa JJ, Gosain A, et al. *Operative Techniques in Plastic Surgery.* Wolters Kluwer; 2020. Tech Figure 1.60.7.

[b]Figure from Chung KC, Disa JJ, Gosain A, et al. *Operative Techniques in Plastic Surgery.* Wolters Kluwer; 2020. Figure 1.70.1.

○ Internal silastic splints can be used for 1 week to compress the septum, provide stability, and prevent development of synechiae between intranasal incisions and septal incisions. This is especially crucial if turbinate work is done (can stick to septum and form scar bands).

○ Patients are advised to keep their head of bed elevated as much as possible; no bending over.

○ Saline sprays can be used for postoperative nasal congestion. Afrin spray can help to reduce light bleeding.

TABLE 60-2 Sutures

Suture technique	Description	Diagram
Transdomal[a]	Horizontal mattress suture across domal segment Narrows dome, corrects asymmetry Mildly increases tip projection Improves definition	
Interdomal[a]	Horizontal mattress suture from one dome to contralateral dome Narrows tip, narrows tip defining points, increases tip projection	
Medial crural suture[a]	Placed between medial crura Can be placed anywhere along sagittal plane depending on desired result Reduces footplate flaring Can stabilize columellar strut graft	
Medial crural septal suture[b]	Any variety of sutures from medial crura to septum. Three point stitch from each medial crus to septum Used to increase/decrease tip projection/rotation depending on bite location and size	

[a]Figures from Thorne CH, ed. *Grabb and Smith's Plastic Surgery*. 7th ed. Lippincott Williams & Wilkins; 2014. Figures 48.31, 48.30, 48.29.
[b]Figure from Chung KC, Disa JJ, Gosain A, et al. *Operative Techniques in Plastic Surgery*. Wolters Kluwer; 2020. Tech Figure 1.60.4A.

COMPLICATIONS

- **Bleeding:** major epistaxis is rare (<1%) and most bleeding can be treated with head elevation, oxymetazoline nasal spray, careful pressure, and occasionally anterior nasal packing with ribbon gauze and silver nitrate.
  - *Hematoma of the septum should be drained to prevent septal perforations and subsequent saddle-nose deformity. Nasal packing or silastic splints are used after drainage to apply compression.
  - Hematoma under the nasal skin will lead to significant fibrosis and distortion.
- **Infection:** acute infection after rhinoplasty is rare (<1%).
  - Some surgeons use prophylactic antibiotics with patients who have risk factors for poor wound healing or if significant grafting was performed.
  - Nasal packing has been implicated in cases of toxic shock syndrome.
- **Airway Obstruction:** bruising and edema are a normal consequence of rhinoplasty and the acute swelling subsides within 3 weeks. Patients should expect transient nasal airway obstruction during this time.
  - **Intranasal decongestants** should not be used for more than 3-5 days due to rebound nasal congestion after cessation (rhinitis medicamentosa).
  - **Persistent obstruction** should lead to consideration of anatomic causes, such as collapse of the internal or external valves and synechiae.
- **Asymmetry:** revision surgery and treatment of mild postoperative obstruction should be delayed for at least 1 year to allow for scar maturation and complete resolution of nasal edema.
  - However, within 10-14 days, if there is obvious acute deformity (eg, deviation and displacement of tip graft), it is far better to reoperate than to wait.
  - Excess scar formation may be treated with triamcinolone injections.

SECONDARY RHINOPLASTY

- **Definition:** technically, secondary rhinoplasty is when the primary rhinoplasty (or multiple other rhinoplasties) is performed by another surgeon, whereas a revision surgery is when you reoperate on your own primary case.
- **How is secondary rhinoplasty different from primary rhinoplasty?**
  - Highly variable nasal anatomy due to distortion by scar tissue.
  - The skin envelope is more limiting due to scarring and adhesions.
  - There is often depletion of septal cartilage for grafting. When this is suspected, make sure to discuss with patient re: using conchal cartilage, or rib (either autologous or cadaveric).
  - Will encounter previous interventions and inherit problems.
  - Patient expectations will be different.
  - Airway problems may have resulted from primary rhinoplasty.
- **Anatomic factors** that, when missed during preoperative evaluation for primary rhinoplasty, predispose secondary rhinoplasty.
  - Low radix or low dorsum
  - Narrow midvault
  - Inadequate tip projection
  - Alar cartilage malposition
  - Alar rim weakness

PRESERVATION RHINOPLASTY

- A philosophy of rhinoplasty that is composed of three primary parts
  - Preservation of the nasal dorsum without creating an open roof deformity
  - Maintaining the alar cartilages, achieving desired goals with suturing as opposed to cartilage excision and grafting
  - Elevation of the soft tissue envelope in the subperichondrial/subperiosteal plane

- Dorsal Preservation
  - Historically, reduction of dorsal humps has classically been performed by excision of prominent cartilage and bone, leading to an open roof requiring midvault reconstruction. Dorsal preservation involves resection of portions of the septum and then osteotomies to bring down the dorsum.
- Soft Tissue Envelope Preservation
  - Reduces swelling, preserves sensation, and avoids long-term thinning of the soft tissue when compared with sub-SMAS dissection
- Alar Cartilage Preservation
  - Preserves the entire alar cartilage to reduce likelihood of eventual tip changes and enhancing function.
  - Further explanation of preservation rhinoplasty is well beyond the scope of this text; however, the basic principles are as enumerated above. Preservation rhinoplasty is a rapidly expanding ideology in recent years with increasing complexity and nuance.

PEARLS

1. Preoperative analysis is key to the successful rhinoplasty. Make sure to perform detailed, systematic evaluation of the nose from all views as well as in context with a total facial analysis to make sure you are addressing all areas and performing a comprehensive surgery.
2. If preexisting airway issues (or rhinosinusitis) are not detected during the preoperative evaluation, a rhinoplasty may result in worsening of this underlying condition. Many patients may benefit from preop saline sprays, sinus rinses, and consideration of Flonase.
3. The nose must be harmonious with the rest of the face. In a patient with an overprojected nose and chin, reduction rhinoplasty will exaggerate the appearance of the already prominent chin.
4. Rhinoplasty is a very complex operation and the anatomy is interconnected. Maneuvers in one region of the nose may affect the appearance and structure of another.
5. Avoid reoperation for a minimum of 1 year after primary rhinoplasty.
6. If a patient appears to be preoccupied with subtle defect causing significant social distress, think of the possibility of BDD. The surgeon should facilitate psychological consultation and inform the patient that such evaluation is necessary prior to further discussion of surgery.

QUESTIONS YOU WILL BE ASKED

1. What could cause nasal deviation?
   Deviated septum, deformity of the ULC, asymmetric nasal bone, prior trauma and scarring, craniofacial abnormality, allergic rhinitis, nonallergic rhinitis, rhinosinusitis, and any mucosal inflammation of any etiology in the nose.
2. What structures does the quadrangular septal cartilage articulate with?
   Inferiorly—the maxillary crest, crest of the palatine bone; superiorly/anteriorly—nasal bone; posteriorly—perpendicular plate of the ethmoid and vomer.
3. What are the major and minor tip support mechanisms?
   Major: medial crura attachment to the septum, strength, quality, shape and resiliency of the LLC, attachment of the ULC and LLC (the scroll).
   Minor: dorsal septum, interdomal ligaments, anterior nasal spine, membranous septum, nasal skin envelope, minor accessory cartilages.
4. What is the relationship between the ULC and the LLC?
   At the scroll area, the caudal end of the ULC is rolled deep to the cephalic end of the LLC. This is one of the three major tip support mechanisms.

5. The attending points to the lateral ala and asks: What cartilage supports this part of the nose?
   None. The alar component of the LLC sweeps superiorly to meet the ULC; thus, the majority of the substance of the ala is without cartilage.
6. What is the ideal angle for the internal valve?
   10°-15°.
7. What is the ideal nasolabial angle?
   95°-100° for women, 90°-95° for men.
8. Describe the fundamental tip suturing techniques as well as the impact they have on tip appearance, rotation, and projection.
   Transdomal, interdomal, medial crural, and medial crural septal sutures. See **Table 60-2.**
9. Should I harvest some septal cartilage and then perform dorsal hump reduction?
   No. Doral hump reduction should be done before septal harvest to ensure that there is a (ideally) 15-mm-wide L-strut to support the nose. Otherwise, potential overre-section may lead to saddle-nose deformity.
10. What is a potential etiology of the following rhinoplasty complications?
    Open roof: failure to close the gap between dorsal septum and lateral nasal wall. Nasal bridge will appear wide, flat, and may have palpable breaks.
    Pollybeak: it is a convexity of the supratip area and loss of the supratip break.
    Inverted-V: sharp transition between caudal border of the nasal bones and the cephalic border of the ULC. Caused by failure to resuspend the ULC to the dorsum, leading to mid vault collapse.
    Bossa: contour irregularities of the tip due to suboptimal healing and scarring.
    Rocker deformity: overly aggressive medial osteotomy leading to a very sharp naso-frontal angle.
    Saddle nose: overresection of the quadrangular cartilage with insufficient dorsal L-strut. Can be caused by many etiologies though (surgical and nonsurgical).

Recommended Readings
1. Brito ÍM, Avashia Y, Rohrich RJ. Evidence-based nasal analysis for rhinoplasty: the 10-7-5 method. *Plast Reconstr Surg Glob Open.* 2020;8(2):e2632.
2. Byrd HS, Hobar PC. Rhinoplasty: a practical guide for surgical planning. *Plast Reconstr Surg.* 1993;91(4):642-654; discussion 655-656.
3. Daniel RK et al. *Preservation Rhinoplasty.* 3rd ed. Septum Publisher; 2020.
4. Gunter JP, Rohrich RJ, Adams WP Jr. *Dallas Rhinoplasty: Nasal Surgery by the Masters.* Quality Medical Publishing; 2007.
5. Oneal RM, Beil RJ. Surgical anatomy of the nose. *Clin Plast Surg.* 2010;37(2):191-211.
6. Rohrich RJ, Ahmad J. Rhinoplasty. *Plast Reconstr Surg.* 2011;128(2):49e-73e.
7. Sieber DA, Rohrich RJ. Finesse in Nasal Tip Refinement. *Plast Reconstr Surg.* 2017;140(2):277e-286e.

61

Face-lift and Neck Lift

Christopher J. Breuler and Rami D. Sherif

OVERVIEW

PRINCIPLES OF FACIAL REJUVENATION

- **Improve the quality of the skin** with chemical peels, laser, and dermabrasion.
- **Address the loss of volume** (both soft tissue and bone) with fat grafting, fillers, bone, or skeletal implants.
  - ○ Atrophy of the fat pads of the face is a key contributor to facial aging.
  - ○ Addressing loss of volume in conjunction with face-lift and neck lift is imperative in restoring a youthful appearance.
- **Return tissues to their original anatomical place** (ie, lift what has fallen and tighten what has become lax).
- **Excise redundant tissue** (eg, facial skin and orbital fat).

ANATOMY

- **Layers of the face (Fig. 61-1):** skin, subcutaneous fat, superficial musculoaponeurotic system (SMAS), facial mimetic muscles (note, the SMAS invests the zygomaticus muscles), and deep facial fascia (parotideomasseteric fascia)
  - ○ In the cheek, the facial nerve, parotid duct, facial vessels, and buccal fat pad are all deep to the parotideomasseteric fascia.
  - ○ **Temporal region**
    - ■ *Three fascial layers: temporoparietal fascia (ie, superficial temporal fascia), superficial layer of deep temporal fascia, and deep layer of deep temporal fascia. Temporalis muscle is deep to all three layers.
    - ■ Superficial and deep layers of deep temporal fascia separated by superficial temporal fat pad.
- **SMAS (Fig. 61-2)**
  - ○ *Thin fascial layer that invests the superficial mimetic muscles and separates the overlying subcutaneous fat from the underlying parotideomasseteric fascia.
  - ○ SMAS is the facial extension of the superficial fascial system present throughout the body.
  - ○ Continuous with the galea, the superficial temporal fascia (temporoparietal fascia), superficial cervical fascia, and the platysma.
- **Facial fat compartments**—studies have shown that facial fat is divided into well-defined compartments.
  - ○ Divided into superficial and deep compartments
    - ■ There are 23 superficial compartments that span the forehead, periorbital, midface, and lower face regions.
    - ■ Deep compartments are located beneath the facial mimetic muscles. These include the medial and lateral suborbicularis oculi fat, deep medial cheek fat, and buccal fat.
  - ○ Fat compartments are divided by various retaining ligaments and interconnections.
  - ○ Knowledge of compartments guides dissection during face-lift.

---

*Denotes common in-service examination topics.

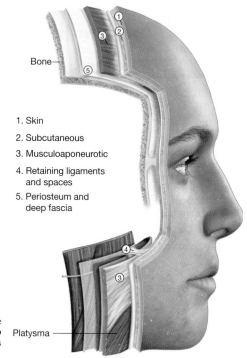

Bone

1. Skin
2. Subcutaneous
3. Musculoaponeurotic
4. Retaining ligaments and spaces
5. Periosteum and deep fascia

Platysma

Figure 61-1 The five layers of the face, analogous to layers of the scalp and neck. The facial nerve travels deep to or within the SMAS layer.

- Compartments atrophy at different time points throughout a person's life. Understanding the temporal pattern of facial fat atrophy and restoring volume in these areas is key to facial rejuvenation.
  - Superficial fat is improved by repositioning, while deep fat is improved by volumetric augmentation.
- **Mimetic muscles: four layers from superficial to deep**
  - Depressor anguli oris, zygomaticus minor, and orbicularis oris
  - Depressor labii inferioris, risorius, platysma (innervated by cervical branch of facial nerve)
  - Zygomaticus major, levator labii superioris alaeque nasi
  - *Deep muscles (innervated on their superficial surface): levator anguli oris, buccinator, and mentalis
- **Parotideomasseteric fascia**
  - Continuous with the deep layer of cervical fascia.
  - Facial nerve branches within the cheek lie just deep to this layer laterally and become more superficial medially.
  - Loré fascia (also known as tympanoparotid fascia, platysma-auricular ligament, and parotid-cutaneous ligament) is an area of dense fibrous tissue in front of the earlobe. Some techniques place anchoring sutures here.
- **Retaining ligaments of the face (Fig. 61-3)**
  - Well-defined ligamentous structures that create areas of fixation and anchor the soft tissues of the face. With time, these ligaments attenuate and, along with fat compartment atrophy and descent, cause many of the stigmata of facial aging.

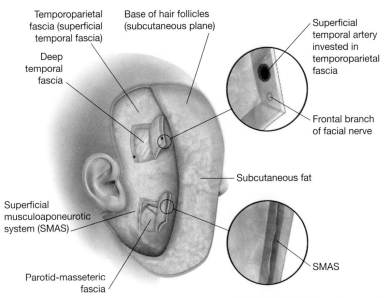

Figure 61-2 The superficial musculoaponeurotic system (SMAS). The SMAS is continuous with the temporoparietal fascia (superficial temporal fascia). Within the temporoparietal fascia runs the superficial temporal artery and the frontal branch of the facial nerve.

- ○ Osteocutaneous ligaments
  - ■ Zygomatic ligaments: arise from lateral zygoma and pass through SMAS and malar fat pad to overlying skin. Support the upper and lateral cheek
  - ■ Mandibular ligaments: arise from the periosteum of the mandible and support the soft tissues of the chin
- ○ Masseteric cutaneous ligaments: arise along anterior border of masseter to support lower cheek and jowl. Exist along the entire anterior border of the masseter; however, are most dense at the superior portion where they coalesce with the zygomatic ligaments.
- ○ Parotid cutaneous ligaments: originate from fascial attachments over parotid gland and support the lateral cheek.
- • **Blood supply**
  - ○ Primarily from branches of external carotid
    - ■ Anterior: facial, labial, supratrochlear, and supraorbital
    - ■ Lateral: submental, zygomatico-orbital, and anterior auricular
    - ■ Forehead and scalp: occipital, superficial temporal, and posterior auricular
  - ○ Rhytidectomy divides fasciocutaneous perforators from lateral facial arteries leaving flap dependent on medially based musculocutaneous perforators.
- • **Nerves and zones of danger of the face (Fig. 61-4)**
  - ○ **Facial nerve (CN VII)**—provides innervation to muscles of facial expression
    - ■ **Five main branches: temporal (frontal), zygomatic, buccal, marginal mandibular, and cervical.**
    - ■ The facial nerve emerges from the stylomastoid foramen and lies between the deep and superficial lobes of the parotid gland where it branches.
    - ■ Branches exit the parotid anteriorly and travel along the superficial surface of the masseter, deep to the parotideomasseteric fascia.

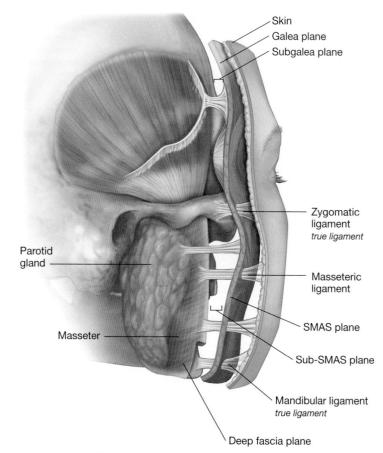

Skin
Galea plane
Subgalea plane

Zygomatic
ligament
true ligament

Masseteric
ligament

SMAS plane

Sub-SMAS plane

Mandibular ligament
true ligament

Parotid
gland

Masseter

Deep fascia plane

Figure 61-3 Retaining ligaments of the face. (From Chung KC, Disa JJ, Gosain A, Lee G, Mehrara B, Thorne CH, van Aalst J, ed. *Operative Techniques in Plastic Surgery*. Wolters Kluwer; 2020. Figure 1.44.4.)

- Anterior and medial to the masseter, the nerve branches lie over the buccal fat pad.
- Branches penetrate the parotideomasseteric fascia to innervate the overlying mimetic muscles.
- Most of the facial muscles lie superficial to the plane of the facial nerve and receive their innervation from their deep surfaces except for the buccinator, levator anguli oris, and mentalis muscles.
- **Frontal branch of the facial nerve:** follows a path from 0.5 cm below the tragus to a point 1.5 cm above the lateral brow, also known as **Pitanguy line.**
  □ The frontal branch is deep to the SMAS at least until the level of the zygomatic arch, where it hugs the periosteum of the arch. Once the frontal branch crosses the zygomatic arch (crosses midway between tragus and lateral canthus), it steadily becomes more superficial to lie within or just deep to the SMAS (temporoparietal fascia). It is here that the nerve is most susceptible to injury during a rhytidectomy.

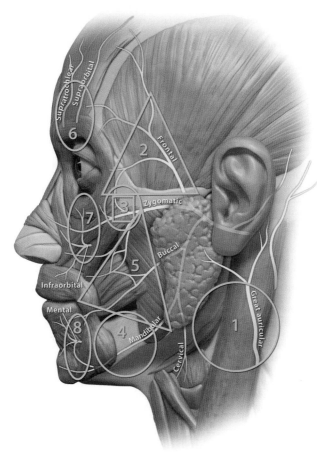

Figure 61-4 Zones of danger of the face. These zones are where the major nerves of the face are most susceptible to injury during face-lift and neck lift dissections. (Adapted by permission from Seckel BR . Facial danger zones: avoiding nerve injury in facial plastic surgery. *Can J Plast Surg.* 1994;2(2):59-66. Copyright © 1994 SAGE Publications.)

- **Zygomatic and buccal branches of the facial nerve:** exist deep to deep fascia upon exit from parotid and overly the masseter.
  - The zygomatic branch is vulnerable during release of the zygomatic retaining ligaments. The buccal branch can be injured during buccal fat pad dissection.
  - Injury to these nerves is rarely symptomatic long term due to multiple interconnections.
- *Marginal mandibular branch of the facial nerve.
  - **Exits the parotid 4 cm below the base of the earlobe** just anterior to the angle of the mandible.
  - **In most cases (81%), the nerve courses above the mandibular border.** It runs superficial to the facial artery and vein and can be identified where the facial vessels cross the mandibular border, just anterior to the insertion of the masseter.
  - Remains deep to deep fascia along most of its, thus injury is quite rare.

- **Cervical branch of the facial nerve:** exits parotid gland just anterior to angle of mandible and penetrates deep fascia to travel in the subplatysmal plane.
  - □ The cervical branch's more superficial nature leads to it being more commonly injured. This can occur during dissection deep to the platysma.
  - □ Cervical branch injury causes weakness of lip depression, which can be distinguished from marginal mandibular nerve injury by the preservation of the ability to evert and purse the lips with cervical branch injury.
- **Great auricular nerve (C2-C3):** provides sensory innervation to lower half of ear including earlobe
  - □ *Crosses the midportion of the sternocleidomastoid muscle 6.5 cm below the external auditory canal (known as McKinney point).
  - □ *Courses in the same plane as the external jugular vein, which is a useful landmark during dissection.
  - □ *Most commonly injured symptomatic nerve during rhytidectomy.
  - □ Division of nerve causes numbness of the posterior ear.
  - □ Most likely to be injured during postauricular dissection over sternocleidomastoid muscle.
- **Auriculotemporal nerve**
  - □ Runs with superficial temporal artery.
  - □ *Division during face-lift can cause Frey syndrome where facial skin receives sympathetic reinnervation causing gustatory sweating.

INDICATIONS AND PATIENT ASSESSMENT

- **Address the specific complaints of each patient** and tailor the operative plan individually.
- **The rhytidectomy preoperative evaluation** includes assessment and documentation of facial asymmetries as well as skin redundancy, abnormal fat accumulations, platysma laxity, and salivary gland laxity. Detailed facial evaluation is critical (see **Chapter 57: Evaluation of Facial Aging**).
- **Special consideration is given to:** the contour of the jawline and neckline, the status of the nasolabial folds, jowling, and facial fat atrophy.
- As with any procedure, detailed preoperative history and physical examination with special considerations to smoking status, hypertension, diabetes, use of anticoagulation/antiplatelet agents, and any other conditions that may increase bleeding risk or wound healing problems.

FACE-LIFT AND NECK-LIFT (RHYTIDECTOMY) TECHNIQUE

INCISION DESIGN

- There are three components to the standard face-lift and neck lift incision: temple, preauricular, and postauricular.
  - ○ Temple: can be either within hair (when minimal excess temporal skin will be excised) or along the temporal hairline (when significant excess temporal skin will be excised). The goal is to preserve a patient's sideburn and temporal hairline.
  - ○ Preauricular: follows the boundary of the ear and the posterior cheek along the contour of the superior helix continuing retrotragally and down to the base of the ear. Some surgeons utilize a pretragal incision in men to avoid bringing hair onto the tragus.
  - ○ Postauricular: generally placed in the retroauricular sulcus and then crosses to follow the occipital hairline. (Note: techniques such as the "short-scar face-lift" avoid the postauricular extension, which can be suitable when minimal neck work is necessary.)
- A submental incision can be added to address the anterior neck per surgeon preference. This should be posterior to the existing submental crease, which should be released with anterior dissection.

OPERATIONS/APPROACHES

- **Subcutaneous rhytidectomy**
  - Described in early 20th century, the first face-lift involved excising skin anterior to the ear and temporal hairline. Further iterations involved more extensive undermining of skin.
  - Has largely fallen out of favor as it relies on skin tension to tighten the underlying soft tissues, which can cause skin necrosis, widened scars, and facial distortion.
  - Occasionally, still has a role in thin patients with skin-only excess and without ptosis of deeper structures. Has the additional benefit as being very safe since there is no risk of nerve injury in the subcutaneous plane.
- **Deep subcutaneous rhytidectomy**
  - Flaps are raised in plane immediately superficial to SMAS, bringing superficial fat compartments up with the skin flap, which is then contoured.
  - Benefits include a more robust flap and a reduction in risk of facial nerve damage by leaving the SMAS down.
- **Subcutaneous rhytidectomy with SMAS plication or SMASectomy (SMAS resection)**
  - Face-lifts involving SMAS plication or SMASectomy are the most widely employed by plastic surgeons.
  - Skin flap dissection is performed in a lateral-to-medial direction, leaving a small layer of fat on the flap. Dissection ends just lateral to the nasolabial folds.
  - The SMAS is then plicated or a narrow ellipse is excised (SMASectomy). Other forms of the operation involve SMAS stacking and imbrication. The direction of pull should be superior and lateral across the midface parallel to the nasolabial fold.
  - The main advantage of this technique is the ability to manipulate the skin and SMAS separately, so that the SMAS can be repositioned vertically and skin can be redraped laterally with minimal tension (**Fig. 61-5**).
  - Manipulation of the SMAS improves longevity of the face-lift.
- **Minimal access cranial suspension lift**
  - A subcutaneous flap is elevated similar to other face-lift methods.
  - The SMAS is elevated by weaving sutures throughout the SMAS that are then anchored to the deep temporal fascia.
- **Deep-plane rhytidectomy**
  - Described by Tord Skoog—a sub-SMAS dissection is extended over the zygomaticus muscles and medially beyond the nasolabial folds, totally releasing all SMAS attachments and creating a thick flap composed of skin, subcutaneous fat, and platysma. **Skin is NOT elevated as a separate layer.**
  - The total release of the SMAS allows all components of the flap to be lifted and advanced back to their original position.
  - The correct plane is below the SMAS and just above the thin parotideomasseteric fascia, which serves to protect the branches of the facial nerve.
  - Modified by Hamra to include the lower lid orbicularis muscle.
  - Expectedly, the deep-plane technique is associated with a slightly higher risk of facial nerve injury.
- **Dual plane/lamellar lift**
  - Broad term for a variety of techniques that involve dissecting a subcutaneous flap and then a separate SMAS flap, which are then repositioned in different vectors.
  - Many different methods described by Barton, Baker, Stuzin, etc., which are beyond the scope of this text but are important to understand for the well-rounded face-lift surgeon.
  - These techniques carry the advantage of allowing tailored movement of SMAS and skin layers permitting creation of ideal facial and neck contours. Additionally, more anterior release of the SMAS has a greater effect in the anterior face. Disadvantages include risk of nerve injury and damage to thin SMAS flap.
- **Subperiosteal rhytidectomy**

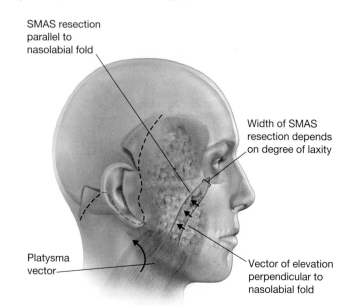

SMAS resection
parallel to
nasolabial fold

Width of SMAS
resection depends
on degree of laxity

Platysma
vector

Vector of elevation
perpendicular to
nasolabial fold

Figure 61-5 Rhytidectomy with SMAS excision or plication. The SMAS and facial fat are repositioned in an upward manner, while the skin is redraped in a more posterior direction.

- Developed by Tessier, this extensive approach can specifically address structural laxity in the midface and involves degloving of the upper face and midface and elevation of tissues in the subperiosteal plane.
- This technique is almost never utilized these days.
- **Midface lift (concentric malar lift)**
  - This technique directly addresses ptosis of the malar fat pad through a lower lid blepharoplasty incision (either subciliary or transconjunctival).
  - Wide subperiosteal dissection over the anterior maxilla from the level of the inferorbital rim is performed.
  - The infraorbital nerve is carefully preserved.
  - The periosteum is released, allowing repositioning and fixation of the cheek mass to the infraorbital rim or the temporalis fascia.
- **Neck lift (Fig. 61-6)**
  - Corrects cervicomental obliquity and platysmal banding.
  - Supra- and subplatysmal fat can be removed by either liposuction or direct excision. Some surgeons will also address prominent submandibular glands and hypertrophy of the anterior belly of the digastric muscles by resecting portions of these structures; however, these techniques carry risks and should only be attempted by experienced surgeons.
  - The platysma can be tightened (platysmaplasty) by plicating it in the midline with or without transecting it inferolaterally or pulling the platysma superolaterally and fixating to Loré fascia. Platysma myotomy can also be performed to address dynamic platysmal banding.
  - Make incision just posterior to submental crease.
- **Adjunctive Procedures**
  - Fat grafting—a critical component of many face-lifts since a distinct part of facial aging is fat compartment atrophy.

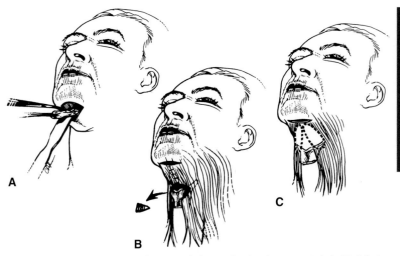

Figure 61-6 Treatment of medial platysma and platysma bands. Alternatives include (**A**) defatting of the anterior platysma without muscle modification; (**B**) midline platysmaplasty with wedge excision and platysmal plication; (**C**) resection of platysmal bands without midline approximation. If a submental incision is elected, option (**B**) is usually the best alternative.

○ Face-lift and neck lift can be combined with blepharoplasty, brow lift, and/or upper lip lift for total facial rejuvenation.
○ Chemical peels and lasers can be used; however, opinions differ regarding safety of use on elevated face-lift flap.

PERIOPERATIVE MANAGEMENT

• Preoperative
  ○ Stop all nonsteroidal anti-inflammatory drugs, aspirin, and supplements that induce bleeding 2 weeks prior to the operation.
  ○ Hypertension must be well-controlled.
  ○ Smoking, poorly controlled diabetes, and uncontrolled hypertension are all contraindications to face-lift/neck lift.
• Intraoperative
  ○ Meticulous hemostasis throughout the operation.
  ○ Careful intraoperative blood pressure control—there are many algorithms described for perioperative blood pressure control in face-lift/neck lift that are beyond the scope of this text; however, many use chlorpromazine and clonidine for intra- and postoperative control.
• Postoperative
  ○ Blood pressure control.
  ○ Most surgeons place a drain that is removed on postoperative day 1.
  ○ Face and neck wrapped with gentle dressing that is also removed on postoperative day 1.
  ○ Avoidance of strenuous activity, heavy lifting, or bending over for 2 weeks.

COMPLICATIONS

• **Hematoma**
  ○ Most common complication and accounts for 70% of all rhytidectomy complications.
  ○ Occurs in 3%-8% of cases depending on the study.

- o More common in men than in women.
- o More common in secondary rhytidectomy.
- o Must be evacuated to prevent overlying skin necrosis and scarring.
- o *Perioperative blood pressure control and avoidance of substances that can interfere with clotting mechanisms (eg, aspirin and nonsteroidal anti-inflammatory drugs) are the most important preventative measures.
- **Flap loss and/or ischemia**, most commonly affecting smokers.
- **Infection** is a rare complication (<1%).
- **Asymmetry:** all preoperative asymmetries should be noted and pointed out to the patient prior to surgery as asymmetries present before surgery will likely be present postoperatively and may possibly be more noticeable.
- **Great auricular nerve injury**
- o Most common *symptomatic* nerve injury after face-lift.
- o Occurs in 7% of cases.
- o *Presents as numbness of the lower ear and earlobe.
- o If inadvertent transection is identified intraoperatively, the nerve should be repaired and good sensory results expected.
- **Facial nerve injury** and palsy
- o Less than 1% in most studies.
- o The most commonly injured branch of the facial nerve is the buccal branch. However, injury is frequently unrecognized due to overlap of innervation with other facial nerve branches.
- o *Injury to a cervical branch can mimic injury to the marginal mandibular branch producing lower lip depressor weakness. However, patients with a marginal mandibular nerve injury cannot purse their lower lip (mentalis and orbicularis function).
- o Spontaneous recovery expected in 80% of patients because most injuries are due to neuropraxia or stretch. Reexploration in the early postoperative period is rarely described, but in individual cases may be warranted if the index of suspicion for a transection is exceedingly high.
- **Excessive scarring or temporal alopecia.**
- **Permanent alopecia occurs in ~3% of cases.**
- **Pixie ear deformity** refers to a lobule that has been pulled inferiorly and anteriorly, caused by insetting the lobule under tension.

FACIAL AUGMENTATION WITH FACIAL IMPLANTS

- The chin is the most commonly augmented site, followed by the malar region (see **Chapter 62: Genioplasty**).
- Augmentation is useful in combination with rhytidectomy to compensate for soft tissue and bony atrophy that occurs with aging.
- **Alloplastic Materials**
- o **Silicone**
  - ▪ The most commonly used material because it is biocompatible, stable, and the shape can be easily modified.
  - ▪ Silicone implants become encased by a tissue capsule and can be easily removed if necessary.
- o **Polyethylene** (Medpor)
  - ▪ Used for rigid skeletal augmentation.
  - ▪ Available in a variety of shapes to augment the orbital rim, malar area, piriform, mandibular angle, chin, and nasal dorsum.
  - ▪ Polyethylene is porous and allows tissue ingrowth with a theoretical advantage of fewer complications from infection, extrusion, and malposition.
  - ▪ For this reason, polyethylene is more difficult to remove than silicone.
- o **Hydroxyapatite:** used for cranial reconstruction, alveolar ridges, and other bony facial structures

- **The ratio of soft tissue response to facial skeletal change is ~0.66.** For example, an implant with 1 cm of projection will usually result in 0.66 cm of soft tissue augmentation projection. In general, chin implants usually provide more reliable projection than malar implants due to their location and surrounding soft tissue contour.
- **Common complications** include hematoma, lower lip dysfunction (mentalis injury), infection, extrusion, malposition, and mental nerve injury.

PEARLS

1. Change to the facial skeleton with aging includes decrease in height of the midface and lower face, increased prominence of the chin, increased prominence of the zygomatic arch, and increased facial depth. These changes must be considered when altering the soft tissue envelope during face-lift surgery.
2. The key to a successful and safe face-lift is a detailed understanding of three-dimensional facial anatomy.
3. Manipulation of the SMAS is critical to correcting stigmata of facial aging and contributing to longevity of face-lift results.
4. Knowledge of facial fat compartments and retaining ligaments is essential to understanding facial aging. Addressing fat atrophy and descent is a foundation of the modern face-lift.
5. Patients should be informed that the effects of face-lifts are considered to last for about 10 years, although this is depend on many factors, such as the age at which the procedure is performed and the general health status of the patient.

QUESTIONS YOU WILL BE ASKED

1. Which muscles are innervated on their superficial surface?
   Levator anguli oris, buccinators, and mentalis muscles.
2. What is the SMAS?
   Superficial musculoaponeurotic system; fascial layer investing the mimetic muscles.
3. What is the most commonly injured branch of the facial nerve?
   Buccal.
4. What is the most common symptomatic nerve injury?
   Great auricular nerve.
5. What complication do you expect when operating on a smoker?
   Skin flap necrosis.
6. How do you avoid a pixie ear deformity?
   Tension-free inset of the lobule.

Recommended Readings
1. Baker DC. Minimal incision rhytidectomy (short scar face lift) with lateral SMASectomy. *Aesthet Surg J*. 2001;21(1):68-79.
2. Hester TR Jr, Codner MA, McCord CD, Nahai F, Giannopoulos A. Evolution of technique of the direct transblepharoplasty approach for the correction of lower lid and midfacial aging: maximizing results and minimizing complications in a 5-year experience. *Plast Reconstr Surg*. 2000;105(1):393-406; discussion 407-408.
3. Mitz V, Peyronie M. The superficial musculo-aponeurotic system (SMAS) in the parotid and cheek area. *Plast Reconstr Surg*. 1976;58(1):80-88.
4. Rohrich RJ, Pessa JE. The fat compartments of the face: anatomy and clinical implications for cosmetic surgery. *Plast Reconstr Surg*. 2007;119(7):2219-2227.
5. Rohrich RJ, Stuzin JM, Dayan E, Ross EV. *Facial Danger Zones: Staying Safe with Surgery, Fillers and Non-Invasive Devices*. Thieme; 2020.
6. Shaw RB Jr, Katzel EB, Koltz PF, et al. Aging of the facial skeleton: aesthetic implications and rejuvenation strategies. *Plast Reconstr Surg*. 2011;127(1):374-383.

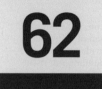

62 Genioplasty

Rami D. Sherif

OVERVIEW

- Genioplasty refers to surgery that repositions the chin either by
  - Augmentation with filler/fat, an implant, or movement of patient's own bone
  - Reduction by movement and/or recontouring the existing bone
- The chin is a critical element of facial aesthetics. Small changes can make relatively large differences in appearance.

RELEVANT ANATOMY

- **Bony Anatomy (Fig. 62-1)**
  - Mental protuberance: triangular bony prominence of lower anterior aspect of the mandible.
  - *Mental foramen: opening through which mental nerve emerges and provides sensation to the chin and lower lip soft tissues. Generally, at the level of the second premolar, halfway between the alveolar crest and the inferior mandibular border.
    - Important to note that the inferior alveolar canal (through which the mental nerve courses) dips inferior to the level of the mental foramen before curving up to the level of the foramen. This is critical in osseous genioplasty— osteotomy should be at least 6 mm below the level of the foramen to ensure protection of the mental nerve.
- **Muscular Anatomy**
  - Mimetic muscles
    - **Mentalis:** paired conical muscle that originates from the incisive fossa of the mandible and inserts into the soft tissue and skin of the chin
      - Assists in lip eversion and pout. Causes wrinkling and dimpling of the overlying chin skin
    - Other muscles that insert around the anterior chin include the orbicularis oris and the depressor anguli oris.
  - Muscles of mastication: geniohyoid and anterior belly of digastric
  - Muscles of deglutition: genioglossus and mylohyoid
- **Nerve Supply**
  - **Mental nerve** terminal branch of inferior alveolar nerve emerges from mental foramen. **Care must be taken to protect this nerve during genioplasty.**
  - Mentalis is supplied by marginal mandibular branch of the facial nerve (CN VII).
- **Vascular Supply**
  - Lower lip and chin skin supplied by inferior labial artery off the facial artery
  - Anterior mandible supplied by both endosteal and periosteal supplies
    - Endosteal—inferior alveolar artery
    - Periosteal—facial artery (buccal surface) and supra/inframylohyoid arteries (lingual surface)

TERMINOLOGY

- Microgenia: vertical chin deficiency.
- Macrogenia: vertical or sagittal chin excess.

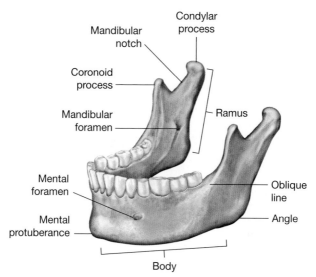

Figure 62-1 Bone anatomy and relationships of the mandible. (From Chung KC, Disa JJ, Gosain A, et al., eds. *Operative Techniques in Plastic Surgery.* Wolters Kluwer; 2020. Figure 1.74.1A.)

- Retrogenia: sagittal chin deficiency.
- Note that micrognathia and retrognathia refer to mandibular size and position and are not terms to describe chin size.

EVALUATION

- **History**
  - Full medical history with specific attention to issues that impair wound healing and may interfere with implants such as diabetes, smoking, disorders, or medications causing immunosuppression. If considering any intraoral approach, **ensure that patient has good dental health and does not have active dental infections.**
- **Physical**
  - Careful examination of the face from frontal and lateral positions allows complete analysis of the chin.
  - **Vertical chin position**
    - Lower face height—the lower third of the face should be equal in height to the middle and upper thirds. If a patient has a short or long lower third, the patient may benefit from a lengthening or reductive genioplasty, respectively.
      - The upper lip height (distance from subnasale to stomion) should be ½ the lower lip/chin height (distance from stomion to menton).
    - If the patient exhibits increased incisal show and mentalis strain, these are signs of vertical maxillary excess and the patient would be better treated with formal orthognathic evaluation and correction.
  - **Sagittal projection**
    - Chin projection: most simply evaluated by drawing Riedel line (**Fig. 62-2**).
      - **Riedel line** describes a line connecting the anterior-most points along the upper and lower lip. The most projected portion of the chin should touch this line.
      - If the chin lies posterior to this line, then the chin needs to be augmented in the horizontal direction.

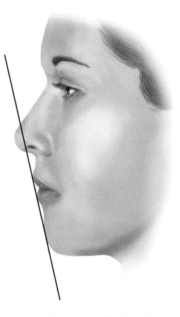

Figure 62-2 Riedel plane. (From Chung KC, Disa JJ, Gosain A, et al., eds. *Operative Techniques in Plastic Surgery.* Wolters Kluwer; 2020. Figure 2.44.3B.)

- Another method of evaluation involves drawing a line perpendicular to the Frankfort horizontal, tangential to the most projecting portion of the upper lip. For males, the chin should touch this line, while for females, the chin should lie 2-3 mm behind this line.
  - **Occlusion:** defined by relationship between maxillary first molar and mandibular first molar
    - Class 1: mesiobuccal cusp of maxillary first molar rests in the buccal groove of mandibular first molar.
    - Class 2: mesiobuccal cusp of maxillary first molar is mesial to buccal groove of mandibular first molar.
    - Class 3: mesiobuccal cusp of maxillary first molar is distal to buccal groove of mandibular first molar.
  - **Labiomental crease:** indentation between the cutaneous lower lip and the skin of the chin pad.
    - Depth should be ~4 mm in women and 6 mm in men.
    - Deep labiomental crease can be due to excessive chin projection, lower incisor flaring, or both.
    - Shallow crease can be due to microgenia, lingually inclined teeth, or both.
  - **Soft tissue:** evaluate thickness of soft tissue pad, lower lip length, mentalis strain, presence of witch's chin deformity.
    - Witch's chin—soft tissue ptosis of the chin pad. Submental crease is exaggerated. Usually due to failure to resuspend the mentalis during closure of an intraoral approach to the chin, but can also occur due to normal aging and descent of soft tissues.
    - Cervicomental angle—angle between chin and neck. Should be 105°-120°.
- **Imaging**
  - Not a critical component of preoperative evaluation; however, essential when more complex deformity suspected or to rule in/out need for more extensive orthognathic intervention. If so, cephalograms and panorex are ideal modalities.
  - Cephalometrics: analysis of lateral cephalograms (XR) of the human skull to evaluate the dental and skeletal relationships.

- ○ Important points in analysis of mandible and chin position include the following:
    - ▪ Menton—most inferior point of chin
    - ▪ Pogonion—most projecting point of mandible
    - ▪ Nasion—nasofrontal junction
    - ▪ A (Subspinale)—columella-labial junction
    - ▪ B (Supramentale)—deepest point between pogonion and incisor
- ○ More detailed analysis of cephalometrics can be found in **Chapter 18: Orthognathic Surgery.**

SURGICAL APPROACH AND OPTIONS

In general, genioplasty can be accomplished through the use of implants or osteotomies and movement of patient's autologous bony tissue. For smaller and more subtle changes, filler or fat grafting can be used to augment the chin.

SURGICAL APPROACH

- Intraoral (**Fig. 62-3**)
    - ○ Works for both osseous and implant-based genioplasty.
    - ○ Provides a "hidden" incision that heals without any visible scars.
    - ○ For implants, some have concern that this introduces higher risk of implant infection due to contamination with oral flora.
    - ○ Additionally, **can predispose to improperly superiorly placed implant.**
    - ○ Approach:
        - ▪ An incision is designed along the lower gingivolabial sulcus.
    - ○ Critical to leave a cuff of mucosa of ~10 mm.
    - ○ Distally, along the level of the mental nerves, the incision is curved closer to the canines and premolars to prevent nerve injury.
    - ○ Incision is carried out through the mucosa with a Bovie (needle point tip is helpful here).
    - ○ The next structure encountered is the mentalis muscle. It is similarly critical to leave a cuff of mentalis for closure.

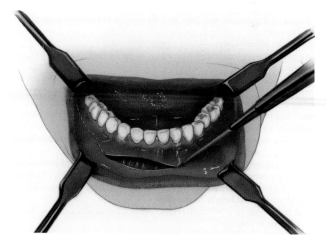

Figure 62-3 Transoral exposure of the mandible with labial sulcus approach, incision placement. (From Mandibular Vestibular Approach. In: Ellis E III, MF. *Surgical Approaches to the Facial Skeleton*. 3rd ed. Wolters Kluwer; 2019:137-150. Figure 8.5.)

- o Incise through mentalis with the Bovie and carry dissection straight down to bone.
- o For implant, decision is made to be pre- or subperiosteal.
  - ▪ If preperiosteal, dissect out pocket to fit implant precisely, taking care to identify and protect mental nerves.
  - ▪ If subperiosteal, then incise the periosteum and elevate to inferior border, identify and protect mental nerves, and create precise pocket for implant.
  - ▪ If osseous genioplasty, then desired osteotomies are carried out followed by movement of the bony segment and fixation.
- Closure
  - o **Imperative to close mentalis and mucosa to prevent development of witch's chin deformity.**
  - o Both layers can be separately approximated using interrupted absorbable sutures, for example, Vicryl.
- Submental approach
  - o Similarly can be used for both implants and osseous genioplasty.
  - o Allows excellent visibility of pocket, which is specifically important in implant-based genioplasty as it allows precise placement of implant under direct visualization. Also some argue that it prevents contamination with oral flora.
  - o This approach does result in an **external scar.**

OSSEOUS GENIOPLASTY

- The mental protuberance is altered by performing osteotomies inferior to the mental foramina and moving the bony segment to achieve alteration of the chin position and appearance.
- **Indications**
  - o Sagittal deficiency or excess
  - o Vertical deficiency or excess
  - o Horizontal asymmetries
  - o Revisions
- Versatile technique that allows correction of all types of chin deformity in three dimensions, in contrast to implant-based genioplasty (**Fig. 62-4**).
- Osteotomies are performed with care to protect the mental nerves. The bony segment is then moved to the desired position, and fixation is performed with plates/screws, lag screws, or wires.
- **Types of osseous genioplasty**
  - o **Sliding genioplasty:** horizontal osteotomy is performed, and bony segment is advanced anteriorly or posteriorly.
    - ▪ For **sagittal (horizontal) deformity.** Can be used to increase or decrease projection
  - o **Jumping genioplasty:** inferior mandibular osteotomy is performed, and the bony segment is advanced anteriorly and superiorly. The piece of bone essentially acts as an implant along the anterior mandible.
    - ▪ For improvement of sagittal chin projection with **simultaneous height reduction.** Larger anterior moves than sliding genioplasty.
  - o **Vertical lengthening:** horizontal osteotomy is performed, and positioned inferiorly to the desired length. If <5 mm, can be positioned with plates, otherwise need to place bone graft or bone substitute in between segment and mandible.
    - ▪ For **short vertical height of the chin**
  - o **Vertical reduction:** two horizontal osteotomies are made, and the intervening bony segment is removed.
    - ▪ For **excessive vertical height of the chin.** Can also address cants/asymmetry if the horizontal lines are adjusted to remove a variable amount of bone on one side vs the other.
  - o **Asymmetric wedge:** a wedge of bone is removed to correct a cant or vertical asymmetry.

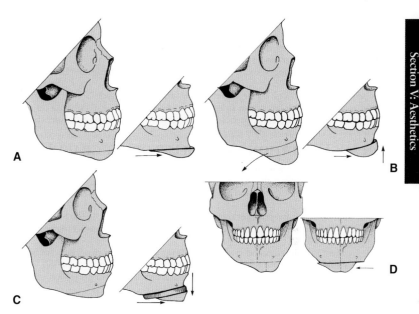

Figure 62-4 A. Standard location and orientation of the advancement osseous genioplasty. Note that the osteotomy is placed well below the mental foramina to avoid injury to the inferior alveolar nerve. The osteotomy extends well posterior to the vicinity of the molar teeth. The angulation of this osteotomy allows forward advancement of the chin without any vertical changes. **B.** Simultaneous advancement and vertical reduction of the chin. Note that the two parallel osteotomies are performed with an intervening ostectomy. **C.** Simultaneous advancement and vertical elongation of the chin. The interpositional material typically employed includes blocks of porous hydroxyapatite. **D.** Lateral shifting of the symphyseal segment to restore lower face symmetry. (From Chung KC, ed. *Grabb and Smith's Plastic Surgery.* 8th ed. Wolters Kluwer; 2020. Figure 54.10.)

- ○ **Narrowing/widening osteotomy**
  - ▪ To narrow the chin, a central segment of bone is removed and the two lateral segments are mobilized with a horizontal osteotomy and they are medialized.
  - ▪ To widen the chin, midline and horizontal osteotomies are made and the two segments are moved laterally. If the central gap is more than 5 mm, it must be filled with bone graft or bone substitute.
- • Expected soft tissue changes (expressed as ratio of soft tissue change:bony movement):
  - ○ 0.9:1 with sagittal advancement
  - ○ 0.8-1:1 with vertical lengthening
  - ○ 0.25:1 with shortening

ALLOPLASTIC GENIOPLASTY

- • An alloplastic implant is placed in a pocket anterior to the mental protuberance to augment the chin.
- • The only indications for this technique are **correction of mild sagittal deficiencies** and **correction of shallow labiomental fold.**
- • Cannot be used for correction of vertical excess, vertical deficiency, or asymmetries.
  - ○ **Perform with caution in smokers or diabetics.**
- • Types of implant
  - ○ Silicone: inert material that is commonly used for implants throughout the body.
    - ▪ Forms a capsule

- ○ Medpor: porous polyethylene that allows tissue ingrowth and implant incorporation.
  - ▪ Theoretically more resistant to infection; however, more difficult to remove than silicone implant due to tissue ingrowth.
- Expected soft tissue changes (expressed as ratio of soft tissue change:implant):
  - ○ 0.7-0.9:1
- Can be performed through either submental or intraoral approach. Some theorize that intraoral approach has higher infection rate; however, the available data do not support this. In the intraoral approach, however, care must be taken to ensure that the implant is not malpositioned superiorly.

CHIN AUGMENTATION USING FILLER OR FAT GRAFTING

- **Fat grafting:** less invasive technique for augmenting the chin by injecting small volumes of fat throughout the chin soft tissue pad.
  - ○ Especially effective for minimal microgenia (chin lies <5 mm posterior to ideal sagittal position).
  - ○ Not appropriate for significant microgenia.
  - ○ Added benefit of restoring volume lost due to facial aging and softening of rhytids in the area.
- **Filler:** augmentation of chin and jawline is performed using filler material. Can be temporary filler (hyaluronic acid) vs permanent filler (calcium hydroxyapatite).
  - ○ Similar to fat grafting—good option for small increases in chin projection or height.
  - ○ Filler genioplasty with temporary hyaluronic filler is a good option for patients who want to "test out" the effect of chin augmentation prior to proceeding with a permanent option such as fat injection or surgical genioplasty.

POSTOPERATIVE CARE

DRESSINGS, CARE, AND RESTRICTIONS

- Patients are placed in a compressive tape dressing over the chin. This reduces swelling and supports the closure. These are kept on for up to a week.
- Peridex rinses.
- Head of bed elevation.
- Some surgeons have patients on a liquid diet for 24-48 hours before advancing to a regular diet.

COMPLICATIONS

- For genioplasty in general
  - ○ Asymmetry
  - ○ Lower lip paresthesias
    - ▪ Usually neuropraxia from traction. Temporary numbness is very common in the immediate postoperative period. Permanent sensory deficits have been cited as high as 10% in some studies.
  - ○ Infection
    - ▪ Approximately 5% in implant genioplasty, slightly lower in osseous genioplasty
  - ○ Lip/chin ptosis
  - ○ Witch's chin
    - ▪ Results from failure to resuspend the mentalis and approximate the soft tissues properly
  - ○ Hematoma
    - ▪ Rare but should be washed out with thorough irrigation to prevent infection.

- Specific to osseous genioplasty
  - Over-advancement or overreduction
  - Dental injury
- Specific to implant-based genioplasty
  - Implant malposition
  - Osseous absorption
    - Some studies have shown that this can be as high as 0.1 mm per year.
  - Implant infection
    - As stated above, occurs ~5% of the time

PEARLS

1. Complete evaluation of the chin requires analysis of the vertical and sagittal position of the chin as well as the overlying soft tissue, including the labiomental fold and cervicomental angle.
2. Depending on the desired effects, genioplasty can be accomplished through bony osteotomies, implants, or filler/fat grafting.
3. Access to the chin can be gained through either an intraoral or submental incision.
4. Reapproximation of the mentalis muscle when using an intraoral approach is critical to prevent witch's chin deformity.
5. Great care must be taken to protect the mental nerve during genioplasty.

QUESTIONS YOU WILL BE ASKED

1. What type of deficiency can be addressed with a silicone chin implants?
   Sagittal deficiency (and shallow labiomental crease).
2. How do you prevent a witch's chin deformity?
   Resuspend the mentalis muscle during closure.
3. Where can you identify the mental nerve?
   Inferior to the second mandibular premolar, approximately halfway between the alveolar crest and the inferior border of the mandible.

Recommended Readings
1. Guyuron B. MOC-PS(SM) CME article: genioplasty. *Plast Reconstr Surg.* 2008;121(4 Suppl):1-7.
2. Rohrich RJ, Sanniec K, Afrooz PN. Autologous fat grafting to the chin: a useful adjunct in complete aesthetic facial rejuvenation. *Plast Reconstr Surg.* 2018;142(4):921-925.
3. Rosen HM. Aesthetic guidelines in genioplasty: the role of facial disproportion. *Plast Reconstr Surg.* 1995;95(3):463-469; discussion 470-472.
4. Rosen HM. Aesthetic refinements in genioplasty: the role of the labiomental fold. *Plast Reconstr Surg.* 1991;88(5):760-767.
5. Sati S, Havlik RJ. An evidence-based approach to genioplasty. *Plast Reconstr Surg.* 2011;127(2):898-904.

63 Gender-Affirming Facial Surgery

Megan Lane

OVERVIEW

- Gender-affirming facial surgery is a collection of operations aimed at altering the soft tissues and bony anatomy of the face to convey a more masculine or feminine appearance.
- As opposed to other types of gender-affirming procedures, the current WPATH Standards of Care (SOC 8) **does not** require a letter from a therapist prior to undergoing gender-affirming facial surgery.
- There are key differences between classically feminine and masculine facial appearances (**Table 63-1**), but there are few individuals who have purely feminine or masculine features.
- Importantly, some patients do not want an entirely feminine or masculine appearance.

EVALUATION

- Evaluation and treatment planning should be focused on shared decision-making and addressing patient's concerns. This chapter will primarily focus on facial feminization, which is more common than facial masculinization.
- There are some changes in facial appearance that can be induced by gender-affirming hormones, specifically improvement in jawline, facial hair growth, and changes in hairline for transmasculine individuals and malar volume for transfeminine individuals.
- **Preoperative Imaging**
    - Preoperative photomanipulation is a useful tool to ensure the operative plan is consistent with a patient's goals for surgery.
    - If planning on performing forehead feminization, obtain head CT to evaluate the location and thickness of the anterior table and location of the frontal sinus.
    - For chondrolaryngoplasty, consider CT of the neck to determine distance from the true vocal chords to the thyroid cartilage.
    - In genioplasty, CT scan can aid in surgical planning of osteotomies.

NON-OPERATIVE AND OPERATIVE TECHNIQUES

NONSURGICAL ADJUNCTS

- Electrolysis and laser hair removal may be helpful for transfeminine individuals with excess facial hair.

FOREHEAD AND EYEBROWS

- **Forehead feminization** is focused on reshaping the contour of the forehead and addressing differences in the hairline.
- Feminine foreheads have a convex shape with minimal frontal bossing. Feminine hairlines are "U" shaped as opposed to "M" shaped with minimal hair loss. Hair lines are typically 5-6 cm above the brow.

---

*Denotes common in-service examination topics.

TABLE 63-1 Key Characteristics of Masculine and Feminine Faces

Feature	Feminine	Masculine	M to F available procedures
Forehead	Rounded forehead without frontal bossing	Frontal bossing with prominent supraorbital rims	Burring of the frontal bone and supraorbital rim, frontal bone osteotomy and frontal sinus setback
Hairline	5-6 cm above the brow, linear hairline or hairline with widow's peak	5-6 cm above the brow, "M"-shaped hairline common due to hair loss	Hairline advancement, hair transplant
Eyebrows	Eyebrows have a gentle curve with the apex of the curve ideally being at the lateral limbus, typically located above orbital rim	Straight eyebrows with little curve, located at orbital rim	Brow lift
Cheeks	Increased soft tissue volume at malar eminence	Decreased soft tissue volume at the malar eminence	Fat grafting, midface osteotomies
Nose	Small nose with gentle sloping of the dorsum, well-defined tip with supratip break	Larger nose with straight dorsum, minimal supratip break	Rhinoplasty
Lips	Larger volume lips with more vermillion show, 2- to 4-mm incisor show	Less vermilion show, 0- to 2-mm incisor show	Filler, fat grafting, potentially lip lift
Mandible	Sloping mandibular angle with a small, rounded chin	Strong mandibular angle with angular, larger chin	Genioplasty, mandibular angle burring
Thyroid cartilage	No prominent thyroid cartilage	Prominent thyroid cartilage ("Adam's apple")	Chondrolaryngoplasty

Adapted from Morrison S, Vyas KS, Motakef S, et al. Facial feminization: systematic review of the literature. *Plast Reconstr Surg.* 2016;137(6):1759-1770.

- **Bony Procedures**
  - Ousterhout organized patients by frontal sinus characteristics and corresponding procedures.
    - Type I: moderate frontal bossing with small to no frontal sinuses → burring can be used
    - Type II: moderate frontal bossing with a thin anterior table and normal frontal sinus size → burring or frontal bone osteotomy can be used
    - Type III: severe frontal bossing with a thin anterior table and normal to large frontal sinus size → frontal bone osteotomy used
    - Type IV: no frontal bossing with underprojection of the brow. Rarely occurs and requires augmentation with fat, filler, or methyl methacrylate
  - **Preoperative CT** aids in evaluation of the anterior table and frontal sinuses.
  - Procedures are typically combined with a hairline advancement, and a pretrichial incision is used.
- **Soft Tissue**
  - **Hairline** advancement is usually performed at the time of any bony forehead recontouring.
  - Hairline advancement includes undermining the scalp in the subgaleal plane, advancing the scalp, and securing with monocortical bone tunnels or reverse Endotines.
  - The shape of the forehead following bony recontouring may additionally be augmented with fat grafting.
  - Please **see Chapter 59: Periocular Rejuvenation: Blepharoplasty, Eyelid Ptosis, and Brow Lift** for brow evaluation and brow lift approaches.
  - Hairline can be augmented with hair transplantation.
    - *The hair life cycle has three stages: anagen (growth, 3-6 years), catagen (hair follicle regression, 1-2 weeks), and anagen (hair loss and resting phase, 3-6 weeks).
    - Male androgenic alopecia or "male-pattern baldness" (balding in the frontotemporal region) is primarily caused by an alteration in the cycle of hair growth.
    - A predominant driving factor of male androgenic baldness is a by-product of testosterone, dihydrotestosterone (DHT). In addition to individuals assigned male at birth, transmasculine individuals on testosterone can experience male-pattern baldness.
    - Medical therapy includes finasteride (5-alpha reductase inhibitor) and minoxidil (vasodilator).
    - Follicular unit transplantation is the most common type of hair transplantation in which hair follicle units are transplanted rather than large areas of hair-bearing scalp.
      - Donor site is commonly occipital scalp.
      - *Micrografting is transplanting one to two hair follicles at a time, and minigrafting is three to four hair follicles at a time.

NOSE

- **Rhinoplasty** in facial feminization follows the same principles and techniques as aesthetic rhinoplasty.
- Aesthetic goals include dorsal hump reduction, definition of the tip and supratip break, and potentially shortening of the nose.
- Please see **Chapter 60: Rhinoplasty** for evaluation and approaches.

CHEEKS AND LIPS

- **Cheek feminization** is aimed at augmenting the malar eminence.
- Facial fat grafting or filler can be used to augment the malar region. Some institutions additionally use implants or zygomatic osteotomies for augmentation.

- **Lip feminization** is aimed at improving the volume of lips and vermillion show.
- Lips can be augmented with hyaluronic acid–based filler or fat grafting. Lip lift may additionally be appropriate in select patients.

MANDIBLE

- **Feminization of the mandible** aims to round and reduce the size of the chin.
  - Sliding genioplasty and genioplasty with T osteotomies are common options.
    - Typically performed through lower buccal sulcus approach.
    - Subperiosteal dissection performed.
    - Care should be taken to preserve the mental nerve, which is located between the first and second premolars.
  - Feminization may additionally include mandibular angle reduction.
- **Mandibular masculinization** is less common than feminization and can include sliding genioplasty, genioplasty with chin implant, and mandibular augmentation with bone grafting or implants.

THYROID CARTILAGE

- Prominent thyroid cartilage is colloquially called an "Adam's apple," and thyroid cartilage reduction (chondrolaryngoplasty) is popularly called a "tracheal shave."
- **Preoperative CT** scan can be used to visualize the distance from the thyroid cartilage to the true vocal cords.
- Aggressive burring can lead to attenuation of the true vocal chords and lowering of the voice.
- Procedure
  - Incision made at the cervicomental angle.
  - Platysma and strap muscles are split and blunt dissection is performed to clear off the thyroid cartilage.
  - Reduction is carried out through burring.
  - Direct visualization via laryngoscopy may be used to ensure burring is not at the level of the true vocal cords.

PEARLS

1. Facial gender-affirming surgery is a collection of operations commonly performed in aesthetic and reconstructive facial surgery. Shared decision-making is critical to developing a surgical plan and specific procedures for a particular patient.
2. The thickness of the anterior table and presence of the frontal sinus determines if frontal bone burring vs osteotomies is indicated in forehead feminization.
3. Burring of the thyroid cartilage can attenuate the true vocal cords and lower a patient's voice.

QUESTIONS YOU WILL BE ASKED

1. Does facial feminization require a letter from a therapist?
   In WPATH guidelines at the time of publication of this book, a letter is not required.
2. Describe the key differences between a feminine and masculine appearing face.
   Please **see Table 63-1**. Feminine foreheads are rounded while masculine hairlines are "M" shaped, and feminine brows have a gentle curve while masculine brows are straight. Masculine jawlines have a pronounced mandibular angle and square chin. Importantly, there are few individuals with purely masculine or feminine features.

Recommended Readings
1. Bellinga RJ, Capitán L, Simon D, Tenório T. Technical and clinical considerations for facial feminization surgery with rhinoplasty and related procedures. *JAMA Facial Plast Surg.* 2017;19(3):175-181.

2. Capitán L, Gutiérrez Santamaría J, Simon D, et al. Facial gender confirmation surgery: a protocol for diagnosis, surgical planning, and postoperative management. *Plast Reconstr Surg.* 2020;145(4):818e-828e.
3. Dechamps-Braly JC. Facial gender affirmation surgery: facial feminization surgery and facial masculinization surgery. *Gender Confirmation Surgery*. Springer-Nature Switzerland; 2020:99-113.
4. Morrison S, Vyas KS, Motakef S, et al. Facial feminization: systematic review of the literature. *Plast Reconstr Surg.* 2016;137(6):1759-1770.
5. Pansritum K. Forehead and hairline surgery for gender affirmation. *Plast Reconstr Surg Glob Open.* 2021;9(3):e3486.

64 Liposuction, Panniculectomy, and Abdominoplasty

Christopher J. Breuler

BODY CONTOURING OVERVIEW

- Body contouring encompasses several procedures aimed at improving aesthetic appearance typically after weight loss, most often through surgical manipulation of skin, adipose tissue, and muscle. These procedures are some of the most common cosmetic surgeries performed.
    - Liposuction: 210 000+ cases each year in the United States
    - Abdominoplasty: 95 000+ cases each year in the United States
- It is important to review the expected outcomes and limitations of these procedures, establish with the patient the areas of greatest concern, and decide which approach to take (liposuction vs excision vs combination of approaches). Thoughtful history and examination are key to determining which procedure(s) are most appropriate for a given patient.
- With the exception of liposuction, in these surgeries, you are typically trading better contour for significant scars.
- The goals of the procedures discussed in this chapter are as follows:
    - **Liposuction:** improve body contour by removing subcutaneous adipose tissue (does not address skin laxity)
    - **Abdominoplasty:** aesthetic procedure to excise excess skin and adipose tissue, with possible rectus plication and/or umbilical transposition, and to improve abdominal contour
    - **Panniculectomy:** functional procedure to remove large overhanging pannus

PATIENT HISTORY

- **The patient's weight should be stable for 3-6 months for optimal results.** History of weight loss and gain should be noted as well as plans for future weight loss.
- **Complete medical and surgical history** should be obtained, including medical comorbidities such as diabetes, heart disease, chronic obstructive pulmonary disease (COPD), and deep venous thrombosis (DVT)/pulmonary embolism (PE) are elicited to determine the risk of surgery. In some cases, such as with massive panniculectomy, the functional benefits of surgery may supersede the risks. Note history of breast cancer in women, as well as prior abdominal surgeries (including bariatric surgery).
- **Number of pregnancies and children** should be elicited as well as any plans for future pregnancies.
- **Social history** includes recent smoking or nicotine use (50% risk of wound healing complications), plans for any future pregnancies, available social support network, and level of physical activity.
- **Medications** that inhibit wound healing (eg, steroids that increase risk of dehiscence) or that increase perioperative risk (eg, hormones and blood thinners) are noted and temporarily discontinued if possible.
- ***All body contouring patients should be screened for unrealistic expectations, unhealthy external motivations, body dysmorphic disorders, eating disorders, and psychiatric history.** Full disclosure regarding the pros and cons of the unique approach for each individual is paramount to success and patient satisfaction.

---

*Denotes common in-service examination topics.

PHYSICAL EXAMINATION

- **Height, Weight, BMI, and Circumferences**
- **Skin Quality:** elasticity, intertriginous rashes or ulcerations, presence of striae
  - In addition, it is important to assess skin laxity between the pubis and umbilicus (this will help determine liposuction vs excise some vs combination).
- **Rectus Diastasis and Hernias** (including ventral and umbilical hernias)
- **Preoperative Abdominal Scars**
  - A subcostal scar (eg, Kocher incision) is a relative contraindication to a full abdominoplasty, as this incision interrupts Huger zone III.
  - A midline abdominal incision disrupts cross-midline perfusion and can result in wound healing complications.
    - Lower scars excised with the pannus have no effect.
    - Upper scars that will be transposed below the umbilicus are a relative contraindication and an absolute contraindication when combined with liposuction.
  - Transverse upper abdominal scars transposed below the umbilicus may limit blood supply with full abdominoplasty.
  - Variations of open appendectomy scars have little effect on surgical planning.
- **Symmetry**
- **Fat Distribution**
  - Epigastric fat will become the entire abdomen with a full abdominoplasty. If prominent, results of abdominoplasty are less favorable. Simultaneous liposuction is high risk and may lead to skin and fat necrosis due to disruption of zone III perfusion.
  - Excess fat and soft tissue over hips that will not be excised during abdominoplasty should be shown to patient.
  - Discussing intra-abdominal fat is an important part of the examination as this will not change following body contouring and can lead to suboptimal outcomes.
- **Pinch Test** (assess thickness of subcutaneous fat)
  - ≥ 3 cm for liposuction of the abdomen/hips/subtrochanteric areas
  - ≥ 2 cm for calves/ankles
- **Overall, the location and degree of adiposity vs skin laxity guides best surgical options—liposuction vs excision (or both). Most patients have mix of adiposity *and* laxity.**

MASSIVE WEIGHT LOSS PATIENTS

- Growing number of patients present after massive weight loss (MWL), either from diet and exercise or bariatric surgery.
- Body contouring may be considered once weight is stable.
- **MWL patients have unique risk factors** that contribute to postoperative complications and inferior aesthetic results.
  - Relative avascularity of adipose tissue.
  - Poor skin quality.
  - Musculofascial laxity. Some patients also have large abdominal hernias that will require repair by general surgery.
  - *Nutritional deficiencies after bariatric surgery, especially protein, calcium, iron (most common), and vitamins A, D, E, K, and B_{12}.
  - Body mass index. Greater risk of complications if BMI is >35.
- Discuss the patient's desires vs likely outcomes and complications.
- Help the patient understand what insurance will and will not cover prior to committing to a surgical plan.
- Intra-op fluids should include maintenance rate 10 mL/kg/h and close monitoring of post-op fluids and urine output.

LIPOSUCTION

OVERVIEW

- **General Considerations**
  - Aspiration of subcutaneous fat using small diameter cannulas connected to source of high vacuum (1 atm or 760 mm Hg, enough to achieve vapor pressure).
  - Adherent fat avulsed by back and forth motion of cannula.
  - Overlying skin shrinks to reduced fat volume.
  - Fibrous stoma containing neurovascular bundles is resistant to suction.
  - Best for fat deposits in patients with good skin elasticity who are unresponsive to diet/exercise.
  - Cannulas
    - Surface irregularities reduced by smaller cannulas
    - Set back cannula holes (prevent suction in superficial compartment)
    - Size range = 1.5-6 mm
    - Three-holed "Mercedes" cannula most popular
- **Adipose Tissue and Cellulite**
  - Adipocytes are produced in utero, early childhood, and early adolescence. After liposuction, adipocytes do not regenerate, but remaining adipocytes can hypertrophy with weight gain.
  - Retinacula cutis
    - Vertical fibrous septa connect the dermis to the underlying fascia, creating a "honeycomb" network to provide support to the fat.
    - Cellulite refers to skin dimpling and irregularity from herniation of adipose tissue through the attenuated retinacula cutis.
      □ Primary cellulite (cellulite of adiposity) results from hypertrophied superficial fat and responds to weight loss.
      □ Secondary cellulite (cellulite of laxity) results from generalized soft tissue redundancy and laxity. This is only correctable surgically.
  - Reserve fat of Illouz
    - Located deep to the superficial fascia (eg, sub-Scarpa fat), this fat has horizontal fibrous septa.
    - Targeting this layer of fat during liposuction improves the overall contour with less risk of focal contour abnormalities.
- Patient Evaluation
  - Best candidates
    - Isolated areas of moderate adiposity, good skin elasticity, and turgor.
    - Skin that does not "snap back" quickly when pinched will show redundancy after liposuction and can worsen the cosmetic appearance.
    - Striae, cellulite, abdominal pannus, and buttock ptosis respond poorly to liposuction and require surgical resection.
- **Wetting Solution**
  - Fluid delivered to the subcutaneous tissues prior to suctioning. It provides both anesthesia and hemostasis.
  - *50 mL of 1% lidocaine and 1 mL of 1:1000 epinephrine per liter of lactated Ringer solution = 0.05% lidocaine with 1:1 000 000 epinephrine (use 30 mL of lidocaine if larger than 4 L liposuction planned).
  - **Wet technique**
    - 200-300 mL of fluid is infiltrated into the area.
    - Blood loss is up to 30% of aspirate.
  - **Super wet technique**
    - 1 mL of infiltrate per 1 mL of aspirate.
    - *Blood loss is ~1% of aspirated volume.
  - **Tumescent technique**
    - *2-3 mL of infiltrate per 1 mL of aspirate.
    - *Blood loss is ~1% of aspirated volume.

- ○ *Lidocaine toxicity
  - ▪ Symptoms include light-headedness, visual disturbance, metallic taste, headache, perioral tingling, tinnitus, and seizure.
  - ▪ To minimize risk of toxicity, the wetting solution dose should be <35 mg/kg (though literature does cite up to 55 mg/kg as safe theoretically).
  - ▪ Timing and peak of absorption vary by body region—above the neck can occur in <6 hours, while thighs can take 12+ hours.
    - □ Patients have reported symptoms starting 8-12 hours after the procedure.
    - □ When infiltrating multiple areas, avoid overlapping phases of absorption (eg, do neck before thighs).
    - □ Lidocaine is not necessarily needed if the patient is under general anesthesia.

TYPES OF LIPOSUCTION

- Suction-assisted liposuction (SAL)
  - ○ **Indications:** excess fatty deposits, often in submental area, abdomen/flanks/lower back, thighs, medial knees, and calf/ankle.
  - ○ **Mechanics:** removal of fat cells by direct mechanical avulsion aided by suction forces.
  - ○ **Cannulas:** blunt tips with lumens ranging from 1.5 to 8 mm. Smaller lumen cannulas are less prone to creating contour irregularities.
  - ○ Technique
    - ▪ **Markings:** with the patient standing, perform pinch test to identify areas of relative fatty excess.
    - ▪ **Tumescent solution** is infiltrated into the area.
    - ▪ **Pretunneling** is performed by passing the cannula multiple times without suction. This establishes a gliding plane at the correct level (deep to the superficial fascia) to prevent contour irregularities.
    - ▪ **Using a crisscross technique** permits smooth transitions and improves contouring (**Fig. 64-1**).
    - ▪ Too many cannula passes at the insertion site under suction can result in a contour depression due to focal overresection.
    - ▪ **SAFELipo technique** ("**Separation, Aspiration, and Fat Equalization**") has been described for use in conjunction with abdominoplasty as a way to minimize damage to flap blood supply.
      - □ It relies on fat separation without suction, which prevents avulsion injury to blood vessels associated with suction.
      - □ Fat is subsequently aspirated with a smaller diameter cannula (less traumatic), with particular care taken in Huger zone III so as not to cause suction avulsion injury to blood vessels supplying the flap.
      - □ Posttunneling is performed to leave behind a layer of separated fat with the goal of reducing contour deformities secondary to scar adhesions.

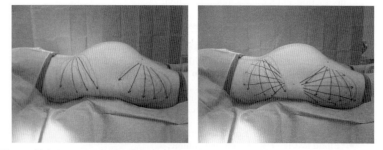

Figure 64-1 Cross-tunneling technique. (From Thorne CH. *Grabb and Smith's Plastic Surgery.* Lippincott Williams & Wilkins; 2014. Figure 65.3.)

- Systemic complications
  - ▪ Fluid imbalance
    - ▫ Hypervolemia and resultant edema are common early.
    - ▫ *Hypovolemia can occur 12-36 hours postoperatively from fluid shifts. The risk is decreased with the use of super wet and tumescent techniques.
    - ▫ Electrolyte disturbances
  - ▪ Pulmonary fat embolus: can be increased in patients with low serum albumin. Highest risk after liposuction with subsequent gluteal fat grafting.
  - ▪ Venous thromboembolic event (deep venous thrombosis and PE): increased risk with larger suction volumes and longer operations. Though rare (occurring in 0.03% of patients), it is most common cause of death.
  - ▪ Lidocaine toxicity (see above).
  - ▪ Other complications: contour irregularities (most common complication of liposuction, reported by as many as 9% of patients), infection (1%-3% complication rate), seroma/hematoma (2% complication rate), abdominal perforation, and skin pigment changes.
- Ultrasound-assisted liposuction
  - Ultrasound-assisted liposuction may be more effective in fibrofatty areas (eg, breast, back, male chest, etc.), and some studies suggest an advantage over SAL in treatment of gynecomastia.
  - Cavitation is created by pulsatile waves of ultrasonic energy, which preferentially liquefies adipocytes during suctioning. Vascular architecture may be better preserved resulting in less blood loss compared to SAL.
  - **An increased rate of seroma formation has been reported vs SAL.**
  - Skin burns can be reduced by using more wetting solution to dissipate heat and avoiding "end" hits against the dermis.
  - Most studies suggest similar aesthetic outcomes and patient satisfaction when compared to SAL.
- Laser-assisted lipolysis
  - Laser-assisted lipolysis has been recommended for areas with skin laxity or potential for poor skin retraction after SAL.
  - Presumably, laser energy delivered to adipose tissue results in thermal lysis. The targeted chromophores are fat and water.
  - Smaller cannula probes are used (1-2 mm), and the most frequent laser is the 1064 nm Nd:YAG.
  - Reported to result in less intraoperative blood loss, less postoperative ecchymoses, and improved skin tightening when compared to SAL.
  - Complications are rare and not unique to the use of the laser, except for thermal injury to the subcutaneous tissues or skin.
- Power-assisted liposuction
  - Power-assisted liposuction is considered for fibrous or technically challenging areas.
  - *This technique can reduce operative time, aspirate more fat per area, and result in less user fatigue.
- Radiofrequency-assisted liposuction (RFAL)
  - RFAL uses bipolar radiofrequency energy to disrupt cell membranes and induce lipolysis.
  - The heat generated by RFAL can also burn the overlying skin.
- Large-volume liposuction (LVL)
  - *Most studies define LVL as removal of 5000 mL or greater of total aspirate.
  - Increasing volumes of lipoaspirate thought to be associated with greater rates of complications.
  - More recent data suggest this procedure may be safe and effective in appropriately selected patients. Larger fluid resuscitation volumes are often needed.
  - Patients undergoing >5000 mL of total aspirate should be admitted to the hospital for observation due to concern for large fluid shifts.

- **Postoperative Care**
  - Patients should wear compression garments at all times (except to shower) for several weeks, typically 2- to 4-week duration; this will help with postoperative edema and reduce contour irregularities.
  - Pain, edema, and ecchymoses are expected in the postoperative setting, and patients should be educated accordingly.
  - **Outcomes**
    - Improved body contour following resolution of ecchymoses and edema.
    - Liposuction does **not** address skin laxity, and performing liposuction in areas with excess laxity will likely only exacerbate the appearance.

ABDOMINOPLASTY

OVERVIEW

- This operation removes redundant abdominal skin and fat between the umbilicus and pubis and can address abdominal wall laxity.
- **Etiology** of laxity in skin, fascia, and muscles of the abdominal wall.
  - Pregnancy: results in abdominal wall laxity, rectus diastasis, and skin excess.
  - Significant weight loss or gain causes dermatolipodystrophy, characterized by cellulite and reduced skin elasticity.
  - Aging causes an increase in visceral fat and skin laxity with a loss of elasticity.
  - Hereditary factors contribute to varying patterns of fat distribution and can predispose to abdominal laxity.
  - Ultraviolet radiation damages skin quality and reduces elasticity.
- **Anatomy**
  - *Layers of the anterior abdominal wall lateral to the rectus muscles are skin, Camper fascia, fat, Scarpa fascia, reserve (subscarpal) fat, external oblique, internal oblique, transversus abdominis, transversalis fascia, and peritoneum.
  - Scarpa fascia is contiguous with the superficial fascia in other regions of the body, forming the superficial fascial system (SFS).
  - Suprascarpal fat is thicker and denser than subscarpal fat.
  - *Vascular anatomy of the abdominal wall (Fig. 64-2).
    - **Huger zone I**
      - Directly over the rectus abdominis
      - Supplied by perforators of the deep superior and inferior epigastric arteries
    - **Huger zone II**
      - Inferolateral abdominal wall (inferior to line between anterior superior iliac spines down to inguinal crease)
      - Supplied by the circumflex iliac system, superficial epigastric, and superficial pudendal arteries
    - **Huger zone III**
      - Lateral over the external obliques
      - Supplied by the segmental lumbar and intercostal perforators. The abdominoplasty flap relies on zone III perfusion (zones I and II are disrupted by abdominoplasty flap elevation and incisions, respectively)
  - **Sensory innervation**
    - **The anterior abdominal wall:** innervated laterally from T6 to L1, which run between the internal oblique and the transversus abdominis muscles.
    - **The lateral femoral cutaneous nerve (L2-L3)**
      - **Provides sensation to the anterolateral thigh.** it is located 1-6 cm medial to the ASIS; it can be injured during abdominoplasty dissection and closure.
      - Leaving fat down on fascia medial to ASIS and not placing plications sutures in this area can help reduce chance for injuring the nerve.
    - **The ilioinguinal (L1) and iliohypogastric (T12-L1) nerves** are mixed sensorimotor nerves that can be injured with deep plication of the inferior

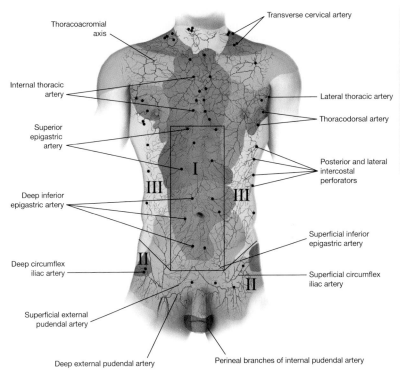

Figure 64-2 Blood supply to the abdominal wall and Huger zones. (From Thorne CH. *Grabb and Smith's Plastic Surgery.* Lippincott Williams & Wilkins; 2014.)

rectus abdominis muscles, sometimes resulting in sensory deficits in their respective distributions.

- □ **Ilioinguinal nerve** provides sensation to upper anteromedial thigh and parts of the genitalia. It pierces the internal oblique to enter the inguinal canal, where it passes through the superficial ring before giving off its terminal sensory branches.
- □ **Iliohypogastric** nerve provides sensation to posterolateral gluteal and suprapubic regions. The **lateral cutaneous branch** pierces the internal and external obliques above the iliac crest before it is distributed to the skin posteriorly. The **anterior cutaneous branch** pierces the aponeurosis of the external oblique 2.5 cm above the superficial inguinal ring.
- ○ **Abdominal wall musculature**
  - ▪ **Vertical layer** (provides vertical pull)
    - □ **Rectus abdominis**
      - ▪ Origin: pubic symphysis/crest
      - ▪ Insertion: xiphoid process, costal cartilages of ribs 5-7
      - ▪ Blood supply: inferior and superior epigastric arteries, as well as posterior intercostal, subcostal, and deep circumflex arteries
      - ▪ Innervation: intercostal (T7-T11) and subcostal (T12) nerves
      - ▪ Action: trunk flexion
    - □ A varying degree of diastasis is normal.

- □ *The arcuate line of Douglas is located halfway between the umbilicus and the pubis: inferior to this landmark, both anterior and posterior rectus fascias fuse and run superficial to the rectus muscles, leaving only transversalis fascia, a thin layer of preperitoneal fat, and parietal peritoneum deep to the rectus muscle.
  - □ **External oblique**
    - ▪ Origin: ribs 5-12
    - ▪ Insertion: linea alba, pubic tubercle, anterior portion of iliac crest
    - ▪ Blood supply: posterior intercostal, subcostal, and deep circumflex iliac arteries
    - ▪ Innervation: intercostal (T7-T11) and subcostal (T12) nerves
    - ▪ Action: trunk flexion/lateral trunk flexion/trunk rotation
- ▪ **Horizontal layer** (provides horizontal pull)
  - □ **Internal oblique**
    - ▪ Origin: inguinal ligament, iliac crest, and thoracolumbar fascia
    - ▪ Insertion: ribs 10-12, linea alba, pubic crest, pectineal line of the pubis
    - ▪ Blood supply: subcostal arteries
    - ▪ Innervation: intercostal (T7-T11), subcostal (T12), ilioinguinal (L1), and iliohypogastric (L1) nerves
    - ▪ Action: trunk flexion/lateral trunk flexion/trunk rotation
  - □ **Transversus abdominis**
    - ▪ Origin: ribs 5-12, thoracolumbar fascia, anterior iliac crest, inguinal ligament and associated fascia
    - ▪ Insertion: linea alba, pubic crest, pectineal line of the pubis, aponeurosis of internal oblique
    - ▪ Blood supply: posterior intercostal, subcostal, superior and inferior epigastric, superficial and deep circumflex, and posterior lumbar arteries
    - ▪ Innervation: intercostal (T7-T11), subcostal (T12), ilioinguinal (L1), and iliohypogastric (L1) nerves. Action: trunk flexion/rotation
    - ▪ Action: compresses abdominal contents/trunk rotation
- ○ **Umbilicus**
  - ▪ Umbilical stalk is dissected out and preserved during abdominoplasty.
  - ▪ Care must be taken to avoid injuring previously undiagnosed umbilical hernias. Small umbilical hernias may be repaired during abdominoplasty.
  - ▪ **Blood supply**
    - □ Subdermal plexus.
    - □ Right and left deep inferior epigastric artery.
    - □ Ligamentum teres.
    - □ Median umbilical ligament.
    - □ **This allows for either preserving the umbilicus on its stalk or transecting it at its base.**
- ○ **Gender differences**
  - ▪ **Men**
    - □ More commonly have subscarpal fat deposits in the flanks, abdomen, and chest (Android distribution).
    - □ Rectus diastasis occurs more in the upper abdomen.
    - □ Redundant skin is less common, unless there has been MWL.
    - □ There is increased intra-abdominal fat with aging.
  - ▪ **Women**
    - □ More commonly have fat deposits in the lower abdomen, hips, and thighs (Gynecoid distribution).
    - □ Rectus diastasis occurs more in the lower abdomen.
    - □ Skin redundancy or striae are more common and are exacerbated by pregnancy and weight loss.

PREOPERATIVE EVALUATION

- **History and physical examination** (see above sections History and Physical Examination for additional details)
    - Of note, patients undergoing abdominoplasty are at relatively high risk for developing venous thromboembolism (VTE) compared to other operations in plastic surgery, with a reported incidence as high as 2%-8%.
        - Part of the preoperative evaluation should thus include risk stratifying patients at risk for VTE.
        - The 2005 Caprini Risk Assessment Model is commonly used to risk stratify patients at risk for developing VTE after surgical procedures (see **Chapter 12: Preoperative Cardiopulmonary Risk Stratification and Prophylaxis**).
        - Current literature suggests strongly considering postoperative chemoprophylaxis in patients with a Caprini score of 7 or higher and in those with individual risk factors.
    - **COPD and other respiratory comorbidities** have unique implications after abdominoplasty. Consider preoperative pulmonary function tests to identify at-risk patients.
        - Increased risk of wound dehiscence with coughing.
        - Baseline pulmonary compromise is worsened by restriction of expansion after rectus plication.
- **Relative Contraindications**
    - **Prior abdominal scars.**
    - **Plans for future pregnancy**, which would cause re-expansion and laxity recurrence. Abdominoplasty will not inhibit the growth of a fetus.
    - **Active changes in weight (ideal stable weight of 3-6 months).**
    - **Chronic medical conditions** (eg, DVT, COPD, DM, etc.) require appropriate medical clearances before surgery.
    - **Obese patients are poor abdominoplasty candidates.** Significant intra-abdominal fat, relative avascularity, and generalized adiposity inhibit closure and predispose to wound healing complications.
    - **Smoking or nicotine use** is a contraindication to most surgeons.
        - Risk of smoking and wound healing deficits after abdominoplasty in smokers: 12%-14%.
        - Cutoff for pack years and risk of infection: 8.5.

SURGICAL TECHNIQUES

- **Full abdominoplasty**
    - Involves removal of excess abdominal skin and fat, rectus plication, and umbilical transposition.
    - For patients with significant skin excess, abdominal wall laxity, and rectus diastasis.
    - Discuss scar placement. **Low transverse incisions** sit at least 5-7 cm above the vaginal introitus/penile base, at the superior level of the pubic hair. Depending on type of pants and undergarment/bathing suit patient prefers, final scar location especially in relation to ASIS should be planned. Patients can bring in undergarments to aid in scar placement.
    - The superior incision is usually made above the umbilicus, which must be exteriorized on a stalk and repositioned. Final resection will depend on the amount of tissue that can safely be removed.
    - Undermine up to costal margins and xiphoid. Avoid dissecting further lateral than is needed so as to maximally preserve blood supply from the intercostal perforators.
    - The anterior rectus abdominis fascia is plicated from xiphoid to pubis to contour the abdominal wall.
    - During closure, the abdominal flap should be pulled medially. This tension will improve aesthetic contour of hips and waist.
    - Postoperative instructions include abdominal compression garments and no heavy lifting for 6 weeks.

- **Miniabdominoplasty**
  - For patients with isolated lower abdominal contour deformity involving central skin excess and fascial laxity.
  - A conservative 6-15 cm ellipse of midline lower abdominal skin is resected without repositioning the umbilicus.
  - Rectus plication is performed inferior to the umbilicus under direct visualization and is optional above umbilicus with use of an endoscope.
- **Vertical component**
  - Adding a vertical component to standard panniculectomy (resulting in a "fleur-de-lis" design) provides improved lateral contouring with the tradeoff of a long vertical midline scar extending to the xiphoid (**Fig. 64-3**).
  - Allows for management of both vertical and horizontal excess.
  - Vertical excision is performed first to prevent over resection.
  - This technique results in a T-shaped scar, with limited blood supply at the junction of the flaps.
  - Minimize lateral undermining of abdominal flaps to preserve blood supply.
  - Particularly useful in MWL patients, as they often have notable horizontal and vertical excess.
  - Important that superior and lateral ends of the excisions are done at sharply acute angles to prevent leaving a standing cutaneous deformity.
- **Panniculectomy**
  - This operation removes a large overhanging pannus ("fatty apron") that can cause functional limitations including wounds, hygiene issues, intertriginous rashes, and interference with activities of daily living, among other things.
  - As alluded to above, this operation is typically performed for functional reasons as opposed to cosmetic.

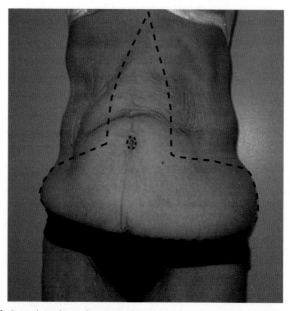

Figure 64-3 General markings for panniculectomy with vertical wedge resection (Fleur-de-lis abdominoplasty). (From Thorne CH. *Grabb and Smith's Plastic Surgery.* Lippincott Williams & Wilkins; 2014.)

- A large soft tissue wedge is designed around the pannus and excised.
- Although similar in concept to abdominoplasty, there is typically no rectus plication or umbilical transposition. Moreover, there is typically no undermining as compared to traditional abdominoplasty procedures.
- Overall, this results in a less complicated procedure that maximizes vascularity to the skin (important as patients often have comorbidities and risk factors for skin necrosis and wound healing complications).
- **Circumferential torsoplasty**
  - This operation removes excess skin and fat circumferentially around the torso, unlike traditional abdominoplasty in which only the anterior abdomen is addressed.
  - Useful for patients following MWL with significant lateral and posterior skin excess.
  - Effectively eliminates dog-ears and improves contour of the abdomen, hips, back, and buttocks.
- **Postoperative Care**
  - Drains are often utilized, and patients should be educated on proper drain care.
  - It is often recommended that patients maintain a flexed position at the hip for several weeks postoperatively (beach chair position) to minimize tension on the abdominal closure. For circumferential truncal contouring, it is recommended that patients maintain neutral position at the hip to minimize tension on the incision posteriorly.
  - A compression garment is worn by the patient for several weeks.
  - The patient should be instructed to avoid strenuous activity or heavy lifting for 6 weeks postoperatively.
  - Early ambulation should be encouraged to reduce the risk of VTE. Chemoprophylaxis should be considered based on individual risk stratification as already discussed.
- **Complications**
  - **The overall complication rate is 30%, with <5% major complications.** Higher rates are seen in male patients. Overall complications are doubled in MWL patients.
  - **Seroma (14%):** patients with diabetes and higher preoperative weight have increased incidence. Use of closed suction drains and progressive advancement suturing help reduce seroma risk.
  - **Delayed wound healing and dehiscence (5%-30%):** associated with smoking, longer OR time, higher preoperative weight, and in bariatric surgery patients.
  - **Abdominal flap necrosis:** more common when abdominoplasty is combined with liposuction.
  - **Infection (1%-7%):** risk is increased with smoking and combined procedures due to longer operative time. Only perioperative antibiotics are indicated.
  - **Hematoma (1%-10%):** drain promptly to avoid flap compromise or infection.
  - **Umbilical necrosis:** usually wounds are allowed to heal secondarily.
  - **DVT and PE (1%):** of all common plastic surgery operations, abdominoplasty carries the highest risk. Risk increases when BMI > 30, when there is >1500 g resection, in combined procedures with longer operative time, and with use of hormone therapy. Risk decreases with use of postoperative DVT prophylaxis.

PEARLS

1. For all body contouring procedures, proper SFS (Scarpa's Fascial System) approximation is a key in providing strength, reducing tension on the closure, and optimizing outcomes.
2. Longer operative time, especially during abdominoplasty and combined procedures, increases the risk of thrombotic events—use prophylactic perioperative anticoagulation for patients in need of multiple procedures.
3. Active smoking results in a significant increase in infections and wound healing complications and is a contraindication to these contouring procedures.

QUESTIONS YOU WILL BE ASKED

1. What is the mechanism for cellulite development?

   The development of cellulite is due to the architectural changes of the superficial tissues. Cellulite fat is no different than subcutaneous fat elsewhere in the body. Superficial fat is separated into small compartments by multiple dense vertical septa. As the fat hypertrophies with weight gain or as skin relaxes with aging, the unyielding septa do not change, and this discrepancy leads to a dimpled appearance on the skin surface.

2. Will fat cells multiply with weight gain after removal (eg, liposuction)?

   Fat cells multiply *in utero* through childhood and adolescence. Once a person is mature, fat cells do not replicate; with weight gain, existing fat cells hypertrophy to accommodate the increase in fat stores. However, in the unique setting of morbid obesity, fat cells may once again divide.

3. How do you determine if a patient needs excision as opposed to liposuction?

   Skin quality. Liposuction will remove the subcutaneous fat but will not address issues with the skin (eg, severe skin excess, thin skin, skin with low elasticity, sun-damaged skin). Therefore, with poor skin quality, the skin will not conform after liposuction and the cosmetic appearance will be worse after surgery. For these patients, it is better to perform a skin resection operation.

4. What is superficial fascia system and its significance?

   It is the layer of horizontal connective tissue with associated vertical and oblique investing septa. Informally, it is the layer fascia found throughout the subcutaneous level in all areas of the body contiguous with Scarpa fascia.

5. Why did I ask this woman about a history of breast cancer if she is here for an abdominoplasty consultation?

   A common donor site for autologous breast reconstruction is the abdominal tissues. Abdominal-based breast reconstruction is precluded after abdominoplasty or panniculectomy because the perforators supplying the abdominal skin and fat are transected during these procedures.

Recommended Readings

1. Ahmad J, Eaves FF 3rd, Rohrich RJ, Kenkel JM. The American Society for Aesthetic Plastic Surgery (ASAPS) survey: current trends in liposuction. *Aesthet Surg J.* 2011;31(2):214-224.
2. Berry MG, Davies D. Liposuction: a review of principles and techniques. *J Plast Reconstr Aesthet Surg.* 2011;64(8):985-992.
3. Buck DW 2nd, Mustoe TA. An evidence-based approach to abdominoplasty. *Plast Reconstr Surg.* 2010;126(6):2189-2195.
4. Chia C, Neinstein R, Theodorou S. Evidence-based medicine: liposuction. *Plast Reconstr Surg.* 2017;139(1):267e-274e.
5. Richter DF, Stoff A, Velasco-Laguardia FJ, Reichenberger MA. Circumferential lower truncal dermatolipectomy. *Clin Plast Surg.* 2008;35(1):53-71. discussion 93.

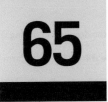

65 Brachioplasty and Thighplasty

Geoffrey E. Hespe

Brachioplasty and thighplasty are key components of body contouring and typically performed in tandem with other procedures (eg, abdominoplasty, mastopexy, etc.) to address concerns of aging and/or massive weight loss.

BRACHIOPLASTY

- Brachioplasty is a surgical procedure to remove excess skin and subcutaneous fat from the upper arm to restore a slimmer, more youthful contour.
- First described in the 1920s by Thorek for obese patients and modernized for aesthetic concerns in the 1950s by Correa-Iturraspe and Fernandez.

PATIENT HISTORY

- Patient's weight should be stable for at least 6 months in order to achieve optimal results.
- Evaluate patient comorbidities, social history (eg, smoking status, future pregnancies, physical activity), medications, and expectations of surgical outcomes (see Chapter 64: Liposuction, Panniculectomy and Abdominoplasty for more details).
  - Physical examination—the patient is examined with arms in the "victory position" (arms abducted 90° at shoulders, flexed 90° at elbows). Excess tissue is evaluated by pinching. Important to evaluate skin quality (eg, thickness, elasticity and striae).
  - Determine whether there is excess skin, adipose tissue, or both.
  - Evaluate whether the excess extends into the axilla.

GOALS

- Optimize scar placement.
  - Patients should be counseled on the visibility of scars and the tendency for them to widen in brachioplasty.
- Resect upper arm dermatolipodystrophy to improve contour.
- Elevate the axillary fold.
- Avoid overresection.

ANATOMY

- Fascia
  - The superficial fascia of the forearm is part of the superficial fascial system.
  - The axillary fascia comprises the floor of the axilla. The axillary vein and medial brachial cutaneous nerve are located just deep to this fascia.
  - Lockwood in the 1990s described the importance of resuspending the superficial fascia system in brachioplasty to improve outcomes.
- Nerves
  - *The medial antebrachial cutaneous (MABC) nerve runs with or just anterior to the basilic vein and becomes superficial to the deep fascia about 14 cm (8-21 cm) proximal to the medial epicondyle. *It is the most commonly injured nerve in brachioplasty.
    - **The MABC provides sensation to the anterior and medial skin of the midarm and forearm.**

---

*Denotes common in-service examination topics.

- Avoid injury to the MABC by leaving a cuff of fat on the deep fascia during dissection.
  ○ The medial brachial cutaneous nerve provides sensation to the medial upper arm and travels posterior to the basilic vein.
  ○ Both the medial brachial cutaneous and MABC nerves run superficial to the deep fascia in the mid/distal upper arm overlying the musculature and originate most commonly from the medial cord of the brachial plexus.
- Lymphatics
  ○ Upper extremity lymph drains within networks around the basilic and cephalic veins and into the axillary nodal basin.
  ○ During brachioplasty, many of these lymphatics are disrupted, and therefore, the patient requires continuous compression wraps for several weeks after surgery to manage edema.

SURGICAL MANAGEMENT

Correct surgical technique depends on the degree of skin vs fat excess on physical examination.
- **Liposuction**
  ○ Appropriate option for patients with mainly excess adiposity and good skin quality.
  ○ *Avoid liposuction in the bicipital groove as it increases the risk of contour deformities.
  ○ Compression is key postoperatively to help with swelling and contour.
  ○ Access for liposuction can typically be at the posterior upper arm just proximal to the elbow.
- **Surgical Resection (Fig. 65-1)**
  ○ Can be used alone (skin excess) or in combination with liposuction (skin and adipose tissue excess).
  ○ The incision is typically placed either in the bicipital groove or posteriorly oriented.
    - When marking, have the arm at 90° angle.
    - The incision can be carried into the axilla and extended onto the chest wall as needed to excise excess skin/soft tissue.
    - Incisions should be kept proximal to the elbow if possible to prevent scar contracture.
    - A Z- or W-plasty can be added to the end of the incision as needed to improve contour.

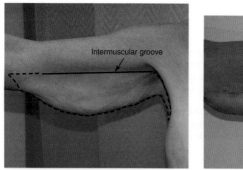
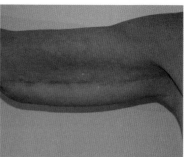

Figure 65-1 Brachioplasty technique. Example of preoperative brachioplasty markings (*left*) and postoperative result (*right*).

○ Limit undermining of remaining tissue to preserve blood and lymphatic supply.
○ **A cuff of adipose tissue should be left on the muscle fascia to prevent injury to the MABC.**
○ Closure and postoperative management
  ▪ To prevent spreading of the incisions and provide lasting results reapproximation of the superficial fascial system and anchoring to the axillary fascia or the fascia of anterior axillary fold is key.
  ▪ In patients with significant laxity, some surgeons will plicate the triceps fascia to the biceps fascia.
  ▪ Use of closed-suction drains is common, especially when skin flaps are undermined.
  ▪ Compression garments for comfort and edema control.

COMPLICATIONS

- The overall complication rate is ~3.5%-29%. Approximately 15%-23% of patients seek revision surgery.
- Rate of complication is increased when combined with other procedures.
- Dehiscence is more frequent when excision is combined with liposuction (~6%).
- Hypertrophic scarring (~10%).
- Seroma (~7%).
- Infection (~3%).
- Nerve injury (1.5%; most often neuropraxia of the MABC; up to 5% permanent risk).
- Lymphedema and lymphocele (~7%; higher rate with use of UAL).

THIGHPLASTY

- Thighplasty is a surgical procedure to remove excess skin and subcutaneous fat of the thigh to improve the contour and appearance.
- Surgical excision is an appropriate option in patients with excess thigh skin and soft tissue who are not good candidates for liposuction.
- Of all the body contouring procedures, thighplasty has the highest rate of complications and lowest satisfaction.

EXAMINATION

- Determine excess skin, adipose tissue, or both.
- Assess skin, including striae, turgor, and elasticity.
- Identify the location of the skin redundancy and laxity; proximal vs distal, and medial vs lateral.
- Evaluation for any venous disease should also be assessed.

ANATOMY

- The medial thigh consists of thin dermis and two layers of underlying adipose tissue with superficial fascia dividing them.
- **Colles Fascia of the Perineum**
  ○ Contiguous with Scarpa fascia of the abdomen
  ○ Fixed through attachments to the ischiopubic rami
  ○ Strongest at junction of perineum and medial thigh
  ○ Lies at deepest lateral-most aspect of vulvar soft tissue near origin of adductor muscles
- Proximally, the posterior thigh has more soft tissue mobility, whereas the distal thigh demonstrates less mobility.
- Femoral Triangle: the borders of the triangle are the inguinal ligament (superiorly), adductor longus (medially), and sartorius (laterally).
  ○ Contents: made up of the femoral nerve, femoral artery, femoral vein, and lymphatics (lateral to medial). **Typically remembered with the pneumonic NAVL**
  ○ Important to protect during surgery to prevent vascular or lymphatic injury

SURGICAL APPROACH

- Can add liposuction to the procedure if excess adipose tissue needs to be removed
- **Upper One-Third Thigh Laxity**
  - ○ Utilizes a groin crease incision and provides a predominately vertical pull.
  - ○ *The closure must be anchored to Colles fascia in perineum for lasting results.
  - ○ Lack of anchoring can lead to
    - ▪ Inferior migration and widening of scars
    - ▪ Lateral traction deformity of the vulva
    - ▪ Early recurrence of ptosis
- **Upper and Lower Thigh Laxity**
  - ○ With significant adiposity and ptosis, consider liposuction first and waiting 6 months to perform medial thigh lift.
  - ○ Significant ptosis requires a longitudinal incision along the length of the medial thigh, achieving circumferential tightening of the soft tissues.
  - ○ In some MWL patients, both vertical and horizontal components (L-shaped incision) are needed.
  - ○ Avoid incisions that cross the knee joint.

COMPLICATIONS

- Overall complication rate is 42% with the most common complications being wound dehiscence (18%) and seroma (8%).
- Also include infection, hematoma, and edema.

QUESTIONS YOU WILL BE ASKED

1. What is superficial fascia system and its significance?
   It is the layer of horizontal connective tissue with associated vertical and oblique investing septa. Informally, it is the layer fascia found throughout the subcutaneous level in all areas of the body contiguous with Scarpa fascia.
2. What is the most commonly injured nerve during brachioplasty and how can you avoid this injury?
   The most commonly injured nerve during brachioplasty is the medial antebrachial cutaneous nerve, which provides sensation to the anterior and medial midarm and forearm. Understanding anatomy is the key at protecting this nerve, which will arise deep fascia about 14 cm (8-21 cm) proximal to the medial epicondyle and thus leaving a cuff on adipose tissue over the muscle will help protect this nerve.
3. How do you prevent vulvar distortion during a medial thigh lift?
   During closure, anchor the thigh flaps to the deep layer of the superficial perineal fascia (Colles fascia).

Recommended Readings
1. El Khatib HA. Classification of brachial ptosis: strategy for treatment. *Plast Reconstr Surg.* 2007;119(4):1337-1342.
2. Knoetgen J III, Moran SL. Long-term outcomes and complications associated with brachioplasty: a retrospective review and cadaveric study. *Plast Reconstr Surg.* 2006;117(7):2219-2223. doi:10.1097/01.prs.0000218707.95410.47
3. Lockwood T. Brachioplasty with superficial fascial system suspension. *Plast Reconstr Surg.* 1995;96(4):912-920.

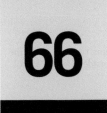

66

How to Excel During Your Plastic Surgery Sub-Internship

Geoffrey E. Hespe and Widya Adidharma

DISCLAIMER: This chapter is a broad overview of helpful pointers for medical students who will be pursuing plastic surgery sub-internships. Not everything discussed in this chapter will apply to every rotation so we recommend checking with the rotation's clerkship director and residents to determine specific expectations.

FINDING THE RIGHT PROGRAM TO VISIT

- Start your search early; most programs will offer away rotations through the AAMC Visiting Student Learning Opportunity (VSLO) program, and spots can fill up quickly once the application window opens.
  - Programs you would like to learn more about (location, training environment, reach programs).
  - Learn about programs from mentors, previous applicants, comedical students.
- Be willing to accept away rotations at the programs you apply to.
  - Don't apply to more rotations than you can do.
- Conduct a sub-internship at your home institution to prepare for an away if possible.

PREPARING FOR YOUR AWAY ROTATION

- Where to Stay: Rotating Room, AirBNB, Friends/Family
- Determine how far away from the hospital or other clinical sites your residence is
- Transportation
  - Do you need a car?
  - Will you need to use a ride-share service?
  - Public transportation

ONCE YOU ARRIVE

- **General Principles**
  - Sub-internships are a demanding, tiring, but tremendously beneficial opportunity to grow as a student before you start residency.
  - Sub-internships can have a huge impact (positive and negative) on your chances of getting an interview/matching at a given program.
    - Doing a great job can open doors for you, whereas a lackluster performance could reduce your chances of getting an interview even if you are a stellar applicant on paper.
  - Sub-internships allow for you to get great insight into the culture and unwritten details of a program since you will typically be there for 2-4 weeks.
    - Remember that programs will also have the same amount of time with you as well.
    - Outstanding qualities and less desirable ones become more apparent.
  - As a sub-intern, you can have the opportunity to contribute at the level of an intern.
    - At the beginning of the rotation, discuss with the intern and team what tasks you can help with throughout the day.
    - Learn to anticipate the needs of your team.

- Other important tips
  - Always be early → nothing is a bigger red flag than being late to rounds, the OR, clinic, etc. Residents understand things happen outside of your control but give yourself a buffer for unexpected events.
  - Be interested.
  - Be helpful.
  - Be available.
  - Be affable.
  - Be prepared—read for everything you can anticipate ahead of time.
- **Rounding Tips**
  - Discuss with the team how you can be helpful on rounds. You may be able to help prepare the morning rounding list—if so, have a systematic way for how you pre-round so you do not miss vital information (overnight events, vitals, cultures, imaging, etc.).
  - Plastic surgery patients often have wounds/incisions that need to be seen on rounds—that means, their dressings will need to be changed. A way you can help make rounds more efficient is to have all the dressing supplies ready.
  - You may be able to help your resident team write patient notes.
  - Some programs may want you to present patients on morning rounds.
- **Operating Room Tips**
  - Always find out which cases you will be attending the next day.
  - Prepare for the case by reading about relevant anatomy and a general overview of the procedure (indications, general steps, complications, etc.).
  - In the operating room, help get the patient in and out of the OR room (eg, help transfer patients, put sequential compression devices on patients, etc.).
  - Take advantage of opportunities to assist during the case whether that is retracting, cutting suture, or helping suture at the end of a case.
  - Be situationally aware (eg, in a challenging part of a case, it may not be the best time to ask a lot of questions).
  - Introduce yourself, where you are from, and what your interest is.
- **Clinic Tips**
  - Clinic is a great time to interact with faculty that is not as high pressure as the OR.
  - If there is time available before clinic, it can be helpful to look over the clinic schedule to see who is coming in so you can read about relevant topics.
  - Depending on the institution/attending, you could be shadowing or seeing patients on your own. If seeing patients on your own, know how to present a patient succinctly and take a stab at offering a reasonable plan.
  - Even if seeing patients with a resident, if you feel comfortable, you may have the opportunity to lead the history taking.
- **Explore the Local Area**
  - Although you will be busy clinically, it is important to spend weekends not on call exploring the local area to see if this is a place you would like to spend the next 6 years.

ONCE YOU LEAVE

- Make a list of the things you like or did not like about the program, city, people, case mix, etc.
- Stay in contact with faculty and residents if you are interested in the program.
- Try to attend journal clubs or other teaching sessions if your time allows to stay connected with programs of interest.

Index

Note: Page numbers followed by an "*f*" denote figures; those followed by a "*t*" denote tables.